Biomarkers in Inborn
Errors of Metabolism

Clinical Aspects and Laboratory Determination of Biomarkers Series

Series Editors: Uttam Garg and Laurie D. Smith

Volume 1
Alcohol and Its Biomarkers: Clinical Aspects and Laboratory Determination

Volume 2
Biomarkers in Inborn Errors of Metabolism: Clinical Aspects and Laboratory Determination

Volume 3
Endocrine Biomarkers: Clinical Aspects and Laboratory Determination

Biomarkers in Inborn Errors of Metabolism

Clinical Aspects and Laboratory Determination

Uttam Garg

Children's Mercy Hospitals and Clinics,
Kansas City, MO, United States;
University of Missouri School of Medicine,
Kansas City, MO, United States

Laurie D. Smith

University of North Carolina School of Medicine,
Chapel Hill, NC, United States

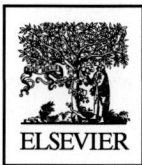

ELSEVIER

Elsevier
Radarweg 29, PO Box 211, 1000 AE Amsterdam, Netherlands
The Boulevard, Langford Lane, Kidlington, Oxford OX5 1GB, United Kingdom
50 Hampshire Street, 5th Floor, Cambridge, MA 02139, United States

Notices

Knowledge and best practice in this field are constantly changing. As new research and experience broaden our understanding, changes in research methods, professional practices, or medical treatment may become necessary.

Practitioners and researchers must always rely on their own experience and knowledge in evaluating and using any information, methods, compounds, or experiments described herein. In using such information or methods they should be mindful of their own safety and the safety of others, including parties for whom they have a professional responsibility.

To the fullest extent of the law, neither the Publisher nor the authors, contributors, or editors, assume any liability for any injury and/or damage to persons or property as a matter of products liability, negligence or otherwise, or from any use or operation of any methods, products, instructions, or ideas contained in the material herein.

British Library Cataloguing-in-Publication Data
A catalogue record for this book is available from the British Library

Library of Congress Cataloging-in-Publication Data
A catalog record for this book is available from the Library of Congress

ISBN: 978-0-12-802896-4

For Information on all Elsevier publications
visit our website at https://www.elsevier.com/books-and-journals

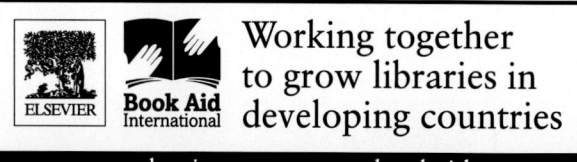

Working together
to grow libraries in
developing countries

www.elsevier.com • www.bookaid.org

Publisher: Mica Haley
Acquisition Editor: Tari Broderick
Editorial Project Manager: Fenton Coulthurst
Production Project Manager: Karen East and Kirsty Halterman
Designer: Mark Rogers

Typeset by MPS Limited, Chennai, India

This book is dedicated to
My family, wife Jyotsna, and daughters Megha and
Mohini who are my inspiration (Uttam Garg).

My family and, most importantly, to the patients and
their parents who have taught me so much by allowing me
to be a part of their lives (Laurie D. Smith).

Contents

CHAPTER 10 Lysosomal storage disorders: sphingolipidoses..**211**
C. Yu

CHAPTER 11 Peroxisomal disorders: clinical and biochemical laboratory aspects...**235**
M. Dasouki

List of Contributors

R. Artuch
Hospital Sant Joan de Déu, Barcelona, Spain

M.J. Bennett
The Children's Hospital of Philadelphia and University of Pennsylvania Perelman School of Medicine, Philadelphia, PA, United States

N. Couser
University of North Carolina, Chapel Hill, NC, United States

M. Dasouki
King Faisal Specialist Hospital and Research Center, Riyadh, Saudi Arabia; University of Kansas Medical Center, Kansas City, KS, United States

P.D. DeArmond
Nationwide Children's Hospital, Columbus, OH, United States

D.J. Dietzen
Washington University School of Medicine, St. Louis, MO, United States; St. Louis Children's Hospital, St. Louis, MO, United States

A.M. Ferguson
University of Missouri School of Medicine, Kansas City, MO, United States; Children's Mercy Hospitals and Clinics, Kansas City, MO, United States

R. Ganetzky
University of Pennsylvania, Philadelphia, PA, United States

A. Garcia-Cazorla
Hospital Sant Joan de Déu, Barcelona, Spain

U. Garg
Children's Mercy Hospitals and Clinics, Kansas City, MO, United States; University of Missouri School of Medicine, Kansas City, MO, United States

M. Gucsavas-Calikoglu
University of North Carolina, Chapel Hill, NC, United States

M. He
University of Pennsylvania, Philadelphia, PA, United States

L. Hubert
Baylor College of Medicine, Houston, TX, United States; Baylor Genetics Laboratories, Houston, TX, United States

P.M. Jones
Children's Medical Center of Dallas and University of Texas Southwestern Medical Center, Dallas, TX, United States

S.F. Lo
Children's Hospital of Wisconsin, Milwaukee, WI, United States

M. Molero-Luis
Hospital Sant Joan de Déu, Barcelona, Spain

M.A. Morrissey
Wadsworth Center, Albany, NY, United States

A. Ormazabal
Hospital Sant Joan de Déu, Barcelona, Spain

A.L. Pyle-Eilola
Nationwide Children's Hospital, Columbus, OH, United States; The Ohio State University, Columbus, OH, United States

F.J. Reynoso
University of Pennsylvania, Philadelphia, PA, United States

L.D. Smith
University of North Carolina School of Medicine, Chapel Hill, NC, United States

Q. Sun
Baylor College of Medicine, Houston, TX, United States

V.R. Sutton
Baylor College of Medicine, Houston, TX, United States; Baylor Genetics Laboratories, Houston, TX, United States; Texas Children's Hospital, Houston, TX, United States

C. Yu
Icahn School of Medicine at Mount Sinai, New York, NY, United States

Biographies

Uttam Garg

Uttam Garg, PhD, is Director of Laboratory Medicine at Children's Mercy Hospital, and Professor of Pathology at the University of Missouri, School of Medicine in Kansas City. Before joining Children's Mercy Hospital, he served as faculty at the New York University Medical Center and the University of Minnesota Medical School. He is board certified in clinical chemistry, and has extensive laboratory experience in the areas of clinical chemistry and biochemical genetics. He served on the Board of Directors of the American Board of Clinical Chemistry and National Registry of Certified Chemists. He is a member of expert panel on newborn screening of Clinical Laboratory Standards Institute. He has published over 150 research papers, review articles, and book chapters in the area of clinical biochemistry, and has edited/coedited 4 books. His research interests include methods development in clinical laboratory diagnosis.

Laurie D. Smith

Laurie D. Smith, MD, PhD, is Associate Professor of Pediatrics at the University of North Carolina in Chapel Hill. She is a board certified pediatrician, clinical geneticist, and clinical biochemical geneticist with extensive experience in the diagnosis and management of patients with inborn errors of metabolism. She serves or has served on a number of national, regional, and state committees and organizations and is a fellow of the American Academy of Pediatrics and the American College of Medical Genetics. She has published numerous research papers and book chapters in the area of metabolic disorders. She has coedited one book.

Preface

Inborn errors of metabolism are biochemical genetic disorders that result from the deficiency of enzymes, membrane transporters, or other functional proteins. Patients with these disorders may present with either acute overwhelming sickness or a prolonged, smoldering illness. For the former, rapid diagnosis is vital in the diagnosis and follow-up of these patients to limit morbidity and mortality. For the latter, diagnosis is important for the initiation of appropriate clinical care. Clinical presentation resulting from these disorders can be quite variable. Therefore, use of laboratory tests and biomarkers are indispensable in the diagnosis and follow-up of these disorders. Rapid tests are generally available for the initial presumptive diagnosis and management of acutely ill patients. Specialized tests involving laboratory biomarkers are not available in most medical centers, and are needed for the confirmation and follow-up of these disorders. Moreover, laboratory biomarkers are used in newborn screening to diagnose biochemical genetic disorders in asymptomatic patients.

In this book, *Biomarkers in Inborn Errors of Metabolism*, the major emphasis is on the test selection and biomarkers used in the diagnosis and follow-up. When possible, biochemical pathways and illustrative chromatograms are provided. In addition, basic information on clinical presentation, pathogenesis, treatment, and prognosis is also presented. Furthermore, confounding factors that may mimic biomarkers used in the diagnosis of inborn error of metabolisms are also covered.

We are indebted to our authors and colleagues for their excellent contributions and making this book possible. We are also thankful to our patients and families who have taught us a lot. Last but not the least, we would like to acknowledge the support of Jeffery Rossetti and Fenton Coulthurst, editorial project managers, for their support during the preparation of this book.

Uttam Garg and Laurie D. Smith

Introduction to laboratory diagnosis and biomarkers in inborn error of metabolism

1

U. Garg[1,3] and L.D. Smith[2]
[1]Children's Mercy Hospitals and Clinics, Kansas City, MO, United States;
[2]University of North Carolina School of Medicine, Chapel Hill, NC, United States;
[3]University of Missouri School of Medicine, Kansas City, MO, United States

1.1 INTRODUCTION

Inborn errors of metabolism (IEM) are genetic disorders of intermediary metabolism. The majority of these disorders are due to single gene defects resulting in the deficiency of an enzyme, membrane transporter, or other functional protein. Timely biochemical genetic testing, and, in many cases, newborn screening are important in early recognition and treatment of these disorders. Often there is accumulation of toxic substrates or metabolites or deficiency of essential products. Clinical presentation resulting from IEM can be quite variable. Broadly, IEM can be divided into those that involve defects in metabolism of complex molecules, those that result in acute intoxication and those that result in energy deficiency.[1,2] Patients with IEM are diagnosed through clinical suspicion or newborn screening. A family history can provide clues but does not exclude an underlying IEM. One of the scenarios that might suggest an IEM in a neonate is an acute sepsis-like illness, poor feeding, lethargy, poor growth, and so on, that does not respond to conventional treatment. In an older child, symptoms such as vomiting, metabolic acidosis, ataxia, or coma might suggest an IEM. Further testing is needed to confirm a clinical suspicion of an IEM. In addition to making a diagnosis of an IEM in a symptomatic patient, a significant number of patients are diagnosed through newborn screening programs. In recent years, newborn screening programs have expanded to include more than 50 inherited metabolic disorders, including aminoacidopathies, organic acidemias, fatty acid oxidation disorders, and lysosomal storage disorders.[3–6] Newborn screening results are considered presumptive positive and are confirmed by more definitive laboratory tests.[6,7] Many of these disorders may present later in life with chronic and progressive multisystem (skeletal muscle, liver, kidneys, gastrointestinal tract, eyes, skin, or central nervous system) symptoms. Lysosomal disorders involving the accumulation of complex molecules may present with behavioral changes, coarsening of facial features, or joint contractures. The IEM can also present with specific organ involvement such as a cardiomyopathy or hepatic dysfunction. Generally, an IEM should be considered in any patient who does not have a clear diagnosis and does not respond

Biomarkers in Inborn Errors of Metabolism. DOI: http://dx.doi.org/10.1016/B978-0-12-802896-4.00001-8

to conventional treatment. Laboratory tests are often needed to confirm clinical suspicion and to make a definitive diagnosis. This chapter covers the basics of laboratory tests and biomarkers in the diagnosis of IEM. A number of excellent publications are available on the clinical aspects of inherited metabolic diseases.[1,8–17]

1.2 LABORATORY BIOMARKERS AND TESTS IN DIAGNOSIS OF IEM

In most IEM, clinical symptoms are nonspecific: vomiting, poor feeding, lethargy, hypotonia, seizure, poor linear growth, poor weight gain. Biochemical genetic testing is essential for the diagnosis and clinical management of patients with IEM. The purpose of testing is to either confirm or exclude the diagnosis of a suspected disorder. Once the diagnosis of a particular disorder is established, specific biomarkers are followed to monitor clinical management of the patient.

Initial laboratory tests such as blood gases, pH, glucose, electrolytes, ammonia, lactate, renal function tests, liver function tests, urinalysis, and basic hematological tests are available in most hospital laboratories. Although these tests are not diagnostic of a specific IEM, they are very helpful in managing the acutely ill patient. These tests can also provide important clues in the differential diagnosis of inherited metabolic disorders. For example, hyperammonemia, lactic acidemia, ketonuria, and hypoglycemia may point toward a metabolic condition, such as an organic acidemia.[10,18] Routine laboratory tests and their association with various diseases are shown in Table 1.1.[19] More specialized tests such as plasma amino acid profiles, urine organic acid profiles, plasma acylcarnitine profiles, free fatty acid profiles, pyruvate, acetoacetate, 3-hydroxybutyrate, mucopolysaccharides, oligosaccharides, enzyme activity assays, functional assays, and mutational analyses are needed to make the definitive diagnosis.[7] Specialized tests are not available in the routine clinical laboratories, and are sent to specialized centers. The GeneTests website (https://www.genetests.org/), supported by National Institutes of Health, is an invaluable source for identifying laboratories experienced with specialized metabolic testing. Some laboratories also perform spot screening tests. These tests can provide quick, useful information when specialized tests are not available. Since these screening tests lack specificity or sensitivity, results of these tests should be interpreted with caution and in context with clinical information. Several screening tests are listed in Table 1.2.[19,20]

Many IEM may only be apparent when a patient is under metabolic stress. When well, the disease markers may be normal or only slightly abnormal providing inconclusive information. It may be necessary to carry out functional tests to artificially create metabolic stress in these patients, although in this era of gene sequencing, functional tests are being used less frequently. In general, in functional testing, the patient is exposed to a high concentration of a specific substrate to cause metabolic stress, and specimens are collected before and after metabolic stress. Functional tests should be carried out only by an experienced care provider as they may lead

Table 1.1 Routine Laboratory Tests/Biomarkers with Commonly Associated Diseases

Test/Biomarker	Disorders
↑ Ammonia	Urea cycle disorders Hyperornithinemia-hyperammonemia-homocitrullinuria (HHH) Dibasic amino aciduria Lysinuric protein intolerance Hyperinsulinism-hyperammonemia Carnitine uptake defect Carnitine palmitoyltransferase-1 (CPT-1) deficiency Acylcarnitine translocase deficiency Maple urine syrup disease (may be) Medium chain acyl-CoA dehydrogenase (MCAD) deficiency Branched chain amino acids organic acidurias (may be) Certain organic acidurias (methylmalonic, propionic, isovaleric) Severe liver disease

Abnormal liver function tests
 	
↑ Aspartate aminotransferase (AST), ↑ Alanine aminotransferase (ALT), ↑ Bilirubin
	Tyrosinemia type 1
	Fatty acid oxidation defects:
	    Carnitine uptake defect
	    Carnitine palmitoyltransferase-1 deficiency
	    Carnitine palmitoyltransferase-2 deficiency
	    Very long chain acyl-CoA dehydrogenase deficiency
	    Medium chain acyl-CoA dehydrogenase deficiency
	    Short chain acyl-CoA dehydrogenase deficiency
	    Long chain 3-hydroxyacyl-CoA dehydrogenase deficiency
	    Multiple acyl-CoA dehydrogenase deficiency
	Carbohydrate metabolism defects:
	    Galactosemia
	    Glycogen storage disease types 1, 3, 6, 9
	    Glycogen synthase deficiency
	    Pyruvate carboxylase deficiency
	    Galactose-1-phosphate uridyltransferase deficiency
	    Hereditary fructose intolerance
	    Fructose-1,6-diphosphatase deficiency
	Lipid metabolism/Lysosomal storage defects:
	    Cholesterol-7-hydroxylase deficiency
	    3-Hydroxy-Δ^5-C27-steroid dehydrogenase deficiency
	    3-Oxo-Δ^4-5β-reductase deficiency
	    3-Hydroxy-3methylglutaryl-CoA synthase deficiency
	    Cholesteryl ester storage disease
	    Gaucher's disease, type 1
	    Niemann-Pick disease, types A and B
	    Acid lipase deficiency/Wolman's disease
	Hyperammonemias
	    Ornithine transcarbamylase deficiency
	    Argininosuccinic aciduria
	    Arginase deficiency
	    Lysinuric protein intolerance
	Hemochromatosis
	Mitochondrial disorders
	α1-antitrypsin deficiency
	Wilson disease
	Wolman's disease
	Zellweger syndrome
	CDG-1e

(Continued)

Table 1.1 Routine Laboratory Tests/Biomarkers with Commonly Associated Diseases (Continued)

Test/Biomarker	Disorders
↑ Cholesterol	Lipoprotein lipase deficiency Dysbetalipoproteinemia Defective apoB-100 Hepatic lipase deficiency Lecithin cholesterol acyltransferase deficiency Sterol 27-hydroxylase deficiency
↓ Cholesterol	Mevalonic aciduria Abetalipoproteinemia Hypobetalipoproteinemia Smith-Lemli-Opitz syndrome Other cholesterol biosynthesis disorders Barth syndrome Glucosyltransferase I deficiency ALG6-CDG (CDG-Ic)

↑ Creatine kinase	Fatty acid oxidation defects:
	    Carnitine palmitoyltransferase-2 deficiency
	    Very long chain acyl-CoA dehydrogenase deficiency
	    Long chain 3-hydroxyacyl-CoA dehydrogenase deficiency
	    Multiple acyl-CoA dehydrogenase deficiency
	Glycogen storage disorders type 2, 3, 5
	ALG6-CDG
	Myoadenylate deaminase deficiency

↓ Creatinine	Creatine synthetic defects
↑ Creatinine/Urea	Lysosomal cystine transport Hyperoxaluria type 1
↓ Glucose	Fatty acids oxidation disorders Glycogen storage disorders Galactosemia Fructose-1,6-diphosphatase deficiency Pyruvate carboxylase deficiency Multiple acyl-CoA dehydrogenase deficiency Hereditary fructose intolerance
↓ Hemoglobin	B12 metabolism deficiency Folate metabolism disorders Glucose-6-phosphate dehydrogenase deficiency 5-Oxoprolinuria Glutathione synthesis defects Glycolysis defects
↑ Ketones	Methylmalonic aciduria Propionic aciduria Isovaleric aciduria Pyruvate carboxylase deficiency Gluconeogenesis defects

(Continued)

Table 1.1 Routine Laboratory Tests/Biomarkers with Commonly Associated Diseases (Continued)

Test/Biomarker	Disorders

↑ Lactate	Glycogen metabolism disorders:
	    Amylo-1,6-glucosidase deficiency
	    Glucose-6-phosphate translocase deficiency
	    Glycogen synthetase deficiency
	    Liver phosphorylase deficiency
	Gluconeogenesis defects:
	    Glucose-6-phosphatase deficiency
	    Fructose 1,6 diphosphatase deficiency
	Lactate/Pyruvate disorders:
	    Pyruvate dehydrogenase deficiency
	    Pyruvate carboxylase deficiency
	Krebs cycle/Respiratory chain/Mitochondrial defects:
	    Ketoglutarate dehydrogenase defect
	    Fumarase defect
	Respiratory chain defects:
	    Complex I (NADH-CoQ oxidoreductase) deficiency
	    Complex II (Succinate-CoQ reductase) deficiency
	    Complex III (CoQ cytochrome C reductase, complex III) deficiency
	    Complex IV (Cytochrome oxidase C) deficiency
	Organic aciduria:
	    Methylmalonic aciduria
	    Propionic aciduria
	    Isovaleric aciduria
	    L-2-Hydroxyglutaric aciduria
	Hyperammonemias
	Biotinidase deficiency
	Holocarboxylase synthetase deficiency
	Fatty acids oxidation defects
	Acquired causes:
	    Hypoxia
	    Drug intoxications—salicylate, cyanide
	    Renal insufficiency
	    Convulsions

↓ pH, Acidosis	Organic acidurias:
	    Methylmalonic aciduria
	    Propionic aciduria
	    Isovaleric aciduria
	    3-Methylcrotonylglycinuria
	    3-Methylglutaconic aciduria
	    3-Hydroxy-3-methylglutaryl-CoA lyase deficiency
	    Biotinidase deficiency
	    Holocarboxylase synthetase deficiency
	    3-Oxothiolase deficiency
	    2-Ketoglutarate dehydrogenase complex deficiency
	    3-Hydroxyisobutyric aciduria

(Continued)

Table 1.1 Routine Laboratory Tests/Biomarkers with Commonly Associated Diseases (Continued)

Test/Biomarker	Disorders
	Maple syrup urine disease
	Mitochondrial disorders
	Fatty acid oxidation defects:
	Carnitine uptake defect
	Carnitine palmitoyltransferase-1 deficiency
	Very long chain acyl-CoA dehydrogenase deficiency
	Medium chain acyl-CoA dehydrogenase deficiency
	Short chain acyl-CoA dehydrogenase deficiency
	Long chain 3-hydroxyacyl-CoA dehydrogenase deficiency
	Multiple acyl-CoA dehydrogenase deficiency
	Carbohydrate metabolism defects:
	Glycogen storage disease types 1, 3, 6, 9
	Glycogen synthase deficiency
	Pyruvate carboxylase deficiency
	Galactosemia
	Fructose-1,6-diphosphatase deficiency
	Glycerol kinase deficiency
↑ Triglycerides	Glycogen storage disease type 1
	Lipoprotein lipase deficiency
	Dysbetalipoproteinemia
	Hepatic lipase deficiency
	Lecithin cholesterol acyltransferase deficiency
↑ Uric acid	Hypoxanthine phosphorybosyl transferase deficiency
	Phosphorybosylpyrophosphate synthetase deficiency
	Glycogen storage disease type 1
↓ Uric acid	Purine nucleoside phosphorylase deficiency
	Molybdenum cofactor deficiency
	Xanthine oxidase deficiency

Modified and Reprinted with permission from Garg U, Smith LD, Heese BA. Introduction to the laboratory diagnosis of inherited metabolic diseases. In: Garg U, Smith LD, Heese BA, eds. Laboratory Diagnosis of Inherited Metabolic Diseases. Washington, DC: AACC Press, 2012:1–12.

to dangerously high levels of toxic metabolites and cause serious complications. In recent years, laboratory diagnostic techniques have improved significantly reducing the need for functional tests. Some functional tests are listed in Table 1.3.[21]

Diagnostic biomarkers for various disorders are given in Table 1.4.[2,9,18,19,22–29]

1.3 SPECIMEN TYPES

Whole blood is collected on filter paper for newborn screening. Commonly used specimens for metabolic testing include serum or plasma, urine and cerebrospinal fluid. Amniotic fluid, fibroblasts, leukocytes, liver and muscle are also used in the diagnosis and confirmation of inherited metabolic diseases. In postmortem investigations, bile

Table 1.2 Urinary Metabolic Screening Tests

Test	Disorder	Substance (s) Detected	Comment
Cyanide nitroprusside (sodium nitroprusside and sodium cyanide)	Cystinuria, homocystinuria, β-mercaptolactate-cysteine disulfiduria	Cystine, homocysteine, glutathione	False positive due to sulfhydryl or disulfide containing compounds such as N-acetylcysteine, 2-Mercaptoethanesulfonate, 2-Mercaptopropionylglycine, captopril, penicillamine
Dinitrophenylhydrazine (DNPH)	Maple syrup urine disease (MSUD), phenylketonuria, tyrosinemia, histidinemia, methionine malabsorption (oasthouse syndrome)	Branched chain 2-ketoacids (2-keto-isovaleric, 2-keto-isocaproic, 2-keto-3-methylvaleric acids), phenylpyruvic acid, 4-hydroxyphenylpyruvic acid	DNPH reacts with 2-ketoacids to form hydrazones, which form precipitates. Radiopaque contrast material will form a precipitate with DNPH.
Reducing substances	Fructose intolerance, Galactosemia, alkaptonuria, tyrosinemia	Fructose, galactose, homogentisic acid, 4-Hydroxyphenylpyruvic acid	Reducing substances reduce copper (cupric ions) to form green to orange color. Many other substances including glucose, lactose, maltose, arabinose, ribose, uric acid, ascorbic acid, cysteine, ketones, sulfanilamide, oxalic acid, hippuric acid, glucuronic acid, formaldehyde, isoniazid, salicylates, cinchophen, and salicyluric acid cause positive test
Sulfite	Sulfite oxidase deficiency, molybdenum cofactor deficiency	Sulfite	Sulfite rapidly oxidizes to sulfate. Therefore, the specimen should be tested freshly

Table 1.3 Functional Tests

Test	Indication
Allopurinol test	Diagnosis of heterozygous or mild cases of ornithine transcarbamylase deficiency. There is increased excretion of urinary orotic acid. Increased urinary orotic acid is also seen in phosphoribosylpyrophosphate synthetase deficiency.
Prolonged fasting test	Prolonged fasting can be life-threatening. The test should be carried out under strict supervision. Diagnosis of hypoglycemia due to disorders of gluconeogenesis, fatty acid oxidation, glycogen metabolism, and ketolysis. The patient is fasted for 12–24 hours, and specimens are collected at 2–4-hour intervals. Additional studies may include lactate/pyruvate ratio, 3-hydroxybutyrate/acetoacetate ratio, ammonia, pH, blood gases, amino acids, urine organic acids, plasma acylcarnitine profile, free fatty acids, insulin, cortisol, adrenocorticotropic hormone (ACTH), and growth hormone. Urine organic acids and plasma acylcarnitines profiles can be carried out to rule out fatty acids oxidation defects.
Fructose intolerance test	Evaluation of hereditary fructose intolerance. Leads to metabolic disturbances such as hypoglycemia, hypophosphatemia, hyperuricemia, hyperlactatemia and ketosis.
Glucagon stimulation test	Diagnosis of glycogen storage disease type 1 (von Gierke disease).
Glucose challenge test	To access aerobic generation of energy and disorders of energy metabolism. Blood sugar will be elevated and lactate should not rise more than 20%.
Leucine challenge test	To detect leucine-sensitive hyperinsulinemia.
Methionine challenge test	Rise in homocysteine indicates reduced remethylation.
Oral galactose loading test	Diagnosis of glycogen storage disease types 0, 1, 3, 6, 9. Lactate increases in these disorders.
Phenylpropionic acid loading test	Increased excretion of phenylpropionylglycine and insufficient excretion of hippuric acid suggest medium-chain acyl-CoA dehydrogenase (MCAD) deficiency.
Tetrahydrobiopterin (BH$_4$)	Identify BH$_4$ responsive phenylketonuria (PKU) patients.

Table 1.4 Diagnostic Biomarkers for Various Disorders

Disorder	Diagnostic Tests/Biomarkers[a]
Amino acid disorders	
Cystinuria	↑Cystine (U), ↑Ornithine (U), ↑Lysine (U), ↑Arginine (U)
Homocystinuria (cystathionine β-synthase deficiency)	↑Homocyst(e)ine (B, U), ↑Methionine (B)
Homocystinuria (methylenetetrahydrofolate reductase/cobalamin deficiency)	↑Homocyst(e)ine (B, U), ↓Methionine (B) (may be)
Lowe (oculocerebrorenal) syndrome	All amino acids (U)
Maple syrup urine disease (MSUD)	↑Valine (B), ↑Leucine (B), ↑Isoleucine (B), ↑Alloisoleucine (B); α-keto-3-methylvaleric (U), α-ketoisocaproate (U), and α-ketoisovaleric (U)
Nonketotic hyperglycinemia	↑Glycine (B, CSF)
Phenylketonuria/Hyperphenylalaninemia	↑Phenylalanine (B), ↓Tyrosine (B), ↑ Phenylalanine:Tyrosine ratio (B)
Proline oxidase deficiency/Hyperprolinemia type 1	↑Proline (U), ↑Hydroxyproline (U), ↑Glycine (U)
Sulfite oxidase deficiency	↑Sulfocysteine (U), ↑Cysteine (U)
Trimethylaminuria, fish odor syndrome	↑Triethylamine (U)
Tyrosinemia type 1 (hepatorenal /fumarylacetoacetate hydrolase deficiency)	↑Tyrosine (B), ↑Succinylacetone (urine/plasma), Tyrosine metabolites (U)
Tyrosinemia type 2 (oculocutaneous /tyrosine aminotransferase deficiency)	↑Tyrosine (B), Tyrosine metabolites (U)
Urea cycle defects/hyperammonemias	
Arginase deficiency	↑Ammonia (B), ↑Arginine (B), ↑Orotic acid (U)
Argininosuccinic aciduria	↑Ammonia (B), ↑Argininosuccinic acid (U,B), ↑Citrulline (U), ↓Arginine (B)
Carbamyl phosphate synthetase (CPS) deficiency	↑Ammonia (B), enzyme/molecular tests
Citrullinemia type 1	↑Ammonia (B), ↑Citrulline (U,B), ↑Orotic acid (U), ↓Arginine (B)
Citrullinemia type 2 (citrin deficiency)	↑Ammonia (B), ↑Threonine:Serine ratio (B), ↑Bilirubin (B)
Hyperornithinemia-hyperammonemia-homocitrullinemia (HHH) syndrome	↑Ammonia (B), ↑Homocitrulline (U), ↑Ornithine (P)
Lysinuric protein intolerance (LPI)	↑Ammonia (B), ↑Dibasic amino acids (U); ↑Orotic acid (U, may be)
Ornithine transcarbamylase (OTC) deficiency	↑Ammonia (B), ↑Orotic acid (U), ↓Citrulline (B)

(Continued)

Table 1.4 Diagnostic Biomarkers for Various Disorders (Continued)

Disorder	Diagnostic Tests/Biomarkers[a]
Organic acidemias	
Alanine: glyoxylate aminotransferase deficiency, primary hyperoxaluria type 1	↑Oxalate (B,U), ↑Glycolate (B,U)
Alkaptonuria	↑Homogentisic acid (U)
Canavan disease (aspartoacylase deficiency)	↑N-acetylaspartic acid (U)
Fumarase deficiency, fumaric aciduria	↑Fumaric acid
Glutaric aciduria type 1	↑Glutaric acid, ↑3-Hydroxyglutaric acid, ↑Glutaconic acid, ↑C5DC (B)
D-Glyceric acidemia	↑D-Glyceric acid (U) (chirality determination is needed)
4-Hydroxybutyric aciduria	↑4-Hydroxybutyric (U)
3-Hydroxyisobutyric aciduria	↑3-Hydroxyisobutyric (U)
D-2-Hydroxyglutaric aciduria	↑D-2-Hydroxyglutaric (U) (chirality determination is needed)
L-2-Hydroxyglutaric aciduria	↑L-2-Hydroxyglutaric (U) (chirality determination is needed)
Isovaleric acidemia	↑Isovalerylglycine (U), ↑3-Hydroxyisovaleric acid (U), ↑4-Hydroxyvaleric acid (U), ↑C5 (B)
2-Ketoglutarate dehydrogenase complex deficiency	↑2-Ketoglutarate (U)
β-Ketothiolase/Mitochondrial acetoacetyl-CoA thiolase deficiency	↑2-Methyl-3-hydroxybutyrate (U), ↑2-Methylacetylacetate (U), ↑Tiglylglycine (U), C5-OH (B)
Malonic aciduria	↑Malonic acid (U)
2-Methylbutyryl-CoA dehydrogenase deficiency, short/branched-chain acyl-CoA dehydrogenase deficiency	↑2-Methylbutyrylglycine (U), ↑C5 (B)
3-Methylcrotonyl CoA carboxylase deficiency (can be benign)	↑3-Hydroxyisovaleric acid (U), ↑3-Methylcrotonylglycine (U), ↑C5-OH (B)
3-Methylglutaconic aciduria	↑3-Methylglutaconic acid (U), ↑3-Methylglutaric acid (U)
Methylmalonic acidemia (mutase deficiency)	↑Methylmalonic acid (U), ↑3-Hydroxypropionic acid (U), ↑Methylcitrate (U), ↑Propionylglycine (U), ↑Tiglylglycine (U), ↑C3 (B)
Methylmalonic aciduria and homocystinuria (cobalamin C and D disease)	↑Methylmalonic acid, ↑Methyl citrate, ↑3-Hydroxypropionic acid, ↑C3, ↑C4DC (B)
Mevalonic aciduria	↑Mevalonic acid (U), ↑Mevalonolactone (U)

(Continued)

Table 1.4 Diagnostic Biomarkers for Various Disorders (Continued)

Disorder	Diagnostic Tests/Biomarkers[a]
Multiple carboxylase/ Holocarboxylase synthetase/ Biotinidase deficiency	↑3-Hydroxyisovaleric acid (U), ↑ Methylcitrate (U), 3-↑Methylcrotonylglycine (U), ↑Propionylglycine (U), ↑C5-OH (B)
Propionic acidemia	↑3-Hydroxypropionic acid (U), ↑Methylcitrate (U), ↑Propionylglycine (U), ↑Tiglylglycine (U), ↑C3 (B)
Disorders of fatty acid oxidation	
Carnitine palmitoyltransferase I (CPT-I) deficiency	↑C0 (B), ↓Long chain acylcarnitines
Carnitine palmitoyltransferase II (CPT-1I) deficiency	↑C16:0, ↑C18:2, ↑C18:1
Carnitine translocase deficiency	↑C16:0, ↑C18:2, ↑C18:1
Carnitine transporter deficiency	↓Total and free carnitine (B), ↑Carnitine (U)
3-Hydroxy-3-methylglutaryl-CoA-lyase deficiency	↑3-Hydroxy-3-methylglutaric (U), ↑3-Hydroxyisovaleric (U), ↑3-Methylglutaconic (U), ↑3-Methylglutaric acids, ↑C5-OH (B), ↑C6DC (B)
Long-chain 3-hydroxyacyl-CoA dehydrogenase (LCHAD) deficiency— trifunctional protein deficiency	↑C16-OH (B), ↑C18-OH (B), ↑C18:1-OH
Medium-chain acyl-CoA dehydrogenase deficiency	↑C6, ↑C8, ↑C10:1
Multiple acyl-CoA dehydrogenase deficiency (MADD)/Glutaric aciduria, type II/Ethylmalonic-adipic aciduria	↑Glutaric acid (U), ↑Isovalerylglycine (U), ↑Hexanoylglycine (U), ↑Suberylglycine (U), ↑Butyryl/isobutyryl glycine (U), ↑2-Methylbutyryl glycine (U), ↑C5 (B), ↑C5-DC (B), ↑C8 (B), ↑C10 (B), ↑C10:1 (B), ↑C14:1 (B)
Short chain acyl-CoA dehydrogenase (SCAD) deficiency	↑Ethylmalonic acid (U), ↑Methylsuccinic acid (U), ↑Butyrylglycine (U), ↑C4 (B)
Very long-chain acyl-CoA dehydrogenase (VLCAD) deficiency	↑C14:0, ↑C14:1 and ↑C14:2
Disorders of carbohydrate metabolism	
Galactosemia	↓GALT (RBC, most cases), ↑Galactose (RBC), ↑Galactose-1-phosphate (RBC), ↑Reducing substances (U)
Glycogen storage disorders	Variable, Common: ↓Glucose (B), ↑Lactate (B), ↑Liver enzymes (B), ↑Uric acid (B)
Hereditary fructose intolerance, aldolase B deficiency	↑Fructose (B, U), ↓Glucose (B), ↓Phosphate (B), ↑Uric acid (B)
Peroxisomal disorders	
X-linked adrenoleukodystrophy	↑VLCFA(B)
Biogenesis defect/Zellweger spectrum	↑VLCFA(B), ↑Pristanic acid (B), ↑Phytanic acid (B), ↓Plasmalogens (RBC), ↑C27 Bile acids, ↑Bilirubin (B)

(Continued)

Table 1.4 Diagnostic Biomarkers for Various Disorders (Continued)

Disorder	Diagnostic Tests/Biomarkers[a]
Rhizomelic Chondrodysplasia Punctata type 1	↓Pristanic acid (B), ↓Plasmalogens (RBC)
Rhizomelic Chondrodysplasia Punctata type 2 and 3	↓Plasmalogens (RBC)
Phytanoyl-CoA-α-hydroxylase deficiency (Refsum disease)	↓Pristanic acid (B), ↑Phytanic acid (B)
2-Methylacyl-CoA racemase deficiency	↑Pristanic acid (B), ↑C27 Bile acids (B)
D-Bifunctional protein deficiency	↑VLCFA(B), ↑Pristanic acid (B), ↑Phytanic acid (B), ↑C27 Bile acids
Sterol carrier protein X deficiency	↑Pristanic acid (B), ↑C27 Bile acids
Purine and pyrimidine metabolism defects	
Adenine phosphoribosyl-transferase (APR1) deficiency	↑Adenine (U), ↑Dehydroxyadenine (U)
Adenosine deaminase deficiency	↑Deoxyadenosine (U)
Adenylosuccinate lyase deficiency	↑Succinyladenosine (U), ↑SAICAR (U)
Dihydropyrimidinase deficiency	↑Uracil (U), ↑Thymine (U), ↑Dehydrouracil (U), ↑Dehydrothymine (U)
Dihydropyrimidine dehydrogenase deficiency	↑Uracil (U), ↑Thymine (U)
Hypoxanthine-guanine-phosphoribosyltransferase deficiency	↑Hypoxanthine (U), ↑Xanthine (U), ↑Uric acid (B,U)
Phosphoribosylpyrophosphate synthetase superactivity	↑Hypoxanthine (U), ↑Uric acid (B,U)
Purine nucleoside phosphorylase deficiency	↑Guanosine (U), ↑Inosine (U), ↑Deoxyguanosine (U), ↑Deoxyinosine (U), ↓Uric acid (B,U)
Uridine 5'-monophosphate synthase deficiency	↑Orotic acid (U)
Ureidopropionase deficiency	↑Uracil (U), ↑Thymine (U), ↑Dehydrouracil (U), ↑Dehydrothymine (U), ↑Ureidopropionic (U), ↑Ureidoisobutyric (U)
Xanthine oxidase deficiency (and molybdenum cofactor deficiency)	↑Hypoxanthine (U), ↑Xanthine (U), ↓Uric acid (B,U)
Lysosomal storage disorders—mucopolysacchridoses	
Type I, Hurler	↑Dermatan sulfate (U), ↑Heparan sulfate (U)
Type II, Hunter	↑Dermatan sulfate (U), ↑Heparan sulfate (U)
Type III, Sanfilippo	↑Heparan sulfate (U)
Type IVA, Morqio A	↑Chondroitin-6-sulfate (U), ↑Keratan sulfate (U)
Type IVB, Morqio B	↑Keratan sulfate (U)
Type VI, Maroteaux-Lamy	↑Dermatan sulfate (U)
TypeVII, Sly	↑Dermatan sulfate (U), ↑Heparan sulfate (U), ↑Chondroitin-6-sulfate (U)

(Continued)

Table 1.4 Diagnostic Biomarkers for Various Disorders (Continued)

Disorder	Diagnostic Tests/Biomarkers[a]
Lysosomal storage disorders—sphingolipidoses and transport disorders	
Fabry disease	↓α-Galactosidase activity (leukocytes, fibroblasts)
α-Fucosidosis	↓α-fucosidase (leukocytes, fibroblasts), ↑Fucose-rich oligosaccharides
Gaucher disease	↓β-Glucocerebrosidase activity (leukocytes, fibroblasts)
GM1 gangliosidosis	↓β-Galactosidase activity (leukocytes, fibroblasts)
GM2 Sandhoff disease	↓β-N-acetyl-hexoaminidase A and B (leukocytes, fibroblasts)
Krabbe disease	↓Galactocerebrosidase (leukocytes, fibroblasts)
Metachromatic leukodystrophy	↓Arylsulfatase A (leukocytes, fibroblasts)
Mucolipidosis type IV	↑Gastrin (P)
Niemann-Pick disease A/B	↓Acid sphingomyelinase activity (leukocytes, fibroblasts)
Niemann-Pick type C disease/cholesterol-processing abnormality	↓Foamy macrophages (B)
Pompe disease (acid maltase deficiency, glycogen storage disease type II)	↓α-Glucosidase (fibroblasts)
Tay-Sachs disease	↓β-N-acetyl-hexoaminidase A (leukocytes, fibroblasts)
Other disorders	
Creatine metabolism—arginine:glycine amidinotransferase (AGAT) deficiency	↓Guanidinoacetate (B,U), ↓Creatine (B,U)
Creatine metabolism—guanidinoacetate methyltransferase (GAMT) deficiency	↓Guanidinoacetate (B), ↓Creatine (B)
Creatine metabolism—guanidinoacetate methyltransferase (GAMT) deficiency	↑Creatine (U)
Menkes disease	↓Copper (B)
Wilson disease	↓Ceruloplasmin (B), Copper (B, U, liver)
Cystinosis	↑Cystine (leukocytes)

B—Blood/Plasma/Serum; U—Urine; CSF—Cerebrospinal fluid; Acylcarnitine. Abbreviations: C0 = Free Carnitine; C3 = Propionylcarnitine; C4 = Isobutyryl/Butyrylcarnitine; C5:1 = Tiglylcarnitine; C5 = Isovaleryl/2-methylbutyryl; C5-OH = 3-OH-Isovaleryl/2-methyl-3-OH-butyrylcarnitines; C5-DC = Glutarylcarnitine; C6 = Hexonylcarnitine; C6-DC = 3-Methyl-glutarylcarnitine; C8 = Octanoylcarnitine; C10:1 = Decenoylcarnitine; C14 = Tetradecanoylcarnitine; C14:1 = Tetradecenoylcarnitine; C14:2 = Tetradecadienoylcarnitine; C16 = Hexadecanoylcarnitine; C16-OH = 3-Hydroxyhexadecanoylcarnitine; C18:1 = Oleylcarnitine; C18:2 = Linoleylcarnitine; C18-OH = 3-Hydroxystearoylcarnitine; C18:1-OH = 3-Hydroxyoleylcarnitine; SAICAR = 5-phosphoribosyl-5-amino-4-imidazole-succinocarboxamide riboside; VLCAD = Very long-chain acyl-CoA dehydrogenase deficiency.
[a]These are common laboratory biomarkers/tests. Details of these biomarkers/tests are provided in individual chapters.

and vitreous fluids have been used in the diagnosis of IEM. For most analyses, serum/ plasma is the specimen of choice since it is less variable as compared to urine. Urine is the specimen of choice for diagnosis of certain disorders such as organic acidurias and renal transport diseases. In these disorders abnormal metabolites concentrate in urine. To normalize for sample dilution and reduce variability, urine results are generally expressed relative to creatinine concentration. CSF is used in the diagnosis of neurotransmitter disorders and certain other diseases such as non-ketotic hyperglycinemia.

1.4 SPECIMEN COLLECTION AND PROCESSING

The importance of correct specimen collection and processing cannot be over emphasized. It is important that the right specimens are collected at the right time. Many tests need special attention during specimen collection. For example, when possible, the best specimen for the diagnosis of the aminoacidopathies is from a fasting patient. Specimens for lactate and ammonia testing should be put on ice immediately after collection. Since many medical centers do not encounter or perform specialized biochemical genetics tests, it is important that instructions for specimen collection and processing from reference laboratories be followed closely. Furthermore, for correct interpretation, it may be necessary to collect additional information such as the patient's clinical status, medications, nutritional status, and so on.

Specimen requirements for commonly used tests are given in Table 1.5.[19]

1.5 SPECIMEN ANALYSIS, QUALITY CONTROL, AND QUALITY ASSURANCE

Specimen analysis, quality control, and quality assurance in the biochemical genetics laboratory can be quite challenging. Unlike routine chemistry laboratory studies, most biochemical genetics tests require quite extensive manual sample preparation. Most methods require specialized techniques such as gas-chromatography mass spectrometry, liquid-chromatography mass spectrometry, and tandem mass spectrometry. Specialized personnel and training are needed to properly operate and troubleshoot these instruments. Furthermore, premade commercial reagents, standards, calibrators, internal standards, and controls are not available for most of the biochemical genetics tests, and the laboratory is responsible for preparing and performing quality control of these reagents. For example, many organic acids and acylcarnitines of clinical interest are not available as pure compounds. Their estimation is based on surrogate calibrators that are semi-quantitative at best. Owing to these challenges, there is significant variability among different labs. This is evident from the College of American Pathologists (CAP) survey results shown in Table 1.6. The coefficient of variation for certain analytes is >100%. In addition, significant variability exists among laboratories in identifying the correct diagnosis (Table 1.7). For some diagnoses, 20–25% laboratories fail to identify the correct diagnosis.

Table 1.5 Specimen Collection and Handling

Analyte	Specimen Type	Storage/Shipping/Comment
Acylcarnitines	Plasma (EDTA or heparin)	Freeze
Acylglycines	Urine	Freeze
Alkaline phosphatase	Serum or plasma (heparin)	Refrigerate if specimen cannot be analyzed in 4 h.
Amino acids	Plasma (heparin) or urine (random), cerebrospinal fluid (CSF)	Refrigerate if done in-house. Freeze for shipping. Fasting blood specimen is preferred.
Ammonia	Plasma (heparin)	Send immediately on ice. Postprandial specimen is preferred. Recollect if specimen is hemolyzed. Freeze plasma if analysis cannot be done in 4 h.
Benzoic acid	Plasma (heparin)	Freeze
Complete blood count (CBC)	Blood (EDTA)	Refrigerate if specimen cannot be analyzed the same day.
Creatine kinase	Serum or plasma (heparin)	Hemolysis will falsely increase creatine kinase. Refrigerate if specimen cannot be analyzed in 4 h.
Creatinine/Urea	Serum or plasma (heparin)	Stable at room temperature for 3 days.
Electrolytes	Serum or plasma (heparin)	Hemolysis will cause increase in potassium.
Glucose	Plasma (fluoride, heparin)	Send as soon as possible. Heparin plasma is acceptable if specimen can be processed and analyzed within 30 min. Fasting specimen when possible.
Lactate	Plasma (heparin or fluoride)	Send immediately on ice. Separate plasma immediately. Freeze if specimen cannot be analyzed within 4 h.
Lactate dehydrogenase	Serum or plasma (heparin)	Hemolysis will cause false increase in lactate dehydrogenase.
Lipids	Serum or plasma (heparin)	Refrigerate
Liver enzymes	Serum or plasma (heparin)	Hemolysis will increase AST.
Mucopolysaccharides	Urine (random)	Refrigerate

(Continued)

Table 1.5 Specimen Collection and Handling (Continued)

Analyte	Specimen Type	Storage/Shipping/Comment
Organic acids	Urine (random)	Refrigerate if done in-house. Freeze for shipping. Scope of testing varies between laboratories.
pH and blood gases	Whole blood (heparin)	Send immediately on ice.
Pyridoxal-5-phosphate	CSF	Freeze
Pyruvate	Whole blood (heparin)	Add specimen to prechilled tube containing perchloric acid.
Sialic acid	Urine	Freeze
Succinyladenosine	CSF	Freeze
Sulfocysteine	Urine	Freeze
Uric acid	Serum or plasma (heparin) Urine (random or timed collection)	A large number of drugs interfere in uric acid methods. Consult laboratory.
Urinalysis	Urine (random or timed)	Tests generally include pH, specific gravity, protein, glucose, bilirubin, urobilinogen, leukocyte esterase, and cell count.

Modified and Reprinted with permission from Garg U, Smith LD, Heese BA. Introduction to the laboratory diagnosis of inherited metabolic diseases. In: Garg U, Smith LD, Heese BA, eds. Laboratory Diagnosis of Inherited Metabolic Diseases. Washington, DC: AACC Press, 2012:1–12. The table provides general information that can vary among laboratories.

Table 1.6 Variability Among Different Labs for Certain Analytes on Recent CAP Surveys (2014/2015)

Survey/Specimen	Disorder	Analyte/Biomarker	% CV[a]
BGL-B (2015)	Tyrosinemia type II (oculocutaneous)	Tyrosine	10
BGL-B (2015)	Medium chain acyl-CoA dehydrogenase deficiency	Octanoylcarnitine	22
		Decenoylcarnitine	29
		Hexanoylcarnitine	22
		Decanoylcarnitine	25
BGL-B (2015)	Maple syrup urine disease	Valine	23
		Leucine	22
		Isoleucine	24
		Alloisoleucine	69
BGL-A (2015)	Citrullinemia	Citrulline	9
		Glutamine	11
		Glutamic acid	19

(Continued)

Table 1.6 Variability Among Different Labs for Certain Analytes on Recent CAP Surveys (2014/2015) (Continued)

Survey/Specimen	Disorder	Analyte/Biomarker	% CV[a]
BGL-A (2015)	Isovaleric acidemia	Isovalerylglycine	65
BGL-A (2015)	Carnitine uptake defect	Free carnitine	17
		Acetylcarnitine	62
BGL-A (2015)	Medium-chain acyl CoA dehydrogenase deficiency	Hexanoylglycine	38
		Adipic	46
		Phenylpropionylglycine	54
		Suberylglycine	82
BGL-B (2014), urine amino acids	Cystinuria	Lysine	29
		Cystine	46
		Arginine	20
		Orinthine	15
BGL-B (2014), urine organic acids	Propionic acidemia	Methylcitric	140
		3-Hyroxypropionic	148
		Propionylglycine	84
		Tigylglycine	48
BGL-B (2014), plasma Acylcarnitine	Glutaric acidemia type II	Decanoylcarnitine	19
		Octanoylcarnitine	18
		Hexadecanoylcarnitine	17
		Dodecanoylcarnitine	24
		Isovalerylcarnitine/2-methyl-butyrylcarnitine	23
		Tetradecenoylcarnitine	19
		Tetradecanoylcarnitine	21
		Hexanoylcarnitine	32
BGL-B (2014), urine organic acids	Phenylketonuria	Phenyllactic	34
		2-Hydroxyphenylacetic	24
		Phenylacetic	55
		Phenylpyruvic	59
BGL-A (2014), plasma amino acids	Arginase deficiency	Arginine	8
		Glutamine	9
BGL-A (2014), urine organic acids	Glutaric acidemia type I	3-Hydroxyglutaric	79
		Glutaric	84
BGL-A (2014), plasma acylcarnitine	Very long chain acyl-CoA dehydrogenase deficiency	Tetradecenoylcarnitine	29
		Tetradecanoylcarnitine	19
		Tetradecadienoylcarnitine	29
		Hexadecanoylcarnitine	21
		Hexadecenoylcarnitine	26
BGL-A (2014), urine organic acids	Neuroblastoma	Homovanillic acid	17
		Vanillylmandelic acid	39

[a]% CV (coefficient of variation) is for all methods.

Table 1.7 Laboratories Reporting Correct Diagnosis on Recent CAP Surveys (2014/2015)

Disorder Class/Disorder	% Correct Diagnosis
Amino Acid	
Tyrosinemia type II (oculocutaneous)	100
Maple syrup urine disease	93
Citrullinemia	97
Cystinuria	94
Arginase deficiency	99
Organic Acid (Urine)	
Normal urine	96
Isovaleric acidemia	97
Propionic acidemia	99
Glutaric acidemia type 2	87
Phenylketonuria	93
Glutaric acidemia type I	80
Mucopolysaccharide (Urine)	
Normal urine	94
Hurler or Hunter syndrome (MPS I or II)	75
Morquio syndrome (type IV A or B)	75
Sanfilippo A, B, C, or D syndrome (type III A, B, C, or D)	93
Acylcarnitine (Plasma)	
Medium chain acyl-CoA dehydrogenase deficiency	100
Carnitine uptake defect	86
Medium chain acyl-CoA dehydrogenase deficiency	89
Glutaric acidemia type II	86
Very long chain acyl-CoA dehydrogenase deficiency	100

Quality control is an integral part of sample analysis. At least two, and generally three, quality control samples are included in the analysis of each batch of clinical samples. Quality control samples have values in the physiological and pathological range. Patient sample results are considered acceptable if concentrations of quality control samples are within the established range. Quality control ranges are generally established by the repeat analysis of the controls and calculating the range from mean ±2 or 3 standard deviations (SDs). Mean ±2 SD range is preferred, but may result in a high rejection rate. On the other hand, mean ±3 SD range will result in high acceptance rate with the possibility of falsely low or high patient results. These quality control schemes work well for methods involving single analytes, but may not work well for the analyses involving multiple analytes such as amino acid, acyl-carnitine, and organic acid profiles. For example, when the 2 SD rule is used, the chances of one quality control sample being within quality control range is 95%, and the probability of two controls being within quality control ranges is $0.95 \times 0.95 = 0.9025$ or 90.25%. The chances of all the controls within control ranges, for a 20-component analysis, is only $(0.95)^{\wedge 20 \times 2} = 0.128$ or 12.8%. Although these calculations assume independent analyses, and therefore overestimate the failure rate, nevertheless, this does make a point that in multicomponent analysis, simple quality control schemes do not work. Therefore, subjectivity is involved in accepting quality controls in multicomponent analysis by a properly trained analyst. In addition, the presence of an analyte, regardless of concentration may be clinically important. For example, detection of a succinylacetone peak on a urine organic acid profile may be clinically significant despite the lack of an acceptable quality control for succinyl-acetone. Therefore, the analyst should be knowledgeable and be able to objectively judge the performance of a method to be acceptable for clinical use.

Another important component of quality assurance is quality assessment through internal or external quality assessment programs. In the United States, specialized biochemical genetics tests are considered high-complexity tests under Clinical Laboratory Improvement Amendments (CLIA) of 1988. Laboratories that perform these tests must meet the CLIA requirements for high-complexity testing. For accreditation and quality control and assurance purposes, laboratories have to develop internal or external quality assessment programs. External quality assessment through proficiency testing, for a limited number of analytes, is available from the CAP[30] and the European Research Network for Evaluation and Improvement of Screening, Diagnosis, and Treatment of Inherited Disorders of Metabolism (ERNDIM).[31] These external proficiency-testing programs provide a glimpse into the challenges in the biochemical genetics laboratory diagnosis. As shown in Table 1.7, correct diagnosis among different labs varied from 75 to 100%.

1.6 METHOD SELECTION AND EVALUATION

Owing to the reasons listed above, method development and ongoing quality control for biochemical testing can be challenging. Before bringing a new method into the laboratory, several considerations including patient care needs, equipment, reagents, staffing, employee competency, quality control, and proficiency testing should be assessed. CLIA regulations and good laboratory practice require the establishment and/or verification of assay performance characteristics that include accuracy, precision, analytical sensitivity, analytical specificity, and reportable range. In addition, method validation may include method comparison with an established method, interferences, recovery, specimen stability, and verification or establishment of reference ranges.[32–36]

Accuracy refers to the closeness of the test result to the true values. There are various ways to determine the accuracy. It can be determined by comparing the results of the method in development with the results from a well-established reference method. In another approach, matrix-matched samples containing known amounts of the analyte are prepared, and the concentrations are compared to the known concentrations of a certified material. When possible, matrix-matched certified materials should be used. A minimum of three, ideally five to six, concentrations that cover the expected concentrations should be used. These specimens are analyzed several times, generally three to five, and the mean is calculated. Accuracy is determined by comparing the measured values with the target values, and is considered acceptable if the bias is within acceptable limits. Deviation of less than 10–20% is generally considered acceptable.

Precision of an analytical method refers to statistics of reproducibility, namely, the closeness of individual results. Precision is generally measured by evaluating imprecision, and expressed as coefficient of variation (CV) that is defined as relative standard deviation (RSD) and is calculated as SD × 100/Mean. Precision studies are generally conducted using quality control materials made from same biological matrix as the intended samples. Two to three concentrations in the expected range are generally used. Both short-term (within-run or within-day) and long-term (between-run or between-days) imprecision should be evaluated. Short-term imprecision can be evaluated by running quality control samples, ~20 times, within a run or within a day. Long-term imprecision is evaluated by analyzing quality control samples, ~20 times, at different days. Long-term imprecision is typically evaluated across users and different instruments. Imprecision of less than 10–20% is generally considered acceptable. Clinical and Laboratory Standards Institute (CLSI) guidelines are available for evaluating and verifying precision.[32,33]

Analytical sensitivity refers to lowest concentration of an analyte that can be measured with confidence. For most clinical assays, the lower limit of detection (LLOD) and lower limit of quantitation (LLOQ) are evaluated. LLOD is the lowest concentration that a method can detect or the lowest concentration that can be differentiated from zero concentration with confidence. LLOD can be calculated by running a blank sample that does not contain an analyte of interest multiple times, and calculating the value from mean + 2 or 3 SD. Since a number of biochemical genetics methods use chromatographic technique, a different approach is generally used to calculate LLOD. In chromatographic techniques, blank samples are spiked with low and varying concentrations of analyte(s) of interest. The lowest concentration that produces a clear peak is considered LLOD. LLOQ is defined as the concentration that can be measured with a defined accuracy and precision. Limit of quantitation can be calculated by analyzing samples of low analyte concentrations. CV is calculated at each concentration. The lowest concentration at which an acceptable CV is obtained is referred as LLOQ.

Analytical specificity, also frequently referred as selectivity, refers to the ability of an assay to measure an analyte of interest only and not other analytes. Ideally, a method should not measure nontarget analytes, but this is often not possible. Analytical specificity of a method is measured by spiking patient samples with potential interferents, and measuring analyte(s) of interest with and without the presence of interferents. It is generally not possible to carry out these studies in detail.

Literature should be consulted for possible interferences and the laboratory should be aware of these interferences, and make sure that the patient results are not affected or reported in case of interferences. In recent years, mass spectrometry assays are increasingly being used in biochemical genetics laboratories. These methods are relatively more specific and less prone to interferences.

Reportable range, also referred as linearity, is the range of analyte concentrations that a method can measure without dilution. In multistandards assay, it is the range between the lowest and highest standards used to produce a calibration curve. Reportable range can be calculated by analyzing four to six concentrations that cover the reportable range, and calculating the measured values with the target values within allowable error. CLSI guidelines are available for evaluating linearity.[37] In a more complex multiple component analysis, it may not be easy or feasible to calculate reportable range for all the analytes. For example, in amino acids analysis, it is difficult to validate very high concentrations of individual amino acids by spiking very high concentrations of individual amino acids. Also, it is not known how a very high concentration of one amino acid can affect the quantitation of another amino acid. To avoid delay in result reporting, it may be acceptable to report an approximate value that is close to an actual value.

Reference intervals also called as "reference values," "normal values," and "expected values," refer to the range of values found in a healthy or reference population. For endogenous compounds, reference intervals are customarily defined as limits covering central 95% of the values or the mean $\pm$ 2 SD (if the data has Gaussian distribution). Reference ranges are either established or taken from the literature and verified. Many factors including age, sex, race, geographic location, fasting, specimen type, and so on can influence reference intervals. Reference intervals must be verified or established using well-defined approaches.[38]

1.7 TREATMENT AND PROGNOSIS

The treatment and prognosis of IEM vary significantly among different disorders. For disorders that present with acute illness, empiric therapeutic management is generally needed before a definitive diagnosis is made. Initial aggressive treatment may be life-saving and avoid long-term sequelae. For example, acidosis is treated with sodium bicarbonate, and seizures with antiepileptic drugs. Long-term therapies include dietary therapy such as protein restriction, avoidance of fasting, or cofactor supplementation. In recent years, more specific treatments such as enzyme replacement therapies and bone marrow transplantation for several of the lysosomal storage diseases or organ transplantation in the urea cycle disorders, or some of the organic acidurias, have become feasible. Efforts to develop treatments through gene therapy are being actively studied, and may provide additional therapeutic possibilities in the future. For many disorders, only supportive and palliative care is available with little effect on final outcomes. Nevertheless, even if no treatment is available, accurate diagnosis, genetic counseling, and prenatal screening can be invaluable.

REFERENCES

1. Saudubray J-M. *Inborn metabolic diseases: diagnosis and treatment*, 5th ed. New York, NY: Springer-Verlag; 2011.
2. Saudubray JM, Desguerre I, Sedel F, Charpentier C. A clinical approach to inherited metabolic diseases. In: Fernandes J, Saudubray JM, van den Berghe G, Walter JH, editors. *Inborn metabolic diseases: diagnosis and treatment* 4th, rev. ed.. Heidelberg: Springer; 2006. p. 3–48.
3. Jacob H. Update on expanded newborn screening. *Arch Dis Child Educ Pract Ed* 2015.
4. Ombrone D, Giocaliere E, Forni G, Malvagia S, la Marca G. Expanded newborn screening by mass spectrometry: new tests, future perspectives. *Mass Spectrom Rev* 2016;**35**(1):71–84.
5. Rinaldo P, Lim JS, Tortorelli S, Gavrilov D, Matern D. Newborn screening of metabolic disorders: recent progress and future developments. *Nestle Nutr Workshop Ser Pediatr Program* 2008;**62**:81–93. discussion 93-6.
6. Dietzen DJ, Rinaldo P, Whitley RJ, et al. National academy of clinical biochemistry laboratory medicine practice guidelines: follow-up testing for metabolic disease identified by expanded newborn screening using tandem mass spectrometry; executive summary. *Clin Chem* 2009;**55**(9):1615–26.
7. Rinaldo P, Hahn S, Matern D. Inborn errors of amino acid, organic acid and fatty acid metabolism. In: Burtis CA, Ashwood ER, Bruns DE, editors. *Tietz textbook of clinical chemistry and molecular diagnostics* 4th ed. St. Louis, MO: Saunders; 2006. p. 2207–47.
8. Hoffmann GF, Zschocke J, Nyhan WL. *Inherited metabolic diseases: a clinical approach*. Heidelberg: Springer; 2010.
9. Clarke JTR. *A clinical guide to inherited metabolic diseases*, 3rd ed. Cambridge, U.K. New York: Cambridge University Press; 2006.
10. Blau N. *Physician's guide to the laboratory diagnosis of metabolic diseases*, 2nd ed. Berlin; New York: Springer; 2003.
11. Genetests. www.genetests.org.
12. Nyhan WL, Barshop BA, Ozand PT. *Atlas of metabolic diseases*, 2nd ed. London: Hodder Arnold; 2005.
13. Scriver CR. *The metabolic & molecular bases of inherited disease*, 8th ed. New York: McGraw-Hill; 2001.
14. Mak CM, Lee HC, Chan AY, Lam CW. Inborn errors of metabolism and expanded newborn screening: review and update. *Crit Rev Clin Lab Sci* 2013;**50**(6):142–62.
15. Miller MJ, Kennedy AD, Eckhart AD, et al. Untargeted metabolomic analysis for the clinical screening of inborn errors of metabolism. *J Inherit Metab Dis* 2015;**38**(6):1029–39.
16. Raghuveer TS, Garg U, Graf WD. Inborn errors of metabolism in infancy and early childhood: an update. *Am Fam Physician* 2006;**73**(11):1981–90.
17. Rinaldo P, Hahn S, Matern D. Clinical biochemical genetics in the twenty-first century. *Acta Paediatr Suppl* 2004;**93**(445):22–6. discussion 27.
18. Blau N, Duran M, Gibson KM. *Laboratory guide to the methods in biochemical genetics*. Berlin: Springer; 2008.
19. Garg U, Smith LD, Heesee BA. Introduction to the laboratory diagnosis of inherited metabolic diseases. In: Garg U, Smith LD, Heesee BA, editors. *Laboratory diagnosis of inherited metabolic diseases*. Washington, DC: AACC Press; 2012. p. 1–12.

20. Gibson KM, Duran M. Simple metabolic screening tests. In: Blau N, Duran M, Gibson KM, editors. *Laboratory guide to the methods in biochemical genetics*. Berlin: Springer; 2008. p. 24–33.

21. Zschocke J. Function testsHoffman G.F.Zschocke J, Nyhan WL, editors. *Inherited metabolic diseases: a clinical approach*, **xiv**. Heidelberg: Springer; 2010. p. 386.

22. Atherton AM, Smith LD, Heesee BA, Garg U. Lysosomal storage disorders: mucopolysaccharidoses and mucolipidoses. In: Garg U, Smith LD, Heesee BA, editors. *Laboratory diagnosis of inherited metabolic diseases*. Washington, DC: AACC Press; 2012. p. 105–17.

23. Atherton AM, Smith LD, Heesee BA, Garg U. Lysosomal storage disorders: sphingolipidoses and lysosomal transport disorders. In: Garg U, Smith LD, Heesee BA, editors. *Laboratory diagnosis of inherited metabolic diseases*. Washington, DC: AACC Press; 2012. p. 119–31.

24. Ferguson AM, Smith LD, Garg U. Disorders of carbohydrate metabolism. In: Garg U, Smith LD, Heesee BA, editors. *Laboratory diagnosis of inherited metabolic diseases*. Washington, DC: AACC Press; 2012. p. 93–103.

25. Heese BA. Disorders of purine and pyrimidine metabolism. In: Garg U, Smith LD, Heesee BA, editors. *Laboratory diagnosis of inherited metabolic diseases*. Washington, DC: AACC Press; 2012. p. 143–56.

26. Jones PM, Bennett MJ. Disorders of the carnitine cycle and mitochondrial fatty acid oxidation. In: Garg U, Smith LD, Heesee BA, editors. *Laboratory diagnosis of inherited metabolic diseases*. Washington DC: AACC Press; 2012. p. 65–91.

27. Lo SF, Scott-Schwoerer JA, Rhead WJ. Organic acid disorders. In: Garg U, Smith LD, Heesee BA, editors. *Laboratory diagnosis of inherited metabolic diseases*. Washington, DC: AACC Press; 2012. p. 37–53.

28. Smith LD, Garg U. Peroxisomal disorders. In: Garg U, Smith LD, Heesee BA, editors. *Laboratory diagnosis of inherited metabolic diseases*. Washington, DC: AACC Press; 2012. p. 133–41.

29. Zhao Z, Leung-Pineda V, Dietzen DJ. Amino acids disorders. In: Garg U, Smith LD, Heesee BA, editors. *Laboratory diagnosis of inherited metabolic diseases*. Washington, DC: AACC Press; 2012. p. 13–35.

30. http://www.cap.org/apps/cap.portal.

31. http://www.erndim.unibas.ch/.

32. Evaluation of Precision of Quantitative Measurement Procedures; Approved Guideline—Third Edition (EP05-A3). ISBN Number: 1-56238-967-X. Wayne, PA: Clinical and laboratory Standards Institute; 2014.

33. User Verification of Precision and Estimation of Bias; Approved Guideline—Third Edition (EP15-A3). ISBN Number: 1-56238-965-3. Wayne, PA: Clinical and laboratory Standards Institute; 2014.

34. Oxyley DK, Garg U, Olsowka ES. Maximizing the information from laboratory tests. In: Jacobs DS, Demott WR, Oxley DK, editors. *Jacobs and Demott laboratory test handbook* 4th ed. Hudson, OH: Lexi-Comp; 2001. p. 15–33.

35. Solber HE. Establishment and use of reference values. In: Burtis CA, Ashwood ER, Bruns DE, editors. *Tietz textbook of clinical chemistry and molecular diagnostics* 5th ed. Elsevier Health Sciences; 2011. p. 425–48.

36. Linnet K, Boyd JC. Selection and analytical evalutation of methods with statistical techniques. In: Burtis CA, Ashwood ER, Bruns DE, editors. *Tietz textbook of clinical chemistry and molecular diagnostics* 4th ed. St. Louis, MO: Saunders; 2006. p. 353–407.

37. Evaluation of the Linearity of Quantitative Measurement Procedures: A Statistical Approach; Approved Guideline. EP06-A. Wayne, PA: Clinical and Laboratory Standards Institute; 2003.

38. Horowitz GL, Altaie S, Boyd JC, et al. *Defining, establishing, and verifying reference intervals in the clinical laboratory: approved guidelines*, 3rd ed. Wayne, PA: Clinical and Laboratory Standards Institute; 2008.

Amino acids disorders

2

P.D. DeArmond[1], D.J. Dietzen[2,3] and A.L. Pyle-Eilola[1,4]

[1]*Nationwide Children's Hospital, Columbus, OH, United States;* [2]*Washington University School of Medicine, St. Louis, MO, United States;* [3]*St. Louis Children's Hospital, St. Louis, MO, United States;* [4]*The Ohio State University, Columbus, OH, United States*

2.1 INTRODUCTION

Inborn errors of amino acid metabolism result from an aberration in the normal breakdown of amino acids in the body: intestinal absorption, renal excretion and reabsorption, synthesis into functional proteins, and metabolism.[1] As a result, amino acids and metabolic intermediates build up in blood and tissues. Symptoms of disease manifest as the result of toxicity of the accumulated intermediates and/or from the lack of downstream metabolic products.

Aminoacidopathies and other inborn errors of metabolism (IEM) may be suspected on the basis of nonspecific symptoms of infants and children, and more rarely in adults, including lethargy, failure to thrive, digestive and neurological problems, movement disorders, and history of metabolic derangement. When a patient presents in the midst of acute symptomology, efforts should be made to obtain urine and blood samples during the critical state, as diagnostic findings may only be detectable from samples obtained during the height of such a presentation. Investigation of IEM may also be prompted on the basis of a previously affected sibling or from abnormal results from a newborn screen (NBS). Measurement of urine organic acids, plasma amino acids, and acylcarnitines are appropriate screening tests for the initial evaluation of these patients. Urine amino acids are particularly useful for renal amino acid transporter deficiencies, such as cystinuria. Common findings in several aminoacidopathies are summarized in Table 2.1.

The gold standard method for plasma amino acid analysis, employed by most clinical laboratories, is a dedicated, quantitative ion-exchange chromatography with postcolumn derivitization with ninhydrin. Dedicated high-performance liquid chromatography (HPLC) amino acid analyzers quantitate 30–40 amino acids in a single analysis, though it can take well over an hour per sample.[1–5] Other body fluids, including urine and cerebrospinal fluid (CSF), as well as dried blood spots can also be analyzed

Table 2.1 Characteristic Biomarkers of Aminoacidopathies

Disease	Amino Acid Findings	Other Markers
Cystinuria	Cys, Orn, Lys, Arg, Hcy (U) ↑	Cystine crystals and stones (U)
Homocystinuria	Hcy (B, U) ↑ Met (B, U) ↑	Cys, cystathionine (B) ↓ Methylmalonic acid (B) NL/↓
Hypermethioninemia	Met (B, U) ↑	S-adenosylhomocysteine (B) ↑ S-adenosylmethionine (B) ↑
Hyperphenylalaninemia (Non-PKU)	Phe (B) ↑	Biopterin (B, U) ↓ neopterin (B, U) ↑/NL/↓ HVA, 5-HIAA (B) NL/↓
Hyperprolinemia	Pro (B, U) ↑	P5-C (U) ↑ (type II)
Maple Syrup Urine Disease	Valine, Isoleucine, Leucine (B) ↑ Allsoisoleucine (B) ↑	Urine organic acid profile: α-hydroxyisocaropic, α-hydroxyisovaleric, α-hydroxy-β-methylvaleric, α-keto-β-methylvaleric, α-ketoisocaproic, and α-ketoisovaleric acids (U) ↑
Nonketotic Hyperglycinemia	Glycine (B, U, CSF) ↑ CSF/plasma glycine ↑	
Phenylketonuria	Phe (B) ↑ Tyr (B) ↓ Phe/Tyr ratio (B) ↑	Urine organic acid profile: Phenylpyruvic, phenylacetic, phenyllactic, 2-hydroxyphenylacetic, N-phenylacetylglutamic acids (U) ↑
Sulfocysteinuria	Cystine (B) ↓	Sulfite (U) ↑
Tyrosinemia Type I	Tyr (B) ↑	Succinylacetone (B) ↑
Tyrosinemia Type II	Tyr (B) ↑↑	4-hydroxyphenyllactate, 4-hydroxyphenylpyruvate (U) ↑
Tyrosinemia Type III	Tyr (B) ↑	Hydroxyphenylpyruvate, hydroxyphenyllactate, homogentisic acid, hawkinsin, 5-oxoproline (U) ↑

B, blood; U, urine; CSF, cerebrospinal fluid; NL, normal; P5-C, pyrroline 5-carboxylate.

by this method. Other methods for amino acid analysis include tandem mass spectrometry (MS/MS), which is commonly used by NBS laboratories, gas chromatography, and reversed-phase chromatography with precolumn derivatization with various reagents.[3] Normal plasma and urine amino acid profiles are shown in Fig. 2.1.

Amino acid profile results can be reported with just the quantitative data and age-appropriate reference interval for each amino acid. Owing to the complexity of these results, an interpretation by a qualified clinical chemist or biochemical geneticist is usually included to provide an explanation of the results and likely causes for the results. If necessary, the interpretation may include recommendations for additional testing, such as molecular or enzyme activity analysis to confirm a diagnosis.

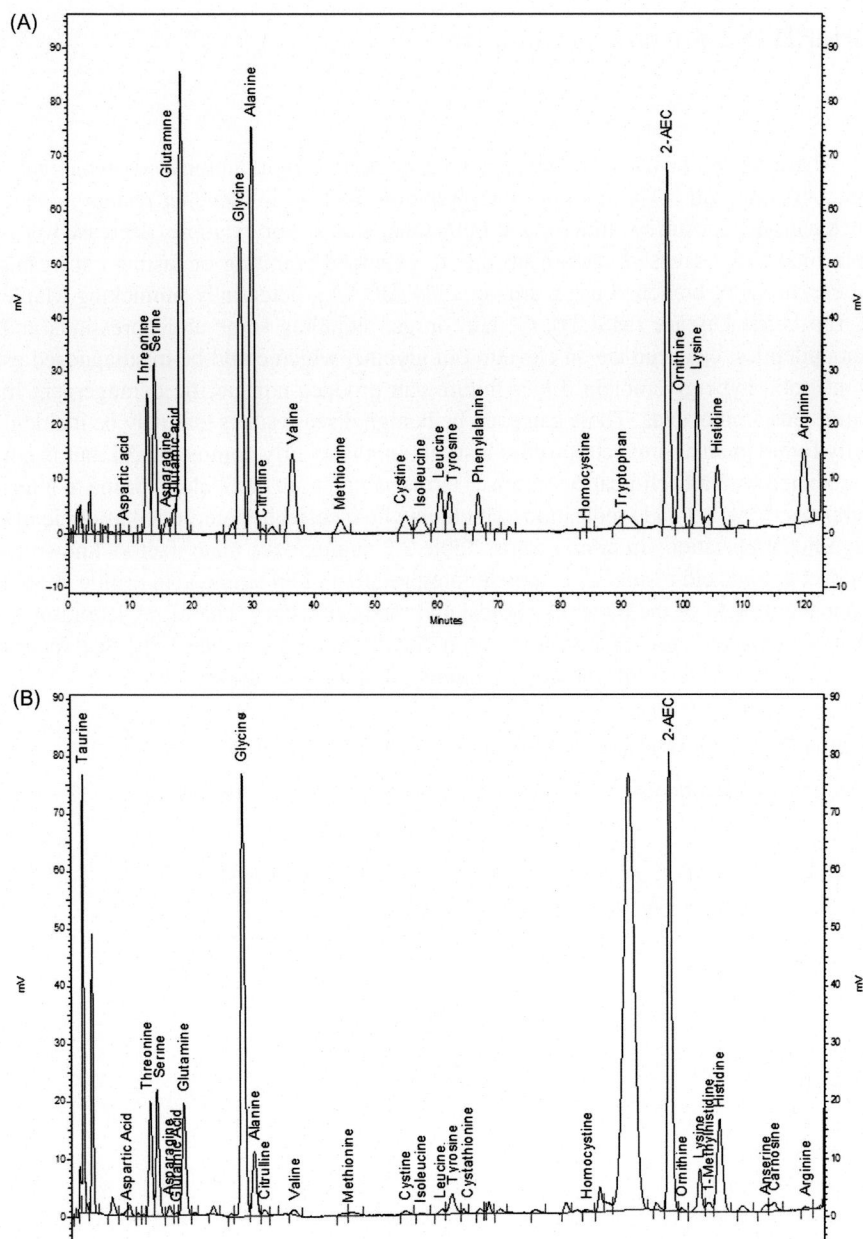

FIGURE 2.1 Plasma and urine amino acid chromatographs from normal individuals.

(A) Normal plasma amino acid chromatograph. (B) Normal urine amino acid chromatograph. Unless otherwise noted, amino acid chromatographs are generated as follows. Samples are spiked with S-(2-aminoethyl)-L-cysteine (2-AEC) then undergo protein precipitation with sulfosalicylic acid, followed by filtration through 0.22 μm membrane. The filtrate was analyzed by Hitachi L-8800 Amino Acid Analyzer. The method is a quantitative, dedicated ion-exchange HPLC with postcolumn ninhydrin derivitization.

There are several causes of nonspecific changes in various amino acids, which may be confusing without a thorough interpretation. Factors influencing results include medications, concurrent illness, and nutritional status. For example, decreased protein intake or increased catabolism due to extended vomiting or fasting can result in elevations of branched chain amino acids (BCAA), potentially mimicking Maple Syrup Urine Disease (MSUD). Certain drugs, including some antidepressants and antiepileptics, can produce an elevation in glycine, which could be misdiagnosed as nonketotic hyperglycinemia. Liver failure can produce nonspecific derangement in numerous amino acids. There can even be benign disease states that may be incidentally found in an amino acid profile: histidinemia is a fairly common IEM, but is not associated with any clinical symptoms.[6] Urine samples are particularly prone to interferences from diet and medication, which may be incorrectly interpreted as clinically significant elevations in amino acids. Table 2.2 summarizes many factors known to impact amino acid results. A complete interpretation of an amino acid profile should be made in light of the patient's clinical and medical history. Therefore, laboratories that do not have access to this information directly through a patient's medical record may require that such information be submitted along with the sample.

Table 2.2 Factors Influencing Amino Acid Profile Interpretation

Preanalytical Condition	Amino Acid Affected	Affect
Hemolysis (B)	Glu, Gly, Asp, Orn	↑
	Gln, Arg	↓
Bacterial contamination (U)	Pro, Ala, Gly	↑
	Phe, Tyr, His, Trp, Ser	↓
Extended storage (B)	Gln, Cys, Hcy	↓
Extended storage (U)	Gln, Asn, phosphoethanolamine	↑
Pregnancy (U)	Arg, His, Thr	↑
Starvation (B)	Gly, Leu, ile, Val	↑
	Ala	↓
Severe burns (B)	Phe	↑
Severe burns (U)	Ala, Gly, Glu, Gln, Orn, Pro, Ser, Thr	↓
Liver dysfunction (B)	Met, Orn, Phe, Tyr	↑
	Leu, Ile, Val	↓
Ketosis (B)	Ile, Leu, Val	↑
Acetaminophen (U)	Phe	↑
Ampicillin/amoxicillin (U)	Met, Phe	↑
Oral contraceptives (B)	Ala, Gly, Leu, Pro, Tyr, Val	↓
Antiepileptics (B, U)	Gly	↑
Infection (B, U)	All amino acids	Varies with degree and type of infection

B, blood; U, urine

2.2 PHENYLKETONURIA (PKU)

2.2.1 BRIEF DESCRIPTION OF THE DISORDER AND PATHWAY

Phenylketonuria (PKU, OMIM: 261600) is the most common inborn error of metabolism of amino acids, affecting approximately 1:15,000 persons in the United States. Incidence is as high as 1:2600 live births in Turkey and as low as 1:200,000 in Finland.[7] There are over 500 known mutations in the phenylalanine hydroxylase (*PAH*) gene that cause PKU, which is inherited in an autosomal recessive manner. The PAH enzyme catalyzes the catabolism of phenylalanine (Phe) to tyrosine (Tyr), so in the absence of fully functional PAH, Phe accumulates while Tyr concentrations fall (Fig. 2.2). Since tetrahydrobiopterin (BH4) is a cofactor required for the conversion of Phe to Tyr, supplementation with BH4 can drive PAH activity in some individuals with certain mutations, lowering plasma Phe.[8]

There are three classes of PKU, each of which can be BH4 responsive or non-responsive: classic, non-PKU hyperphenylalaninemia (HPA), and variant PKU.[9,10] Children with classic, untreated PKU demonstrate microcephaly, significant intellectual and developmental delay, epilepsy, and behavioral problems. Excess Phe in body fluids produces a musty or mousy odor in sweat, cerumen, and urine, and causes eczematous rashes. Lack of Tyr results in decreased melanin synthesis, so patients may have fair hair and skin. Even with rapid initiation of treatment after birth, patients with PKU are more likely to develop neurological sequelae, psychiatric disturbances, and low bone mineral density and osteopenia in later decades.[7,11–14] Fortunately, with the introduction of NBS to identify and treat PKU in early life, highly symptomatic PKU is increasingly rare. Individuals with non-PKU HPA, generally have lower concentrations of plasma Phe on a normal diet and lower incidence of developmental impairment than those with classic PKU (see section "Non-PKU Hyperphenylalaninemias").[15]

2.2.2 BRIEF DESCRIPTION OF TREATMENT

Treatment of PKU centers on lowering the plasma concentrations of Phe and increasing Tyr, thereby preventing neurological, developmental, and psychological sequelae.[16] Therefore, a life-long Phe-restricted, Tyr-supplemented diet is recommended. Women should have Phe levels within the recommended treatment range for at least three months prior to conception as well as during gestation. This is achieved by following a low-protein diet supplemented with Phe-free medical beverages. Diet should be adjusted during times of high growth, stress, activity, or illness, times when body stores of protein may be metabolized for energy, thus increasing plasma Phe. Therefore, particular care should be made during times of stress to maintain Phe and Tyr concentrations within the recommended treatment range.[17]

BH4 supplementation with the synthetic BH4 drug sapropterin dihydrochloride (brand name: Kuvan), can be beneficial for those individuals with BH4-responsive HPA. It has been estimated that 25–50% of individuals with HPA are BH4-responsive,

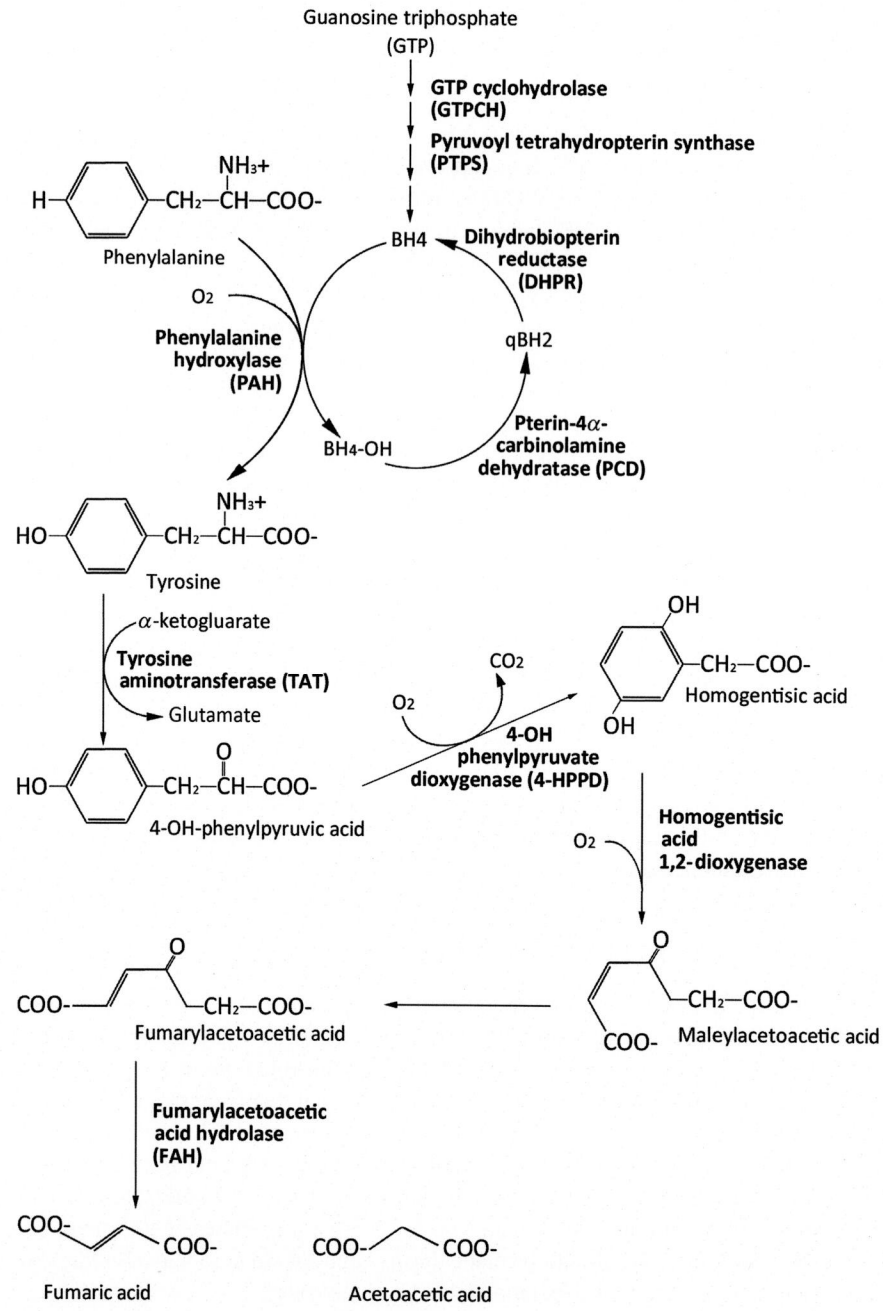

FIGURE 2.2 Phenylalanine and tyrosine metabolic pathway.

Absence of function PAH causes PKU. Non-PKU hyperphenlylaninemia results from failure in BH4 biosynthesis due to mutations in GTPCH, PTPS, DHPR, or PCD. Defects in FAH, TAT, and 4-HPPD cause tyrosinemias type I, II, and III, respectively.

and those with mild HPA are more likely to be responsive.[18] These patients may be able to relax their protein restriction with BH4 supplementation, and some may be able to end dietary restrictions all together while maintaining appropriate Phe and Tyr concentrations. For some patients, this greatly improves treatment compliance and quality of life.[19]

2.2.3 BIOMARKERS FOR DIAGNOSIS

Elevated Phe, specifically with an elevated Phe:Tyr ratio is central for the diagnosis of PKU (Fig. 2.3). There are several methods for measuring these amino acids, but the most common are HPLC-based methods and LC/MS, either as part of a full amino acid profile or targeted quantitation of Phe and Tyr. Testing may be routinely performed on plasma or dried blood spots. Diagnosis of HPA is made on the basis of a plasma Phe concentration >120 μmol/L, or a Phe/Tyr ratio >3.[7,20] Untreated classic PKU is usually associated with Phe >1000 μmol/L.[7] On urine organic acid analysis, patients with PKU will show elevations in phenylpyruvic, phenylacetic, phenyllactic, 2-hydroxyphenylacetic, and N-phenylacetylglutamic acids.[21] Full gene sequencing, duplication/deletion testing, or targeted mutation analysis of the PAH gene may be

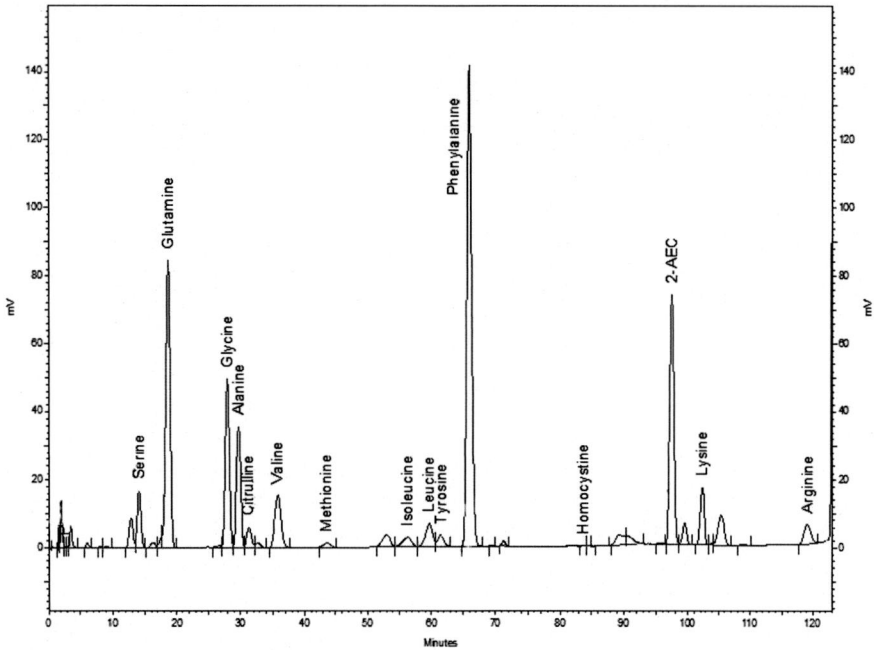

FIGURE 2.3 Plasma amino acid profile from a patient with phenylketonuria.

Patient was doing well, but presented with elevated Phe during acute illness. Phe is 1014 μmol/L, Tyr is 26 μmol/L.

used to confirm a diagnosis of PKU. However, there are over 600 known mutations in PAH, with varying degrees of disease severity. While individuals with similar genotypes do not always have the same phenotype, genotype remains a major determinant of clinical outcome.[18]

In the 1960s, PKU became the first disease to be universally screened in the United States for newborns by the "Guthrie method" of bacterial growth in the presence of high concentration of Phe.[22] By the mid-1970s, PKU was part of the NBS for most countries worldwide. Currently, most NBS methods are based on the MS quantitation of amino acids from a dried blood spot.

2.2.4 BIOMARKERS FOLLOWED FOR TREATMENT EFFICACY

Individuals with PKU have Phe and Tyr routinely monitored, to ensure optimal dietary control of the disease. The National Institutes of Health (NIH) Consensus Development Conference on PKU recommends weekly testing during the first year of life, every two weeks from 1 to 12 years of age, and monthly thereafter, and diet tailored to maintain plasma Phe between 120 and 360 μmol/L. Tyr supplementation is targeted to maintain blood Tyr concentrations within the normal reference interval.[23]

To determine which individuals are responsive to BH4, patients may be given a sapropterin challenge in which plasma Phe is measured at baseline and at several intervals after a 20 mg/kg dose, usually one day, one week, and two weeks. During this time, no dietary changes should be made. A decrease in Phe by at least 30% is considered evidence of BH4 responsiveness. [18]

2.3 NON-PKU HYPERPHENYLALANINEMIAS

2.3.1 BRIEF DESCRIPTION OF THE DISORDER AND PATHWAY

In addition to defects in PAH, accumulation of Phe in blood and tissues can result from defects in synthesis of tetrahydrobiopterin (BH_4), a cofactor for PAH activity. Other BH4-dependent enzymes include nitric oxide synthase, tryptophan hydroxylase, and tyrosine hydroxylase.

Deficits in four enzymes involved in BH4 synthesis and regeneration are responsible for non-PKU hyperphenylalaninemias, and account for only 1–3% of total cases of HPA. These enzymes are guanosine triphosphate cyclohydrolase (GTPCH, OMIM: 266910), pyruvoyl tetrahydropterin synthase (PTPS, OMIM: 261640), dihydrobiopterin reductase (DHPR, OMIM: 264070), and pterin-4α-carbinolamine dehydratase (PCD, OMIM: 261630) (Fig. 2.2). PTPS is the most common of the BH4 deficiencies, accounting for 61% of cases, followed by DHPR at 31%, and GTPCH and PCD at 4% each.[24] In these patients, plasma Phe is elevated, though usually not to the same degree as in PKU, and central nervous system amine deficiency impairs neurotransmitter function. Unlike PKU, which has a Phe:Tyr ratio >3, non-PKU HPA usually has a ratio ≤2.1. The clinical presentation depends on the specific mutation and ranges in severity. PTPS deficiency has two clinical presentations: 80% of patients with PTPS demonstrate the severe form, and 20% have the mild or peripheral form. The severe form presents with truncal hypotonia with increased limb tone, which is often preceded by loss of head control. Peripheral forms of PTPS may be normal early in life, but low levels of CSF neurotransmitters may present neurological abnormalities in the first years. Symptoms of GTPCH deficiency include seizures, mental retardation, hypotonia, temperature instability, and feeding difficulties in infancy. DHPR deficiency is the most severe of the non-PKU HPA diseases, and is similar to the severe presentations of GTPCH and PTPS, with the addition of abnormal vascular and neuronal calcification. PCD deficiency is essentially benign, though some transient neonatal hypotonia has been noted.

2.3.2 BRIEF DESCRIPTION OF TREATMENT

The aim of treatment is generally to control Phe concentration. BH4 administration is the best means of controlling Phe levels in patients with non-PKU HPA. Additionally, 5-hydroxytryptophan, L-dopa, and other neurotransmitter-inducing drugs may be administered to maintain appropriate levels of neurotransmitters.

2.3.3 BIOMARKERS FOR DIAGNOSIS

Plasma or dried blood spot Phe elevation is usually the first indication of an abnormality. However, unlike PKU, untreated non-PKU HPA patients may have only slightly elevated Phe. Therefore, all elevated Phe values from NBS should be investigated.[24]

Urine and blood pterin profiles are central in the diagnosis of non-PKU HPA, whereas these will be normal to elevated in PKU, biopterin is low in PTPS, GTPCH, DHPR, and PCD deficiencies. Neopterin is low with GTPCH deficiency, high in PTPS and PCD deficiencies, and normal to high in DHPR deficiency. Primapterin is notably elevated only in PCD-deficient patients. These findings are summarized in Table 2.3.

The measurement of markers of specific neurotransmitters in CSF, 5-hydroxyindoleacetic acid (5-HIAA) and homovanillic acid (HVA) is also central to the diagnosis. These neurotransmitters are normal in PKU and PCD deficiency, but are below the normal range in PTPS, GTPCH, and DHPR deficiencies.[25]

Enzyme activity assays are available for PTPS, GTPCH, and DHPR. Additionally, gene sequencing may be used to finalize a diagnosis. If there is an affected sibling with a known diagnosis, prenatal diagnosis of a fetus may be achieved by measurement of pterins in amniotic fluid or mutational analysis following chorionic villus sampling if the mutation is known. Enzyme analysis of DHPR or PTPS in fetal erthyrocytes or amniocytes can also be used for diagnosis. However, since GTPCH is only expressed in fetal liver, GTPCH enzyme activity cannot be assessed prenatally.[25]

Table 2.3 Interpretation in the Laboratory Investigation of HPA

Gene	Blood Phe (µmol/L)	Neopterin (B, U)	Biopterin (B, U)	Primapterin (B, U)	HVA, 5-HIAA (CSF)	BH4-Loading Test Phe Response
PTPS	90–1200	↑↑	↓↓	NL	↓	Normalization of Phe w/in 4–8h of administration
GTPCH	240–2500	↓↓	↓↓	NL	↓	
PCD	180–1200	↑	↓	↑↑	NL	
DHPR	180–2500	NL to ↑	↓↓	NL	↓	Near-noramlization
PAH	>120	↑	↑	NL	NL	>30% reduction of Phe in responsive PKU

B, blood; U, urine; CSF, cerebrospinal fluid; PAH, phenylalanine hydroxylase; PTPS, pyruvoyl-tetrahydropterin synthase; GTPCH, guanosine triphosphate cyclohydrolase; DHPR, dihydrobiopterin reductase; PCD, pterin-4α-carbinolamine dehydratase; HVA, homovanillic acid; 5-HIAA, 5-hydroxyindole acetic acid; Phe, phenylalanine; NL, normal.

2.3.4 BIOMARKERS FOLLOWED FOR TREATMENT EFFICACY

Plasma or dried blood spot Phe and pterins may be followed to monitor treatment efficacy in non-PKU HPA patients. Likewise, CSF measurement of HVA and 5-HIAA may also be used to assess adequacy of L-dopa and other neurotransmitter supplementation. Since prolactin is also regulated by dopamine, serum prolactin has been suggested as a marker for monitoring L-dopa treatment.

2.4 TYROSINEMIAS

2.4.1 BRIEF DESCRIPTION OF THE DISORDER AND PATHWAY

Tyrosine is ordinarily a nonessential amino acid with a phenolic side chain. It becomes essential in conditions such as phenylketonuria and defective biopterin metabolism when hydroxylation of the phenyl ring of phenylalanine is impaired. Peptide-bound tyrosine plays an important role in enzyme catalysis and in signaling cascades. Tyrosyl hydrogen bonds aid in stabilizing secondary and tertiary protein structure and also contribute to active-site substrate (e.g., carboxypeptidase A) or coenzyme binding (e.g., lactate dehydrogenase). Phosphorylation of peptide-bound tyrosine residues regulates a number of transmembrane signaling pathways important for cell growth (e.g., mitogen-activated protein (MAP), Janus kinase (JAK) pathways). Tyrosine is also a precursor for a number of important biologic molecules, including thyroxine, dopamine, adrenaline, and melanin. Defects in tyrosine catabolism, therefore, have a broad physiologic impact.

Tyrosine is ultimately catabolized to fumarate and acetoacetate through a series of five enzymatic steps (Fig. 2.2). Tyrosine is, therefore, an anaplerotic, ketogenic, and glucogenic amino acid. Following transamination, the alpha carbon and phenyl ring are oxidized by 4-hydroxyphenlpyruvate dioxygenase (4-HPPD) to form homogentisic acid. The phenyl ring is then broken to successively form maleylacetoacetate and fumarylacetoacetate. Final hydrolysis is achieved by fumarylacetoacetate hydrolase (FAH). Defects in FAH are responsible for tyrosinemia type I. Defects in tyrosine aminotransferase (TAT) and 4-HPPD are responsible for types II and III tyrosinemia, respectively.[26]

Although the various forms of tyrosinemia arise from defects in the same metabolic pathway, these disorders are clinically distinct. Biochemical distinction, therefore, takes on added importance.

Type I (OMIM 276700). Type I disease (also known as hepatorenal tyrosinemia) has an estimated incidence of 1:100,000 and presents in infancy after a brief asymptomatic period. The disorder is primarily characterized by acute hepatic and renal failure. Sequelae include encephalopathy, coagulopathy, and neurologic crises that resemble porphyria. Longer term consequences include nodular liver cirrhosis, often with progression to hepatocellular carcinoma, and rickets. Left untreated, death usually occurs by one year of age.

Type II (OMIM 276600). Type II disease (also known as oculocutaneous tyrosinemia) has an estimated incidence of 1:250,000 and typically presents between the ages of two and four years with painful papular lesions on the digits, palms, and soles, as well as photophobia, vision loss, physical, and developmental delay.

Type III (OMIM 276710). Patients with type III disease present in early infancy. The natural history of this disorder is not well understood because of its rarity but reported phenotypes vary from very mild to developmental delay and seizures. Liver function is notably normal.

A small subset of mutations in 4-HPPD results in an autosomal dominant condition termed *Hawkinsinuria* (OMIM: 140350). The clinical phenotype ranges from very mild to infantile metabolic acidosis and failure to thrive.

2.4.2 BIOMARKERS FOR DIAGNOSIS

Increased plasma tyrosine is observed in all three types of tyrosine catabolic defects. Tyrosine concentrations in type I disease are often modest (100–500 μM) and sometimes within the normal reference interval (<150 μM). The type I defect affects the fourth step in the pathway. While the initial transamination step is readily reversible, subsequent reactions through FAH are less so, resulting in a blunted accumulation of tyrosine. Defective activity of FAH leads to accumulation of fumarylacetoacetate, which is converted to succinylacetoacetate and succinylacetone in successive nonenzymatic reactions. Succinylacetone and related metabolites may exert toxic effects via glutathione depletion and formation of amino acid–adducts.[27,28] The resulting renal Fanconi syndrome can lead to growth failure and rickets.[29] Succinylacetone also inhibits δ-aminolevulinate dehydratase and leads to the porphyria-like crises in affected patients.[30] The mechanisms responsible for nodular liver regeneration and eventual hepatocellular carcinoma are not well defined. Thus, increased tyrosine is a sensitive but not very specific indicator of disease. Detectable quantities of succinylacetone in blood and urine are pathognomonic for the disturbance. Diagnoses are often confirmed by genetic analysis. An amino acid profile from a patient with tyrosinemia I is shown in Fig. 2.4.

Type II tyrosinemia is a defect in the initial step of tyrosine catabolism and typically results in massive hypertyrosinemia of 1000–3000 μM upon initial diagnosis. The skin lesions, photophobia, and vision loss are thought to be directly related to tissue deposition of tyrosine crystals.[31] Extreme tyrosine concentrations are virtually diagnostic of this disorder, which is also characterized by paradoxical urinary excretion of the transaminated tyrosine metabolites, 4-hydroxyphenyllactate and 4-hydroxyphenylpyruvate. These metabolites likely arise from cross reactivity with other aminotransferase activities despite the loss of the tyrosine-specific enzyme. Accumulation of these hydroxyphenyl derivatives is not specific to type II tyrosinemia.

Type III tyrosinemia is characterized by tyrosine concentrations ranging from 300 to 1000 μM and significant urinary excretion of hydroxyphenylpyruvate and hydroxyphenyllactate. Other unusual metabolites that may be detected with this disorder are thought to arise from an epoxide intermediate from the conversion of 4-hydroxyphenylpyruvate

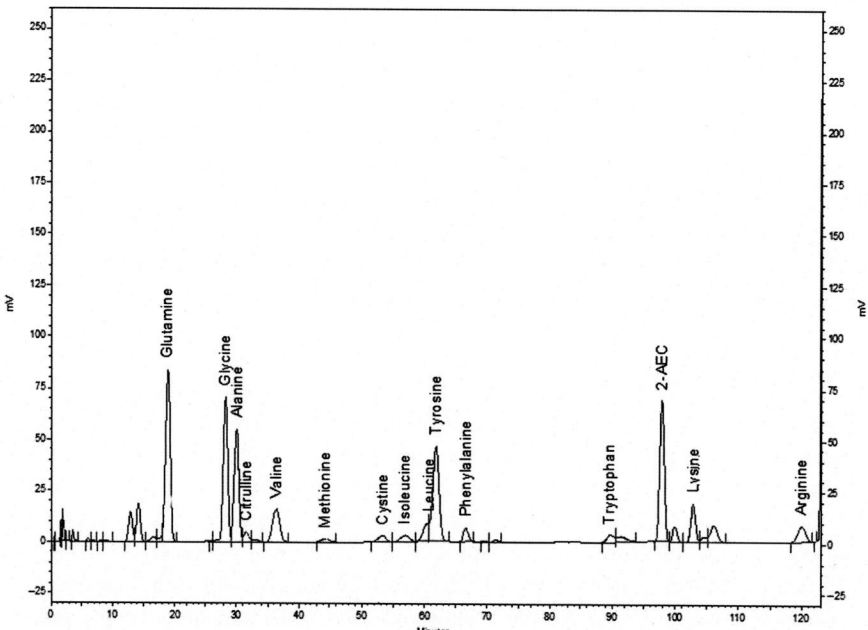

FIGURE 2.4 Plasma amino acid profile from a patient with tyrosinemia I.

This patient has a fairly well-controlled disease; succinylacetone was not detected by a specific assay. Even though well controlled, Tyr is still quite high at 418 μmol/L.

to homogentisic acid. Direct hydrolysis of the epoxide leads to the formation of 4-hydroxycyclohexylacetate. Reaction of the epoxide with glutathione yields an unusual amino acid termed *Hawkinsin* (2-L-cystein-S-yl-1,4-dihydroxycyclohex-5-en-1-yl acetic acid).[32] Another intermediate of the glutathione cycle, 5-oxoproline (pyroglutamic acid), may also be increased in type III disease. Hawkinsin is also detected in the urine of Hawkinsinuria patients, despite a lack of symptoms.

2.4.3 BIOMARKERS FOLLOWED FOR TREATMENT EFFICACY

Restriction of dietary phenylalanine and tyrosine is a mainstay of treatment for all three types of hypertyrosinemia. The goal of such treatment is to maintain tyrosine concentrations less than approximately 500–600 µM to prevent tissue deposition of tyrosine. In addition to dietary restriction, treatment of type I disease employs NTBC (2-[2-nitro-4-(trifluoromethyl)benzoyl]cyclohexane-1,3-dione), a competitive inhibitor of the 4-HPPD reaction.[33] NTBC treatment blocks tyrosine catabolism at a step prior to FAH, preventing accumulation of succinylacetone and the development of hepatic and renal complications. If treatment of type I tyrosinemia fails or is delayed, liver transplantation is the option of last resort. Thus, dietary therapy is primarily monitored by assessment of circulating phenylalanine and tyrosine concentrations. The sufficiency of NTBC therapy in type I disease is monitored by periodic evaluation of succinylacetone and α-fetoprotein (a marker of hepatocellular carcinoma).

2.4.4 CONFOUNDING CONDITIONS

Tyrosine accumulation occurs in circumstances other than congenital genetic–metabolic defects. A transient, benign hypertyrosinemia attributed to slow expression of 4-HPPD often occurs in the newborn period and is responsible for a large fraction of false-positive NBS results for tyrosinemia. Nonspecific tyrosine accumulation also occurs in compromised liver function secondary to a number of other congenital disorders. Acute neonatal liver failure also occurs in galactosemia, hereditary fructose intolerance, viral hepatitis, neonatal hemochromatosis, hemophagocytic lymphohistiocytosis (HLH), and primary mitochondrial pathology. In these situations, elevated tyrosine is also commonly accompanied by dramatically increased concentrations of other amino acids, most notably, methionine.

2.5 NONKETOTIC HYPERGLYCINEMIA (GLYCINE ENCEPHALOPATHY)

2.5.1 BRIEF DESCRIPTION OF THE DISORDER AND PATHWAY

Nonketotoic hyperglycinemia (NKH, OMIM: 605899), also known as glycine encephalopathy, results from the accumulation of glycine in all body tissues, due to inactivity of the glycine cleavage system (GCS). NKH is inherited in an autosomal

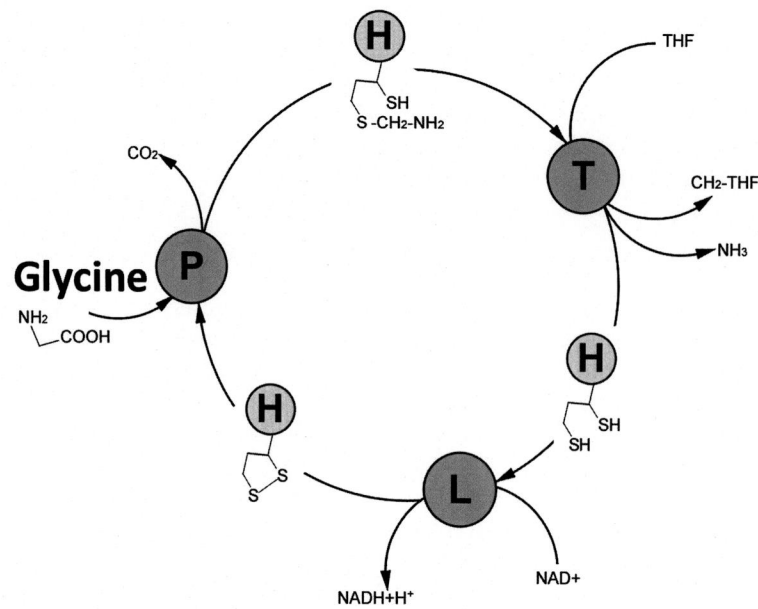

FIGURE 2.5 The glycine cleavage system.

The glycine cleavage system is comprised of four proteins, P-, H-, T-, and L-proteins, and function together to decarboxylate and break down glycine. The H-protein is the nonenzymatic component that shuttles intermediates through the three enzymatic protein steps. THF: tetrahydrofolate, CH3-THF: 5,10-methylene-tetrahydrofolate; NAD: nicotine adenine dinucleotide, P: P-protein, H: H-protein, T: T-protein, L: L-protein.

recessive pattern, and with an estimated incidence as high as 1 in 60,000 in Finland and British Columbia, Canada.[34] It is the second most common disorder of amino acid metabolism.[35] The GCS is a mitochondrial complex consisting of four components: P-protein, T-protein, H-protein, and L-protein. Mutations have been described in the P-, T-, and H-proteins, with as many as 80% of NKH cases possessing P-protein mutations, and 20% with T-protein mutations, while a few H-protein mutations have been described.[35,36] The GCS converts two-carbon glycine into ammonia and carbon dioxide, and transfers one-carbon unit to folate as methylenetetrahydrofolate. Without a fully functional GCS, glycine accumulates in tissue, plasma, urine, and CSF[37] (Fig. 2.5).

The accumulation of glycine in the brain and neuronal tissue is responsible for many of the clinical signs and symptoms of NKH. Glycine is both an excitatory and inhibitory neurotransmitter, and has an excitatory effect when bound to the N-methyl-D-aspartate (NMDA) receptor. The excitatory actions cause seizures, while the inhibitory actions cause hypotonia and lethargy. Classical NKH presents most frequently in the neonatal period (less than one week of age) and less often in the infantile stage (over one week of age). Regardless of the age of presentation, disease severity can be severe or attenuated. Neonatal NKH presents with hypotonia, lethargy, myoclonic jerks, and apnea. Without intervention and ventilation, this presentation is generally fatal. Survivors have profound neurological deficit and intractable seizures. Infantile NKH is hallmarked by hypotonia, seizures, and developmental delay. There are descriptions of mild to severe, atypical forms of NKH that present from late infancy to adulthood.[38] A burst suppression pattern on electroencephalogram is commonly seen in NKH.[39] Recent studies have shown a predictable relationship between prognosis/response to medical intervention and genotype phenotype, and central nervous system malformations.[40]

2.5.2 BRIEF DESCRIPTION OF TREATMENT

Treatment for NKH is aimed at modulating the concentration of glycine in the body and controlling specific symptoms; there is no treatment that prevents or repairs neurological damage.[36,41] High-dose benzoic acid treatment may be used to decrease the accumulation of glycine. Benzoic acid conjugates with glycine, forming hippuric acid, which is freely excreted. NMDA receptor antagonists, including felbamate, ketamine, and dextromethorphan, are also routinely employed to manage symptoms. Therapy efficacy is assessed by the reduction of concentration of plasma glycine and seizure frequency. [36,42,43]

2.5.3 BIOMARKERS FOR DIAGNOSIS

The diagnosis of NKH relies on amino acid analysis, which should reveal an elevation of glycine in plasma, urine, and CSF (Fig. 2.6). However, due to diurnal variation and differences in disease severity, plasma glycine may not be significantly elevated in all cases. With the exception of some mild late-onset cases of NKH, glycine is always elevated in CSF. Therefore, an elevated CSF:plasma ratio, usually greater than 0.08 in classical NKH, and greater than 0.04 in atypical NKH can be used for diagnosis.[11,44] However, there have been rare cases of atypical NKH without this elevation.[45] Urine organic acid and plasma acylcarnitine profiles are normal.[11,46,47]

Although NKH is not a disease recommended for uniform NBS across the United States, as glycine can be measured by the (MS/MS) used for NBS, it can still be detected.[48,49] However, depending on the cut-off used to define a normal glycine result, cases of NKH may be missed.[49,50]

An NKH diagnosis can also be made based on molecular and/or enzymatic studies. For molecular studies, all three genes coding for the P-, T-, and H-proteins, *GLDC, AMT,* and *GCSH*, respectively, should be analyzed, either by sequencing or by targeted mutational analysis.[44,51] Molecular testing may reveal mutations of unknown significance or may miss a mutation or deletion in an unanalyzed region. Therefore, ultimate confirmation of an NKH diagnosis can be made by measuring GCS activity in liver tissue obtained by either biopsy or autopsy.[44] In cases of suspected NKH during pregnancy, enzyme analysis or molecular testing may be conducted on tissue for chorionic villus sampling.[52]

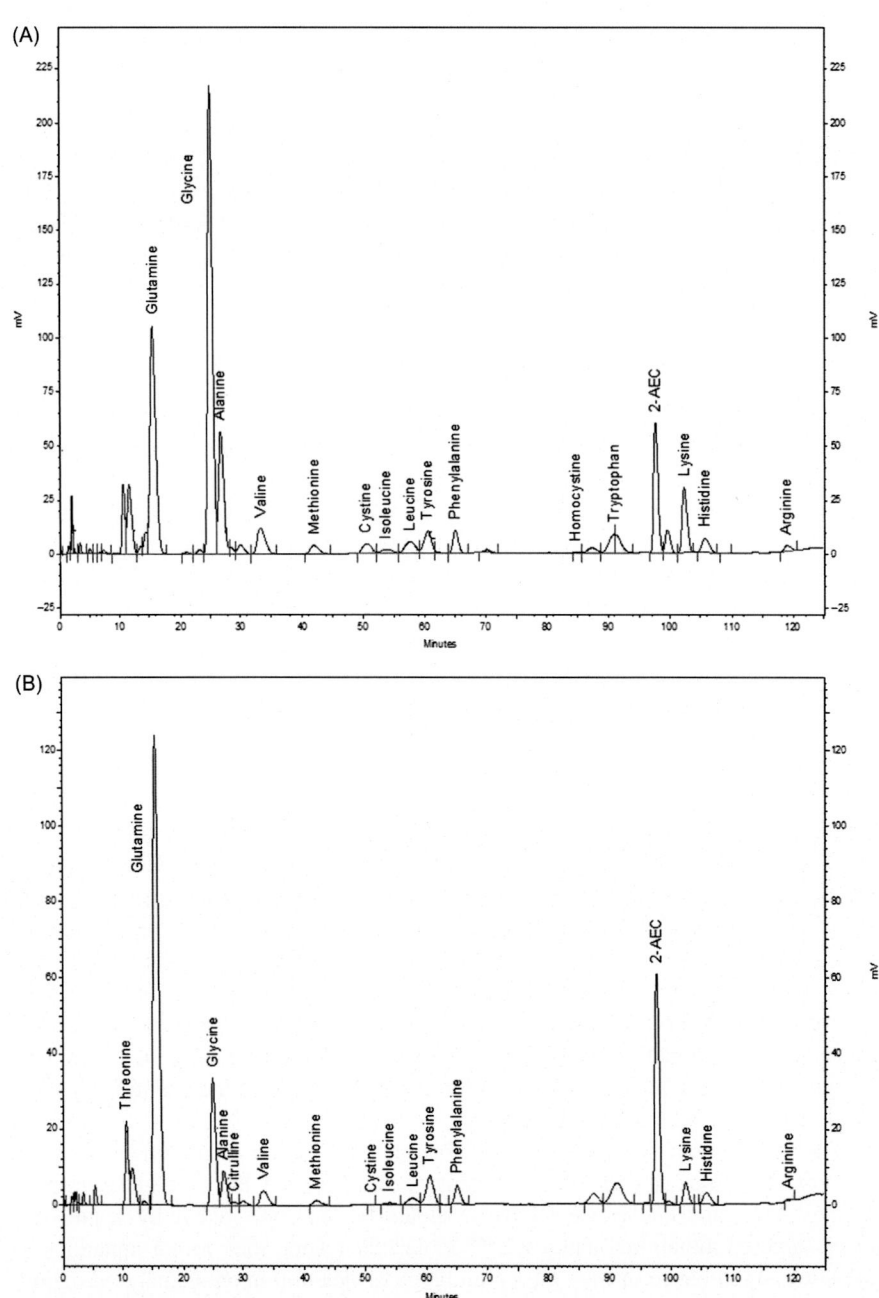

FIGURE 2.6 Amino acid profiles from a patient with NKH.

Plasma (A) and CSF (B) amino acid profiles from a patient with an initial presentation for NKH showing elevated glycine. CSF:plasma ratio is 0.14.

2.5.4 BIOMARKERS FOLLOWED FOR TREATMENT EFFICACY

Since the goal of benzoic acid therapy is to lower body glycine loads, plasma glycine concentration is followed to target a normal value. However, CSF glycine is not normalized by this treatment, and so should not be used to follow treatment.[11,35,44]

Measurement of plasma benzoic acid may also be used to assure that the drug dosage is therapeutic but that it is not dangerously high.[36] High doses of benzoic acid have been associated with fatal renal damage, and so kidney function should also be monitored in these patients.

2.5.5 OTHER BIOMARKERS

A ^{13}C-glycine breath test has been proposed for the use of diagnosing NKH. In this test, after a baseline breath collection, ^{13}C-labeled glycine is given orally or through a gastric tube to patients, followed by additional breath collections in the subsequent five hours. In the presence of a functional GCS, the ^{13}C on the glycine is cleaved to $^{13}CO_2$, which is expelled in the breath. The change from baseline in $^{13}CO_2$ is measured. Breath $^{13}CO_2$ is significantly lower in NKH patients than in normal controls.[51,53]

2.6 MAPLE SYRUP URINE DISEASE

2.6.1 BRIEF DESCRIPTION OF THE DISORDER AND PATHWAY

Maple syrup urine disease (MSUD, OMIM: 248600) arises from a defect in the catabolism of the BCAA valine, leucine, and isoleucine. As a result, these amino acids, their α-keto-acids and α-hydroxy-acid metabolites, and alloisoleucine accumulate in biological fluids.[54,55]

The disorder was first described in 1954 by Menkes et al. with four cases of a progressive infantile disease that was characterized by seizures, respiratory distress, and the smell of maple syrup to the urine.[56] The urinary odor was later attributed to the high concentration of α-keto-acids and α-hydroxy-acids, metabolites of valine, leucine, and isoleucine, which were also shown to be elevated in the blood and urine of these patients.[57] The estimated worldwide prevalence is approximately 1 in 100,000–200,000 births, but may be much higher in certain communities, such as the Mennonites of Pennsylvania, which have an incidence of 1 in 200.[58–60]

MSUD is caused by the inactivity of the branched-chain ketoacid dehydrogenase complex (BCKDC), which decarboxylates the α-keto-acids of valine, leucine, and isoleucine, α-keto$-\beta$-methylvaleric acid, α-ketoisocaproic acid, and α-ketoisovaleric acids, respectively, to α-methylbutyryl-CoA, isovaleryl-CoA, and isobytyryl-CoA. These compounds are further catabolized by multiple enzymatic steps to acetoacetate, acetyl-CoA, and succinyl-CoA, and subsequently feed into the Krebs cycle (Fig. 2.7).[54] BCKDC is a complex of an E1 decarboxylase component (heterodimer comprised of E1α and E1β subunits), an E2 transacylase, and an E3 component and relies on several cofactors for optimal functioning: thiamine pyrophosphate, coenzyme A, flavin

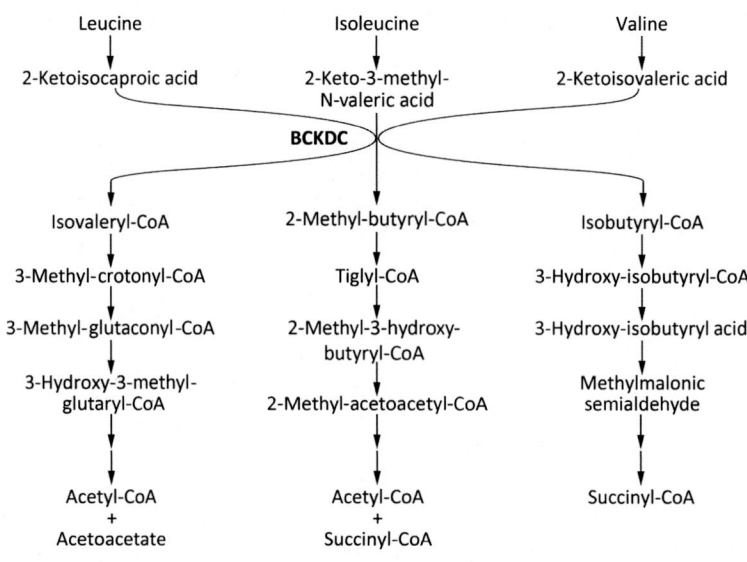

FIGURE 2.7 **Branched-chain amino acid metabolism.**

The branched-chain ketoacid dehydrogenase complex (BCKDC) is defective in MSUD.

adenine dinucleotide (FAD), and nicotinamide adenine dinucleotide (NAD).[54] MSUD may be caused by a mutation in any one of the four genes that code for the BCKDC components, though the majority of cases are caused by mutations in E1α and E1β subunits.[61,62] The E3 component is shared with α-ketoglutarate and pyruvate dehydrogenase complexes. Therefore, deficiency in this component causes a more severe clinical phenotype (dihydrolipoamide dehydrogenase deficiency, OMIM: 246900). In the absence of functional BCKDC, the α-keto-acids (BCKAs) convert to their corresponding α-hydroxy-acids (BCHAs), α-hydroxyisocaropic acid, α-hydroxyisovaleric acid, and α-hydroxy-β-methylvaleric acid.

The clinical signs and symptoms of MSUD are the result of the accumulation of the toxic metabolites, especially α-ketoisocapric acid, the α-keto acid of leucine. Studies have demonstrated that it impairs neural energy metabolism by reducing neuronal respiration and increasing apoptosis.[63,64]

There are five clinical presentations of MSUD that are distinguished based on age and severity of presentation, biochemical profile, and BCKDC activity.[65]

1. Classical MSUD: though normal at birth, within 3–5 days, babies present with poor feeding, irritability, and stupor. Metabolic acidosis, ketonuria, and hypoglycemia are also common. Without treatment, progressive neurological degeneration occurs, manifesting as myoclonus, alternating hyper- and hypotonia, seizures, coma, and even death. Individuals treated early in life that progress to adulthood often have neuropsychiatric issues, including

attention-deficit hyperactivity disorder, depression, and anxiety disorders.[66] Classical MSUD accounts for approximately 75% of cases.

2. Intermediate MSUD: slowly developing decline, leading to failure to thrive, developmental delay, mental retardation, and seizures.
3. Intermittent MSUD: patients are generally normal and lack biochemical evidence of MSUD, until an event, such as acute illness or increased protein intake precipitates metabolic decompensation, ataxia, seizures, and coma.
4. Thiamin-responsive MSUD: similar to intermediate or intermittent MSUD, but treatment with high doses of thiamin normalizes BCAA levels.
5. E3-deficient MSUD: manifests after infancy with metabolic acidosis, hypotonia, developmental delay, movement disorders, and progressive neurological degeneration.

2.6.2 BRIEF DESCRIPTION OF TREATMENT

The goal of treatment for MSUD is to decrease the concentration of BCAAs and their toxic intermediates. In the acutely decompensating patient, protein catabolism must be slowed by encouraging the building of new proteins. This is accomplished by supplying high concentrations of intravenous glucose and fat, as well as a mix of amino acids that lack BCAAs. In patients with very high concentrations of BCAAs, hemodialysis may be used to decrease the toxic compounds in circulation.[67,68]

Long-term treatment focuses on dietary restriction of BCAAs with BCAA-free medical foods and careful supplementation of isoleucine and valine. In cases of illness or other stressors, metabolic decompensation may be prevented by maintaining high carbohydrate supply and BCAA-free amino acids to encourage protein synthesis. Liver transplantation has been successful in treating MSUD and can grant patients restoration of normal BCAA levels, prevention of metabolic crises, and easing of dietary restrictions, as the allograft is believed to manage the BCAA metabolism demands for the body.[69–71]

2.6.3 BIOMARKERS FOR DIAGNOSIS

Diagnosis of MSUD is based on significant elevations of BCAAs, especially leucine, by quantitative plasma amino acid analysis (Fig. 2.8). The elevation of alloisoleucine is pathognomonic for MSUD, though it may not be detected by all amino acid analysis methods.[54,72] Urinary organic acid analysis demonstrates high concentrations of BCKAs and BCHAs. The E3 subunit deficiency also has increased plasma alanine, pyruvate, and lactate, as well as urinary α-ketoglutarate.

MSUD is a core condition recommended for inclusion in a uniform NBS panel by the Health Resources and Services Administration (HRSA).[48] NBS for MSUD is accomplished by (MS/MS) analysis of leucine and isoleucine. Since hydroxyproline is not readily distinguished from leucine and isoleucine by this method, individuals with hydroxyprolinemia may present as a false-positive MSUD.[49]

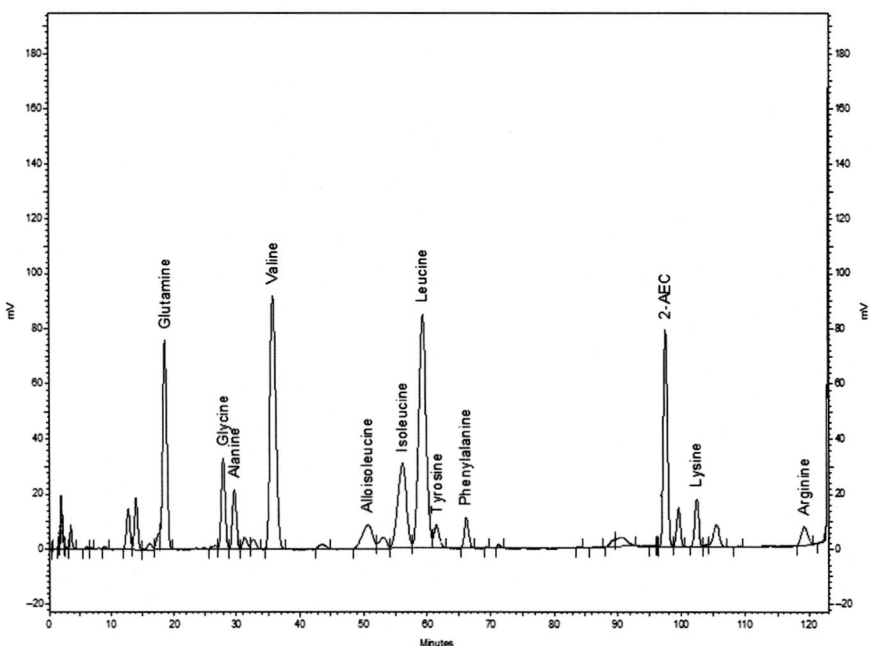

FIGURE 2.8 Plasma amino acid profile from a patient with MSUD.

In a patient with known MSUD and acute illness, alloisoleucine is present; leucine is 911 μmol/L (3.4 times upper limit of normal), valine is 858 μmol/L (2.8 times upper limit of normal), and isoleucine is 430 μmol/L (3.6 times upper limit of normal).

Biochemical testing is generally sufficient for diagnosis for MSUD. However, enzyme activity assessment and molecular genetic testing may be used to confirm a diagnosis. This may be particularly useful in cases of nonclassical MSUD, testing patients with affected family members, and for genetic counseling or carrier testing.[61,73]

2.6.4 BIOMARKERS FOLLOWED FOR TREATMENT EFFICACY

Serial plasma amino acid measurements should be used to monitor dietary compliance with the BCAA-restricted medical foods. The frequency of monitoring varies with age, compliance, and disease severity, but it may be conducted as frequently as weekly for rapidly growing infants.[66] For convenience, many laboratories offer testing of BCAAs from dried blood spots so that families can collect samples routinely at home and mail them in for analysis. Isoleucine and valine supplementation is titrated to maintain a plasma leucine-to-valine ratio of less than 0.5 mol:mol and a leucine-to-isoleucine ratio of approximately 2.0 mol:mol. Leucine concentrations should be targeted to 150–300 μmol/L.

2.6.5 BIOMARKERS FOLLOWED FOR DISEASE PROGRESSION

In acute illness or cases of other physiological stress, intake of BCAAs, other amino acids, glucose, and insulin must be closely monitored to prevent metabolic decompensation. Plasma amino acid analysis may be used to monitor the concentrations of isoleucine, valine, glutamine, alanine, and tyrosine.[73]

2.6.6 OTHER BIOMARKERS: LESS ESTABLISHED, FUTURE

Dinitrophenylhydrazine (DNPH) is an orange-red solid, which in solution will react with the carbonyl group of aldehydes and ketones to form a yellow–white precipitate. The formation of the precipitate has been used as a qualitative or semi-quantitative method of keto acids. This test has been used as an at-home means to monitor urinary keto acids. However, due to the explosive nature of solid DNPH and the availability of an alternate method, home-use urine ketone test strips, the use of DNPH is less common.[73]

2.7 HOMOCYSTINURIA

2.7.1 BRIEF DESCRIPTION OF THE DISORDER AND PATHWAY

Classical homocystinuria is an autosomal recessive deficiency of cystathione β-synthase (CBS, OMIM: 236200), a homotetrameric enzyme that converts homocysteine to cystathionine in the transsulfuration pathway, which contributes to the removal of sulfur-containing amino acids. Homocysteine (Hcy) is synthesized in the metabolism of methionine in the transmethylation cycle via the transfer of methyl groups from tetrahydrofolate (THF), or in the remethylation cycle (Fig. 2.9). Once Hcy is generated, it can be converted back into methionine via betaine-homocysteine methyltransferase (BHMT) in the presence of betaine. However, this pathway is not present in the brain. Hcy can be metabolized in the transsulfuration pathway, the first step of which is CBS. In the absence of functional CBS, Hcy metabolism is impaired and accumulates.

CBS-deficiency is one of the most commonly inherited disorders of amino acid metabolism and the most common disorder of sulfur metabolism, though deficiencies in other enzymes involved with sulfur metabolism, such as methylenetetrahydrofolate reductase (MTHFR, OMIM: 236250), can also cause homocystinuria. CBS-deficient patients can contain as high as 500 µmol/L Hcy, around 50 times the upper limit of normal. Those homozygous for an MTHFR mutation may have a mild elevation in Hcy.[74,75] The disorder is characterized by myopia, osteoporosis, mental retardation, decreased pigmentation of hair and skin, ectopia lentis, dolichostenomelia, and an increased risk of stroke and psychosis.[76][74,77–79] The worldwide prevalence of CBS deficiency is estimated at approximately 1 in 100,000–344,000 births.[58,80] Several hundred mutations have been described for CBS and MTHFR genes, and the clinical presentation and severity may depend upon the specific mutation.[75,80]

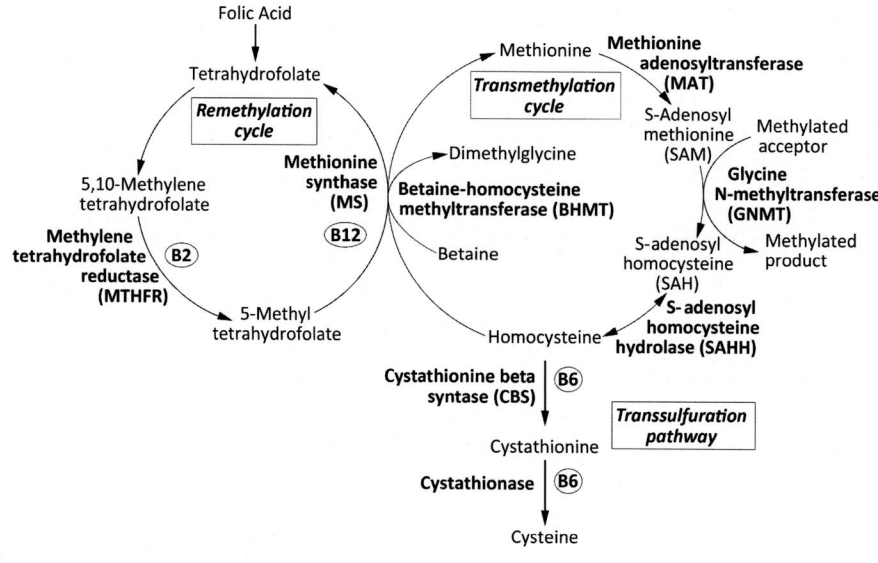

FIGURE 2.9 Transsulfuration pathway.

2.7.2 BRIEF DESCRIPTION OF TREATMENT

The goal of treatment for homocystinuria is to reduce plasma Hcy. Since the transsulfuration, trans- and re-methylation pathways utilize folate, betaine, and B-vitamins as co-factors and substrates, administration of these compounds may drive the pathways past a partially defective enzyme. However, a more severe B6-nonresponsive phenotype has been described. Since BHMT is not present in the brain, the conversion of Hcy back into methionine in the brain is dependent upon methionine synthase and on cobalamin (vitamin B_{12}) and folate.[74,75] Therefore, supplementation with vitamin B_{12} and betaine concurrent with pyridoxine and folate is a common approach, and is especially important for B6-nonresponsive patients. They have also been shown to successfully treat psychosis in a CBS-deficient patient after antipsychotic drugs did not work.[78] Additionally, a methionine-low or free diet supplemented with cysteine may be prescribed to regulate amino acid profiles.[76]

2.7.3 BIOMARKERS FOR DIAGNOSIS

The biomarkers for the diagnosis of CBS-deficiency include increased plasma and urine homocysteine and methionine as well as decreased cysteine, cystathionine, and normal to low methylmalonic acid (Fig. 2.10).[75,78] Classic homocystinuria is frequently diagnosed, based on an abnormal NBS. By most current state screening processes, these patients are flagged for an elevated methionine. Follow-up testing of plasma amino acids and plasma total homocysteine is recommended. An elevated homocysteine along with an elevated methionine is indicative of homocystinuria.

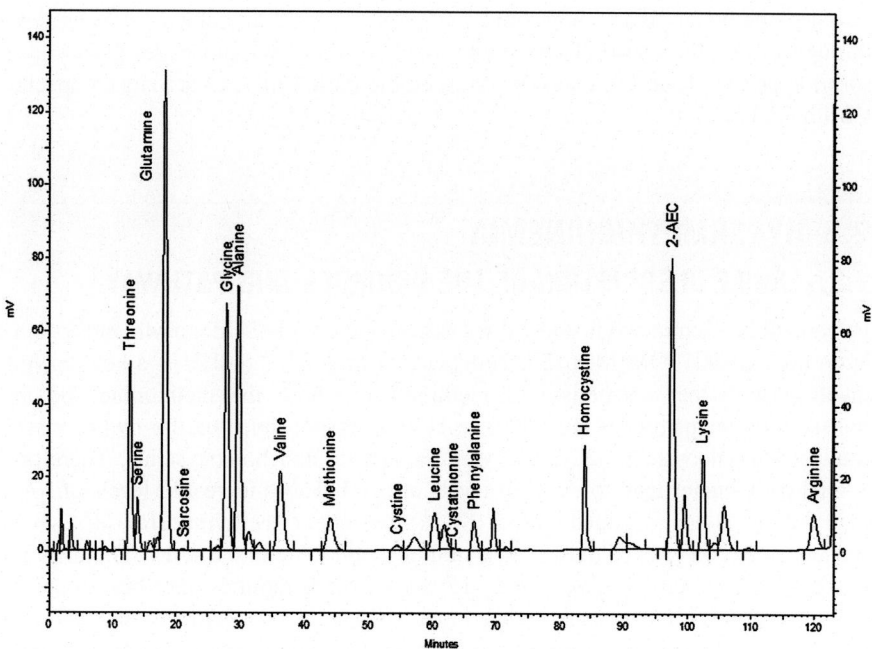

FIGURE 2.10 Plasma amino acid profile from a patient with CBS deficiency.

This amino acid profile is from a patient with poorly controlled CBS deficiency. Total homocysteine is 227 µmol/L (111 times upper limit of normal), methionine is 91 µmol/L (1.7 times upper limit of normal), and cystine is 11 µmol/L (normal range: 7–54 µmol/L).

Cultured skin fibroblasts can be used to assay CBS activity to confirm the diagnosis, or molecular genetic testing can be used to identify mutations in the CBS or MTHFR genes.[75] Of note, moderate-to-severe vitamin B12 deficiency can also cause moderate-to-severe elevations in Hcy, which could be misleading toward a diagnosis of homocystinuria. However, in vitamin B12 deficiency, methylmalonic acid is also elevated, which is not the case in homocystinuria.[74]

2.7.4 BIOMARKERS FOLLOWED FOR TREATMENT EFFICACY

Homocysteine, methionine, and cystine in plasma and urine are followed for treatment (pyridoxine) efficiency.[78,80] The plasma concentrations of folate and vitamin B12 can also be monitored to evaluate the effectiveness of the treatment.[79]

2.7.5 OTHER BIOMARKERS: LESS ESTABLISHED, FUTURE

High homocysteine levels have been shown to affect DNA methylation; therefore, an array-based analysis of DNA could reveal unique methylation patterns of DNA in CBS-deficient patients.[75]

Also, potential treatments could envision rescuing misfolded CBS proteins through osmolytic chemical chaperones such as dimethyl sulfoxide, glycerol, or sorbitol, as they have been shown to rescue the partial in vitro activity of specific CBS mutations.[81,82]

2.8 HYPERMETHIONINEMIA

2.8.1 BRIEF DESCRIPTION OF THE DISORDER AND PATHWAY

Hypermethioninemia was first identified as a disorder due to S-adenosylhomocysteine hydrolase (SAHH, OMIM: 613752) deficiency in 2004.[83] SAHH is a key enzyme involved with the metabolism of methionine in both the methionine and the transsulfuration pathways (Fig. 2.9). SAHH is responsible for the hydrolysis of S-adenosylhomocysteine (SAH) to yield adenosine and homocysteine. Therefore, SAHH deficiencies lead to elevated levels of SAH. These increased levels of SAH then inhibit S-adenosylmethionine (SAM)-dependent methyltransferases, which subsequently downregulate the conversion of methionine into SAM.[83] The disorder is considered extremely rare, as only 12 cases from 6 families have been reported in the literature. It has been speculated that the disease is underdiagnosed, and that previously reported cases of hypermethioninemia with no known cause may actually be due to SAHH deficiency.[83–85]

The disorder affects the muscle, liver, and brain and is characterized by psychomotor development delay, low IQ, unusual facial features, neurological problems, and hypotonia as well as chronic inflammation and fibrosis of the liver.[83] Cases may be asymptomatic until early adulthood, depending on the severity of the mutation. Elevated SAM levels have been associated with liver cancer in animal models, and one SAHH-deficient patient died from hepatocellular carcinoma.[84]

The disorder is most often due to nonconservative mutations in *AHCY*, which encodes SAHH. The severity and age of onset of the disease is likely related to the specific mutation. One reported mutation, a missense mutation R49H in the binding domain, resulted in a mild phenotype likely due to the similarity between arginine and histidine.[84] Other reported mutations include R49C, Y143C, D86G, G71S, Y328D, and premature stop codon W112X.

2.8.2 BRIEF DESCRIPTION OF TREATMENT

Since it is so rare, it still remains somewhat unclear as to what treatments are most effective. The main goals of treatment are to reduce the accumulation of SAH, which inhibits the majority of SAM-dependent methyltransferases, and replenish creatine and phosphatidylcholine. Creatine and phosphatidylcholine are two dominant products of SAM-dependent methyltransferases and play roles in brain and muscle structure and function. Therefore, a low-methionine diet that is supplemented with creatine and phosphatidylcholine is typically administered for SAHH-deficient patients.[84,86] Dietary methionine restrictions have decreased circulating methionine levels; however, this treatment has not always improved the clinical course of the disease.[84] Liver transplantation was performed in a 40-month-old patient with severe SAHH deficiency. Following transplantation, the patient's plasma amino acids became normal on an unrestricted diet, and he showed significant improvement in growth and development.[87]

2.8.3 BIOMARKERS FOR DIAGNOSIS

A key biomarker of SAHH deficiency is elevated serum methionine using standard biochemical methods, and is the marker by which NBS programs would detect SAHH deficiency.[88] However, this is nonspecific, as there are many disorders that can cause hypermethioninemia (e.g., homocystinuria, tyrosinemia, galactosinemia, methionine adenosyltransferase deficiency, glycine N-methyltransferase deficiency, Fig. 2.11). Elevated methionine may not be evident in the neonatal period; one patient did not demonstrate elevated methionine until after she was eight months old.[89] Therefore, elevated serum concentrations of SAH and SAM are highly suggestive of this disorder. Also, the SAM:SAH molar concentration ratio is also distinctively low in SAHH-deficient patients. Measurement of plasma/serum SAH and

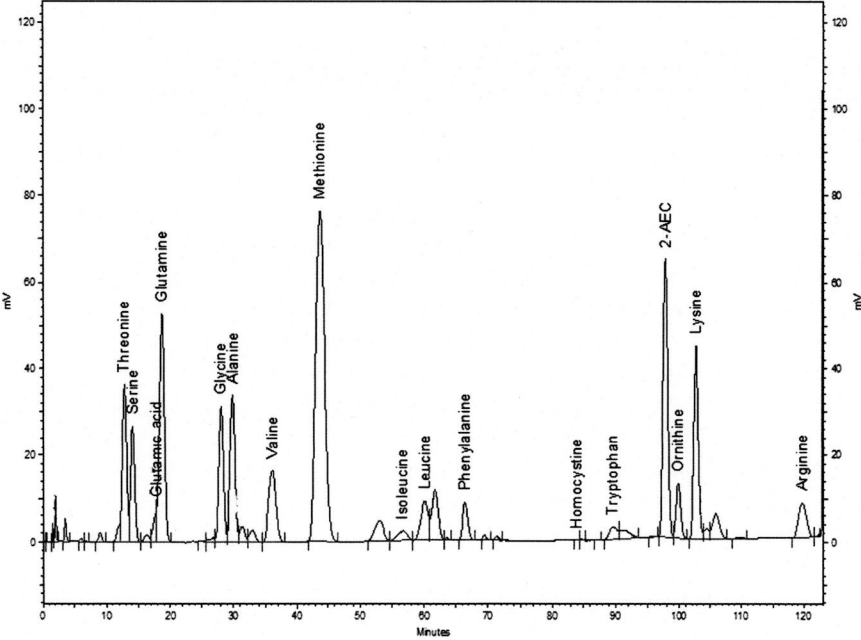

FIGURE 2.11 Plasma amino acid profile from a patient with hypermethioninemia.

This patient's plasma amino acid profile shows a marked elevation in methionine, which is 913 μmol/L (17 times upper limit of normal).

SAM by LC-MS/MS is the most current approach to analysis, though a method for derivatization followed by fluorescent spectroscopy has also been reported.[84,87,90] Elevated aminotransferase and creatine kinase activity, indicative of tissue disease, is commonly used to support the diagnosis. SAHH enzyme activity assays or genetic testing can be used to definitively confirm the diagnosis.

2.8.4 BIOMARKERS FOLLOWED FOR TREATMENT EFFICACY

Biomarkers followed for treatment efficacy predominantly include monitoring liver function with liver function tests and methionine, Hcy, SAH, and SAM levels[84]. Other reported biomarkers include elevated betaine, methylation cycle substrates/products (e.g., creatine, phosphatidylcholine, and guanidinoacetate), and plasma concentrations of BCAAs and other amino acids, especially tryptophan.[87]

2.8.5 BIOMARKERS FOLLOWED FOR DISEASE PROGRESSION

Since SAH inhibits many methyltransferases, the activity of tissue methyltransferases can be analyzed to evaluate disease progression. In particular, the ratio of betaine/dimethylglycine has been used as an indicator of impaired betaine homocysteine methyltransferase.[87] Elevation in liver function tests is suggestive of progression in liver disease.

2.8.6 CONFOUNDING CONDITIONS THAT CAN CAUSE HYPERMETHIONINEMIA

Other causes of hypermethioninemia include deficiencies in the other enzymes in the pathway from methionine to Hcy: methionine adenosyltransferase (MAT, OMIM: 250850) and glycine N-methyltransferase (GNMT, OMIM: 606664) (Fig. 2.9). Deficiency in MAT is generally asymptomatic and is notable only for isolated hypermethioninemia. However, for a small subset of patients, mental retardation, dystonia, and evidence of demyelination has been reported.[91] GNMT deficiency is rare and newly described, and demonstrated elevated plasma methionine, mild transaminitis, and hepatomegaly in the three reported cases.[92,93]

Many of the clinical features of SAHH deficiency resemble those of phosphomannomutase 2 deficiency, including hypotonia, psychomotor delay, strabism, microcephaly, hepatopathy, and coagulopathy. The correct diagnosis may be initially confounded because methionine levels may be within the normal reference range for SAHH-deficient neonates.[89]

2.8.7 OTHER BIOMARKERS: LESS ESTABLISHED, FUTURE

A broad range of other biomarkers may also be useful in determining a course of action during treatment. Other biomarkers that have been monitored include albumin levels (are typically decreased relative to normal), cystathionine (elevated), and free choline (decreased).[83,87]

2.9 HYPERPROLINEMIA

2.9.1 BRIEF DESCRIPTION OF THE DISORDER AND PATHWAY

There are two mutations resulting in hyperprolinemia (HPI): a mutation in the proline dehydrogenase gene causes HPI type I (PRODH, OMIM: 239500) and a mutation in pyrroline 5-carboxylate dehydrogenase (P5-CDH, OMIM: 239510) that causes HPI type II.

Proline is a nonessential amino acid, and along with hydroxyproline, is the only amino acid without a primary amino group, and therefore has a unique metabolic pathway in the mitochondria. Once in the mitochondria, proline is oxidized to pyrroline 5-carboxylate (P5-C) by proline oxidase. P5-C can be recycled to proline or converted to glutamine-γ-semialdehyde, then glutamine by P5-CDH (Fig. 2.12).

Both types of HPI are very rare, and so a consistent clinical presentation is not well defined. HPI type I has been associated with developmental delay, mental retardation, epilepsy, and schizophrenia. Clinical presentation may correlate with the severity of enzyme dysfunction.[94–97] Type II HPI has been associated with seizures and cognitive delay. However, this association may be coincidental and HPI type II is believed to be asymptomatic in many patients.[96]

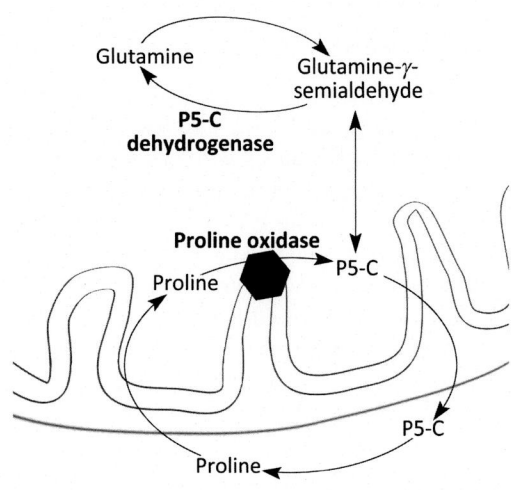

FIGURE 2.12 Proline metabolism pathway.

Deficiency of functional of the mitochondrial inner membrane enzyme, proline oxidase prevents the conversion of proline to pyrroline 5-carboxylate (P5-C) and is the cause of hyperprolinemia type I. Mutations in P5-C dehydrogenase causes hyperprolinemia type II.

2.9.2 BRIEF DESCRIPTION OF TREATMENT

Dietary restriction of proline does little to control plasma proline concentration and has not been shown to impact clinical symptoms. For type II affected individuals with epilepsy, seizure control is critical, especially during infantile illness. Some studies suggest that vitamin B6 supplementation may prevent seizures in HPI type II.[96,98]

2.9.3 BIOMARKERS FOR DIAGNOSIS

The primary marker for diagnosis for HPI is an elevated proline in plasma or urine amino acid profiles (Fig. 2.13). HPI type I heterozygotes may also have elevated proline levels.[96] Of note, for amino acid methods using ninhydrin detection, proline and hydroxyproline are best detected at 440 nm wavelength, rather than 570 nm used for other amino acids. The secondary amine structure of these amino acids confers a different reaction to ninhydrin, which produces a yellow, not purple color.[99]

Biochemical differentiation between HPI types I and II may be made on the presence of P5-C in a urine organic acid screen, which is indicative of HPI type II.[96]

Finally, an HPI diagnosis can be confirmed by mutation analysis and/or sequencing of the affected genes. PRODH is coded for by the *PRODH* gene and has several described mutations and deletions, as does the *ALDH4A1* gene, which codes for 5P-CDH.

2.10 SULFOCYSTEINURIA

2.10.1 BRIEF DESCRIPTION OF THE DISORDER AND PATHWAY

First described in 1967, sulfocysteinuria is a disorder caused by isolated sulfite oxidase (SUOX) deficiency (OMIM: 272300).[100] Sulfocysteinuria is a rare autosomal recessive IEM that presents in early infancy with uncontrollable seizures and severe psychomotor delay, often resulting in brain atrophy and premature death.[101] Most patients develop microcephaly, feeding difficulties, and dislocated ocular lenses. Milder phenotypes (e.g., intermittent ataxia and ectopia lentis) have also been reported, and these phenotypes can have a later onset.[102]

The disorder results from an impaired ability to oxidize sulfite to sulfate during cysteine catabolism due to a deficiency in SUOX, which uses molybdenum as a cofactor (Fig. 2.14). This should not be confused with molybdenum cofactor deficiency.[103] Sulfocysteinuria is caused by a mutation in the *SUOX* gene.[104,105]

2.10.2 BRIEF DESCRIPTION OF TREATMENT

While severe cases of sulfocysteinuria have been traditionally been viewed as untreatable, the typical treatment for mild sulfocysteinuria includes severe dietary protein restrictions consisting of a low-protein diet that is restricted in both methionine and cysteine.[101,106] Additionally, symptomatic treatments can be used to treat seizures.[107]

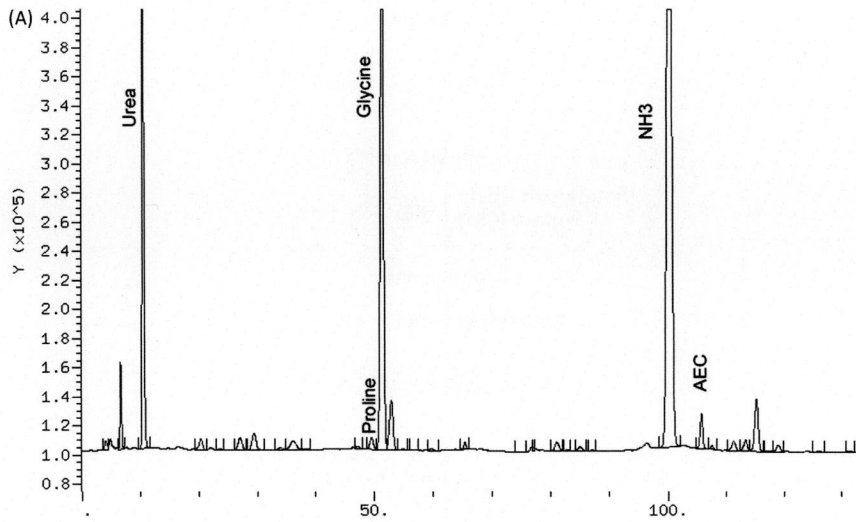

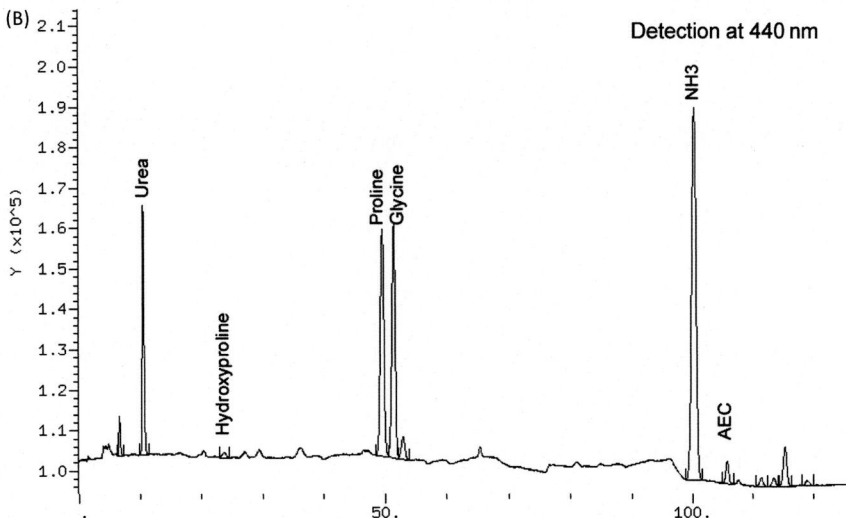

FIGURE 2.13 Urine amino acid profiles from a patient with hyperprolinemia.

Urine sample from a patient with hyperprolinemia. Proline is 5173 µmol/g creatinine (36 times upper limit of normal) and hydroxyproline is 202 µmol/gl creatinine (2.2 times upper limit of normal). Note: While most amino acids are detected at 570 nm (panel A), proline and hydroxyproline are best detected with light at 440 nm (panel B). In this figure, the samples were prepared as in the other figures, but run on a Biochrom 30 amino acid analyzer with ion-exchange chromatography, lithium-citrate buffered mobile phases, and postcolumn ninhydrin derivatization.

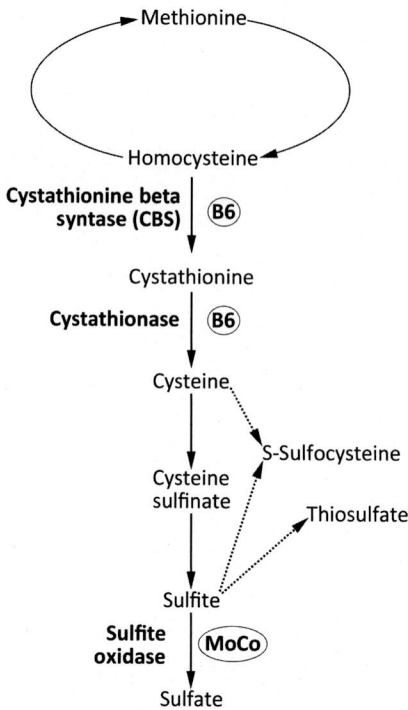

FIGURE 2.14 Sulfur-containing amino acid metabolism to sulfate.

Deficiency of sulfite oxidase leads to an accumulation of sulfite, which in high concentrations is converted to S-sulfocysteine and thiosulfate. Sulfite oxidase is dependent upon molybdenum cofactor (MoCo) to be fully functional.

Enzyme replacement therapies have also been proposed as a potential treatment for sulfocysteinuria.[108]

2.10.3 BIOMARKERS FOR DIAGNOSIS

Quantitation of plasma total homocysteine should be used to screen for the disorder. If homocysteine levels are low, urinary sulfite, sulfite intermediates, and thiosulfates would be elevated with isolated sulfocysteinuria.[109] Sulfite is commonly measured using a dipstick format, but requires that urine be very fresh, and ideally testing should be done at the time of collection. When performing the sulfite stick test, both bacterial degradation of the urine sample and sulfur-containing drugs have been reported to produce false positives.[107,110] Thiosulfate can be measured using derivatization and HPLC-UV detection or by ion chromatography.[109,111] Elevated S-sulfocysteine and taurine, and very low plasma cystine may be noted by amino acid analysis.[112,102,106] Follow-up genetic testing can confirm mutation in the *SUOX* gene, as can fibroblast homogenate SUOX activity analysis.[101,107] Normal blood and urine concentrations of uric acid and lack of xanthinuria distinguish an isolated superoxide dismutase (SOD) mutation from a molybdenum cofactor deficiency.

2.10.4 BIOMARKERS FOLLOWED FOR TREATMENT EFFICACY

Plasma amino acid profiles are monitored to evaluate and adjust dietary therapy, especially homocysteine, taurine, cystine, methionine, and S-sulfocysteine.

2.10.5 CONFOUNDING CONDITIONS

Molybdenum cofactor deficiency (MoCoD, OMIM: 252150), a related IEM caused by defects in the biosynthesis of the molybdenum cofactor used by molybdenum enzymes, is nearly clinically indistinguishable from sulfocysteinuria. As the conversion of hypoxanthine to xanthine to uric acid uses molybdenum cofactor-dependent enzymes, MoCoD can be distinguished from sulfocysteinuria due to low uric acid levels in urine and serum as well as elevated xanthine and hypoxanthine levels. Molecular genetic analysis can also be used for a definitive diagnosis.

2.11 CYSTINURIA (OMIM: 220100)

2.11.1 BRIEF DESCRIPTION OF THE DISORDER AND PATHWAY

Cystinuria is caused by a mutation in the transporter protein of dibasic amino acids in the renal proximal tubules and small bowel, resulting in the accumulation of cystine, lysine, arginine, and ornithine in urine. The accumulation of cystine causes renal stones due to its low solubility in forming urine.[113] The disorder can be classified genetically into type A, type B, and type AB. Cystinuria type A is caused by an autosomal recessive mutation in the *SLC3A1* gene on chromosome 2, which encodes the heavy subunit of the renal amino acid transporter. Cystinuria type B is caused by a mutation in the *SLC7A9* gene on chromosome 19, which encodes the light subunit of the renal amino acid transporter and which is the catalytic component of the transporter. Type B is inherited in an autosomal recessive or autosomal dominant with incomplete penetrance pattern. Last, type AB is caused by a mutation on both genes.[114–117] Clinically, however, cystinuria is classified into type I (normal cystine excretion) and nontype I (i.e., elevated cystine excretion).[117] There exist associations between the above genetic and biochemical phenotype classifications, though the genetic variations span a wide spectrum in terms of functional consequences. Cystinuria usually presents itself clinically before age 30, but one study showed that the presentation of clinical symptoms occurred after age 40 in 21% of the cystinuric patients studied.[118] The clinical symptoms of cystinuria include the formation of cystine stones that can cause serious damage to the kidneys.

2.11.2 BRIEF DESCRIPTION OF TREATMENT

Current treatment concepts include increased fluid intake, limiting sodium and protein intake, and alkalinization of the urine with potassium citrate for mild cases and the use of cystine-binding drugs, including penicillamine and tiopronin, for more severe cases.[119] Surgical removal of stones is also warranted in many cases using techniques such as percutaneous nephrolithotomy and ureterorenoscopic stone removal.[120]

2.11.3 BIOMARKERS FOR DIAGNOSIS

Following assessment of urinary cystine stones and crystals, the diagnosis of cystinuria is typically confirmed by urinary analysis. Urine markers for the disease include increased levels of ornithine, lysine, arginine, cystine, cysteine, and homocystine. Fig. 2.15 shows the urine amino acid profile from a patient with cystinuria. Genetic analysis is not typically performed to confirm the diagnosis.[120]

2.11.4 BIOMARKERS FOLLOWED FOR TREATMENT EFFICACY

Treatment efficacy is monitored by measuring urinary pH and urinary cystine excretion by HPLC. It should be noted that the analytical approach must be able to

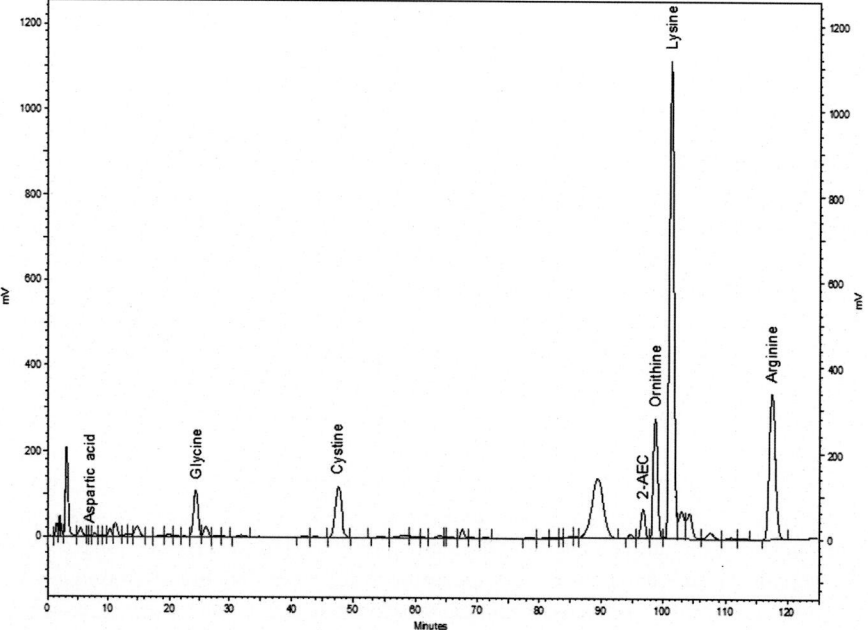

FIGURE 2.15 Urine amino acid profile from a patient with cystinuria.

The urine shows marked elevation in lysine, arginine, ornithine, and cystine.

distinguish cystine from thiol-cysteine drug complexes when using thiol-containing drugs, and certain derivatization procedures can disrupt disulfide bonds, including those of cysteine-drug complexes.[120] Therefore, a solid-phase assay called "cystine capacity" was developed to accurately measure urinary cystine supersaturation in the presence of cystine-binding drugs.[121]

2.11.5 BIOMARKERS FOLLOWED FOR DISEASE PROGRESSION

Routine analysis of urinary cystine is performed to monitor disease progression in addition to biomarkers of liver disease, hematologic complications, and proteinuria.[120]

2.11.6 OTHER BIOMARKERS: LESS ESTABLISHED, FUTURE

Using an untargeted metabolomic LC-MS/MS approach, Janeckova et al. identified cysteinyl-glycine as an additional biomarker in the urine of cystinuria patients.[122] Additionally, a proteomic profile of cystinuric patients showed increased levels of ceruloplasmin, neutrophil gelatinase-associated lipocalin, and vitamin D-binding protein and decreased osteopontin and uromodulin levels.[123]

ACKNOWLEDGMENT

The authors wish to thank Timothy Rhyand for his assistance in gathering patient amino acid chromatographs for the figures.

REFERENCES

1. Rinaldo P, Hahn S, Matern D. Inborn errors of amino acid, organic acid, and fatty acid metabolism. In: Burtis ERA Carl A, Bruns David E, editors. *Tietz textbook of clinical chemistry and molecular diagnostics*. Elsevier Saunders; 2006.
2. Le Boucher J, Charret C, Coudray-Lucas C, Giboudeau J, Cynober L. Amino acid determination in biological fluids by automated ion-exchange chromatography: performance of Hitachi L-8500A. *Clin Chem* 1997;**43**(8 Pt 1):1421–8.
3. Cowan TM, Yu C. Laboratory investigations of inborn errors of metabolism. In: Sarafoglou K, editor. *Pediatric endocrinology and inborn errors of metabolism*. McGraw Hill; 2009.
4. Fekkes D, van Dalen A, Edelman M, Voskuilen A. Validation of the determination of amino acids in plasma by high-performance liquid chromatography using automated pre-column derivatization with o-phthaldialdehyde. *J Chromatogr B Biomed Appl* 1995;**669**(2):177–86.
5. Qu Y, Slocum RH, Fu J, Rasmussen WE, Rector HD, Miller JB, et al. Quantitative amino acid analysis using a Beckman system gold HPLC 126AA analyzer. *Clin Chim Acta* 2001;**312**(1–2):153–62.
6. Widhalm K, Virmani K. Long-term follow-up of 58 patients with histidinemia treated with a histidine-restricted diet: no effect of therapy. *Pediatrics* 1994;**94**(6 Pt 1):861–6.

7. Mitchell JJ, Trakadis YJ, Scriver CR. Phenylalanine hydroxylase deficiency. *Genet Med* 2011;**13**(8):697–707.
8. Zurfluh MR, Zschocke J, Lindner M, Feillet F, Chery C, Burlina A, et al. Molecular genetics of tetrahydrobiopterin-responsive phenylalanine hydroxylase deficiency. *Hum Mutat* 2008;**29**(1):167–75.
9. Kayaalp E, Treacy E, Waters PJ, Byck S, Nowacki P, Scriver CR. Human phenylalanine hydroxylase mutations and hyperphenylalaninemia phenotypes: a metanalysis of genotype-phenotype correlations. *Am J Hum Genet* 1997;**61**(6):1309–17.
10. Bernegger C, Blau N. High frequency of tetrahydrobiopterin-responsiveness among hyperphenylalaninemias: a study of 1,919 patients observed from 1988 to 2002. *Mol Genet Metab* 2002;**77**(4):304–13.
11. Burgard P, Luo X, Hoffmann GF. Phenylketonuria. In: Sarafoglou K, editor. *Pediatric endocrinology and inborn errors of metabolism.* McGraw Hill; 2009.
12. Bone A, Kuehl AK, Angelino AF. A neuropsychiatric perspective of phenylketonuria I: overview of phenylketonuria and its neuropsychiatric sequelae. *Psychosomatics* 2012;**53**(6):517–23.
13. Berry SA, Brown C, Grant M, Greene CL, Jurecki E, Koch J, et al. Newborn screening 50 years later: access issues faced by adults with PKU. *Genet Med* 2013;**15**(8):591–9.
14. Demirdas S, Coakley KE, Bisschop PH, Hollak CE, Bosch AM, Singh RH. Bone health in phenylketonuria: a systematic review and meta-analysis. *Orphanet J Rare Dis* 2015;**10**:17.
15. Mitchell JJ. Phenylalanine hydroxylase deficiency. In: Pagon RA, Adam MP, Ardinger HH, Wallace SE, Amemiya A, Bean LJH, editors. *GeneReviews(R).* Seattle, WA: University of Washington, Seattle; 1993.
16. Al Hafid N, Christodoulou J. Phenylketonuria: a review of current and future treatments. *Translational pediatrics* 2015;**4**(4):304–17.
17. Burgard P, Bremer HJ, Buhrdel P, Clemens PC, Monch E, Przyrembel H, et al. Rationale for the German recommendations for phenylalanine level control in phenylketonuria 1997. *Eur J Pediatr* 1999;**158**(1):46–54.
18. Vockley J, Andersson HC, Antshel KM, Braverman NE, Burton BK, Frazier DM, et al. Phenylalanine hydroxylase deficiency: diagnosis and management guideline. *Genet Med* 2014;**16**(2):188–200.
19. Thiele AG, Rohde C, Mutze U, Arelin M, Ceglarek U, Thiery J, et al. The challenge of long-term tetrahydrobiopterin (BH4) therapy in phenylketonuria: Effects on metabolic control, nutritional habits and nutrient supply. *Mol Genet Metab Rep* 2015;**4**:62–7.
20. Peat J, Garg U. Determination of phenylalanine and tyrosine by high performance liquid chromatography-tandem mass spectrometry. *Methods mol biol* 2016;**1378**:219–25.
21. Xiong X, Sheng X, Liu D, Zeng T, Peng Y, Wang Y. A GC/MS-based metabolomic approach for reliable diagnosis of phenylketonuria. *Anal bioanal chem* 2015;**407**(29):8825–33.
22. Guthrie R, Susi A. A simple phenylalanine method for detecting phenylketonuria in large populations of newborn infants. *Pediatrics* 1963;**32**:338–43.
23. Bross R, Ball RO, Clarke JTR, Pencharz PB. Tyrosine requirements in children with classical PKU determined by indicator amino acid oxidation. *Am J Physiol Endocrinol Metab* 2000;**278**(2):E195–201.
24. Blau N, Thony B. Hyperphenylalaninemias: disorders of tetrahydrobiopterin metabolism. In: Sarafoglou K, editor. *Pediatric endocrinology and inborn errors of metabolism.* McGraw Hill; 2009.

25. Walter JH, Lackmann RH, Burgard P. Hyperphenylalaninaemia. In: Saudubray J-M, van den Berghe G, Walter JH, editors. *Inborn metabolic diseases: diagnosis and treatment* 5th ed. Springer; 2012.
26. Mitchell GA, Grompe M, Lambert M, Tanguay RM. Hypertyrosinemias. In: Valle D, editor. *The online metabolic and molecular bases of inherited disease*. New York, NY: McGraw-Hill; 2014.
27. Jorquera R, Tanguay RM. The mutagenicity of the tyrosine metabolite, fumarylacetoacetate, is enhanced by glutathione depletion. *Biochem Biophys Res Commun* 1997;**232**(1):42–8.
28. Manabe S, Sassa S, Kappas A. Hereditary tyrosinemia. Formation of succinylacetone-amino acid adducts. *J Exp Med* 1985;**162**(3):1060–74.
29. Kumar G, Kamath N, Phadke KD, Iyengar A. The case mid R: a challenging case of severe rickets. *Kidney Int* 2012;**82**(6):725–6.
30. Sassa S, Kappas A. Hereditary tyrosinemia and the heme biosynthetic pathway. Profound inhibition of delta-aminolevulinic acid dehydratase activity by succinylacetone. *J Clin Invest* 1983;**71**(3):625–34.
31. Driscoll DJ, Jabs EW, Alcorn D, Maumenee IH, Brusilow SW, Valle D. Corneal tyrosine crystals in transient neonatal tyrosinemia. *J Pediatr* 1988;**113**(1 Pt 1):91–3.
32. Niederwieser A, Matasovic A, Tippett P, Danks DM. A new sulfur amino acid, named hawkinsin, identified in a baby with transient tyrosinemia and her mother. *Clin Chim Acta* 1977;**76**(3):345–56.
33. Lindstedt S, Holme E, Lock EA, Hjalmarson O, Strandvik B. Treatment of hereditary tyrosinaemia type I by inhibition of 4-hydroxyphenylpyruvate dioxygenase. *Lancet* 1992;**340**(8823):813–17.
34. Applegarth DA, Toone JR. Nonketotic hyperglycinemia (glycine encephalopathy): laboratory diagnosis. *Mol Genet Metab* 2001;**74**(1-2):139–46.
35. Hennermann JB, Berger JM, Grieben U, Scharer G, Van Hove JL. Prediction of long-term outcome in glycine encephalopathy: a clinical survey. *J Inherit Metab Dis* 2012;**35**(2):253–61.
36. Van Hove JL, Vande Kerckhove K, Hennermann JB, Mahieu V, Declercq P, Mertens S, et al. Benzoate treatment and the glycine index in nonketotic hyperglycinaemia. *J Inherit Metab Dis* 2005;**28**(5):651–63.
37. Kikuchi G, Motokawa Y, Yoshida T, Hiraga K. Glycine cleavage system: reaction mechanism, physiological significance, and hyperglycinemia. *Proc Jpn Acad Ser B Phys Biol Sci* 2008;**84**(7):246–63.
38. Dinopoulos A, Matsubara Y, Kure S. Atypical variants of nonketotic hyperglycinemia. *Mol Genet Metab* 2005;**86**(1–2):61–9.
39. Dhamija R, Mack KJ. A 2-day-old baby girl with encephalopathy and burst suppression on EEG. Nonketotic hyperglycinemia. *Neurology* 2011;**77**(3):e16–19.
40. Swanson MA, Coughlin Jr. CR, Scharer GH, Szerlong HJ, Bjoraker KJ, Spector EB, et al. Biochemical and molecular predictors for prognosis in nonketotic hyperglycinemia. *Ann Neurol* 2015;**78**(4):606–18.
41. Suzuki Y, Kure S, Oota M, Hino H, Fukuda M. Nonketotic hyperglycinemia: proposal of a diagnostic and treatment strategy. *Pediatr Neurol* 2010;**43**(3):221–4.
42. Boneh A, Degani Y, Harari M. Prognostic clues and outcome of early treatment of nonketotic hyperglycinemia. *Pediatr Neurol* 1996;**15**(2):137–41.
43. Hamosh A, Maher JF, Bellus GA, Rasmussen SA, Johnston MV. Long-term use of high-dose benzoate and dextromethorphan for the treatment of nonketotic hyperglycinemia. *J Pediatr* 1998;**132**(4):709–13.

44. Van Hove J, Coughlin II C, Scharer G. Glycine encephalopathy. In: Pagon RA, Adam MP, Ardinger HH, Wallace SE, Amemiya A, Bean LJH, editors. *GeneReviews(R)*. Seattle, WA: University of Washington, Seattle; 2002.
45. Jackson AH, Applegarth DA, Toone JR, Kure S, Levy HL. Atypical nonketotic hyperglycinemia with normal cerebrospinal fluid to plasma glycine ratio. *J Child Neurol* 1999;**14**(7):464–7.
46. Van Hove JL, Kishnani P, Muenzer J, Wenstrup RJ, Summar ML, Brummond MR, et al. Benzoate therapy and carnitine deficiency in non-ketotic hyperglycinemia. *Am J Med Genet* 1995;**59**(4):444–53.
47. Wei SH, Weng WC, Lee NC, Hwu WL, Lee WT. Unusual spinal cord lesions in late-onset non-ketotic hyperglycinemia. *J Child Neurol* 2011;**26**(7):900–3.
48. Centers for Disease Control and Prevention (CDC). Good laboratory practices for biochemical genetic testing and newborn screening for inherited metabolic disorders. *MMWR Recomm Rep* 2012; **61**(RR-2):1–44.
49. Chace DH, Kalas TA, Naylor EW. Use of tandem mass spectrometry for multianalyte screening of dried blood specimens from newborns. *Clin Chem* 2003;**49**(11):1797–817.
50. Tan ES, Wiley V, Carpenter K, Wilcken B. Non-ketotic hyperglycinemia is usually not detectable by tandem mass spectrometry newborn screening. *Mol Genet Metab* 2007;**90**(4):446–8.
51. Kure S. Two novel laboratory tests facilitating diagnosis of glycine encephalopathy (nonketotic hyperglycinemia). *Brain Dev* 2011;**33**(9):753–7.
52. Applegarth DA, Rolland MO, Toone JR, Coulter-Mackie M, Saura R. Molecular prenatal diagnosis of non-ketotic hyperglycinemia (glycine encephalopathy). *Prenat Diagn* 2002;**22**(3):266–7.
53. Kure S, Korman SH, Kanno J, Narisawa A, Kubota M, Takayanagi T, et al. Rapid diagnosis of glycine encephalopathy by 13C-glycine breath test. *Ann Neurology* 2006;**59**(5):862–7.
54. Burrage LC, Nagamani SC, Campeau PM, Lee BH. Branched-chain amino acid metabolism: from rare Mendelian diseases to more common disorders. *Hum Mol Genet* 2014;**23**(R1):R1–R8.
55. Wang XL, Li CJ, Xing Y, Yang YH, Jia JP. Hypervalinemia and hyperleucine-isoleucinemia caused by mutations in the branched-chain-amino-acid aminotransferase gene. *J Inherit Metab Dis* 2015;**38**(5):855–61.
56. Menkes JH, Hurst PL, Craig JM. A new syndrome: progressive familial infantile cerebral dysfunction associated with an unusual urinary substance. *Pediatrics* 1954;**14**(5):462–7.
57. Mackenzie DY, Woolf LI. Maple syrup urine disease: an inborn error of the metabolism of valine, leucine, and isoleucine associated with gross mental deficiency. *Br Med J* 1959;**1**(5114):90–1.
58. Moorthie S, Cameron L, Sagoo GS, Bonham JR, Burton H. Systematic review and meta-analysis to estimate the birth prevalence of five inherited metabolic diseases. *J Inherit Metab Dis* 2014;**37**(6):889–98.
59. Naylor EW, Guthrie R. Newborn screening for maple syrup urine disease (branched-chain ketoaciduria). *Pediatrics* 1978;**61**(2):262–6.
60. Morton DH, Strauss KA, Robinson DL, Puffenberger EG, Kelley RI. Diagnosis and treatment of maple syrup disease: a study of 36 patients. *Pediatrics* 2002;**109**(6):999–1008.
61. Nellis MM, Kasinski A, Carlson M, Allen R, Schaefer AM, Schwartz EM, et al. Relationship of causative genetic mutations in maple syrup urine disease with their clinical expression. *Mol Genet Metab* 2003;**80**(1-2):189–95.

62. Nellis MM, Danner DJ. Gene preference in maple syrup urine disease. *Am J Hum Genet* 2001;**68**(1):232–7.

63. Jouvet P, Rustin P, Taylor DL, Pocock JM, Felderhoff-Mueser U, Mazarakis ND, et al. Branched chain amino acids induce apoptosis in neural cells without mitochondrial membrane depolarization or cytochrome c release: implications for neurological impairment associated with maple syrup urine disease. *Mol Biol Cell* 2000;**11**(5):1919–32.

64. Sgaravatti AM, Rosa RB, Schuck PF, Ribeiro CA, Wannmacher CM, Wyse AT, et al. Inhibition of brain energy metabolism by the alpha-keto acids accumulating in maple syrup urine disease. *Biochim Biophys Acta* 2003;**1639**(3):232–8.

65. Chuang JL, Wynn RM, Moss CC, Song JL, Li J, Awad N, et al. Structural and biochemical basis for novel mutations in homozygous Israeli maple syrup urine disease patients: a proposed mechanism for the thiamin-responsive phenotype. *J Biol Chem* 2004;**279**(17):17792–800.

66. Muelly ER, Moore GJ, Bunce SC, Mack J, Bigler DC, Morton DH, et al. Biochemical correlates of neuropsychiatric illness in maple syrup urine disease. *J Clin Invest* 2013;**123**(4):1809–20.

67. Atwal PS, Macmurdo C, Grimm PC. Haemodialysis is an effective treatment in acute metabolic decompensation of maple syrup urine disease. *Mol Genet Metab Rep* 2015;**4**:46–8.

68. Hoffmann GF, Schulze A. Organic aciduria. In: Sarafoglou K, editor. *Pediatric endocrinology and inborn errors of metabolism*. McGraw Hill; 2009.

69. Shellmer DA, DeVito Dabbs A, Dew MA, Noll RB, Feldman H, Strauss KA, et al. Cognitive and adaptive functioning after liver transplantation for maple syrup urine disease: a case series. *Pediatr Transplant* 2011;**15**(1):58–64.

70. Mazariegos GV, Morton DH, Sindhi R, Soltys K, Nayyar N, Bond G, et al. Liver transplantation for classical maple syrup urine disease: long-term follow-up in 37 patients and comparative United Network for Organ Sharing experience. *J Pediatr* 2012;**160**(1): 116–21.e1.

71. Strauss KA, Mazariegos GV, Sindhi R, Squires R, Finegold DN, Vockley G, et al. Elective liver transplantation for the treatment of classical maple syrup urine disease. *Am J Transplant* 2006;**6**(3):557–64.

72. Schadewaldt P, Bodner-Leidecker A, Hammen H-W, Wendel U. Significance of l-alloisoleucine in plasma for diagnosis of maple syrup urine disease. *Clin Chem* 1999;**45**(10):1734–40.

73. Strauss KA, Puffenberger EG, Morton DH. Maple syrup urine disease. In: Pagon RA, Adam MP, Ardinger HH, Wallace SE, Amemiya A, Bean LJH, et al., editors. *GeneReviews(R)*. Seattle, WA; 2006.

74. Petras M, Tatarkova Z, Kovalska M, Mokra D, Dobrota D, Lehotsky J, et al. Hyperhomocysteinemia as a risk factor for the neuronal system disorders. *J Physiol Pharmacol* 2014;**65**(1):15–23.

75. Iacobazzi V, Infantino V, Castegna A, Andria G. Hyperhomocysteinemia: related genetic diseases and congenital defects, abnormal DNA methylation and newborn screening issues. *Mol Genet Metab* 2014;**113**(1–2):27–33.

76. Testai FD, Gorelick PB. Inherited metabolic disorders and stroke part 2: homocystinuria, organic acidurias, and urea cycle disorders. *Arch Neurol* 2010;**67**(2):148–53.

77. Rahman T, Cole EF. Capgras syndrome in homocystinuria. *Biol Psychiatry* 2014; **76**(6):e11–12.

78. Colafrancesco G, Di Marzio GM, Abbracciavento G, Stoppioni V, Leuzzi V, Ferrara M. Acute psychosis in an adolescent with undiagnosed homocystinuria. *Eur J Pediatr* 2015;**174**(9):1263–6.

79. Elsaid MF, Bener A, Lindner M, Alzyoud M, Shahbek N, Abdelrahman MO, et al. Are heterocygotes for classical homocystinuria at risk of vitamin B12 and folic acid deficiency? *Mol Genet Metab* 2007;**92**(1–2):100–3.
80. Casique L, Kabil O, Banerjee R, Martinez JC, De Lucca M. Characterization of two pathogenic mutations in cystathionine beta-synthase: different intracellular locations for wild-type and mutant proteins. *Gene* 2013;**531**(1):117–24.
81. Kožich V, Sokolová J, Klatovská V, Krijt J, Janošík M, Jelínek K, et al. Cystathionine β-synthase mutations: effect of mutation topology on folding and activity. *Human Mutation* 2010;**31**(7):809–19.
82. Singh LR, Chen X, Kožich V, Kruger WD. Chemical chaperone rescue of mutant human cystathionine β-synthase. *Mol Genet Metab* 2007;**91**(4):335–42.
83. Baric I, Fumic K, Glenn B, Cuk M, Schulze A, Finkelstein JD, et al. S-adenosylhomocysteine hydrolase deficiency in a human: a genetic disorder of methionine metabolism. *Proc Natl Acad Sci U S A* 2004;**101**(12):4234–9.
84. Stender S, Chakrabarti RS, Xing C, Gotway G, Cohen JC, Hobbs HH. Adult-onset liver disease and hepatocellular carcinoma in S-adenosylhomocysteine hydrolase deficiency. *Mol Genet Metab* 2015;**116**(4):269–74.
85. Gaull GE, Bender AN, Vulovic D, Tallan HH, Schaffner F. Methioninemia and myopathy: a new disorder. *Ann Neurol* 1981;**9**(5):423–32.
86. Barić I, Ćuk M, Fumić K, Vugrek O, Allen RH, Glenn B, et al. S-adenosylhomocysteine hydrolase deficiency: a second patient, the younger brother of the index patient, and outcomes during therapy. *J Inherit Metab Dis* 2005;**28**(6):885–902.
87. Strauss KA, Ferreira C, Bottiglieri T, Zhao X, Arning E, Zhang S, et al. Liver transplantation for treatment of severe S-adenosylhomocysteine hydrolase deficiency. *Mol Genet Metab* 2015;**116**(1–2):44–52.
88. Huemer M, Kozich V, Rinaldo P, Baumgartner MR, Merinero B, Pasquini E, et al. Newborn screening for homocystinurias and methylation disorders: systematic review and proposed guidelines. *J Inherit Metab Dis* 2015;**38**(6):1007–19.
89. Honzik T, Magner M, Krijt J, Sokolova J, Vugrek O, Beluzic R, et al. Clinical picture of S-adenosylhomocysteine hydrolase deficiency resembles phosphomannomutase 2 deficiency. *Mol Genet Metab* 2012;**107**(3):611–13.
90. Capdevila A, Wagner C. Measurement of plasma S-adenosylmethionine and S-adenosylhomocysteine as their fluorescent isoindoles. *Anal Biochem* 1998;**264**(2):180–4.
91. Mudd SH, Levy HL, Tangerman A, Boujet C, Buist N, Davidson-Mundt A, et al. Isolated persistent hypermethioninemia. *Am J Hum Genet* 1995;**57**(4):882–92.
92. Augoustides-Savvopoulou P, Luka Z, Karyda S, Stabler SP, Allen RH, Patsiaoura K, et al. Glycine N-methyltransferase deficiency: a new patient with a novel mutation. *J Inherit Metab Dis* 2003;**26**(8):745–59.
93. Mudd SH, Cerone R, Schiaffino MC, Fantasia AR, Minniti G, Caruso U, et al. Glycine N-methyltransferase deficiency: a novel inborn error causing persistent isolated hypermethioninaemia. *J Inherit Metab Dis* 2001;**24**(4):448–64.
94. Efron ML. Familial hyperprolinemia. *N Engl J Med* 1965;**272**(24):1243–54.
95. Afenjar A, Moutard M-L, Doummar D, Guët A, Rabier D, Vermersch A-I, et al. Early neurological phenotype in 4 children with biallelic PRODH mutations. *Brain Dev* 2007;**29**(9):547–52.
96. Mitsubuchi H, Nakamura K, Matsumoto S, Endo F. Biochemical and clinical features of hereditary hyperprolinemia. *Pediatr Int* 2014;**56**(4):492–6.
97. Guilmatre A, Legallic S, Steel G, Willis A, Di Rosa G, Goldenberg A, et al. Type I hyperprolinemia: genotype/phenotype correlations. *Hum Mutat* 2010;**31**(8):961–5.

98. Farrant RD, Walker V, Mills GA, Mellor JM, Langley GJ. Pyridoxal phosphate deactivation by pyrroline-5-carboxylic acid. Increased risk of vitamin B6 deficiency and seizures in hyperprolinemia type II. *J Biol Chem* 2001;**276**(18):15107–16.

99. Friedman M. Applications of the ninhydrin reaction for analysis of amino acids, peptides, and proteins to agricultural and biomedical sciences. *J Agric Food Chem* 2004;**52**(3):385–406.

100. Mudd SH, Irreverre F, Laster L. Sulfite oxidase deficiency in man: demonstration of the enzymatic defect. *Science* 1967;**156**(3782):1599–602.

101. Del Rizzo M, Burlina AP, Sass JO, Beermann F, Zanco C, Cazzorla C, et al. Metabolic stroke in a late-onset form of isolated sulfite oxidase deficiency. *Mol Genet Metab* 2013;**108**(4):263–6.

102. Rocha S, Ferreira AC, Dias AI, Vieira JP, Sequeira S. Sulfite oxidase deficiency – an unusual late and mild presentation. *Brain Dev* 2014;**36**(2):176–9.

103. Johnson JL, Rajagopalan KV. Human sulfite oxidase deficiency. Characterization of the molecular defect in a multicomponent system. *J Clin Invest* 1976;**58**(3):551–6.

104. Kisker C, Schindelin H, Pacheco A, Wehbi WA, Garrett RM, Rajagopalan KV, et al. Molecular basis of sulfite oxidase deficiency from the structure of sulfite oxidase. *Cell* 1997;**91**(7):973–83.

105. Johnson JL, Coyne KE, Garrett RM, Zabot MT, Dorche C, Kisker C, et al. Isolated sulfite oxidase deficiency: identification of 12 novel SUOX mutations in 10 patients. *Hum Mutat* 2002;**20**(1):74.

106. Touati G, Rusthoven E, Depondt E, Dorche C, Duran M, Heron B, et al. Dietary therapy in two patients with a mild form of sulfite oxidase deficiency. Evidence for clinical and biological improvement. *J Inherit Metab Dis* 2000;**23**(1):45–53.

107. Sass JO, Gunduz A, Araujo Rodrigues Funayama C, Korkmaz B, Dantas Pinto KG, Tuysuz B, et al. Functional deficiencies of sulfite oxidase: differential diagnoses in neonates presenting with intractable seizures and cystic encephalomalacia. *Brain Dev* 2010;**32**(7):544–9.

108. Belaidi Abdel A, Röper J, Arjune S, Krizowski S, Trifunovic A, Schwarz G. Oxygen reactivity of mammalian sulfite oxidase provides a concept for the treatment of sulfite oxidase deficiency. *Biochem J* 2015;**469**(2):211–21.

109. Cole DEC, Evrovski J. Quantitation of sulfate and thiosulfate in clinical samples by ion chromatography. *J Chromatogr A* 1997;**789**(1–2):221–32.

110. Duran M, Aarsen G, Fokkens RH, Nibbering NM, Cats BP, de Bree PK, et al. 2-Mercaptoethanesulfonate-cysteine disulfide excretion following the administration of 2-mercaptoethanesulfonate—a pitfall in the diagnosis of sulfite oxidase deficiency. *Clin Chim Acta* 1981;**111**(1):47–53.

111. Chwatko G, Bald E. Determination of thiosulfate in human urine by high performance liquid chromatography. *Talanta* 2009;**79**(2):229–34.

112. Poretti A, Blaser SI, Lequin MH, Fatemi A, Meoded A, Northington FJ, et al. Neonatal neuroimaging findings in inborn errors of metabolism. *J Magn Reson Imaging* 2013;**37**(2):294–312.

113. Thomas K, Wong K, Withington J, Bultitude M, Doherty A. Cystinuria—a urologist's perspective. *Nat Rev Urol* 2014;**11**(5):270–7.

114. Barbosa M, Lopes A, Mota C, Martins E, Oliveira J, Alves S, et al. Clinical, biochemical and molecular characterization of Cystinuria in a cohort of 12 patients. *Clinical Genetics* 2012;**81**(1):47–55.

115. Font-Llitjos M, Jimenez-Vidal M, Bisceglia L, Di Perna M, de Sanctis L, Rousaud F, et al. New insights into cystinuria: 40 new mutations, genotype-phenotype correlation, and digenic inheritance causing partial phenotype. *J Med Genet* 2005;**42**(1):58–68.

116. Dello Strologo L, Pras E, Pontesilli C, Beccia E, Ricci-Barbini V, de Sanctis L, et al. Comparison between SLC3A1 and SLC7A9 cystinuria patients and carriers: a need for a new classification. *J Am Soc Nephrol* 2002;**13**(10):2547–53.

117. Eggermann T, Venghaus A, Zerres K. Cystinuria: an inborn cause of urolithiasis. *Orphanet J Rare Dis* 2012;**7**

118. Rhodes HL, Yarram-Smith L, Rice SJ, Tabaksert A, Edwards N, Hartley A, et al. Clinical and genetic analysis of patients with cystinuria in the United Kingdom. *Clin J Am Soc Nephrol* 2015;**10**(7):1235–45.

119. Moe OW, Pearle MS, Sakhaee K. Pharmacotherapy of urolithiasis: evidence from clinical trials. *Kidney Int* 2011;**79**(4):385–92.

120. Andreassen KH, Pedersen KV, Osther SS, Jung HU, Lildal SK, Osther PJS. How should patients with cystine stone disease be evaluated and treated in the twenty-first century? *Urolithiasis* 2015;**44**(1):65–76.

121. Coe FL, Clark C, Parks JH, Asplin JR. Solid phase assay of urine cystine supersaturation in the presence of cystine binding drugs. *J Urol* 2001;**166**(2):688–93.

122. Janeckova H, Kalivodova A, Najdekr L, Friedecky D, Hron K, Bruheim P, et al. Untargeted metabolomic analysis of urine samples in the diagnosis of some inherited metabolic disorders. *Biomed Pap Med Fac Univ Palacky Olomouc Czech Repub* 2015;**159**(4):582–5.

123. Kovacevic L, Lu H, Goldfarb DS, Lakshmanan Y, Caruso JA. Urine proteomic analysis in cystinuric children with renal stones. *J Pediatr Urol* 2015;**11**(4):217 e1–6.

Organic acid disorders

3

S.F. Lo

Children's Hospital of Wisconsin, Milwaukee, WI, United States

3.1 INTRODUCTION

Diagnosis and monitoring of organic acidemia disorders requires urine organic acid testing. Analysis by a gas chromatography/mass spectrometry (GC/MS) instrument using a capillary column method represents the standard of analysis and quantitation of organic acids in urine. While there are several methods to identify organic acids in urine, the most commonly used extraction method[2] requires extraction with an organic solvent, such as ethyl acetate, followed by chemical derivation into volatile trimethylsilyl (TMS) compounds. The capillary GC column is used to separate the TMS compounds that flow into the MS for fragmentation. Each compound is identified by their retention time and characteristic fragmentation pattern. Mass spectra libraries assist in identifying compound fragmentation patterns. Unfortunately, many neutral and positively charged compounds of interest to metabolic physicians and biochemical geneticists are not detected using this classical technique.

A second method for organic acid identification utilizes the enzyme urease.[3,4] Pretreatment of urine samples with urease permits TMS derivatization of virtually all organic molecules in urine and other body fluids. In this method, the urine is treated with urease to remove urea, the most abundant compound in urine. Then the urease and other proteins are precipitated and the remaining sample is derivatized into volatile TMS compounds. Samples and eleven deuterated organic acid, amino acid and carbohydrate internal standards are introduced into the GC/MS (Fig. 3.1) and identification is accomplished with the assistance of mass spectral libraries. This method can quantitate 55 organic acid metabolites, 39 amino acids, 10 acylglycines, 12 sugars and carbohydrates, 7 neurotransmitters, and 5 purines and pyrimidines during a single 45-minute run. While the method is very laborious, the value in identifying many more biochemical compounds warrants that this method be seriously considered for organic acid testing.

For the ethyl acetate extraction and urease methods, identification of fragmentation patterns of different compounds utilizes one or more mass spectral libraries. Samples collected during periods of acute metabolic decompensation or acute illness have the advantage of being more informative as abnormal organic acid profiles are

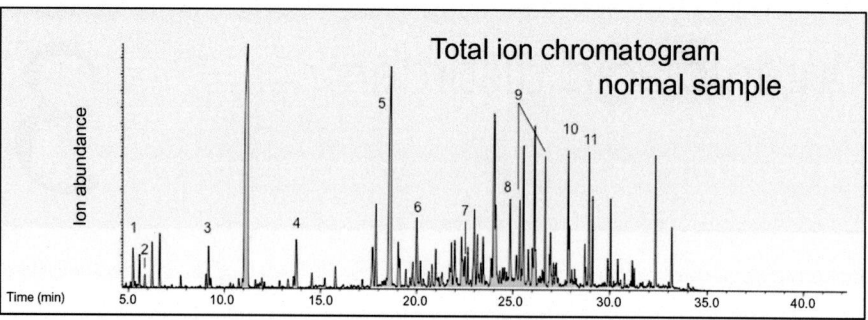

FIGURE 3.1

GC/MS total ion chromatogram of normal patient. Internal standards, in order of elution: 1. L-lactate-d_3, 2. Pyruvate-$^{13}C_3$, 3. Methyl-d_3-malonic acid, 4. DL-serine-d_3, 5. Creatine-d_3, 6. L-phenyl-d_5-alanine, 7. Orotic-$^{15}N_2$ acid, 8. Sebacic-d_4 acid, 9. D-glucose-$^{13}C_6$ (2 peaks), 10. Myo-inositol-d_6, 11. L-tryptophan-d_5.

more likely. Analysis of urine is most common. Rarely is blood or cerebrospinal fluid used for the diagnosis of an organic acidemia.

Newborns typically present within 1–2 weeks of age. While the pregnancy is typically unremarkable, a careful family history may suggest an inborn error. Poor feeding, vomiting, and increasing lethargy are commonly observed. Diagnosis is not limited to the newborn period. Many variants of these disorders can be identified beyond infancy into childhood, and sometimes adulthood. Although their presentation is more variable, the symptoms are similar. Typically an acute decompensation occurs in tandem with an illness that develops a metabolic acidosis with an increased anion gap, ketosis, and hyperammonemia.

3.2 SELECTED ORGANIC ACID DISORDERS

3.2.1 PROPIONIC ACIDEMIA (PA)

The enzyme propionyl-coenzyme A (CoA) carboxylase converts propionyl-CoA to D-methylmalonyl-CoA (Fig. 3.2). A deficiency in the enzymatic activity of propionyl-CoA carboxylase results in the accumulation of propionyl-CoA, a catabolic product of the amino acids isoleucine, valine, methionine, and threonine. A minor pathway generating propionyl-CoA is derived from cholesterol and odd chain fatty acids. Propionic acidemia (PA) has a prevalence of about 1 in 100,000 live births. PA is an autosomal recessive disease. Mutations involve either of the two genes encoding PCC, *PCCA or PCCB*. Mutations in these genes lead to decreased enzymatic activity of propionyl-CoA carboxylase resulting in the accumulation of propionyl-CoA. Propionyl-CoA carboxylase is a biotin-dependent enzyme, thus defects in the biotin utilization pathway involving biotinidase and holocarboxylase synthase will have a clinical and biochemical overlap with PA.

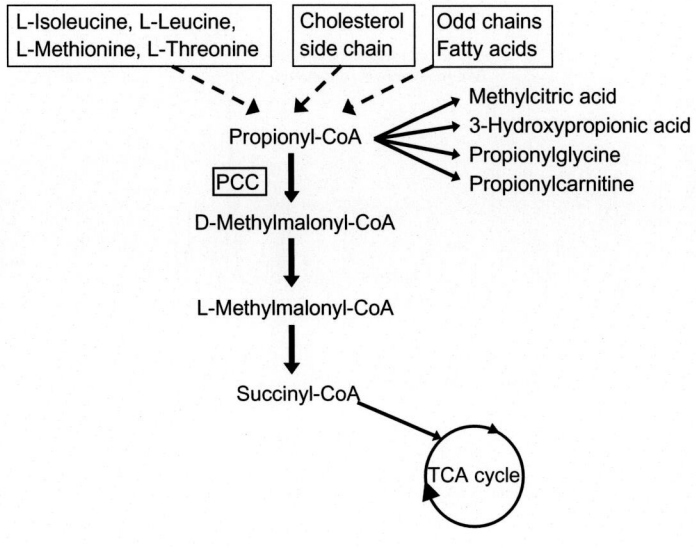

FIGURE 3.2

Pathway involving propionyl-CoA carboxylase. PCC, Propionyl-CoA carboxylase.

PA, also called propionyl-CoA carboxylase (PCC) deficiency, is characterized by massive metabolic decompensation.[5] Most commonly occurring in the neonatal period, these decompensations are rapid and severe, if not fatal, if left undiagnosed and untreated. The presentation is nonspecific and includes lethargy, poor feeding, vomiting, and hypotonia. Hyperammonemia, lactic and metabolic acidosis, increased plasma glycine and alanine, and ketosis are usually present. Outside the neonatal period, frequent metabolic decompensations occur as well as seizures, vomiting, and hepatomegaly. Children with the later-onset form may experience poor growth, developmental delay, or varying forms of intellectual disability.

Newborn screening can identify patients with PA. Elevations in C3 acylcarnitine indicate a positive screen, though not specific for PA, requiring follow-up confirmatory testing. Follow-up testing through urine organic acid testing should reveal increased levels of 3-hydroxypropionic acid, methyl citrate, propionylglycine (Fig. 3.3), and tiglylglycine in PA. Plasma glycine levels are commonly increased, as well as lactic acid and ammonia. Plasma acylcarnitine testing will show increased C3 acylcarnitine, consistent with the newborn screen. Confirmatory testing may be accomplished by enzyme analysis in fibroblasts or leukocytes, as well as sequencing of *PCCA* and *PCCB*, which is becoming the confirmatory test of choice.

Treatment utilizes a highly modified protein-restricted diet supplemented with PA-precursor depleted amino acid supplements, L-carnitine, and biotin supplementation.[6] The protein-restricted diet limits the abnormal accumulation of propionyl-CoA. Carnitine assists in promoting the excretion of propionyl-CoA as propionylcarnitine.

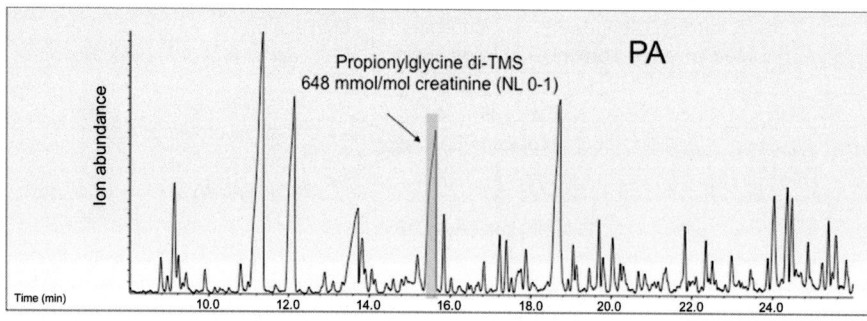

FIGURE 3.3

GC/MS total ion chromatogram of PA patient.

Since propionyl-CoA carboxylase requires biotin as a cofactor, a cofactor found in other carboxylases, PA may be identified in patients with multiple carboxylase deficiency. Not all PAs are responsive to biotin, in which case the modified diet is the only treatment. Although outcomes are generally poor, patients identified and treated earlier have a better prognosis than those diagnosed later. Survival of the early-onset group is not as good as in the late-onset group. The Surtees study, completed in 1992, identified the median survival age of the early-onset group at 3 years of age.[7] Improvement in patient outcomes remains poor despite earlier identification and more aggressive interventions.[8] Unfortunately, those identified with late-onset disease typically acquired neurologic damage.

3.2.2 METHYLMALONIC ACIDEMIA

A heterogeneous group of disorders are classified by the impairment of methylmalonic acid metabolism or methylmalonic acidurias (MMAs) include methylmalonyl-CoA mutase deficiency, 5′-deoxyadenosylcobalamin metabolic defects, and vitamin B12 deficiency.[5] Absence of methylmalonyl-CoA mutase (MMM) does not allow methylmalonyl-CoA to be converted to succinyl-CoA (MUT[0]). The result of this blockage is an increase in the production of methylmalonic acid and propionic acid, a precursor of methylmalonic acid (Fig. 3.4). Other MMM mutations that result in lesser reductions in enzymatic activity constitutes another category of mutase deficiency termed MUT[−]. Defects in the synthesis of 5′-deoxyadenosylcobalamin, a cofactor for the mutase enzyme, will also present at MMA and are classified into several complementary classes (Fig. 3.5). CblA, CblB, and CblH involve defects in adenosylcobalamin synthesis resulting in a similar biochemical presentation as observed in mutase deficiency. CblC and CblD are involved in cobalamin reduction resulting in decreased mutase activity and decreased methionine synthase activity. Methionine synthase converts homocystine to methionine using the methylcobalamin as cofactor, and thus these defects produce both MMA and homocystinemia. Mutations CblF

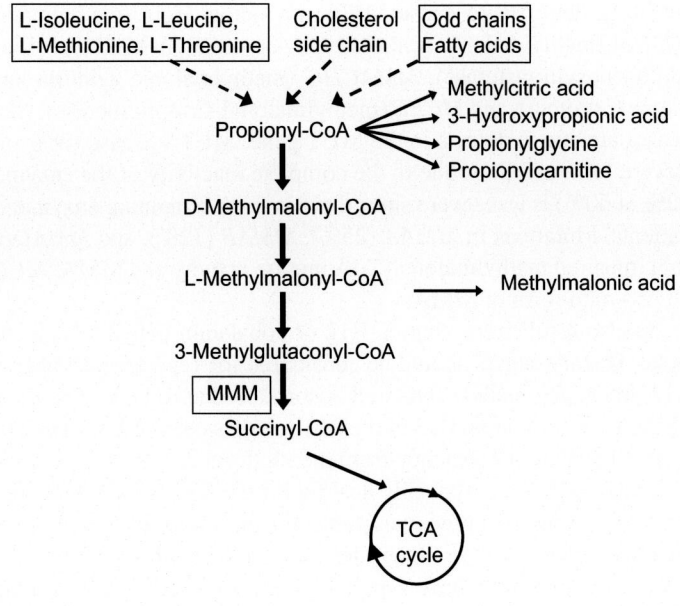

FIGURE 3.4

Pathway involving methylmalonyl-CoA mutase. MMM, methylmalonyl-CoA mutase.

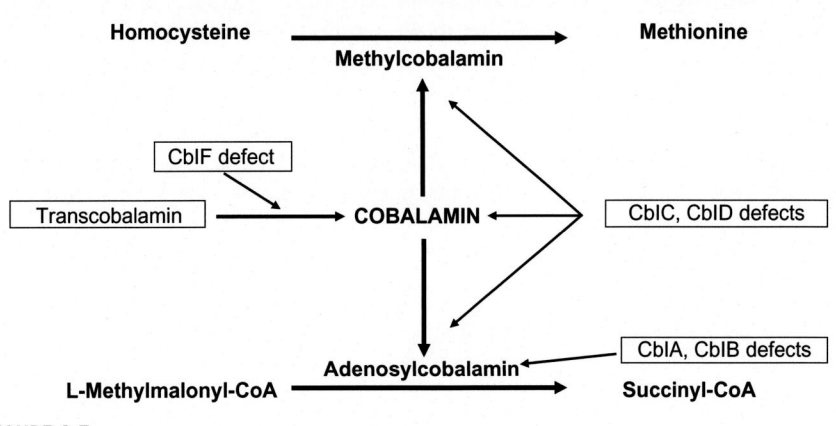

FIGURE 3.5

Cobalamin and localization of cobalamin defects.

and CblJ are due to defects in transcobalamin degradation, which prevent cobalamin from being transported from lysosomes for recycling in the cytoplasm.

The prevalence of MMA is suspected to be between 1 in 50,000 and 1 in 100,000 live births.[9] MMA is inherited in an autosomal recessive manner. Several genes have been identified to cause MMA, including *MUT* (methylmalonyl-CoA mutase), *MMAA* (methylmalonic aciduria type A protein), *MMAB* (cob(l)yrinic acid a,c-diamide adenosyltransferase), *MMACHC* (methylmalonic aciduria and homocystinuria type C protein), and *MCEE* (methylmalonyl-CoA epimerase). Nearly 60% of MMA cases are due to defects in the MUT gene. MUT^0 disease (78% of 60%) is the most severe form of MMA due to the complete inactivity of the enzyme. MUT^- disease (22% of 60%) is less severe since there is some remaining enzymatic activity in these patients. Mutations in *MMAA* (25%), *MMAB* (12%), and *MMADHC* genes also result in impaired methylmalonyl-CoA mutase activity and MMA. *MCEE* mutations result in a mild form of MMA.

MMA can also result from vitamin B12 or cobalamin deficiency due to limited dietary intake. Dietary causes should be considered for vegetarians. Other causes of vitamin B12 deficiency include impaired absorption due to lack of intrinsic factor. Transient MMA due to vitamin B12 of the newborn has been observed due to vertical transmission of cobalamin deficiency from the mother.

Newborns with MMA are typically healthy for the first 1–2 weeks of life. MUT^0 and severe MUT^--affected individuals typically present with hypotonia, lethargy, and poor feeding. Older infants and children with milder MUT^- mutations will present with poor growth or only have symptoms during periods of intervening illness. Symptoms include lethargy, seizures, and hypoglycemia. The CblC form of MMA may present with symptoms related to homocystinuria, which included progressive myopathy, thrombosis, and retinal findings.

Newborn screening can identify patients with MMA. Elevations in C3 acylcarnitine signal a positive screen, similar to PA, requiring follow-up confirmatory testing. Follow-up testing for MMA should reveal elevations in methylmalonic acid (Fig. 3.6), methyl citrate, and 3-hydroxypropionic acid. Increases in propionylglycine and propionylcarnitine may also be observed. Determination of the different enzymatic subtypes requires additional studies in vitamin B12 responsiveness, ^{14}C-propionate incorporation, and cobalamin distribution assays.[8] Confirmatory

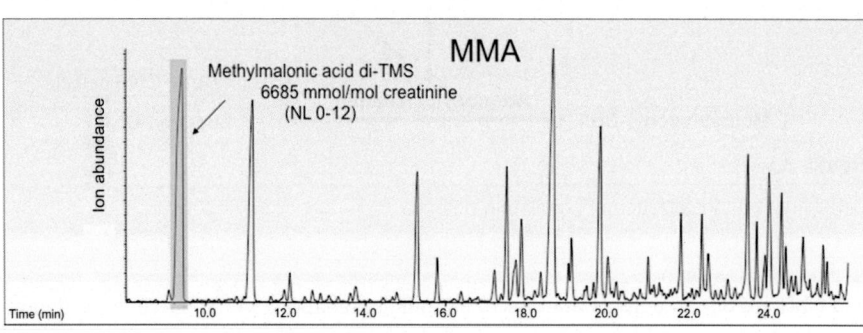

FIGURE 3.6

GC/MS total ion chromatogram of MMA patient.

testing is also accomplished through complementation studies. Sequencing of *MUT* and other genes for disorders of cobalamin metabolism may also be done.

Treatment for MMA involves a highly modified protein-restricted diet supplemented with PA-precursor depleted amino acid supplements, adjusted for age and weight. Cobalamin (cyano- or hydoxycobalamin) and L-carnitine supplementation may also be provided. Prolonged periods of fasting should be avoided. Prognosis is related to response to treatment and outcome is dependent upon disease subtype where MUT[0] has the worst prognosis and CblA has the best prognosis. The severity of the other classes range between these two defects. In a study by Nicolaides et al., early-onset cobalamin nonresponders had a median survival of roughly 6 years.[10]

3.2.3 ISOVALERIC ACIDEMIA

Isovaleric acidemia (IVA) is caused by a deficiency of the enzyme isovaleryl-CoA dehydrogenase (IVD), a mitochondrial flavoenzyme. Loss of IVD function results in the accumulation of isovaleryl-CoA by preventing its oxidation to 3-methylcrotonyl-CoA (Fig. 3.7). This catalytic step is part of the catabolic pathway of leucine. IVA is the first organic acidemia diagnosed by GC/MS,[11] and is readily detected with tandem MS.[12]

IVA has a prevalence of 1 in 250,000 and is an autosomal recessive disorder characterized by mutations in the IVD gene. The protein product is a homotetramer. IVD is initially synthesized in the cytoplasm as a 45 kDa precursor. Upon posttranslational modification and transfer into the mitochondria, a 43 kDa mature protein is created. The combination of four mature polypeptides forms IVD. The molecular

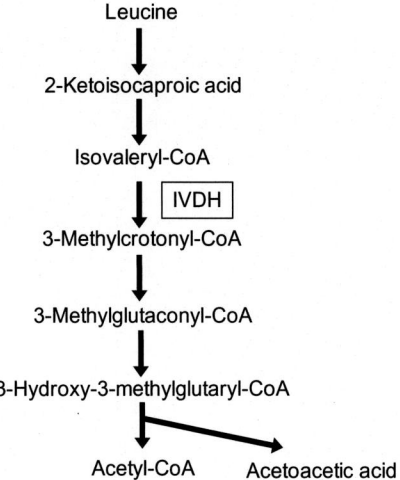

FIGURE 3.7

Leucine metabolism involving IVDH. IVDH, isovaleryl-CoA dehydrogenase.

heterogeneity of IVD has been classified into six classes. Class I mutations generate a mixture of the precursor and mature peptides, suggesting the presence of point mutations and normal processing. Classes II, III, and IV mutations generate smaller proteins of the precursor and mature forms, suggesting the presence of point mutations and deletions. Classes V and VI do not form any detectable protein product due to either an inability to translate mRNA, and the formation of unstable mRNA, or defective transcription.

There are two forms of IVA, an acute neonatal form and a chronic intermittent form. The biochemical defect is the same for both. The difference in clinical presentation is not only determined by the causative mutation, but is also a consequence of catabolic stress and other factors.[13] Neonates with the acute form begin to exhibit signs and symptoms within the first few days of life. Poor feeding, vomiting, and lethargy is apparent and the foul "odor of sweaty feet" is commonly found. Lab findings demonstrate increased ketones, metabolic acidosis, increased lactate, and hyperammonemia. Other findings include thrombocytopenia, neutropenia, pancytopenia, and hypocalcemia.[14–17] Neonates that survive the acute episode will then fall into the chronic intermittent form of disease and their development may be normal.[16–18]

In the chronic intermittent form of IVA, presentation occurs within the first year of life. Similar to the acute form, vomiting, lethargy, acidosis with ketonuria, and the "odor of sweaty feet" is commonly found at presentation. It is common for patients with IVA to have some form of developmental delay and mental retardation, along with an aversion to protein-rich foods.[19] With the improvements in early diagnosis, normal development of individuals with IVA is more common than in the past.

Newborn screening using tandem MS is used to detect elevations in C5 acylcarnitine. While the characteristic "odor of sweaty feet" due to increased concentrations of isovaleric acid is commonly identified during acute episodes, it is not completely specific for IVA, since a similar odor is identifiable in glutaric acidemia type 2 (GA2; multiple acyl-CoA dehydrogenase deficiency). In IVA, GC/MS for urine organic acid testing will specifically identify isovalerylglycine (Fig. 3.8). During acute episodes, concentrations of urinary isovalerylglycine are 100–500 times normal. In remission,

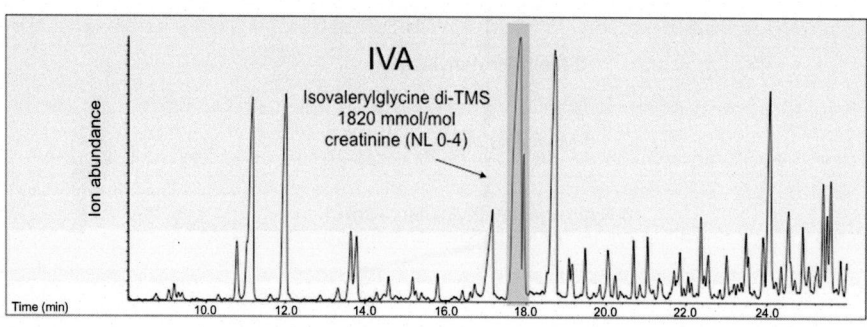

FIGURE 3.8

GC/MS total ion chromatogram of IVA patient.

concentrations range from normal to 10 times normal. Plasma acylcarnitine analysis is a complementary test for IVA diagnosis. Identification of C5 acylcarnitine suggests the presence of isovalerylcarnitine, though an isobaric isomer, 2-methylbutyrylcarnitine, may also be present. However, the isomer is typically accompanied with increased C4- and C16-acylcarnitines if GA2 (multiple acyl-CoA dehydrogenase deficiency) is present. DNA analysis for specific IVD mutations, as well as sequencing is available for confirmatory testing. Confirmatory testing by enzymatic analysis on fibroblasts can also be done.

If no neurological damage has occurred before the initiation of treatment with a leucine restricted diet, and glycine and/or carnitine, then prognosis for normal development is good.

3.2.4 MULTIPLE CARBOXYLASE DEFICIENCY (HOLOENZYME SYNTHETASE AND BIOTINIDASE)

Multiple carboxylase deficiency includes more than one disorder due to the utilization of biotin as a cofactor for several enzymes.[20] Specifically the enzymes pyruvate carboxylase, propionyl-CoA carboxylase, 3-methylcrotonyl-CoA carboxylase, and acetyl-CoA carboxylase require biotin as an essential, covalently bound cofactor. When the synthesis of biotin cofactor is disrupted, the functional activity of these enzymes is decreased or eliminated, and consequently will have effects on fatty acid synthesis, gluconeogenesis, pyruvate metabolism, and amino acid catabolism. Biotin itself is a water-soluble vitamin derived primarily from diet. Errors in the metabolism of biotin result in two types of disorders, holocarboxylase synthetase deficiency, and biotinidase deficiency.

Typical clinical symptoms of holocarboxylase synthetase deficiency include lethargy, hypotonia, seizures, and difficulty feeding and breathing. Other findings include ketoacidosis, hypoglycemia, hyperammonemia, skin rash, and alopecia.[21] Onset of symptoms for holocarboxylase synthetase deficiency typically occurs during the neonatal period, although later presentations are common. In biotinidase deficiency, clinical features typically include neurological, dermatological, immunological, and ophthalmological symptoms.[22] The onset of symptoms of biotinidase-deficient individuals usually appears during infancy. While the onset of symptoms for both disorders is usually different, there is considerable temporal and clinical overlap.

Multiple mutations have been found in the genes for holocarboxylase synthetase and biotinidase. The prevalence of holocarboxylase synthetase deficiency is about 1 in 87,000 and for biotinidase it is roughly 1 in 60,000 live births.[23] The inheritance pattern of these disorders is autosomal recessive. The mutations in these genes result in defective enzymes involved in the utilization of biotin. Consequently, enzymes requiring biotin as a cofactor decrease their activity or become inactive.

The biotin cycle is the process by which biotin is utilized and recycled. Enzymes that require biotin as a cofactor, the apocarboxylases, require biotin to be covalently attached through a lysine residue, thereby forming the fully active holocarboxylases (pyruvate carboxylase, propionyl-CoA carboxylase, 3-methylcrotonyl-CoA carboxylase, and acetyl-CoA carboxylase). The enzyme responsible for covalently attaching biotin to the apocarboxylases is holocarboxylase synthetase. The biotin cycle involves recycling biotin from the holocarboxylases by proteolytic degradation by which the biotin is cleaved from the lysine side chain by the enzyme biotinidase, resulting in the release of free biotin for use in holocarboxylase synthesis.

Newborn screening for biotinidase deficiency is available.[24,25] Screening of holocarboxylase synthetase deficiency can be identified by elevations of C5-hydroxyacylcarnitine. Follow-up testing using urine organic acid analysis will reveal increases in 3-hydroxyisovaleric acid, methylcitric acid, 3-methylcrotonylglycine, and propionylglycine. Confirmatory testing is done either by determining enzymatic activity, DNA sequence analysis, or targeted mutation analysis of either enzyme.

Fortunately, patients with either holocarboxylase synthetase deficiency or biotinidase deficiency can both be treated with oral biotin. Most patients are responsive to biotin, resulting in the reversal of symptoms. If treatment is initiated before the onset of neurological symptoms, prognosis is very good. Unfortunately, once vision and hearing symptoms are present, they are usually irreversible.

3.2.5 GLUTARIC ACIDEMIA, TYPE 1

Glutaric acidemia type 1 (GA1), also called glutaryl-CoA dehydrogenase deficiency, is a disorder of the catabolic pathways of lysine, hydroxylysine, and tryptophan (Fig. 3.9). Increased concentrations of these amino acids and their breakdown products can cause damage to the basal ganglia, leading to dystonia and dyskinesia.[26]

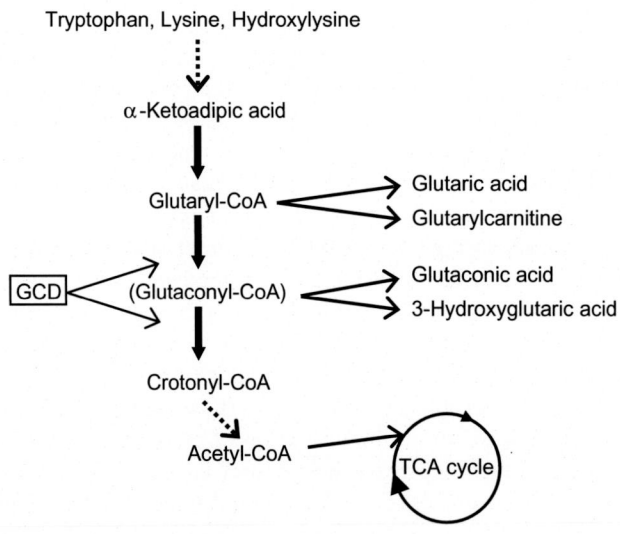

FIGURE 3.9

Catabolism of tryptophan, lysine and hydroxylysine involving glutaryl-CoA dehydrogenase. GCD, glutaryl-CoA dehydrogenase.

This condition is inherited in an autosomal recessive fashion and occurs in roughly 1 in 30,000 to 1 in 100,000 births. In some homogeneous populations, the incidence of disease can be as frequent as 1 in 225 births.[27] Heterozygous carriers are essentially normal. Mutations in the glutaryl-CoA dehydrogenase gene (*GCDH*) prevent the catabolism of lysine, hydroxylysine, and tryptophan. Decreased enzymatic activity leads to the accumulation of glutaric acid, 3-hydroxyglutaric acid, glutaconic acid, and glutarylcarnitine. *GCDH* is about 7 kb long and has 11 exons.[28] The protein product is about 4.5 kDa. Over 100 mutations have been identified and enzymatic activity typically ranges from 0% to 10% in GA1 tissues from GA1 patients. No correlation between specific mutations and clinical severity has been demonstrated.

Unlike the previous organic acidemias, development can be normal throughout the first year of life, but macrocephaly is commonly present. Noticeable chronic symptoms may include difficulty feeding and irritability. Initial presentation, typically between 4 and 18 months, is usually an acute, irreversible, encephalopathic, stroke-like episode acquired concurrent with another illness, infection, fasting, or minor trauma. Loss of head control, hypotonia, and seizures can evolve rapidly. Other irreversible neurological symptoms follow including dystonia, opisthotonus, and rigidity. These symptoms previously suggested cerebral palsy, but with the development of newborn screening for GA1, this catastrophic presentation is less common. After 5 years of age, onset of symptoms is rare. If metabolic crises recur, dyskinesia and dystonia may worsen and become very severe. Unfortunately for the affected individual, regardless of neurological symptoms, intellect is generally preserved. Individuals with GA1 exhibit a wide range of neurological complications.

Diagnosis can be made by detecting increased glutaric acid and 3-hydroxyglutaric acid in urine organic acid analysis (Fig. 3.10). 3-Hydroxyglutaric acid is usually but not always detectable, but if identified, it is pathognomic for GA1. Complementary testing using tandem MS for plasma acylcarnitines reveals increased C5-DC acylcarnitine. This method is also used to detect glutarylcarnitine in dried blood spots for newborn screening. Confirmatory testing can be done by enzymatic analysis using ^{14}C-labeled glutaryl-CoA and measuring the release of $^{14}CO_2$.[29] Specific mutation detection and genetic sequencing of *GCDH* is also available for confirmatory testing.

Treatment uses carnitine supplementation, as well as immediate and vigorous treatment of illnesses with antipyretics, fluids, insulin, and glucose. When treated properly, greater than 80% of GA1 patients developed normally.[30] It is unclear if dietary restriction of protein, lysine, and tryptophan provides any benefit, although many centers restrict dietary intake of these amino acids.

3.2.6 3-METHYLCROTONYL-CoA CARBOXYLASE DEFICIENCY

As with other biotin-dependent carboxylases, the isolated deficiency of 3-methylcrotonyl-CoA carboxylase (3-MCC) must be distinguished from the biotin-responsive disorders holocarboxylase synthetase or biotinidase deficiencies, as well as other isolated carboxylase deficiencies. In isolated 3-MCC deficiency, also called 3-methylcrotonylglycinuria, the catabolism of leucine is impaired and this enzyme is unable to convert 3-methylcrotonyl-CoA to 3-methylglutaconyl-CoA (Fig. 3.11).

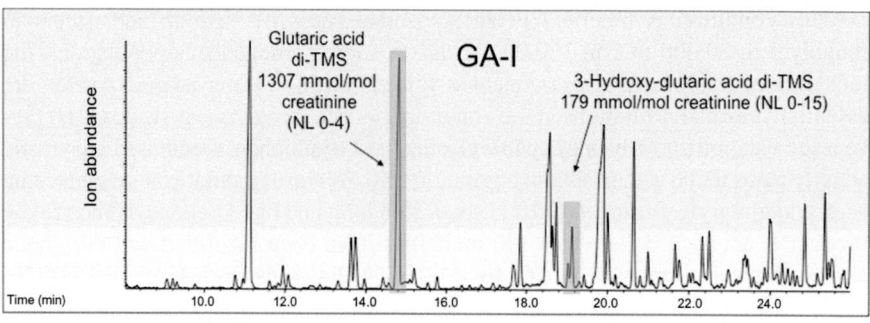

FIGURE 3.10

GC/MS total ion chromatogram of GA-I patient.

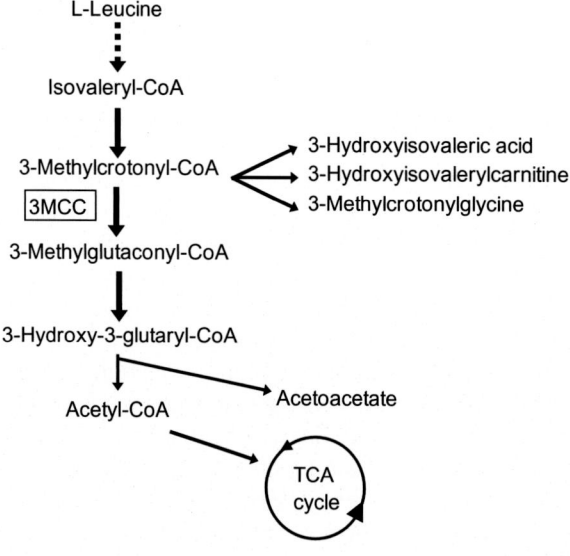

FIGURE 3.11

Leucine metabolism involving 3MCC. 3MCC, 3-methylcrotonyl-CoA carboxylase

Prevalence is about 1 in 50,000 live births. Inheritance of this disorder is autosomal recessive. 3-MCC is comprised of two subunits encoded by two genes. The gene *MCCC1* codes for methylcrotonyl-CoA carboxylase subunit alpha, and *MCCC2* codes for methylcrotonyl-CoA carboxylase subunit beta.

There is a large range of clinical presentations for 3-MCC, ranging from clinically benign to severe disease and death. The most severely affected patients can present with metabolic acidosis, hypoglycemia, and hyperammonemia.[13] Other

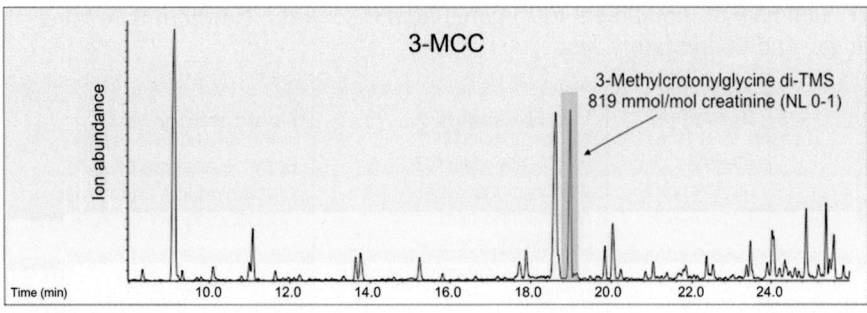

FIGURE 3.12

GC/MS total ion chromatogram of 3-MCC patient.

laboratory findings include elevated hepatic transaminases, moderate ketonuria, and plasma carnitine deficiency.[31] Initial signs may include poor feeding, vomiting, and lethargy. Untreated 3-MCC patients may present with failure to thrive, Reye-like symptoms, hypotonia, seizures, coma, developmental delay, and possibly death. With the expansion of newborn screening to include 3-MCC and additional studies to assess its impact, it has been observed that less than 10% of screen-positive individuals develop symptoms. It appears that 3-MCC deficiency is predominantly a benign disease. Consequently, Germany does not screen for 3-MCC deficiency.[32]

Newborn screening with tandem MS can identify 3-MCC by detecting isobaric isomers of C5-hydroxyacylcarnitine. Since five metabolic diseases can generate high concentrations of an isobaric acylcarnitine with the same mass as 3-methylcrotonyl-carnitine on tandem MS screening, follow-up testing is required to determine which disorder is responsible for the positive screen. Diagnosis is made by urine organic acid testing demonstrating increased concentrations of 3-hydroxyisovaleric acid and 3-methylcrotonylglycine (Fig. 3.12). If methyl citrate, 3-hydroxypropionic acid, and lactate are present, multiple carboxylase deficiency must be considered. Diagnosis of isolated 3-MCC may also be confirmed by plasma acylcarnitine analysis and the identification of significant elevations of 3-hydroxyisovalerylcarnitine.[33] Confirmatory testing is done by enzyme activity analysis of 3-MCC in leukocytes. To distinguish 3-MCC from multiple carboxylase deficiency, normal activity of at least one carboxylase should be demonstrated. Genetic sequencing of *MCCC1* and *MCCC2* may also be used for confirmatory testing.

The spectrum of clinical disease is broad. Most individuals remain asymptomatic throughout their lifetime. Others begin to have symptoms as early as 3 months of age and commonly before 3 years of age. Treatment may require the restriction of leucine and carnitine supplementation since carnitine deficiency occurs secondary to urinary loss of 3-methylcrotonyl-carnitine. Glycine may also be administered to remove 3-MCC as 3-methylcrotonylglycine.[34] Development is typically normal with treatment (Table 3.1).

Table 3.1 Summary of Biomarkers for Organic Acid Disorders—Newborn Screening, Lab Findings, and Confirmatory Test

Disorder	Newborn Screening	Lab Findings	Confirmatory Test
Propionic acidemia	Elevated C3 acylcarnitine	PAC—elevated C3 acylcarnitine; UOA—methylcitric acid, 3-hydroxypropionic acid, propionylglycine, tiglylglycine	Enzyme analysis of propionyl-CoA carboxylase. Sequencing of *PCCA/PCCB*
Methylmalonic acidemia	Elevated C3 acylcarnitine	PAC—elevated C3 acylcarnitine; UOA—methylmalonic acid, methylcitric acid, 3-hydroxypropionic acid	Complementation studies. Sequencing of MUT/genes for disorders of cobalamin metabolism
Multiple carboxylase deficiencies			
A. Holocarboxylase synthetase deficiency	Elevated C5-OH acylcarnitine	PAC—mild elevations in C3, C5-OH acylcarnitine; UOA—3-hydroxyisovaleric acid, methylcitric acid, 3-methylcrotonylglycine, propionylglycine	Enzyme analysis of holocarboxylase synthetase. Sequencing of *HLCS*
B. Biotinidase	Enzyme analysis		Enzyme analysis of biotinidase. Targeted mutation analysis or sequencing of *BTD*
Isovaleric acidemia	Elevated C5 acylcarnitine	PAC—elevated C5 acylcarnitine; UOA—isovalerylglycine, 3-hydroxyisovaleric acid, 4-hydroxyvaleric acid	Targeted mutation analysis or sequencing of *IVA*
Glutaric acidemia type 1	Elevated C5-DC acylcarnitine	PAC & UAC—elevated C5-DC acylcarnitine; UOA—3-hydroxyglutaric acid, glutaric acid	Enzyme analysis of glutaryl-CoA dehydrogenase. Targeted mutation analysis or sequencing of *GCDH*
3-Methylcrotonyl-CoA carboxylase deficiency	Elevated C5-OH acylcarnitine	PAC & UAC—elevated C5-OH acylcarnitine; UOA—3-methylcrotonylglycine, 3-hydroxyisovaleric acid	Enzyme analysis of 3-methylcrotonyl-CoA carboxylase. sequencing of *MCCC1/MCCC2*

PAC—plasma acylcarnitine (profile); UAC—urine acylcarnitine (specific acylcarnitine tested); UOA—urine organic acids.

3.3 OTHER ORGANIC ACID DISORDERS

Many other organic disorders have been identified and are not discussed in this chapter. A few of these less prevalent disorders are shown in Tables 3.2 and 3.3.

Table 3.2 Summary of Other Organic Acid Disorders—Major Clinical Findings, Enzyme and Biological Function, and Gene

Disorder	Major Clinical Findings	Enzyme and Biological Function	Gene
Beta-ketothiolase deficiency (T2)[35]	Episodic severe ketoacidosis usually with stress, possible hyperlacticacidemia	Mitochondrial acetoacetyl-CoA thiolase—involved in ketogenesis and ketolysis, involved in catabolism of isoleucine	ACAT1
3-Methylglutaconic aciduria[36]—Type I[37]	Variable—developmental delay, failure to thrive—neurological, no hyperammonemia, no acidosis	3-Methylglutaconic dehydratase—involved in leucine degradation	AUH
3-Methylglutaconic aciduria—Type II (Barth syndrome)[37,38]	Dilated cardiomyopathy, skeletal myopathy, neutropenia, growth deficiency	Protein predicted to be acyltransferases involved in remodeling of cardiolipin	TAZ (Tafzzin)
3-Methylglutaconic aciduria—Type III (Costeff syndrome)[37,39]	Optic atrophy, choreoathetoid movements	Optic atrophy 3 protein—unknown function	OPA3
3-Methylglutaconic aciduria—Type IV[37]	Variable neurologic features, cardiomyopathy.	Unknown	Unknown
3-Methylglutaconic aciduria—Type V[37]	Dilated cardiomyopathy, ataxia	Unknown	DNAJC19
2-Methylbutyryl-CoA dehydrogenase deficiency, acyl-CoA dehydrogenase short/branched-chain[40]	Variable presentation from asymptomatic to life threatening, poor feeding, lethargy, vomiting, irritable, difficulty breathing, seizures, and coma. Increase frequency in Hmong population.	2-Methylbutyryl-CoA dehydrogenase—involved in degradation of isoleucine	ACADSB (or SBCAD)

(Continued)

Table 3.2 Summary of Other Organic Acid Disorders—Major Clinical Findings, Enzyme and Biological Function, and Gene (Continued)

Disorder	Major Clinical Findings	Enzyme and Biological Function	Gene
Fumarase deficiency, fumaric aciduria[41]	Severe neurological abnormalities—brain malformations, developmental delay, hypotonia, microcephaly, failure to thrive. Minor seizures, unusual facial features, hepatosplenomegaly, polycythemia, leukopenia; no acute crises	Fumarate hydratase/fumarase—catalyzes the conversion of fumarate to malate within the citric acid cycle	*FH*
Malonic aciduria[42–44]	Variable presentation—developmental delay, hypotonia, seizures, diarrhea, vomiting, hypoglycemia, acidosis, cardiomyopathy	Malonyl-CoA decarboxylase—first step in fatty acid biosynthesis	*MLYCD*
L-2-hydroxyglutaric aciduria[36]	Abnormalities in cerebellum, seizures, intellectual disability, macrocephaly	L-2-hydroxyglutarate dehydrogenase; toxic effect of L-2-hydroxyglutarate on central nervous system	*L2HGDH*
D-2-hydroxyglutaric aciduria[36]	Variable presentation (mild and severe), developmental delay, seizures, hypotonia, abnormalities in the cerebrum, cardiomyopathy	D-2-hydroxyglutarate dehydrogenase	*D2HGDH*
Canavan disease (ASPA deficiency or aspartoacylase deficiency)[36,44]	Developmental delay, macrocephaly, lack of head control, hypotonia, blindness	Aspartoacylase—catalyzes the conversion of N-acetylaspartic acid to aspartic acid and acetate	*ASPA*

Table 3.3 Summary of Biomarkers for Other Organic Acid Disorders—Lab Findings and Treatment

Disorder	Lab Findings	Treatment
Beta-ketothiolase deficiency (T2)[34]	UOA: 2-methyl-3-hydroxybutyrate, 2-methylacetylacetate, tiglylglycine. PAC: elevated C5-OH (3-hydroxyisovalerylcarnitine) Enzyme: Confirm with enzyme testing on fibroblast. Molecular DNA testing available	Acute—glucose infusion and treat acidosis but beware of hypernatremia with aggressive alkanization. Chronic—mild protein restriction, avoid fasting and early treatment with illness, carnitine if low
3-Methylglutaconic aciduria[35]—Type I[36]	UOA: 3-methylglutaconic acid, 3-methylglutaric acid; Type 1 also has elevation in 3-hydroxyisovaleric acid. Molecular DNA testing available	Type 1—consider leucine restriction, carnitine supplementation
3-Methylglutaconic aciduria—Type II (Barth syndrome)[35,36]	UOA: 3-methylglutaconic acid, 3-methylglutaric acid. Molecular DNA testing available	No specific treatment (fatty acid therapy under investigation)
3-Methylglutaconic aciduria—Type III (Costeff syndrome)[36,38]	UOA: 3-methylglutaconic acid, 3-methylglutaric acid. Molecular DNA testing available	No specific treatment
3-Methylglutaconic aciduria—Type IV[36]	UOA: 3-methylglutaconic acid, 3-methylglutaric acid	No specific treatment
3-Methylglutaconic aciduria—Type V[36]	UOA: 3-methylglutaconic acid, 3-methylglutaric acid. Molecular DNA testing available	No specific treatment
2-Methylbutyryl-CoA dehydrogenase deficiency, acyl-CoA dehydrogenase short/branched-chain[39]	UOA: 2-methylbutyrylglycine. PAC: elevated C5 (2-methylbutyrylcarnitine)	Variable—no treatment to avoid prolonged periods of time without eating, low-protein diet, restricted isoleucine intake, carnitine
Fumarase deficiency, fumaric aciduria[40]	UOA: fumaric acid. Enzyme: activity assay from fibroblasts, lymphoblasts or white blood cells. Molecular genetic testing available	No specific treatment
Malonic aciduria[41–43]	UOA: malonic acid. Pac: C3DC (malonylcarnitine). Molecular DNA testing available	No consensus for dietary treatment. Long-chain triglyceride restricted/medium-chain triglyceride supplemented diet has been suggested

(Continued)

Table 3.3 Summary of Biomarkers for Other Organic Acid Disorders—Lab Findings and Treatment (Continued)

Disorder	Lab Findings	Treatment
L-2-hydroxyglutaric aciduria[36]	UOA: 2-hydroxyglutaric acid (chirality not determined)	No specific treatment
D-2-hydroxyglutaric aciduria[36]	UOA: 2-hydroxyglutaric acid (chirality not determined)	No specific treatment
Canavan disease (ASPA deficiency or aspartoacylase deficiency)[36,44]	UOA: N-acetylaspartic acid. Molecular DNA testing for ASPA available	No specific treatment
PAC—plasma acylcarnitine (profile) UOA—urine organic acids		

3.3.1 SPURIOUS ORGANIC ACIDS

While the biomarkers used to identify and diagnose specific organic acid disorders are known, the actual process of interpreting an organic acid results profile is confounded by the excretion of organic acids from sources other than an inborn error. For example, while the presence of 3-hydroxypropionic acid is consistent with biotinidase deficiency, holocarboxylase synthetase deficiency, methylmalonic aciduria, and PA, it is also considered a source of bacterial overgrowth. The possibility of extended specimen storage, lactic acidosis, or overgrowth in the small intestine should be considered. 3-Hydroxyisovalerate is commonly present is several disorders including isovaleric acidemia, multicarboxylase deficiency, and 3-methylcrotonyl-CoA carboxylase deficiency, but is also indicative of Reye and Reye-like syndromes, valproate treatment, and ketosis. Methylmalonic acid is present in noninborn errors of metabolism including vitamin B12 deficiency, bacterial gut metabolism, gastroenteritis of newborn infants, short bowel syndrome, and malnutrition. For additional sources of spurious organic acids, the reader is referred to Kumps et al.[45]

REFERENCES

1. Seashore MR. The Organic Acidemias: An Overview. In: Pagon RA, Adam MP, Ardinger HH, Wallace SE, Amemiya A, Bean LJ, Bird TD, Dolan CR, Fong C, Smith RJ, Stephens K, editors. *GeneReviews*. Seattle: University of Washington; 2009.
2. Sweetman L. *Organic acid analysis. Techniques in diagnostic human biochemical genetics. A laboratory manual.* New York: Wiley-Liss; 1991.

3. Shoemaker J, Elliot W. Automated screening of urine samples for carbohydrates, organic and amino acids after treatment with urcasc. *J Chromatography* 1991;**562**:125–38.

4. Lo SF, Young V, Rhead WJ. Identification of urine organic acids for the detection of inborn errors of metabolism using urease and gas chromatograph-mass spectrometry (GC-MS)Garg U.Hammett-Stabler CA, editors. *Clinical Applications of Mass Spectrometry, Methods in Molecular Biology*, **603**. New York: Humana Press; 2010. p. 433–43.

5. Fenton WA, Gravel RA, Rosenblatt DS. In: Valle D, Beaudet AL, Vogelstein B, Kinzler KW, Antonarakis SE, Ballabio A, Gibson K, Mitchell G, editors. *Disorders of Propionate and Methylmalonate Metabolism*. New York, NY: McGraw-Hill; 2014. http://ommbid.mhmedical.com/content.aspx?bookid=971&Sectionid=62677098. Accessed May 2016.

6. Standing Committee on the Scientific Evaluation of Dietary Reference Intakes. Dietary Reference Intakes for Thiamin, Riboflavin, Niacin, Vitamin B6, Folate, Vitamin B12, Pantothenic Acid, Biotin, and Choline. 1999;245–54.

7. Surtees RA, Matthews EE, Leonard JV. Neurologic outcome of propionic acidemia. *Pediatr Neurol* 1992;**8**(5):333–7.

8. Baumgartner MR, Horster F, Dionisi-Vici C, Haliloglu G, Karall D, Chapman KA, et al. Proposed guidelines for the diagnosis and management of methylmalonic and propionic acidemia. *Orphanet J Rare Diseases* 2014;**9**:130. http://www.ojrd/content/9/1/130.

9. Manoli I, Venditti CP. Methylmalonic Acidemia. In: GeneReviews at GeneTests: Medical Genetics Information Resource [database online]. Copyright, University of Washington, Seattle, 1993-2016. Available at http://www.genetest.org. Accessed May 2016.

10. Nicolaides P, Leonard J. Surtees. Neurological outcome of methylmalonic acidemia. *Arch Dis Child* 1998;**78**(6):508–12.

11. Millington DS, Kodo N, Norwood DL, Roe CR. Tandem mass spectrometry. A new method for acylcarnitine profiling with potential for neonatal screening for inborn errors of metabolism. *J Inherit Metab Dis* 1990;**13**:321.

12. Vockley J, Zschocke J, Knerr I, Vockley C, Michael Gibson KK.. In: Valle D, Beaudet AL, Vogelstein B, Kinzler KW, Antonarakis SE, Ballabio A, Gibson K, Mitchell G, editors. *Branched Chain Organic Acidurias*. New York, NY: McGraw-Hill; 2014. http://ommbid.mhmedical.com/content.aspx?bookid=971&Sectionid=62676787. Accessed May 2016.

13. Fischer AQ, Challa VR, Burton BK, McLean WT. Cerebellar hemorrhage complicating isovaleric acidemia A case report. *Neurology* 1981;**31**:746.

14. Mendiola J, Robotham JL, Liehr JG, Williams JC. Neonatal lethargy due to isovaleric acidemia and hyperammonemia. *Texas Med* 1984;**80**:52.

15. Wilson WG, Audenaert SM, Squillaro EJ. Hyperammonemia in a preterm infant with isovaleric acidemia. *J Inherit Metab Dis* 1984;**7**:71.

16. Kelleher JF, Yudkoff M, Hutchison R, August CS, Cohn RM. The pancytopenia of isovaleric acidemia. *Pediatrics* 1980;**65**:1023.

17. Cohn RM, Yudkoff M, Rothman R, Segal S. Isovaleric acidemia. Use of glycine therapy in neonates. *N Engl J Med* 1978;**299**:996.

18. Gerdes AM, Gregersen N, Ludvigsson P, Guttler F. A Scandinavian case of isovaleric acidemia. *J Inherit Metab Dis* 1988;**11**:218.

19. Goodman SI, Frerman FE. In: Valle D, Beaudet AL, Vogelstein B, Kinzler KW, Antonarakis SE, Ballabio A, Gibson K, Mitchell G, editors. *Organic Acidemias Due to Defects in Lysine Oxidation: 2-Ketoadipic Acidemia and Glutaric Acidemia*. New York,

NY: McGraw-Hill; 2014. http://ommbid.mhmedical.com/content.aspx?bookid=971&Sectionid=62677296. Accessed May 2016.

20. Zempleni J, Barshop BA, Cordonier EL, Baier SR, Gertsman I.. In: Valle D, Beaudet AL, Vogelstein B, Kinzler KW, Antonarakis SE, Ballabio A, Gibson K, Mitchell G, editors. *Disorders of Biotin Metabolism*. New York, NY: McGraw-Hill; 2014. http://ommbid.mhmedical.com/content.aspx?bookid=971&Sectionid=62646613. Accessed May 2016.

21. Roth KS, Rang W, Foremann JW, Rothman R, Segal S. Holocarboxylase synthetase deficiency: a biotin-responsive organic acidemia. *J Pediatr* 1980;**96**(5):845–9.

22. Wolf B. Biotinidase deficiency. In: GeneReviews at GeneTests: Medical Genetics Information Resource [database online]. Copyright, University of Washington, Seattle, 1993-2016. Available at http://www.genetest.org. Accessed August 2011.

23. Heard GS, Secor Mcvoy JR, Wolf B. A screening method for biotinidase deficiency in newborns. *Clin Chem* 1984;**30**:125–7.

24. Pettit DA, Amador PS, Wolf B. The quantitation of biotinidase activity in dried blood spots using microtiter transfer plates identification of biotinidase-deficient and heterozygous individuals. *Anal Biochem* 1989;**179**:371.

25. Sweetman L. Organic acid analysis. In: Hommes FA, editor. *Techniques in Diagnostic Human Biochemical Genetics: A Laboratory Manual*. New York: Wiley-Liss; 1991.

26. Greenberg CR, Reimer D, Singal R, Triggs-Raine B, Chudley AE, Dilling LA, et al. A G-to-T transversion at the + 5 position of intron 1 in the glutaryl-CoA dehydrogenase gene is associated with the Island Lake variant of glutaric acidemia type 1. *Hum Mol Genet* 1995;**4**:493.

27. Biery BJ, Stein DE, Morton DH, Goodman SI. Gene structure and mutations of glutaryl-coenzyme A dehydrogenase. Impaired association of enzyme subunits due to an A421V substitution causes glutaric acidemia (type I) in the Amish. *Am J Human Genet* 1996;**59**:1006.

28. Besrat A, Polan CE, Henderson LM. Mammalian metabolism of glutaric acid. *J Biol Chem* 1969;**244**:1461.

29. Hoffmann GF, Athanassopoulos S, Burlina AB, Duran M, de Klerk JBC, Lehnert W, et al. Clinical course, early diagnosis, treatment, and prevention of disease in glutaryl-CoA dehydrogenase deficiency. *Neuropediatrics* 1996;**27**:115.

30. Tsai MY, Johnson DD, Sweetman L, Berry SA. Two siblings with biotin-resistant 3-methylcrotonyl-coenzyme A carboxylase deficiency. *J Pediatr* 1989;**115**:110.

31. van Hove JLK, Rutledge SL, Nada MA, Kahler SG, Millington DS. 3-Hydroxyisovalerylcarnitine in 3-methylcrotonyl-CoA carboxylase deficiency. *J Inherit Metab Dis* 1995;**18**:592.

32. Stadler SC, Polanetz R, Maier EM, Heidenreich SC, Niederer B, Mayerhofer PU, et al. Newborn screening for 3-methylcrotonly-CoA carboxylase deficiency: population heterogeneity of MCCA and MCCB mutations and impact on risk assessment. *Hum Mutat* 2006;**27**:748.

33. Rolland MO, Divry P, Zabot MT, Guibaud P, Gomez S, Lachaux A, et al. Isolated 3-methylcrotonyl-CoA carboxylase deficiency in a 16-month-old child. *J Inherit Metab Dis* 1991;**14**:838.

34. Fukao, T. Beta-ketothiolase deficiency. Orphanet encyclopedia. http://www.orpha.net/consor/cgi-bin/OC_Exp.php?lng=EN&Expert=134. Accessed May 2016.

35. Gunay-Aygun M. 3-Methylglutaconic aciduria: A common biochemical marker in various syndromes with diverse clinical features. *Mol Gene Met* 2005;**84**:1–3.

36. Online Mendelian Inheritance in Man, OMIM®, McKusick-Nathans Institute of Genetic Medicine, Johns Hopkins University, Baltimore, MD. January 2012. World Wide Web URL: http://omim.org/.

37. Barth PG, Valianpour F, Bowen VM, Jam J, Duran M, Vaz FM, et al. X-linked Cardioskeletal myopathy and neutropenia (Barth Syndrome): an update. *Am. J Med. Genet.* 2004;**126A**:349–54.

38. Gunay-Aygun M, Gahl W, Anikster Y. *OPA3*-Related 3-Methglutaconic Aciduria Type 3. In: GeneReviews at GeneTests: Medical Genetics Information Resource [database online]. Copyright, University of Washington, Seattle, 1993–2016. Available at http://www.genetest.org. Accessed May 2016.

39. Matern D, He M, Berry SA, Rinaldo P, Whitley CB, Madsen PP, et al. Prospective diagnosis of 2-methylbutyryl-CoA dehydrogenase deficiency in the Hmong population by newborn screening using tandem mass spectrometry. *Pediatrics* 2003;**112**:74–8.

40. Ewbank C, Kerrigan JF, Aleck K. Fumarate Hydratase Deficiency. In: GeneReviews at GeneTests: Medical Genetics Information Resource [database online]. Copyright, University of Washington, Seattle, 1993–2016. Available at http://www.genetest.org. Accessed May 2016.

41. Salomons GS. Clinical, enzymatic and molecular characterization of nine new patients with malonyl-coenzyme A decarboxylase deficiency. *J Inherit Metab Dis* 2007;**30**:23–8.

42. Zammitt VA. The malonyl-CoA-long chain acyl-CoA axis in the maintenance of mammalian cell function. *Biochem J* 1999;**343**:505–15.

43. Footitt EJ, Stafford J, Dixon M, Burch M, Jakobs C, Salomons GS, Cleary MA. Use of a long-chain triglyceride-restricted/medium-chain triglyceride-supplemented diet in a case of malonyl-CoA decarboxylase deficiency with cardiomyopathy. [Epub] *J Inherit Metab Dis*. June 15, 2010 as http://dx.doi.org/10.1007/s10545-010-9137-z.

44. Matalon R, Michals-Matalon K. Canavan Disease. In: GeneReviews at GeneTests: Medical Genetics Information Resource [database online]. Copyright, University of Washington, Seattle, 1993–2016. Available at http://www.genetest.org. Accessed May 2016.

45. Kumps A, Duez P, Mardens Y. Metabolic, nutritional, iatrogenic and artefactual sources of urinary organic acids: a comprehensive table. *Clin Chem* 2002;**45**:708–17.

Disorders of mitochondrial fatty acid β-oxidation

4

P.M. Jones[1] and M.J. Bennett[2]

[1]*Children's Medical Center of Dallas and University of Texas Southwestern Medical Center, Dallas, TX, United States;* [2]*The Children's Hospital of Philadelphia and University of Pennsylvania Perelman School of Medicine, Philadelphia, PA, United States*

4.1 INTRODUCTION

Mitochondrial fatty acid β-oxidation (FAO) is a four-step cyclical pathway, which occurs in the mitochondria and results in the production of reducing equivalents that are then used to produce adenosine triphosphate (ATP) by the process known as oxidative phosphorylation. Each cycle through the pathway also results in the production of acetyl-CoA and a fatty acid with a carbon chain, which is two carbons shorter than at the start of the cycle. FAO is a primary means of producing energy for the body in those tissues that specifically need the amount of energy supplied by oxidative phosphorylation rather than glycolysis, such as cardiac and skeletal muscle. FAO is also critically important during times when there is an increased need for energy and during times when glucose is low or unavailable for use. Glycolysis is considered to produce roughly 38 mol of ATP from a mole of glucose. FAO will produce an equivalent of 129 mol of ATP from a mole of palmitate.[1] Thus disorders that affect the function of the FAO pathway are regarded as disorders of fasting intolerance or increased energy demand, which may disrupt the energy source for many tissues in the body, as well as disrupting the body's ability to produce energy when glucose is in short supply. FAO is also required for the generation of ketone bodies (acetoacetate and 3-hydroxybutyrate) by the liver as a source of energy for tissues that cannot directly oxidize fatty acids such as brain.

Generally also included in chapters on FAO disorders are the defects that occur in the transport system that moves fatty acids into the mitochondria, the carnitine transport system or carnitine shuttle, because of the intricate connection between the carnitine shuttle and mitochondrial FAO. This chapter will be divided into two main sections, one covering the disorders of the carnitine transport system and one covering the disorders of FAO. Descriptions of disorder presentation and treatment in this chapter are intended to touch on high points rather than being all-inclusive. References containing in-depth descriptions of the disorders of the carnitine shuttle and FAO are available.[2–4]

Biomarkers in Inborn Errors of Metabolism. DOI: http://dx.doi.org/10.1016/B978-0-12-802896-4.00005-5

4.2 DISORDERS OF CARNITINE TRANSPORT

FAO occurs inside the mitochondria where the generated reducing equivalents are readily available to the respiratory chain for oxidative phosphorylation. While short- and medium-chain fatty acids, C4 to C12, appear to be capable of crossing into the mitochondria without the involvement of carnitine, long-chain fatty acids (LCFA; primarily C16 and C18), which provide the great majority of fatty acid substrates, must be transported across the mitochondrial membranes via the carnitine shuttle system (Fig. 4.1). Disorders in this system are presented in the following sections.

4.2.1 CARNITINE TRANSPORTER DEFECT

The carnitine transporter defect is also known as carnitine uptake defect and as primary carnitine deficiency. This disorder is caused by a defect in the energy-dependent carnitine transporter protein in the plasma membrane (see Fig. 4.1). The defect results in low plasma and tissue levels of carnitine, which impairs the carnitine shuttle and subsequent transport of LCFA into the mitochondria for oxidation. The disorder is also associated with massive renal loss of carnitine. The primary defect thus impairs FAO secondarily to a lack of carnitine. The gene associated with this disorder is *SLC22A5*, and the disorder is inherited in an autosomal recessive fashion.[5]

If not identified on newborn screening (NBS), this disorder presents clinically most often in the first year of life with progressive hypotonia, cardiomyopathy, and

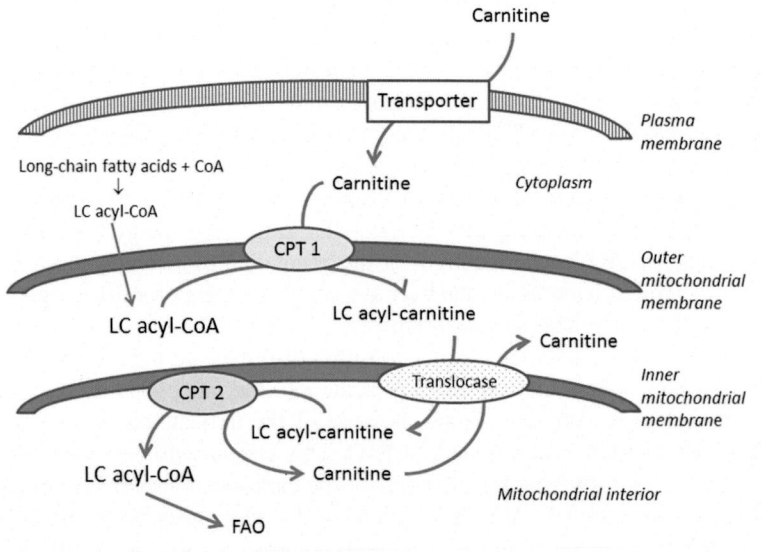

FIGURE 4.1

The carnitine transport system.

muscle weakness. Very rarely it may present as acute liver failure along with hypoketotic hypoglycemia often leading to coma and death. If undiagnosed, most children die in the first few years of life from cardiac failure.[6]

Treatment for this disorder involves carnitine supplementation. Although many FAO disorders are treated with carnitine supplementation, the carnitine transporter defect is the only defect that has been demonstrated to conclusively benefit from this treatment. Infants diagnosed quickly and receiving carnitine may be asymptomatic throughout their lives. Symptomatic infants and children started on carnitine supplementation often see reversal of early effects, although some neurological damage may remain if hypoglycemia was prolonged. Prognosis is excellent when treatment is started early.

This disorder is detected by NBS programs that monitor free carnitine, as the free carnitine levels are very low.[7] The hallmark biomarkers of carnitine transporter defect are low free and total carnitine levels, often accompanied by overall low acylcarnitines (see Table 4.1). Patients with this disorder are routinely monitored by measuring free and total carnitine at intervals. Definitive diagnosis is generally accomplished by genetic testing.[6]

4.2.2 CARNITINE PALMITOYLTRANSFERASE 1 DEFICIENCY

Carnitine palmitoyltransferase 1 (CPT1) is the enzyme in the outer mitochondrial membrane that converts long-chain acyl-CoA species to their corresponding long-chain acyl-carnitines for transport into the mitochondria (see Fig. 4.1). The enzyme is known to exist in three different isoforms: CPT1A is expressed in liver and kidney, CPT1B in cardiac and skeletal muscle, and CPT1C in the brain. To date, only defects in CPT1A have been clinically defined.[8] CPT1A deficiency is caused by a defect in the *CPT1A* gene resulting in the inability of the enzyme to transfer LCFA from their CoA species to acylcarnitines, resulting in increased amounts of free carnitine, low LC-acylcarnitines, and often low generalized acylcarnitines, in particular acetylcarnitine.

CPT1A deficiency presents clinically as fasting intolerance, with lethargy and a Reye-like picture of hepatic failure associated with hypoglycemia and failure of ketone production. Presentation is usually precipitated by conditions that require fatty acids for energy, such as prolonged fasting, starvation, or gastrointestinal illnesses that result in insufficient caloric intake or caloric losses. Although CPT1A deficiency is a disorder of LCFA metabolism, CPT1A is expressed primarily in liver and kidney, thus there are no skeletal muscle symptoms and cardiac muscle symptoms are rare with this disorder, unlike most LCFA disorders. Patients may present with renal tubular acidosis in addition to the hepatic disease.

Treatment for this disorder, as with all FAO disorders involves preventing flux through the FAO pathway as much as possible by preventing fasting and supplying carbohydrate support when necessary. Although cases that have been precipitated by a metabolic decompensation may have liver damage and the severe hypoglycemia may

Table 4.1 Biomarkers for FAO Disorders

Disorder	Primary Acylcarnitine Biomarkers	Other Acylcarnitine Abnormalities	Primary Organic Acid Biomarkers	Other Biomarkers
Carnitine uptake defect	↓ C0; very low free carnitine	↓ Total carnitine	NA	↓ Glucose and ketones (fasting); ↑ CK
Carnitine/acylcarnitine translocase	↑ C16; ↑ C18; ↑ C18:1	↑ C18:2; ↑ C14; ↓ Carnitine	NA	↑ NH₄; ↑ transaminases; ↓ Glucose, ketones (fasting)
Carnitine palmitoyltransferase 1	↑ C0; ↓ C16; ↓ C18; ↑ C0/(C16 + C18)	↓ Overall acylcarnitines	NA	↓ Glucose, ketones (fasting) ↑ NH₄
Carnitine palmitoyltransferase 2	↑ C16; ↑ C18; ↑ C18:1	↑ C16:1; ↑ C18:2; ↑ C14:1; ↑ C14	NA	↑↑ CK; ↑ myoglobin in urine
Very long-chain acyl-CoA dehydrogenase	↑ C14:1; ↑ C14:2	↑ C14; ↑ C16; ↑ C18:1, ↑ C18:2	NA	↑ NH₄, ↑↑ CK, ↑ myoglobin in urine ↓ Glucose and ketones (fasting)
Medium-chain acyl-CoA dehydrogenase	↑ C8; ↑ C10:1; ↑ C10	↑ C6	Hexanoylglycine, suberylglycine Dicarboxylic acids	
Short-chain acyl-CoA dehydrogenase	↑ C4		Ethylmalonic acid, methylsuccinic acid, butyrylglycine	
Long-chain L-3-hydroxyacyl-CoA dehydrogenase/mitochondrial trifunctional protein	↑ C16-OH; ↑ C18-OH; ↑ C18:1-OH		C10 to C14 3-hydroxy-dicarboxylic acids	↑ Long-chain serum 3-OH-fatty acids; ↑ NH₄
Medium/short-chain L-3-hydroxyacyl-CoA dehydrogenase	↑ C4-OH		3-OH-glutarate	↑ Medium/short-chain serum 3-OH-fatty acids serum; ↑ insulin
Multiple acyl-CoA dehydrogenase	↑ C5; ↑ C5-DC; ↑ C8; ↑ C14:1	↑ C4-C8	Glutaric acid, ethylmalonic acid, many acylglycines (isovaleryl, hexanoyl, suberyl, isobutyryl, butyrl, 2-methylbutyryl); dicarboxylic acids	↓ Glucose and ketones (fasting)

result in neurological damage, if diagnosed early and managed appropriately, patients with CPT1A deficiency have good outcomes and can be mostly symptom-free.[9]

This disorder is detected on NBS, with a high free carnitine, low long-chain acyl-carnitines (C16 and C18) and an increased ratio of free to long-chain species. These are the hallmark biomarkers of CPT1 (see Table 4.1). No other FAO disorders show elevated total carnitine concentrations. Definitive diagnosis can be accomplished by enzyme analysis. In general, molecular/genetic diagnosis is difficult because no single mutation is predominant and functional testing may be required to establish pathogenicity.[6]

4.2.3 CARNITINE/ACYLCARNITINE TRANSLOCASE DEFECT

Carnitine/acylcarnitine translocase deficiency (CACT) is caused by a defect in the translocase protein in the inner mitochondrial membrane (see Fig. 4.1) that transports longchain acyl-carnitine into the mitochondrial matrix in exchange for transporting free carnitine out of the mitochondria. Defects in this translocase result in a failure to get LCFAs into the mitochondria for oxidation. The disorder is inherited in an autosomal recessive manner and the gene associated with this disorder is the *SLC25A20* or *CACT* gene.

CACT is a transporter protein that is expressed in all tissues, thus CACT defects classically present with multisystem involvement, including those tissues that are most dependent on fatty acid oxidation for energy such as cardiac and skeletal muscle. Liver involvement is usually also key to the presentation and patients may show a Reye-like illness of hepatic encephalopathy that is usually fasting-induced. Liver biopsy demonstrates steatosis in this and all other FAO disorders. Fasting-induced hypoglycemia and low ketones and persistently elevated ammonia are also present. Cardiomyopathy is often seen, with ventricular tachycardia being present. Milder forms of CACT deficiency have also been described, with more modest liver disease and muscle weakness.[8]

Treatment for CACT deficiency involves attempting to prevent fluxes through the carnitine transport and FAO pathways, especially in times of fasting, febrile illness or gastrointestinal (GI) caloric loss. Calories are provided as carbohydrates to prevent stress on the system, which cannot break down LCFA for energy. Prognosis is generally poor for severe CACT deficiency, as high ammonia levels are difficult to control.

This disorder may be detected on NBS, but cannot be differentiated from carnitine palmitoyltransferase 2 (CPT2) deficiency, as both disorders show accumulation of the same long-chain acylcarnitine species, C14, C16, C18:1, and C18:2 carnitines (see Table 4.1). There is no single good hallmark biomarker of CACT deficiency. Following up a positive NBS result in cases of CACT deficiency by assaying acyl-carnitines will usually show the same pattern as seen on the NBS. Differentiating between CACT and CPT2 deficiency and making the laboratory diagnosis requires functional assays for both proteins or sequencing of the genes for both proteins.[6]

4.2.4 CARNITINE PALMITOYLTRANSFERASE 2 DEFICIENCY

CPT2 deficiency is caused by defects in the *CPT2* gene. CPT2 is a membrane-bound protein in the inner mitochondrial membrane, which converts acylcarnitines back to acyl-CoAs within the mitochondrial matrix, making them accessible for FAO. It is an enzyme that it ubiquitous and expressed in all cell types. Defects in CPT2 result in decreased conversion of long-chain acylcarnitines to acyl-CoAs, the required substrates for fatty acid oxidation (Fig. 4.1).

CPT2 deficiency has a variety of presentations that include three basic phenotypes. Presentations in the newborn period are often fatal and include acute multiorgan failure, especially cardiac and liver failure. Developmental abnormalities, including cystic lesions in the brain and kidneys are often present. Later onset infantile CPT2 deficiency generally presents with multiorgan failure, which is induced by fasting. Hypertrophic cardiomyopthy, skeletal myopathy, and hepatic encephalopathy are common findings but this form of CPT2 deficiency lacks developmental abnormalities. The late childhood or adult-onset CPT2 deficiency is myopathic only and often presents as exercise-induced myopathy, exercise intolerance, or rhabdomyolysis. Cardiac and liver symptoms are generally not seen in this form of CPT2 deficiency but rhabdomyolysis may cause renal failure due to excess myoglobin release from muscle.

Treatment for this disorder depends on the phenotype. For the severe newborn form, prognosis is generally very poor. For the intermediate form, treatment involves management to avoid metabolic decompensation due to increased caloric demands. This management seems to be helpful for some patients with CPT2 deficiency while other patients have frequent metabolic decompensations with multiorgan involvement. Prognosis seems to be almost patient-specific; however, for both types of patients, progressive cardiac disease often occurs, along with skeletal myopathy and a propensity for hepatic disease.[10] Treatment for the late-onset form is to avoid excessive exercise, and depending on circumstances, may also include intravenous (IV) fluids with high carbohydrate concentrations or dietary supplementation with medium-chain triglycerides (MCTs) to provide energy from fatty acids while bypassing the metabolic block. The prognosis in late-onset patients is good.

As described previously for CACT deficiency, this disorder is identified on NBS with elevated concentrations of C16, C18:1, and C18:2-carnitines. These are the hallmark biomarkers of CPT2 deficiency, just as they are of CACT deficiency (Table 4.1). However, this pattern of elevations may be masked by elevations in other long-chain-acylcarnitine species in very ill infants, especially in the severe forms of CPT2 deficiency. In addition, the later onset forms may not be identified on NBS, or may show an initial positive screen, followed by a negative second screen if the infant is feeding well. Thus an initial positive screen should be followed up by enzyme analysis or gene sequencing, even if the follow-up acylcarnitine profile is normal. Diagnosis and differentiating between CPT2 and CACT deficiencies requires either enzyme analysis or gene sequencing.[6]

4.3 DISORDERS OF FATTY ACID OXIDATION

FAO is a four-step cyclical pathway that shortens LCFAs predominantly by two carbons for every cycle, and produces acetyl-CoA and reducing equivalents for oxidative phosphorylation. The basic pathway is shown in Fig. 4.2. Each enzymatic step in
the cycle is accomplished by enzymes with different chain-length specificities. The
cycle is started by acyl-CoA dehydrogenases that act on straight-chain, saturated
fatty acids to remove two hydrogens, and create a double bond between carbons 2
and 3. The hydrogens as reducing equivalents are transferred to the electron transfer
chain at the level of coenzyme Q by the action of electron transfer flavoprotein and
electron transfer flavoprotein dehydrogenase. The second enzymatic step for FAO
involves enoyl-CoA hydratases, which add a water molecule across the double bond,
creating an L-hydroxyl group on carbon 3. The third enzymatic step involves the L-3
hydroxyacyl-CoA dehydrogenases, which remove two additional hydrogens, resulting in a keto-group on carbon 3 and the conversion of NAD (nicotinamide adenine
dinucleotide) to NADH (nicotinamide adenine dinucleotide + hydrogen) and electron transfer at complex 1 of the respiratory chain. The final enzymatic step involves
3-keto acyl-CoA thiolases that cleave across the 2,3 position, forming acetyl-CoA
and an acyl-CoA, which is two carbons shorter and which is recycled through the

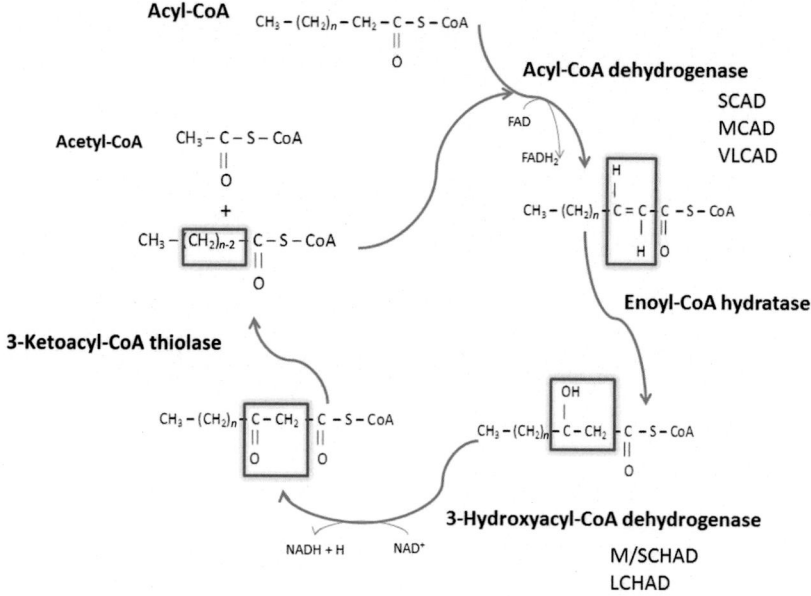

FIGURE 4.2

Fatty acid β-oxidation.

FAO pathway. The acetyl-CoA can be utilized directly in the tricarboxylic acid (TCA) cycle as an energy source.

Although FAO has chain-length specific enzymes, there is some overlap in the enzyme specificity for the various chain lengths, at least when measured *in vitro*. Basically, short- and medium-chain acyl-CoAs of 4–12 carbons in length are metabolized by short- and medium-chain enzymes, which are found in the mitochondrial matrix. Long-chain acyl-CoAs are metabolized by enzymes that are bound to the inner mitochondrial membrane. The last three of the four long-chain enzymes are organized into an octomeric multienzyme complex called the mitochondrial trifunctional protein (MTP), which contains four alpha subunits containing hydratase and long-chain 3-hydroxyacyl-CoA dehydrogenase (LCHAD) activity and four beta subunits containing the ketothiolase activity. Fig. 4.3 shows the enzyme organization in the mitochondria.

Short- and medium-chain fatty acids enter the mitochondria independently of the carnitine cycle, a mechanism that may explain the benefits of MCTs as energy sources in infants failing to thrive.

Disorders of this pathway are described as follows.

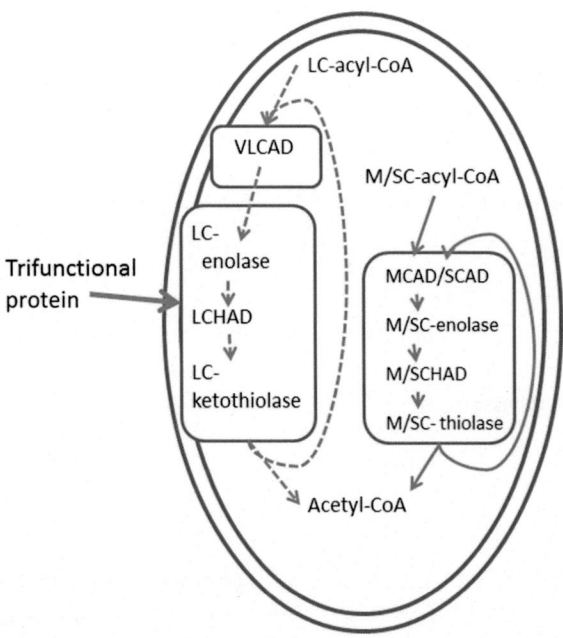

FIGURE 4.3

Mitochondrial fatty acid β-oxidation showing location of matrix medium/short-chain enzymes and membrane-bound long-chain enzymes.

4.4 VERY LONG-CHAIN ACYL-CoA DEHYDROGENASE DEFICIENCY

Very long-chain acyl-CoA dehydrogenase (VLCAD) is the enzyme involved in the first step of FAO, utilizing fatty acids with 14–18 carbons. It is in physical proximity to CPT2. VLCAD deficiency is caused by mutations in the *ACADVL* gene. More than 150 different mutations have been found across all 20 of the gene's exons. The only single prevalent mutation that has been identified is the S113L mutation, which results in late-onset myopathic disease. LCFAs that have been transported into the mitochondrial matrix and converted to the respective long-chain acyl-CoAs via the carnitine shuttle are the substrates for this enzyme (Figs. 4.2 and 4.3). When the enzyme is deficient, long-chain acyl-CoAs cannot be oxidized resulting in a lack of energy from the major source in tissues such as cardiac and skeletal muscle. There is also an accumulation of long-chain metabolic intermediates such as the CoA esters and acylcarnitines which maybe toxic. In particular, long-chain acylcarnitines may have an arrhythmic effect on cardiac muscle.[11]

VLCAD deficiency presents clinically very much like CPT2 deficiency, with three distinct phenotypes, a severe neonatal presentation without developmental abnormalities, a milder multisystemic presentation in childhood and an adult-onset cardiac and skeletal myopathic presentation.[12] In the most severe form of VLCAD deficiency, cardiomyopathy and hepatomegaly are the most common findings and this type of presentation is often fatal. Presentation later in childhood is less frequently fatal and may depend on the degree of caloric restriction catabolism. All forms of VLCAD deficiency demonstrate similar metabolic decompensation with hypoketotic hypoglycemia and liver failure demonstrating raised levels of transaminases, hyperammonemia, and reduced clotting factors. The childhood-onset form may show progressive cardiomyopathy and/or muscle symptoms such as rhabdomyolysis with markedly elevated creatine kinase (CK) levels. Late-onset VLCAD deficiency presents as muscle pain and rhabdomyolysis with elevated plasma CK and myoglobinuria, which may be significant enough to lead to acute renal damage.

Treatment for this disorder involves reducing LCFAs in the diet and supplementing energy requirements by adding medium-chain fatty acids in the form of MCTs that work by by-passing the metabolic block. Preventing fasting, and thus fatty acid breakdown is also important, especially in severe VLCAD deficiency, in which even a mild hypoglycemia may cause a significant metabolic decompensation. Metabolic decompensations that do occur are generally treated with IV glucose. In the adult-onset and more myopathic forms of VLCAD deficiency, avoiding exercise extremes that can cause decompensation is a major treatment. Prognosis is very good for the milder forms of this deficiency, and if diagnosed promptly and treated aggressively, the severe neonatal form can be controlled as well with a relatively good prognosis.

VLCAD deficiency is identified on NBS, with the hallmark biomarker being an elevated C14:1-carnitine, usually accompanied by an elevated C14:2-carnitine (Table 4.1). Other long-chain acylcarnitine species may be also present, as there may be considerable overlap especially between the elevated long-chain species for VLCAD, CPT2, and CACT deficiencies. In addition, the acylcarnitine profile may be normal when the patient is well and metabolically stable. In the later childhood and adult-onset cases of VLCAD deficiency, measuring CK and urine myoglobin may be helpful for monitoring the disease.[4,6]

4.5 MEDIUM-CHAIN ACYL-CoA DEHYDROGENASE DEFICIENCY

Medium-chain acyl-CoA dehydrogenase (MCAD) deficiency is caused by a defect in the *ACADM* gene. Homozygosity for a common mutation that causes an amino acid substitution (K304E) accounts for most of the disease seen, especially in the northern European population. MCAD deficiency is the most common FAO disorder and results in the inability to oxidize and utilize acyl-CoAs with chain lengths of 8–12 carbons (Fig. 4.3).

Before this disorder was added to NBS programs, presentation was similar to that seen with CPT1A deficiency: fasting from any cause resulted in hypoketotic hypoglycemia with hepatic failure and hepatic encephalopathy. Coma and death occurred very quickly in some cases, often leading to a misdiagnosis of Sudden Infant Death Syndrome. With NBS, MCAD deficiency is usually diagnosed before adverse events occur, treatment is begun early, and acute metabolic decompensations are rare. There remain a few cases of infants who present clinically in the perinatal period before results of a NBS are available. Often, these are tragic cases in which the newborn is being exclusively breast-fed but the mother is unable to provide sufficient milk to prevent a fasting crisis.[13]

Treatment for this disorder involves prevention of fasting. With the above proviso, MCAD deficiency is the ideal NBS success disorder. Before NBS and without diagnosis, patients with MCAD deficiency frequently died suddenly upon fasting. Since NBS, and proper prevention of fasting, there are few sequelae to the disorder whatsoever and patients lead a normal life. Upon diagnosis in the newborn, treatment involves routine feeding, including through the night. Prognosis is exceptionally good[14] with improvement of fasting tolerance over time.

This disorder is included on NBS and was the disorder that initiated the move toward expanding NBS programs to include FAO disorders. The hallmark biomarkers of MCAD deficiency include elevated C6-, C8-, C10-, and C10:1-carnitines (Table 4.1). A urine organic acid analysis will show hexanoylglycine and suberylglycine, along with dicarboxylic acids when the patient is metabolically decompensated or fasting; however, when well and fed, these biomarkers may not be readily detectable. Prior to the introduction of NBS using tandem mass spectrometry (MS) for acylcarnitine analysis, diagnosis of MCAD deficiency was often missed if the patient was treated with glucose and no longer fasted before collecting the urine for analysis of organic acids and acylglycines. In addition, MCTs in the diet result in the excretion of C6–C10 dicarboxylic acids in the urine, which may confound the diagnosis in a urine organic acid analysis. The pattern of excretion, however, is distinct with MCT supplementation versus MCAD deficiency. In MCT supplementation the pattern will show increasing concentrations from C6 to C10, or may show C6 excretion, lesser C8 excretion, and greater C10 excretion. C10 excretion is almost always in the greatest concentration. In contrast, with disorders of FAO, the pattern is reversed, with C6 always excreted in the highest concentration, followed by decreasing amounts of C8 and C10.

4.6 SHORT-CHAIN ACYL-CoA DEHYDROGENASE DEFICIENCY

Short-chain acyl-CoA dehydrogenase (SCAD) is the enzyme that catalyzes the first step of FAO utilizing acyl-CoAs with 4–6 carbons. SCAD deficiency is poorly understood due to the high prevalence of polymorphic sequence variations in the *ACADS* gene that are found in patients who have biomarkers of the disorder. In addition, many individuals with defects, either polymorphisms or distinct variants in *ACADS*, have no symptoms and appear to do well with no therapeutic interventions. Thus, it may be that factors other than or along with genetic mutations are necessary for the disorder to present itself.[15]

This disorder may or may not be included in NBS programs. Owing to the increasing number of asymptomatic individuals found with an elevated butyrylcarnitine upon NBS, SCAD deficiency is considered by many investigators to be a benign condition. The hallmark biomarker of SCAD deficiency is an elevated butyrylcarnitine on acylcarnitine profiling. Urine organic acids often demonstrate an elevated excretion of ethylmalonic acid and methylsuccinate and may also include butyrylglycine (see Table 4.1).

4.7 LONG-CHAIN L-3-HYDROXYACYL-CoA DEHYDROGENASE AND MITOCHONDRIAL TRIFUNCTIONAL PROTEIN DEFICIENCIES

The MTP is a multienzyme complex on the inner mitochondrial membrane that is made up of the last three long-chain enzymes of the FAO pathway (Fig. 4.3). LCHAD is one of those three enzymes and thus LCHAD deficiency is a form of MTP deficiency. LCHAD deficiency involves mutations that only affect the LCHAD enzyme on the alpha subunit while MTP deficiency results from alpha- and beta-chain mutations that affect all three enzymes. LCHAD deficiency has a common mutation occurring at G1528C that occurs as homozygous alleles in 65% of LCHAD deficient individuals, and heterozygously in the remaining 35%.

Individuals with these disorders present with heterogeneous phenotypes, with symptoms ranging from feeding difficulty and poor growth and poor weight gain, to hepatic failure and a Reye-like picture, to cardiac arrest and sudden death. Unique among FAO disorders, patients with LCHAD deficiency have chronic progressive liver disease, peripheral neuropathies, and degenerative and progressive opthalm-alogical abnormalities leading to blindness.[16] In addition, LCHAD deficiency has been associated with maternal liver disease when the mother is carrying an affected fetus, including acute fatty liver of pregnancy (AFLP) and the HELLP (hemoly-sis, elevated liver enzymes, low platelet) syndrome.[17,18] MTP deficiency, like other long-chain FAO disorders, has three main phenotypic presentations, a severe neona-tal multisystemic disease, a milder fasting-induced childhood presentation and an essentially myopathic later onset form. MTP deficiency most commonly presents with muscle symptoms, usually exercise-induced, after childhood. Severely present-ing MTP though is associated with sudden death, often cardiac, and may be indistin-guishable from LCHAD deficiency.

Treatment for this disorder involves avoidance of fasting, decreasing LCFAs in the diet, and the dietary supplementation of medium-chain fatty acids in the form of MCTs in order to provide energy from fatty acids for high-energy requiring tissues thus bypassing the long-chain block of oxidation. In addition, MCT supplementation seems to decrease the accumulation of long-chain 3-hydroxy-metabolites, which are believed to be toxic and responsible for the clinical symptoms. Prognosis with this disorder is not very good, with a high mortality in severe presentations, and signifi-cant morbidity, even when milder presentations are aggressively treated.

LCHAD deficiency can be detected by NBS. The hallmark biomarkers of LCHAD deficiency are elevated concentrations of C16-OH-, C18-OH-, and C18:1-OH-acylcarnitines (Table 4.1). Like other long-chain disorders, the acylcarnitine profile in these patients may be normal when the individual is metabolically stable. Other biomarkers that may be useful include measuring 3-OH-fatty acids in serum as these long-chain (C14 to C18) species are always elevated in LCHAD deficiency.[19]

4.8 MEDIUM/SHORT-CHAIN L-3-HYDROXY-ACYL-CoA DEHYDROGENASE

Medium/short-chain L-3-hydroxy-acyl-CoA dehydrogenase (M/SCHAD) deficiency is also known as SCHAD deficiency. The defect affects the mitochondrial matrix L-3 hydroxy acyl-CoA dehydrogenase, which has a broad chain-length specificity for short- and medium-chain-length fatty acids from 4 to 14 carbons. M/SCHAD deficiency is caused by a defect in the gene variously called SCHAD, HADH, or HAD1, and the defect results in the inability to adequately oxidize medium- and short-chain fatty acids (Fig. 4.3).

This disorder is a rare disorder of FAO, with only about 14 cases reported. The clinical presentation is variable and not clearly defined due to the few cases. The disorder has been shown to result in Sudden Infant Death Syndrome,[20] and has also been demonstrated to be a rare cause of congenital hyperinsulinism.[21] It may also present with fulminant liver failure, or with hypotonia, hypoglycemia, and hepatic steatosis. Skeletal and cardiac muscle abnormalities have not been associated with SCHAD deficiency.

Treatment for this disorder involves prevention of fasting, and, if associated with hyperinsulinism, treatment with diazoxide, appears to be effective in preventing hyperinsulinism and hypoglycemia. If these episodes can be controlled, prognosis is good.

SCHAD deficiency is considered a secondary target of the NBS panel. It is not diagnosed as a primary target but should be picked up in the follow-up testing for disorders that are detected on NBS. The main biochemical abnormality, and possibly the only biochemical abnormality, is an elevated C4-OH-carnitine (Table 4.1). Urine organic acid analysis may or may not show elevated 3-hydroxyglutarate. Short- and medium-chain serum 3-hydroxy-fatty acids are elevated, but these findings are also seen with ketosis and in individuals with MCTs in their diet. Hyperinsulinism is seen in those patients with *HADH1* mutations that result in no or reduced amounts of protein. Western blot analysis is an important diagnostic requirement to predict those patients who might be responsive to diazoxide therapy.

4.9 MULTIPLE ACYL-CoA DEHYDROGENASE DEFICIENCY

Multiple acyl-CoA dehydrogenase deficiency (MADD) is also known as glutaric acidemia, type 2 (GA2). This disorder is caused by a defect or defects in the mitochondrial matrix protein ETF (electron-transferring flavoprotein) or the mitochondrial membrane protein ETF-QO (electron transfer flavoprotein-ubiquinone oxidoreductase; ETF dehydrogenase) of the electron transport system of the oxidative phosphorylation pathway. ETF transfers electrons from reducing equivalents produced by multiple pathways to ETF-QO, which then transfers them into the electron transport chain. Defects in the system affect a multitude of dehydrogenase enzymes, including the three major acyl-CoA dehydrogenases. Three genes are responsible for MADD, the genes for the alpha and beta subunits of ETF and the gene for ETF-QO. Truncation or null mutations in any of these genes can result in severe phenotypes, while missense mutations tend to occur in the milder forms of the disorder.[22]

MADD shows three different clinical presentations. Type 1 is severe and often fatal and presents in the neonatal period with multisystem failure, often accompanied by polycystic alterations in the brain and kidneys, a similar phenotype to that seen in neonatal CPT2 deficiency. Type 2 is also an infantile presentation, lacking developmental abnormalities but with severe metabolic decompensations and multisystem failure, including liver failure, cardiac and skeletal myopathies, and renal tubular acidosis. Both infantile forms also present with an unusual odor identical to that of isovaleric acidemia, arising from the functional defect in isovaleryl-CoA dehydrogenase. The third type of MADD is a later onset form, which demonstrates a milder phenotype most often precipitated by catabolic stress. Progressive cardiomyopathy and mild skeletal myopathy usually occur, as does hepatic encephalopathy.

Because of the multiple dehydrogenases and pathways affected by this disorder there is no good treatment. Individuals with type 1 MADD, in general, do not survive the neonatal period and type 2 individuals also do very poorly. ETF and ETF-QO are flavoproteins, thus type 3 and surviving type 2 are often treated with high-dose riboflavin, even though outcomes are rarely shown to be improved.

MADD may be picked up on NBS, although unfortunately for the severe forms, the presentation often pre-dates the screening results. The acylcarnitine profile will show elevations of intermediates of several pathways including isovaleryl- (C5), glutaryl- (C5-DC), C8- and C14:1-carnitines (Table 4.1). Urine organic acid analysis will show multiple acylglycines, although a quantitative urine acylglycine analysis may be necessary to detect low levels that may not be apparent on a normal organic acid analysis. A combination of enzyme analysis and genetic analysis is required for definitive diagnosis. No common mutations are found, with most mutations being private, necessitating a need for sequencing of all three genes. Riboflavin deficiency may demonstrate the same acylcarnitine pattern of abnormalities as MADD, confounding the diagnosis. However, riboflavin deficiency is easily treated with oral riboflavin, resulting in the resolution of abnormal biochemical and clinical findings.

REFERENCES

1. Baynes JW. Oxidative metabolism of lipids in liver and muscle. In: Baynes JW, Dominiczak MH, editors. *Medical biochemistry* 3rd ed. Philadelphia: Mosby/Elsevier; 2009. p. 185–93. Chapter 15.
2. Rinaldo P, Matern D, Bennett MJ. Fatty acid oxidation disorders. *Annu Rev Physiol* 2002;**64**:477–502.
3. Strauss AW, Andresen BS, Bennett MJ. Mitochondrial fatty acid oxidation defects. In: Sarafoglou K, Hoffmann GF, Roth KS, editors. *Pediatric endocrinology and inborn errors of metabolism*. New York: McGraw Hill; 2009. p. 51–70.
4. Vockley J, Bennett MJ, Gillingham MB. Mitochondrial fatty acid oxidation disorders. In: Valle D, Beaudet AL, Vogelstein B, Kinzler KW, Antonarakis SE, Ballabio A, Gibson KM, Mitchell G, editors. *Scriver's online metabolic & molecular bases of inherited disease*. McGraw Hill; April 2016. http://www.ommbid.com [accessed 10.05.16].
5. Stanley CA, Bennett MJ, Longo N. Plasma membrane carnitine transporter defect. In: Valle D, Beaudet AL, Vogelstein B, Kinzler KW, Antonarakis SE, Ballabio A, editors. *Scriver's online metabolic & molecular bases of inherited disease*. McGraw Hill; November 2011. http://www.ommbid.com [accessed 10.02.16].
6. Jones PM, Bennett MJ. Disorders of the carnitine cycle and mitochondrial fatty acid oxidation. In: Garg U, Smith L, Heese B, editors. *Laboratory diagnosis of inherited metabolic diseases*. Washington DC: AACC Press; 2012. p. 65–91. Chapter 5.
7. Schimmenti LA, Crombez EA, Schwahn BC, et al. Expanded newborn screening identifies maternal primary carnitine deficiency. *Mol Genet Metab* 2007;**90**:441–5.
8. Stanley CA, Palmieri F, Bennett MJ. Disorders of the mitochondrial carnitine shuttle. In: Valle D, Beaudet AL, Vogelstein B, Kinzler KW, Antonarakis SE, Ballabio A, editors. *Scriver's online metabolic & molecular bases of inherited disease*. McGraw Hill; November 2011. http://www.ommbid.com [accessed 10.02.16].
9. Bennett MJ, Narayan SB, Santani A. Carnitine palmitoyltransferase 1A deficiency (Updated March 7, 2013) in: GeneReviews at GeneTests: Medical Genetics Information Resource [database online]. Copyright, University of Washington, Seattle, 1993–2016. Available at http://www.genetests.org. [accessed 11.02.16].

10. Weiser T. Carnitine palmitoyltransferase II deficiency (Updated May 15, 2014) in: GeneReviews at GeneTests: Medical Genetics Information Resource [database online]. Copyright, University of Washington, Seattle, 1993–2016. Available at http://www.genetests.org. [accessed 11.02.16].

11. Bonnet D, Martin D, de Lonlay P, Villain E, Jouvet P, Rabier D, et al. Arrhythmias and conduction defects as presenting symptoms of fatty acid oxidation disorders in children. *Circulation* 1999;**100**:2248–53.

12. Leslie ND, Valencia CA, Strauss AW, Connor J, Zhang K. Very long-chain acyl-Coenzyme A dehydrogenase deficiency. (Updated Sept 11, 2014) in: GeneReviews at GeneTests: Medical Genetics Information Resource [database online]. Copyright, University of Washington, Seattle, 1993–2016. Available at http://www.genetests.org. [accessed 11.02.16].

13. Soler-Alfonso C, Bennett MJ, Ficicioglu C. Screening for medium-chain acyl CoA dehydrogenase deficiency: current perspectives. *Res Rep Neonatol* 2015;**5**:1–10.

14. Matern D, Rinaldo P. Medium-chain acyl-Coenzyme A dehydrogenase deficiency. (Updated March 5, 2015) in: GeneReviews at GeneTests: Medical Genetics Information Resource [database online]. Copyright, University of Washington, Seattle, 1993–2016. Available at http://www.genetests.org. [accessed 11.02.16].

15. Wolfe L, Jethva R, Oglesbee D, Vockley J. Short-chain acyl-Coenzyme A dehydrogenase deficiency. (Updated August 7, 2014) in: GeneReviews at GeneTests: Medical Genetics Information Resource [database online]. Copyright, University of Washington, Seattle, 1993–2016. Available at http://www.genetests.org. [accessed 11.02.16].

16. Harding CO, Gillingham MB, van Calcar SC, Wolff JA, Verhoeve JN, Mills MD. Docosahexaenoic acid and retinal function in children with long-chain 3-hydroxyacyl-CoA dehydrogenase deficiency. *J Inher Metab Dis* 1999;**22**(3):276–80.

17. Treem WR, Rinaldo P, Hale DE, Stanley CA, Millington DS, Hyams JS, et al. Acute fatty liver of pregnancy and long-chain hydroxyacyl-coenzyme A dehydrogenase deficiency. *Hepatology* 1994;**19**:339–45.

18. Ibdah JA, Bennett MJ, Rinaldo P, Zhao Y, Gibson B, Sims HF, et al. A fetal fatty-acid oxidation disorder as a cause of liver disease in pregnant women. *New Eng J Med* 1999;**340**:1723–31.

19. Jones PM, Quinn R, Fennessey PV, Tjoa S, Goodman SI, Fiore S, et al. Improved stable isotope dilution-gas chromatography-mass spectrometry method for serum or plasma free 3-hydroxy-fatty acids and its utility for the study of disorders of mitochondrial fatty acid β-oxidation. *Clin Chem* 2000;**46**:149–55.

20. Bennett MJ, Spotswood SD, Ross KF, Comfort S, Koonce R, Boriack RL, et al. Fatal hepatic short-chain L-3-hydroxyacyl-coenzyme A dehydrogenase deficiency: clinical, biochemical, and pathological studies on three subjects with this recently identified disorder of mitochondrial beta-oxidation. *Pediat Dev Path* 1999;**2**:337–45.

21. Li C, Chen P, Palladino A, Narayan S, Russell LK, Chen J, et al. Mechanism of hyperinsulinism in short-chain 3-hydroxyacyl-CoA dehydrogenase deficiency involves activation of glutamate dehydrogenase. *J Biol Chem* 2010;**285**:31806–18.

22. Frerman FE, Goodman SI. Defects of electron transfer flavoprotein and electron transfer protein ubiquinone oxidoreductase: Glutaric academia, type 2. In: Scriver CR, Beaudet AL, Sly WS, Valle D, editors. *The metabolic & molecular bases of inherited disease* 8th ed. New York: McGraw Hill; 2001. p. 2357–65.

Urea cycle and other disorders of hyperammonemia

5

L.D. Smith[1] and U. Garg[2,3]

[1]*University of North Carolina School of Medicine, Chapel Hill, NC, United States;*
[2]*Children's Mercy Hospitals and Clinics, Kansas City, MO, United States;*
[3]*University of Missouri School of Medicine, Kansas City, MO, United States*

5.1 INTRODUCTION

Hyperammonemia is characterized by an excess of ammonia in the blood. It is a symptomatic condition, not a clinical diagnosis, and can be life-threatening. As with nonspecific clinical and laboratory findings, hyperammonemia can result from multiple conditions. While impaired detoxification of ammonia comes immediately to mind in pediatric cases, increased production of ammonia is probably a more common cause of hyperammonemia, especially in the adult population.[1] Hyperammonemia can be either primary or secondary. The former is related to any defect of any of the enzymes or transporters necessary for function of the urea cycle (Fig. 5.1). The latter, while caused by urea cycle dysfunction, results from inhibition of the cycle by either toxic metabolites or substrate deficiency.[2]

Increased production of ammonia is associated with intestinal bacterial overgrowth, neurogenic bladder, drugs (valproic acid (VPA), L-asparaginase, chemotherapeutic agents), infections (cytomegalovirus (CMV), herpes simplex virus (HSV)), structural defects (Allagille syndrome, vascular malformation with portosystemic shunting) or provision of total parenteral nutrition. Impaired detoxification can be either primary (a defect in the urea cycle) or secondary (inhibition of N-acetylglutamate synthase (NAGS) and/or carbamoylphosphate synthetase (CPS1) by methylcitrate, propionyl-CoA or isovaleryl-CoA in the organic acidemias). Substrate deficiencies, as those seen in specific transporter defects, result in dysfunction of the urea cycle and diminished detoxification. The classic urea cycle defects result in hyperammonemia specifically related to the inability of the cycle to function due to an enzymatic block.[2]

By and large, the clinical presentation of hyperammonemia is similar, whatever the underlying pathologic etiology and is related to its toxicity. The exception is arginase deficiency, which presents as a subacute or chronic syndrome with cognitive impairment and spasticity. Acute hyperammonemic crisis is a medical emergency that can have an initial presentation at any age. Acute crisis classically presents in the

Biomarkers in Inborn Errors of Metabolism. DOI: http://dx.doi.org/10.1016/B978-0-12-802896-4.00004-3

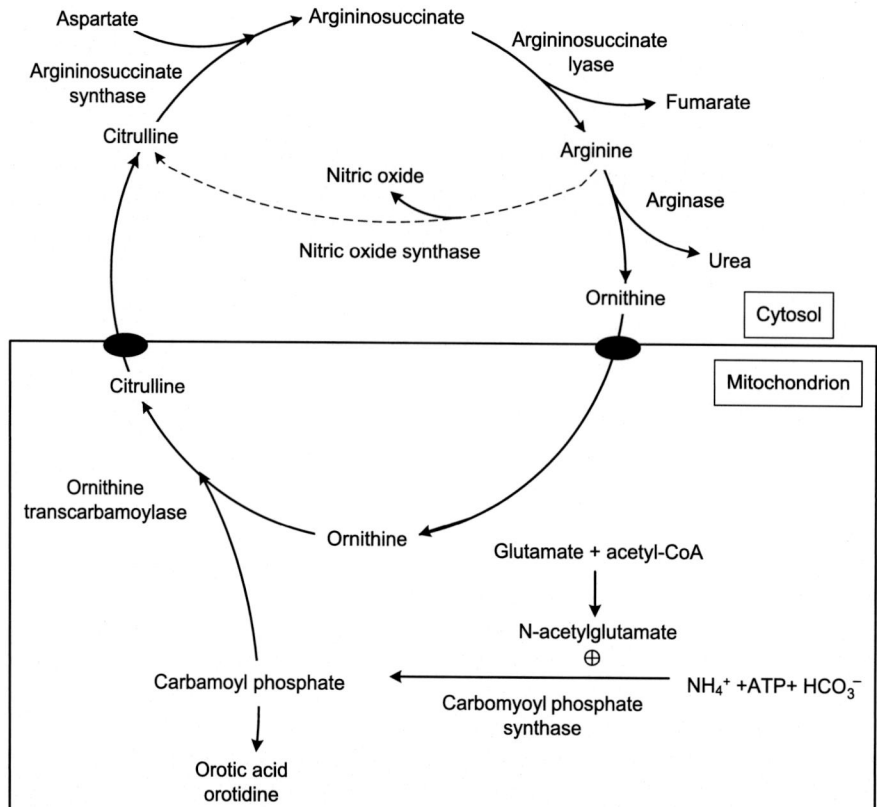

FIGURE 5.1

Urea cycle.

Modified and reprinted with permission from Smith LD, Garg U. The urea cycle disorders and hyperammonemias. In: Garg U, Smith LD, Heese BA, editors. Laboratory diagnosis of inherited metabolic diseases. Washington, DC: AACC Press; 2012. pp. 55–64.

newborn period with poor feeding, lethargy, irritability, and tachypnea, and can rapidly progress to seizures, obtundation, respiratory insufficiency, vasomotor instability and death without urgent intervention. Subacute chronic hyperammonemia may present as a neurobehavioral disorder, as failure to thrive with self-imposed protein restriction, as severe liver disease or as an acute or chronic encephalopathy.

In order to understand hyperammonemic conditions, it is essential to have a basic understanding of the mechanisms of detoxification. First and foremost, the cycle mainly occurs in the periportal hepatocytes in the liver, thus liver disease can result in urea cycle dysfunction separate from a specific defect in the urea cycle. The pathway begins with protein catabolism and ammonia generation.

5.2 BRIEF DESCRIPTION OF CLINICAL PRESENTATION

Clinically, hyperammonemic conditions present in either one of two ways: a rapid, acute decompensation during the newborn period or an indolent chronic condition associated with multiple systemic complaints. While inborn errors of metabolism, including both primary dysfunction of the cycle and secondary inhibition of the cycle by metabolites, are the most common causes of hyperammonemia in the pediatric population, liver disease tends to be the most common underlying pathologic mechanism in the adult population. It is now recognized, however, that inborn errors of the urea cycle are not always rapidly progressive and identifiable as such in the newborn period, but can present later in life as protein avoidance, failure to thrive, intermittent ataxia, episodic headaches, intellectual impairment, behavior disturbances, seizures, and recurrent Reye syndrome. While these presentations should be obviated by the expansion of newborn screening and subsequent identification of affected infants, it is important to keep these conditions in mind, as there is an inherent false negative rate in any screening technique.

Thus, presentation of hyperammonemic conditions has classically been divided into the aforementioned acute and chronic presentations. Acute presentation, is generally described as the case of the well neonate who becomes symptomatic on the second or third day of life with lethargy, poor feeding, vomiting, and irritability that may progress to hyperventilation with accompanying transient metabolic alkalosis, grunting respirations, seizures, coma, and death. Those who survive the initial hyperammonemic episode are at risk of developing recurrent hyperammonemic episodes that present very similarly although the ventilatory abnormalities are generally not seen and ataxia and behavioral changes tend to be more prominent. Again, as mentioned previously, recurrent episodes can also present with intermittent ataxia, headaches, emesis, and anorexia, and may progress to coma and death without intervention.

The more chronic presentation, as is often seen with liver dysfunction and failure, ultimately results in hepatic encephalopathy. A grading system has been devised for the symptoms associated with hepatic encephalopathy. Briefly, the West Haven classification system identifies four grades of symptoms (Table 5.1), ranging from minimal symptoms to overt coma.[3–5]

5.3 UREA CYCLE DISORDERS

The urea cycle is the main system for the clearance of nitrogen waste produced by protein metabolism in the form of free ammonia. It involves five enzymes: CPS1, ornithine transcarbamoylase (OTC), argininosuccinate synthetase, argininosuccinate lyase (ASL), and arginase. It also involves one cofactor, N-acetylglutamate (NAG), producing reaction. NAG is a cofactor for CPS1. In addition, two mitochondrial membrane transporters, the ornithine transporter and the aspartate-glutamate carrier (citrin), are also required for proper functioning of the urea cycle. Hyperammonemia

Table 5.1 Grades of Hepatic Encephalopathy

Grade	Symptoms
0	"Covert" hepatic encephalopathy
	No detectable changes in personality or behavior
	Minimal changes in memory, concentration, intellectual function, and coordination
	No asterixis
1	"Covert" hepatic encephalopathy
	Trivial lack of awareness
	Shortened attention span
	Impaired ability to perform simple mental tasks (addition/subtraction)
	Hypersomnia
	Insomnia or inversion of sleep pattern
	Euphoria, depression, or irritability
	Mild confusion
2	Lethargy or apathy
	Disorientation
	Inappropriate behavior
	Slurred speech
	Asterixis
	Gross deficits in ability to perform mental tasks
	Obvious personality changes
3	Somnolent but arousable
	Unable to perform mental tasks
	Disorientation about time and place
	Marked confusion
	Amnesia
	Rage outbursts
	Incomprehensible speech
4	Coma with or without response to painful stimuli

results from partial or complete deficiency of any of these enzymes or transporters. Deficiencies of these enzymes or transporters are discussed as follows.

5.3.1 N-ACETYLGLUTAMATE SYNTHASE (NAGS) DEFICIENCY

NAGS deficiency is the rarest of all the urea cycle defects. The enzyme is primarily expressed in the liver and intestine, and catalyzes the formation of NAG from glutamate and acetyl-CoA. NAG is the essential allosteric cofactor for CPS1, the first and rate-limiting enzyme of urea cycle. Inhibition of NAGS by various organic and fatty acids metabolites is a common cause of secondary hyperammonemia. This knowledge has provided the basis for the use of N-carbamylglutamate (NCG), an analogue of NAG,[6] as a specific treatment for NAGS deficiency, along with possible treatment for other causes of hyperammonemia related to NAGS inhibition.

Dercksen et al.[7] investigated the inhibition of NAGS by various monocarboxylic and dicarboxylic short-chain coenzyme A esters. Propionyl-CoA and butyryl-CoA were the most powerful inhibitors of NAGS, hence the often observed hyperammonemia associated with organic acidemias and fatty acid oxidation disorders. Branched-chain amino acid related CoAs, isovaleryl-CoA, 3-methylcrotonyl-CoA, isobutyryl-CoA, were less pronounced in the inhibition of NAGS, consistent with irregular occurrence of hyperammonemia in disorders of branched-chain amino acid degradation. Dicarboxylic short-chain acyl-CoAs, methylmalonyl-CoA, succinyl-CoA, glutaryl-CoA had the least inhibitory effect. Furthermore, they identified the glutamate derivatives N-isovalerylglutamate, N-3-methylcrotonylglutamate, and N-isobutyrylglutamate in the urine of patients with different organic acidemias. Oxypurines, xanthine, and uric acid, have been shown to inhibit NAGS.[8] Hence, there is substantial interest in determining efficacy of the use of NCG in liver disease, organic acidurias, and other urea cycle disorders.

5.3.2 CARBAMOYLPHOSPHATE SYNTHETASE (CPS1) DEFICIENCY

CPS1 facilitates the conversion of two ammonia molecules, bicarbonate, and two ATPs to carbamoylphosphate, which is the first step in the urea cycle. When faced with a high nitrogen load, ammonia combines with bicarbonate to generate carbamoylphosphate. This rate-limiting reaction requires the mitochondrial enzyme CPS1 and N-acetylglutamate (discussed earlier), as an allosteric activator. Dysfunction of CPS1 or impairment in the synthesis of NAG disrupts overall function of the urea cycle, since carbamoylphosphate cannot be generated, depriving the cycle of its initial substrate. In general, for all the identified defects of urea cycle function, not only does ammonia concentration increase, but the plasma concentrations of glutamine and alanine also increase since both amino acids are important for maintaining ammonium in the organic form and for its transfer to the liver. Plasma levels of urea cycle intermediates, particularly citrulline, as well as blood urea nitrogen, are decreased and related to the inability of the cycle to complete anapleurotic reactions. Urinary orotic acid concentration is either normal or decreased as it is generated from the condensation of carbamoyl phosphate with aspartic acid. CPS1 deficiency is estimated to occur in 1 of every 65,000 births.

Although it is thought that the most common cause of secondary hyperammonemia is due to inhibition of NAGS, recently hyperammonemia due to inhibition of CPS1 by carboplatin has been reported in a 2-year-old patient.[9]

5.3.3 ORNITHINE TRANSCARBAMYLASE (OTC) DEFICIENCY

OTC, within the mitochondrion, catalyzes the reaction between carbamoylphosphate and ornithine to form citrulline. OTC deficiency is the most commonly diagnosed urea cycle disorder, occurring in 1:15,000 births. The gene for this enzyme (OTC) is located on the X-chromosome and is the only enzyme in the pathway that exhibits X-linked inheritance. While males tend to be more severely affected by OTC deficiency, the phenotype of female carriers may range from completely asymptomatic to completely symptomatic, depending upon random X-inactivation. Deficient enzyme activity results in elevated plasma alanine and glutamine levels as well as highly elevated urine orotic acid levels. Plasma citrulline, arginine, and blood urea nitrogen levels are also decreased. Carrier females with OTC deficiency may have normal biochemical markers, and may need molecular testing or an allopurinol loading test for diagnosis, although the latter is considered to be relatively less reliable than the former.[10]

5.3.4 ARGININOSUCCINATE SYNTHETASE DEFICIENCY

In the cytoplasm, citrulline condenses with aspartic acid to form argininosuccinic acid (ASA), through the action of argininosuccinate synthetase. Transfer of an ammonia group from glutamate to aspartate, and subsequent generation of ASA are responsible for the consumption of a second ammonia group in the urea cycle. Deficiency of this enzyme results in citrullinemia type I, with accumulation of very high concentrations of plasma and urine citrulline, as well as hyperammonemia and orotic aciduria. Arginine concentrations are decreased as ASA and arginine cannot be generated in the absence of the enzyme. In addition to its role in urea cycle, argininosuccinate synthetase is involved in the production of nitric oxide in the cycling of arginine and citrulline.

5.3.5 ARGININOSUCCINATE LYASE DEFICIENCY

Still in the cytoplasm, arginosuccinate lyase cleaves argininosuccinate to form arginine and fumaric acid. Fumaric acid is an important constituent of the Kreb cycle, thus linking the two cycles together. Arginine is converted to ornithine in the next step of the urea cycle. Deficiency of ASL occurs in about 1:70,000 births. It is unique in that deficiency tends to have more systemic effects, particularly in the pathway of nitric oxide generation and vasodilitation with resultant persistent hypertension despite liver transplantation.[11] Unique to and pathognomonic for this deficiency is the elevation of ASA in plasma and urine samples. Plasma glutamine and alanine concentrations are elevated, while arginine levels are diminished. Orotic acid is elevated on urine organic acid profile.

5.3.6 ARGINASE DEFICIENCY

In the final step of the urea cycle, which is also a cytoplasmic reaction, arginine is hydrolyzed via manganese-dependent arginase, to urea and ornithine. Urea (which is the basis for measurement of blood urea nitrogen) is filtered and excreted by the kidney, while ornithine is recycled by the urea cycle by transport across the mitochondrial membrane. Arginase deficiency is quite rare. As would be expected, plasma arginine levels and urine orotic acid levels are elevated in this disorder.

5.3.7 MITOCHONDRIAL ORNITHINE TRANSPORTER (*SLC25A15*) DEFECT

The urea cycle is a compartmentalized cycle, with reactions occurring in both the cytoplasm and the mitochondrion. The enzyme OTC functions within the mitochondrion but ornithine is synthesized in the cytoplasm, allowing for tight regulation of the entire system.[12] Ornithine must be transported across the mitochondrial membrane for the cycle to continue. This is accomplished by ornithine translocase. Mutations in *SLC25A15*, which codes for the solute carrier family 25 (mitochondrial carrier, ornithine transporter) protein, result in deficiency of the transporter and accumulation of cytoplasmic ornithine. The resulting syndrome is known as HHH syndrome (hyperammonemia-hyperornithinemia-homocitrullinemia syndrome). Ammonia accumulates because the urea cycle cannot function secondary to intramitochondrial ornithine depletion. Hyperornithinemia results secondary to increased cytoplasmic ornithine levels. While it is not immediately clear why homocitrulline levels increase, it has been suggested that OTC may lead to its formation from carbamoylphosphate and lysine in the absence of ornithine.[13]

5.3.8 MITOCHONDRIAL ASPARTATE-GLUTAMATE CARRIER (*CITRIN; SLC25A13*) DEFECT/CITRULLINEMIA TYPE 2

Citrulline crosses the mitochondrial membrane passively via a respiration independent process[14] where it undergoes condensation with aspartic acid to form ASA, as discussed earlier. Aspartic acid must be transported across the mitochondrial membrane via an aspartate-glutamate carrier, citrin, which, if deficient, results in diminished cytosolic aspartic acid levels, decreased production of ASA and urea cycle dysfunction. This subsequently leads to elevated plasma glutamine, alanine, citrulline, and ammonia levels, with a concomitant decrease in plasma arginine levels. Citrullinemia type 2 while rare, occurs more frequently in the Japanese population.

5.4 OTHER INBORN DEFECTS ASSOCIATED WITH HYPERAMMONEMIA

5.4.1 LYSINURIC PROTEIN INTOLERANCE

This disorder is caused by impaired transport of the dibasic amino acids lysine, ornithine, and arginine across the intestinal mucosa and renal tubules. Underlying defects in *SLC7A7* that encodes the y+ L amino acid transporter are causative of this autosomal recessive disorder. The incidence of this disorder is highest in those of Finnish (1:60,000) or Japanese (1:57,000) descent. Symptoms are typical of those seen with the urea cycle disorders due to substrate deficiencies of ornithine and arginine, usually appearing during infancy as postprandial hyperammonemia after switching from lower protein containing breast milk to formula feeding. Patients typically have an aversion to high protein foods. They may experience vomiting, diarrhea, hepatomegaly, and lethargy. Additionally, they may have poor growth and intellectual disability. Two very rare medical complications may also be seen in this disorder: alveolar proteinosis and hemophagocytic lymphohistiocytosis. The full natural history and the phenotypic variability of this disorder have yet to be described. In addition to hyperammonemia, urinary lysine, ornithine, and arginine concentrations are highly elevated, while plasma levels may be low or in the low normal range. Interestingly, plasma ferritin, zinc, and lactate dehydrogenase levels are also elevated, with normal serum iron and transferrin levels. Growth retardation is most likely related to lysine deficiency, while intellectual disability is more likely related to recurrent episodes of hyperammonemia and urea cycle dysfunction. Carnitine deficiency also develops, in part due to lysine deficiency.

5.4.2 DISORDERS OF ORNITHINE METABOLISM

In addition to the previously discussed OTC deficiency and HHH syndrome, two other disorders of ornithine metabolism are associated with hyperammonemic states. The first, gyrate atrophy of the choroid and retina and its neonatal form with failure to thrive and encephalopathy, is an autosomal recessive condition caused by deficiency of the pyridoxal phosphate-dependent enzyme, ornithine-δ-aminotransferase (OAT). This enzyme is located in the mitochondrial matrix and, similarly to OTC, requires transport of ornithine across the mitochondrial membrane to function. Since OAT is a freely reversible enzymatic reaction, perinatally, when arginine levels are low, the net flux is toward ornithine, and subsequent arginine, biosynthesis. Flux then switches toward arginine removal that is achieved through the action of Δ^1-pyrroline-5-carboxylate synthase (P5CS), deficiency of which results in the second disorder. While OAT deficiency typically presents as myopia progressing to night blindness in early to mid-childhood, it can present as a more severe neonatal form with hyperammonemia and orotic aciduria. Plasma ornithine, citrulline, and arginine levels are low in the neonatal form. In the later onset form, plasma ornithine is elevated. In both forms, plasma proline levels are normal. On the other hand, P5CS deficiency, also inherited in an autosomal recessive fashion, presents with intellectual disability, lax and wrinkled skin, joint laxity, bilateral cataracts, and a peripheral neuropathy. Plasma citrulline, arginine, ornithine, and proline concentrations are low and there is fasting, rather than postprandial hyperammonemia, secondary to relative deficiency of these intermediates during periods of fasting.[15]

5.4.3 PYRUVATE CARBOXYLASE DEFICIENCY, FRENCH FORM

Pyruvate carboxylase is a biotinylated mitochondrial matrix protein important in the conversion of carbon dioxide and pyruvate to oxaloacetate. It is involved in gluconeogenesis since oxaloacetate is gluconeogenic, whereas pyruvate is formed by an irreversible reaction in glycolysis. It performs an anapleurotic function by generating Kreb cycle intermediates from oxaloacetate and additionally is involved in lipogenesis. There are three recognized phenotypic forms of pyruvate carboxylase deficiency—types A, B, and C. Type A (North American phenotype) presents with lactic acidemia and intellectual disability. Cross-reacting material is identifiable in Type A. Type C is considered a benign variant. Type B, also known as the French phenotype, has complete absence of pyruvate carboxylase mRNA and corresponding protein. Type B is characterized by severe neonatal lactic acidosis, hyperammonemia, and hyperketonemia. This autosomal recessive disorder is rapidly fatal.

5.4.4 HYPERINSULINISM–HYPERAMMONEMIA

The hyperinsulinism–hyperammonemia syndrome is a congenital disorder of hyperinsulinism. The underlying cause of hyperinsulinism–hyperammonemia is mutations in the mitochondrial enzyme glutamate dehydrogenase (GDH) gene (*GLUD1* gene) that lead to increased enzyme activity.[16] The disorder is caused by dominant mutations in *GLUD1* that impair sensitivity to the allosteric inhibitor, guanosine-5′-triphosphate (GTP).[17] However, approximately 80% of the cases are due to *de novo* mutations. Patients with this disorder are characterized by uncontrolled insulin secretion, hyperammonemia, and recurrent episodes of hypoglycemia induced by fasting and a protein-rich diet.[18] The ammonia levels are two to five times the upper limit of normal, but are not associated with lethargy, irritability, and coma.[6] The underlying mechanism of hyperammonia is increased GDH activity that is responsible for conversion of glutamate into α-ketoglutarate and ammonia using NAD^+ and/or $NADP^+$ as a cofactor.

5.4.5 ORGANIC ACIDURIAS

Certain organic acidemias such as isovaleric, methylmalonic, and propionic acidemias cause hyperammonemia, secondary to inhibition of NAGS and/or CPS1 by various organic acids metabolic intermediates. As previously discussed, Dercksen et al.[7] showed that various metabolic intermediates inhibit NAGS to varying degrees. They identified the glutamate derivatives N-isovalerylglutamate, N-3-methylcrotonylglutamate, and N-isobutyrylglutamate in the urine of patients with different organic acidurias. Since organic acidurias lead to NAG deficiency, NCG, an analogue of NAG has been used in the treatment of hyperammonemia due to organic acidurias.[6,19]

5.4.6 FATTY ACID OXIDATION DEFECTS

As discussed previously, hyperammonemia can be seen in many of the fatty acid oxidation defects (carnitine uptake deficiency, carnitine palmitoyltransferase 1 deficiency, carnitine acylcarnitine carrier defect, very long chain acyl-CoA dehydrogenase (VLCAD) deficiency, medium-chain acyl-CoA dehydrogenase (MCAD) deficiency, long-chain 3-hydroxyacyl-CoA dehydrogenase deficiency, multiple acyl-CoA dehydrogenation defect), in which case, it is usually related to mild hepatic dysfunction rather than the inborn error of metabolism.

5.4.7 OTHER

van Karnebeek et al.[20] reported four children who presented with lethargy, hyperlactatemia, and hyperammonemia of unexplained origin. The metabolite profiles in the affected individuals suggested carbonic anhydrase-VA deficiency. Pathways involving bicarbonate and CPS1, pyruvate carboxylase, propionyl-CoA carboxylase, and 3-methylcrotonyl-CoA carboxylase were impaired.

5.5 CONFOUNDING CONDITIONS THAT CAN CAUSE HYPERAMMONEMIA

5.5.1 LIVER DISEASE

Liver is the major organ of ammonia detoxification. Disorders leading to liver failure result in hyperammonemia, as discussed earlier.

5.5.2 TRANSIENT HYPERAMMONEMIA OF THE NEWBORN (THAN)

This condition, observed mostly in premature infants, is characterized by increased ammonia within 24 hours of life and respiratory distress. The ammonia levels can be extremely high (>2,000 μmol/L) requiring vigorous medical intervention. Underlying pathogenesis of transient hyperammonemia of the newborn (THAN) is not well understood, although it is felt to be related to portosystemic shunting resulting in inadequate ammonia filtration.[21] Survivors of THAN do not experience recurrent episodes of hyperammonemia.[21]

5.5.3 DRUG THERAPY

Various drugs can lead to hyperammonemia either by exerting a direct affect on ammonia metabolism or through hepatotoxicity. Valproic acid (VPA) is well known to cause hyperammonemia.[22] One of mechanisms by which valproate causes hyperammonemia is through reduction of acetyl-CoA synthesis by inhibition of fatty acid oxidation. Decreased acetyl-CoA synthesis leads to reduced synthesis of N-acetylglutamate, an activator of carbamoyl phosphate synthetase. VPA is also known to cause carnitine deficiency by directly binding to carnitine. This results in fatty acid oxidation inhibition and reduced synthesis of acetyl-CoA. Hyperammonemic affects of VPA are exaggerated by coadministration of other drugs (such as phenytoin, phenobarbital, and carbamazepine) that induce hepatic enzymes.[23]

Topiramate can also cause hyperammonemia by reducing synthesis of bicarbonate by inhibiting carbonic anhydrase. Bicarbonate is required for synthesis of carbamoyl phosphate from ammonia (Fig. 5.1). Agents used in the treatment of leukemia, including asparaginase, can result in hyperammonemia. Drugs, such as acetaminophen, isoniazid, rifampin, that can cause liver dysfunction may also result in hyperammonemia.

5.5.4 OTHER CONDITIONS

Many other conditions that result in increased production of ammonia are associated with hyperammonemia. Intestinal bacterial overgrowth and urease producing microorganisms (*Proteus*, *Klebsiella*) result in increased ammonia production. Other conditions resulting in hyperammonemia include gastrointestinal bleeding, gastric by-pass, infections (CMV, HSV), increased protein load, severe exercise, burns, structural defects (Allagille syndrome, vascular malformation with portosystemic shunting), or provision of total parenteral nutrition. A high-protein diet for the treatment of anorexia has been shown to cause hyperammonemia.[24] Two anorexic patients treated with a high-protein diet developed altered mental status. This was attributed to high ammonia levels from the high-protein diet. Removal of the high-protein diet resulted in reversal of the symptoms and normalization of the ammonia level.

Table 5.2 lists the various causes of hyperammonemia.

5.6 BIOMARKERS FOR DIFFERENTIAL DIAGNOSIS OF HYPERAMMONEMIA

Developing a differential diagnosis of hyperammonemia requires measurement and interpretation of plasma ammonia level, electrolytes, plasma/urinary amino acid profiles, and urinary organic acid profiles. See Table 5.3 for the differential diagnosis of hyperammonemia.

5.6.1 PLASMA AMMONIA

This is the most important biomarker in the diagnosis of hyperammonemia. Careful sample collection, transportation, and processing are very important to avoid spurious increases in ammonia that can cause false-positive results. Blood samples for ammonia testing should be collected without a tourniquet from a stasis-free vein. The sample should be immediately placed and transported to the laboratory on ice. Once received in the laboratory, plasma should be separated and analyzed within 30 minutes. If analysis cannot be performed immediately, the plasma should be frozen. Icteric, hemolyzed, or lipemic samples should be rejected. Acutely ill patients with urea cycle disorders will usually have significantly higher ammonia levels ($>150\,\mu\text{mol/L}$).

5.6.2 PLASMA AND URINE AMINO ACID PROFILES

Several plasma amino acids are important biomarkers in the differential diagnosis of hyperammonemia, particularly for elucidation of hyperammonemia due to urea cycle defects. For proper interpretation, samples for plasma amino acid profiles should be collected after fasting. The blood sample is collected in a heparin or ethylenediaminetetraacetic acid (EDTA)-containing tube. Plasma should be separated from

Table 5.2 Causes of Hyperammonemia

Hyperammonemia due to urea cycle disorders (see Table 5.3 for biomarkers):

- N-acetylglutamate synthase (NAGS) deficiency
- Carbamoylphosphate synthetase (CPS1) deficiency
- Ornithine transcarbamylase (OTC) deficiency
- Argininosuccinate synthetase deficiency
- Argininosuccinate lyase (ASL) deficiency
- Arginase 1 deficiency
- Mitochondrial ornithine transporter (SLC25A15) defect
- Mitochondrial aspartate-glutamate carrier (Citrin; SLC25A13) defect

Hyperammonemia due to other metabolic defects:

- Lysinuric protein intolerance (LPI)
- Ornithine-δ-aminotransferase (OAT) deficiency
- Pyruvate carboxylase deficiency, French form
- Hyperinsulinism–hyperammonemia syndrome
- Propionic acidemia (Biomarkers on UOA: 3-Hydroxypropionic acid, propionylglycine, methylcitrate)
- Methylmalonic acidemias (Biomarkers on UOA: Methylmalonic acid, 3-hydroxypropionic acid, propionylglycine, methylcitrate)
- Isovaleric acidemia (Biomarkers on UOA: 3-Hydroxyisovaleric acid, isovalerylglycine, methylcitrate)
- 3-Hydroxy-3-methylglutaryl-CoA-lyase deficiency (3-OH-3-methylglutaric, 3-methyl-glutaconic, 3-methylglutaric, 3-hydroxyisovaleric)
- Fatty acid oxidation and carnitine cycle defects

Other causes of hyperammonemia:

- Liver disease
- Open ductus venosus
- Transient hyperammonemia of the newborn
- Valproate therapy
- Topiramate treatment
- Carbamazepine
- Carboplatin
- Aspariginase-5-fluorouracil
- Anorexia
- Intestinal bacterial overgrowth and urease producing microorganisms
- Gastrointestinal bleed
- Gastric by-pass

cells within 1–2 hours of collection and stored frozen. Approximate fasting times in different age groups are: 3 hours in 0–6 months; 3–6 hours in 6–12 months; 6–12 hours in >12 months.[25] Glutamine is generally elevated in all forms of hyperammonemia due to increased production of glutamine from glutamate. Often, alanine and asparagine are also elevated as they serve as reservoirs for waste nitrogen. Diagnostic amino acids biomarkers for hyperammonemia include ornithine, citrulline, ASA, arginine, homocitrulline, lysine, and ornithine (Table 5.3). Various amino acid profiles in several urea cycle defects are shown in Figs. 5.2–5.7.

Table 5.3 Amino Acids Changes in Various Hyperammonemia Disorders

Disorder	Ornithine (P)	Citrulline (P/U)	Argininosuccinic (U)	Arginine (P)	Homocitrulline (U)	Dibasic Amino Acids (U)
NAGS deficiency		↓-N		↓		↑
CPS1		↓-N		↓-N		
OTC		↓-N		↓		
Citrullinemia I		↓↓↓		↓↓		
Citrin deficiency (CTLN2)		↑	↑	N-↓		
Argininosuccinic aciduria		↑	↑↑↑	↓		
Arginase deficiency		↑	↑	↑↑↑		↑
LPI	↓	↑		↓		↑↑
HHH	↑	Normal		Normal	↑↑	

Citrin deficiency: increased threonine:serine ratio, increased pancreatic secretory trypsin inhibitor, secondary deficiency of ASS, neonatal intrahepatic cholestasis, increase galactose, methionine, phenylalanine, threonine, tyrosine, total/direct bilirubin, total bile acids, plasma α-fetoprotein.

LPI: decreased plasma lysine, arginine and ornithine levels; increased plasma glutamine, alanine, serine, proline, citrulline, glycine; increased urine orotic acid, serum lactate dehydrogenase activity, serum ferritin, thyroxin-binding globulin.

HHH: increased lactic, increased lactate:pyruvate ratio, postprandial hyperammonemia, glutamine may paradoxically be elevated with protein restriction.

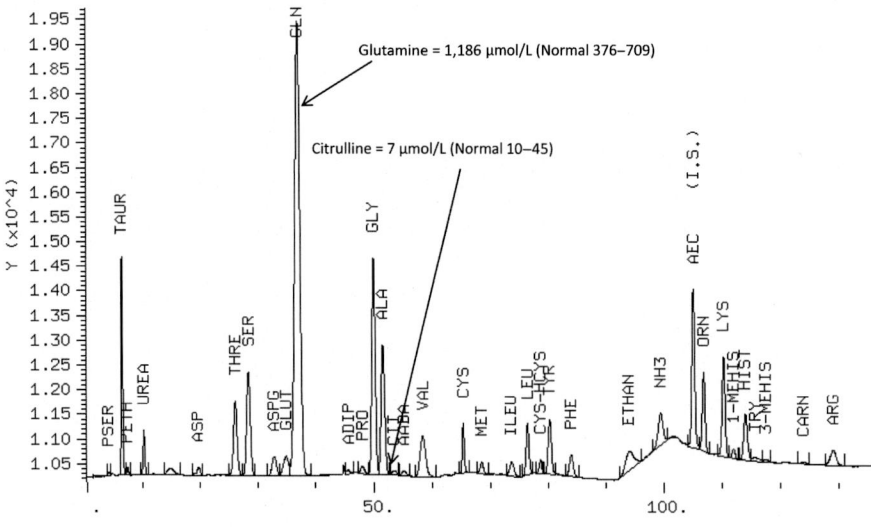

FIGURE 5.2

Plasma amino acids profile from a patient with OTC. Glutamine is elevated and citrulline is low. The sample preparation involved the addition of internal standard S-(2-aminoethyl)-L-cysteine to the sample. Proteins were precipitated using sulfosalicylic acid. The mixture was centrifuged and the supernatant was analyzed using Biochrom 30 amino acid analyzer that involves ion-exchange column, lithium-citrate buffered mobile phases, and postcolumn derivatization with ninhydrin.

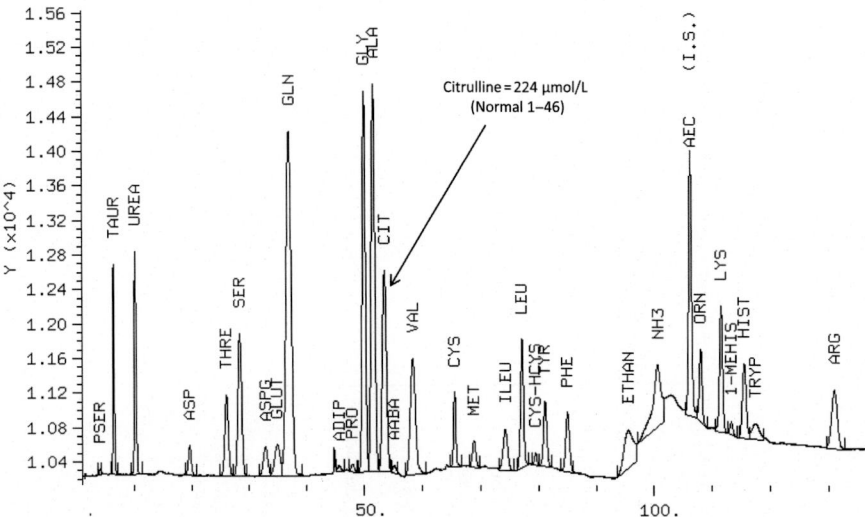

FIGURE 5.3

Plasma amino acids profile from a patient with argininosuccinate synthetase deficiency/citrullinemia type 1. Brief description of sample preparation and analysis is given in Fig. 5.2.

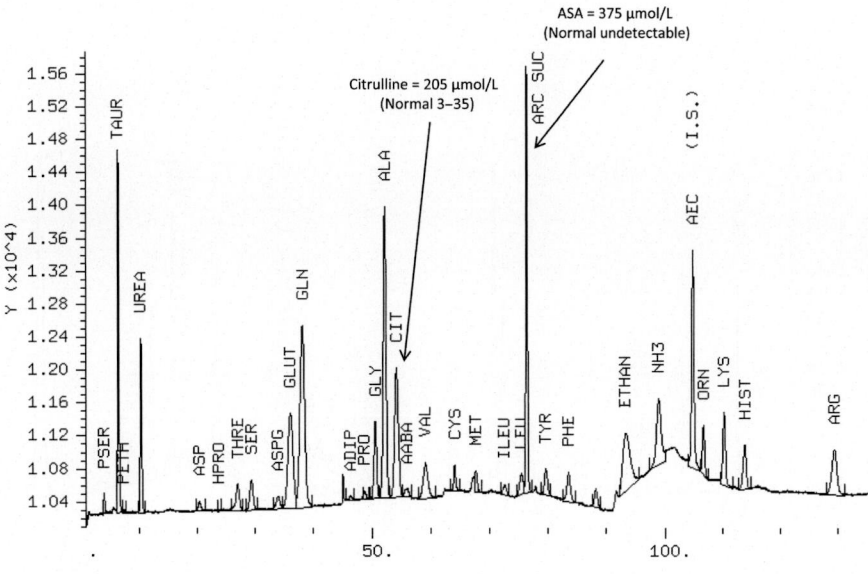

FIGURE 5.4

Plasma amino acids profile from a patient with argininosuccinate lyase deficiency. Brief description of sample preparation and analysis is given in Fig. 5.2.

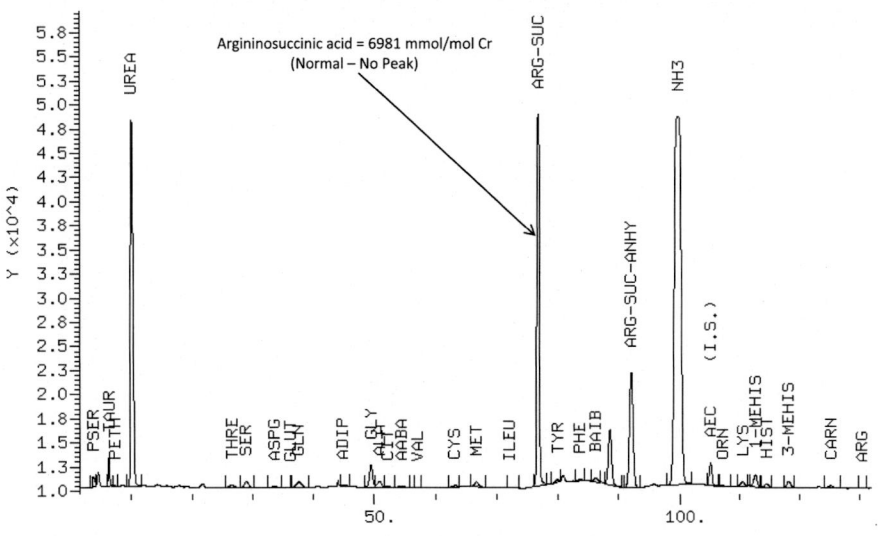

FIGURE 5.5

Urine amino acids profile in a patient with argininosuccinic aciduria. In addition to argininosuccinic acid peak, argininosuccinic anhydride peak is also seen. Brief description of sample preparation and analysis is given in Fig. 5.2.

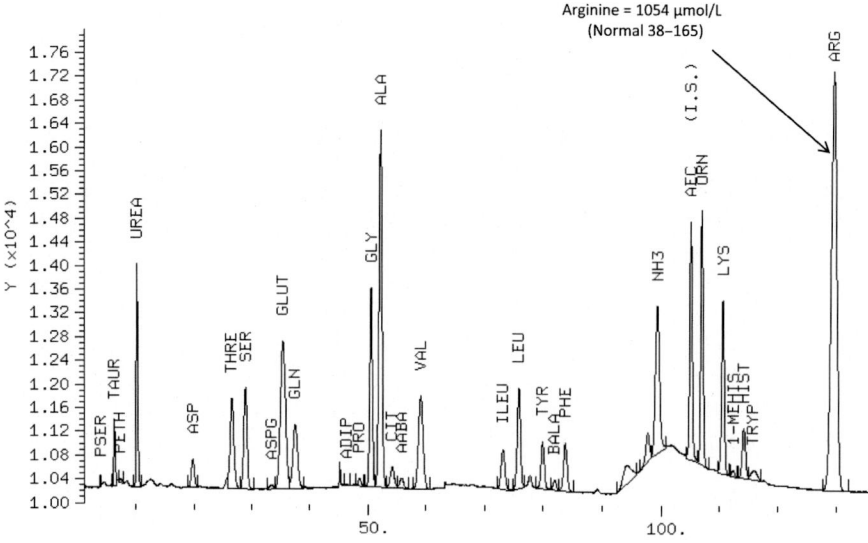

FIGURE 5.6

Plasma amino acids profile from a patient with arginase deficiency. Brief description of sample preparation and analysis is given in Fig. 5.2.

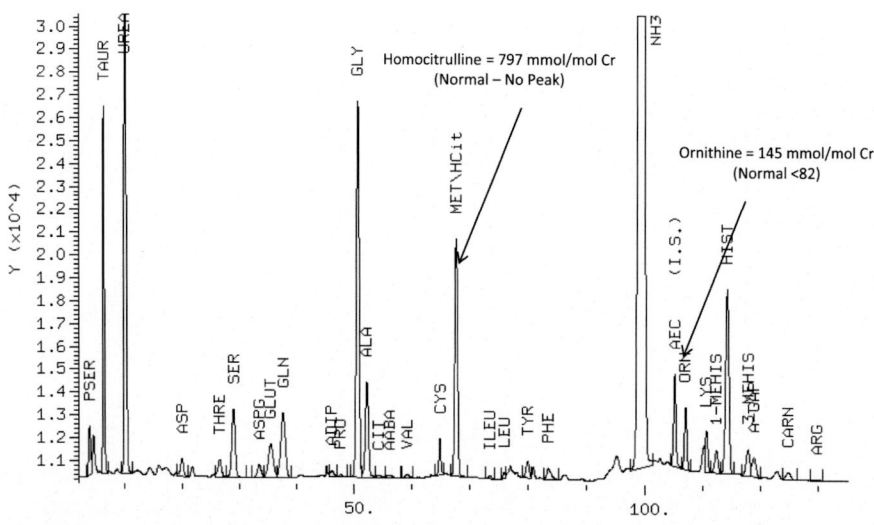

FIGURE 5.7

Urine amino acids profile from a patient with HHH syndrome. Methionine and homocitrulline co-elute. Brief description of sample preparation and analysis is given in Fig. 5.2.

5.6.3 URINE ORGANIC ACID AND ACYLCARNITINE PROFILES

Certain organic acidurias such as propionic, methylmalonic, and congenital lactic acidurias can cause hyperammonemia. Organic acids biomarkers that are elevated in these disorders are shown in Table 5.2. Measurement of pH and calculation of anion gap can help distinguish hyperammonemias due to organic acidemias from urea cycle defects. Generally, pH is low and anion gap is high in organic acidurias as opposed to urea cycle defects where pH is normal or even elevated and anion gap is generally normal. Orotic acid is an important biomarker in the diagnosis of various urea cycle defects. It is elevated in OTC deficiency (Fig. 5.8), citrullinemia, ASA synthase, lysinuric protein intolerance (LPI), and HHH syndrome. It may also be minimally elevated in ASL deficiency.

The acylcarnitine profile is useful in the diagnosis of various organic acidemias leading to hyperammonemia. Acylcarnitine profiles are also useful in the diagnosis of fatty acids oxidation disorders such as MCAD and VLCAD deficiencies, and carnitine deficiency that often lead to hyperammonemia.

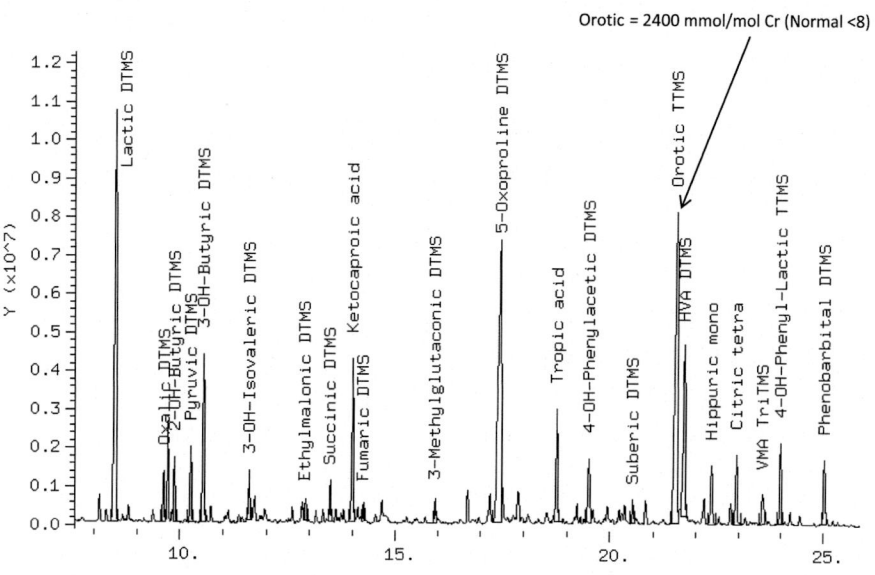

FIGURE 5.8

Urine organic acids profile from a patient with OTC deficiency. The sample preparation involved addition of internal standards, tropic and ketocaproic acids. The urine was alkalinized and oxime derivatives of the ketoacids were prepared using hydroxylamine. The mixture was acidified and organic acids were extracted using ethylacetate. The extract was dried and trimethylsilyl (TMS) derivatives of organic acids were prepared using N,O-bis(trimethylsilyl)trifluoroacetamide (BTSFA)/trimethylchlorosilane (TMCS) and pyridine. The analysis was performed using gas-chromatography mass-spectrometry.

5.7 BIOMARKERS FOLLOWED FOR TREATMENT EFFICACY AND DISEASE PROGRESSION

5.7.1 AMMONIA

Once the diagnosis of hyperammonemia is made, ammonia remains an important biomarker in the follow-up of treatment efficacy. This is particularly important in the beginning of the treatment and in acute crisis management. Individuals who suffer from urea cycle disorders often have and tolerate higher baseline ammonia levels than those with other causes of hyperammonemia. Baseline levels in these individuals are typically less than 105 μmol/L and often do not completely normalize despite medical management.

5.7.2 PLASMA AMINO ACID PROFILE

Since therapy of hyperammonemia includes dietary protein restriction and supplementation of essential amino acids or urea cycle intermediates (citrulline and arginine depending on the defect), plasma amino acid profiles are needed to ensure the appropriate plasma concentrations of various amino acids and to avoid deficiency of essential amino acids.

5.7.3 CARNITINE

Patients with organic acidurias and fatty acid oxidation defects excrete pathologic acylcarnitines leading to carnitine deficiency, as carnitine is used by the body as a metabolic and free oxygen radical scavenger.[26] Periodic assessment of free and total carnitine levels is helpful to ensure adequate levels of carnitine.

5.7.4 OTHER BIOMARKERS

To ensure proper growth in a patient on a protein restricted diet, measurement of total protein, albumin, prealbumin, and transferrin may be performed. Laboratory evaluation may also include liver function tests and hematocrit.

5.8 BRIEF DESCRIPTION OF TREATMENT

A full discussion of the management of hyperammonemia and interventions for specific disorders is beyond the scope of this chapter, but excellent reviews are available on this topic.[27,28] Acute management requires discontinuation of oral protein intake or amino acid infusions and provision of high energy intake as 10–15% glucose orally, if tolerated. If not tolerated, then intravenous glucose should be given at 8–10 mg/kg body weight/minute with the addition of insulin, if necessary. Except in the case of arginase deficiency, L-arginine-HCl should be provided at 2 mmol/kg body weight as a loading dose over 90 minutes, and then as a continuous infusion over 24 hours. Nitrogen scavengers, such as Ammonul (sodium phenylacetate and benzoate) should be used. If hyperammonemia is the result of NAGS or CPS1 deficiency, carbamylglutamate can be considered. Hemodialysis should be considered if the initial ammonia level is >500 μmol/L or if ammonia levels do not respond to treatment with fluids and nitrogen scavengers. Since hemodialysis can be challenging in infants and young children, continuous renal replacement therapy (CRRT) in the mode of continuous venovenous hemodiafiltration has also been used in the treatment of hyperammonemia.[29–31] However, due to small body size and difficult vascular access, performing continuous veno-venous hemofiltration (CVVH) newborns can also be challenging.

In general, long-term management of hyperammonemic conditions relies on restriction of protein, provision of deficient intermediate substrates, and detoxification. Liver transplantation has been successful in treating several of the urea cycle disorders.[32]

5.9 CONCLUSIONS

Hyperammonemias are a diverse group of disorders. Most severe are the ones that are due to defects in urea cycle enzymes or transporters. Several other inherited metabolic disorders such as certain organic acidurias and fatty acid oxidation disorders can also lead to hyperammonemia. Acquired causes of hyperammonia include liver dysfunction, certain drugs, intestinal bacterial overgrowth, and obstruction in blood flow to the liver.

Plasma ammonia is the first and most important test for the diagnosis of hyperammonemia. Plasma and urine amino acids, urine organic acids, and plasma acylcarnitines are used as biomarkers in the differential diagnosis of hyperammonemia. These biomarkers and many other routine laboratory tests are needed in the diagnosis, treatment, and follow-up of patients with hyperammonemia.

ACKNOWLEDGMENT

The authors thank David Scott for help in creating figures for this chapter.

REFERENCES

1. Laish I, Ben Ari Z. Noncirrhotic hyperammonaemic encephalopathy. *Liver Int* 2011;**31**(9):1259–70.
2. Haberle J. Clinical and biochemical aspects of primary and secondary hyperammonemic disorders. *Arch Biochem Biophys* 2013;**536**(2):101–8.
3. Blei AT, Cordoba J. Hepatic Encephalopathy. *Am J Gastroenterol* 2001;**96**(7):1968–76.
4. Kappus MR, Bajaj JS. Covert hepatic encephalopathy: not as minimal as you might think. *Clin Gastroenterol Hepatol* 2012;**10**(11):1208–19.

5. Bajaj JS, Cordoba J, Mullen KD, et al. Review article: the design of clinical trials in hepatic encephalopathy--an International Society for Hepatic Encephalopathy and Nitrogen Metabolism (ISHEN) consensus statement. *Aliment Pharmacol Ther* 2011;**33**(7):739–47.

6. Daniotti M, la Marca G, Fiorini P, Filippi L. New developments in the treatment of hyperammonemia: emerging use of carglumic acid. *Int J Gen Med* 2011;**4**:21–8.

7. Dercksen M, IJlst L, Duran M, et al. Inhibition of N-acetylglutamate synthase by various monocarboxylic and dicarboxylic short-chain coenzyme A esters and the production of alternative glutamate esters. *Biochim Biophys Acta* 2014;**1842**(12 Pt A):2510–6.

8. Nissim I, Horyn O, Nissim I, et al. Down-regulation of hepatic urea synthesis by oxypurines: xanthine and uric acid inhibit N-acetylglutamate synthase. *J Biol Chem* 2011;**286**(25):22055–68.

9. Laemmle A, Hahn D, Hu L, et al. Fatal hyperammonemia and carbamoyl phosphate synthetase 1 (CPS1) deficiency following high-dose chemotherapy and autologous hematopoietic stem cell transplantation. *Mol Genet Metab* 2015;**114**(3):438–44.

10. Grunewald S, Fairbanks L, Genet S, et al. How reliable is the allopurinol load in detecting carriers for ornithine transcarbamylase deficiency? *Journal of Inherited Metabolic Disease* 2004;**27**(2):179–86.

11. Brunetti-Pierri N, Erez A, Shchelochkov O, Craigen W, Lee B. Systemic hypertension in two patients with ASL deficiency: a result of nitric oxide deficiency? *Mol Genet Metab* 2009;**98**(1–2):195–7.

12. Watford M. The urea cycle: a two-compartment system. *Essays Biochem* 1991;**26**:49–58.

13. Kato T, Sano M, Mizutani N. Homocitrullinuria and homoargininuria in lysinuric protein intolerance. *Journal of Inherited Metabolic Disease* 1989;**12**(2):157–61.

14. Gamble JG, Lehninger AL. Transport of ornithine and citrulline across the mitochondrial membrane. *J Biol Chem* 1973;**248**(2):610–8.

15. Baumgartner MR, Hu CA, Almashanu S, et al. Hyperammonemia with reduced ornithine, citrulline, arginine and proline: a new inborn error caused by a mutation in the gene encoding delta(1)-pyrroline-5-carboxylate synthase. *Hum Mol Genet* 2000;**9**(19):2853–8.

16. Huijmans JG, Duran M, de Klerk JB, Rovers MJ, Scholte HR. Functional hyperactivity of hepatic glutamate dehydrogenase as a cause of the hyperinsulinism/hyperammonemia syndrome: effect of treatment. *Pediatrics* 2000;**106**(3):596–600.

17. MacMullen C, Fang J, Hsu BY, et al. Hyperinsulinism/hyperammonemia syndrome in children with regulatory mutations in the inhibitory guanosine triphosphate-binding domain of glutamate dehydrogenase. *J Clin Endocrinol Metab* 2001;**86**(4):1782–7.

18. Hsu BY, Kelly A, Thornton PS, Greenberg CR, Dilling LA, Stanley CA. Protein-sensitive and fasting hypoglycemia in children with the hyperinsulinism/hyperammonemia syndrome. *J Pediatr* 2001;**138**(3):383–9.

19. Soyucen E, Demirci E, Aydin A. Outpatient treatment of propionic acidemia-associated hyperammonemia with N-carbamoyl-L-glutamate in an infant. *Clin Ther* 2010;**32**(4):710–3.

20. van Karnebeek CD, Sly WS, Ross CJ, et al. Mitochondrial carbonic anhydrase VA deficiency resulting from CA5A alterations presents with hyperammonemia in early childhood. *Am J Hum Genet* 2014;**94**(3):453–61.

21. Tuchman M, Georgieff MK. Transient hyperammonemia of the newborn: a vascular complication of prematurity? *J Perinatol* 1992;**12**(3):234–6.

22. Yamamoto Y, Takahashi Y, Imai K, et al. Risk factors for hyperammonemia in pediatric patients with epilepsy. *Epilepsia* 2013;**54**(6):983–9.
23. Yamamoto Y, Takahashi Y, Suzuki E, et al. Risk factors for hyperammonemia associated with valproic acid therapy in adult epilepsy patients. *Epilepsy Res* 2012;**101**(3):202–9.
24. Welsh E, Kucera J, Perloff MD. Iatrogenic hyperammonemia after anorexia. *Arch Intern Med* 2010;**170**(5):486–8.
25. Smith L, Garg U. The urea cycle disorders and hyperammonemias. In: Garg U, Smith L, Heese B, editors. *Laboratory Diagnosis of Inherited Metabolic Diseases*. Washington DC: AACC Press; 2012. p. 55–64.
26. Ribas GS, Vargas CR, Wajner M. L-carnitine supplementation as a potential antioxidant therapy for inherited neurometabolic disorders. *Gene* 2014;**533**(2):469–76.
27. Adam S, Almeida MF, Assoun M, et al. Dietary management of urea cycle disorders: European practice. *Mol Genet Metab* 2013;**110**(4):439–45.
28. Adam S, Champion H, Daly A, et al. Dietary management of urea cycle disorders: UK practice. *J Hum Nutr Diet* 2012;**25**(4):398–404.
29. Kim HJ, Park SJ, Park KI, et al. Acute treatment of hyperammonemia by continuous renal replacement therapy in a newborn patient with ornithine transcarbamylase deficiency. *Korean J Pediatr* 2011;**54**(10):425–8.
30. Pirojsakul K, Tangnararatchakit K, Vaewpanich J, et al. Successful continuous venovenous hemofiltration in a neonate with hyperammonemia from ornithine transcabamylase deficiency. *J Med Assoc Thai* 2013;**96**(11):1512–7.
31. Westrope C, Morris K, Burford D, Morrison G. Continuous hemofiltration in the control of neonatal hyperammonemia: a 10-year experience. *Pediatr Nephrol* 2010;**25**(9):1725–30.
32. Foschi FG, Morelli MC, Savini S, et al. Urea cycle disorders: a case report of a successful treatment with liver transplant and a literature review. *World J Gastroenterol* 2015;**21**(13):4063–8.

Newborn screening

M.A. Morrissey

Wadsworth Center, Albany, NY, United States

6.1 NEWBORN SCREENING

Every year approximately 10 million newborn babies worldwide are screened for up to 50 genetic and metabolic disorders. The objective of newborn screening (NBS) is to identify those children who are at risk and who may need further testing to confirm the presence of one of these disorders. Analysis and reporting must be done in a timely manner so as not to delay potentially life-saving treatment. A typical NBS laboratory must analyze and evaluate several hundred to a few thousand samples for up to 50 different disorders each day.

In 2006, the American College of Medical Genetics (ACMG) made an official statement recommending 29 core conditions that should be screened by all programs and 25 secondary target conditions.[1] As of March 2015 the recommended uniform screening panel (RUSP) comprises 32 core conditions and 26 secondary targets. Of these conditions on the RUSP, 22 of the core conditions and 24 of the secondary targets are inherited metabolic disorders (IMDs).[2] The metabolic disorders may be divided into disorders of amino acid metabolism, organic acidemias, and fatty acid oxidation disorders. These three classes of metabolic disorders are detectable by tandem mass spectrometry (MS/MS). Galactosemia and biotinidase deficiency, two additional metabolic disorders, are detectable by wet-chemical methods with spectrophotometric or fluorescence detection.

To collect a screening sample, a small skin puncture is made in the baby's heel.[3] A few drops of blood from the heel stick are collected on a filter paper form. The sample is often called the Guthrie spot, to recognize the role of Robert Guthrie in NBS. Patient demographic information is attached to the same form as the filter paper sample. The baby's primary care provider or the hospital of birth forwards the dried blood spot (DBS) samples, by courier or mail, to an NBS laboratory. Once at the laboratory the samples are accessioned, demographic data is entered into a database, and samples are taken from the blood spots as a 1/8 inch or 3.2 mm paper punch from a DBS sample analysis; however, different size punches may be required for different methods. Multiple punches from the DBS samples are necessary to run all the tests recommended by the ACMG.

Many of the IMDs are detected by MS/MS of two classes of molecules: amino acids and acylcarnitines. NBS by MS/MS involves the extraction of biomarkers from a DBS sample and detection of the biomarkers by MS/MS. The mass spectrometer (1) produces ions from the compounds in the samples, (2) selects precursor ions (also known as parent ions) according to their mass in the first analyzer of the instrument (Q1), (3) fragments the mass selected precursor ions, by colliding them with argon gas in the collision cell (Q2), to yield product ions (also called daughter ions), and (4) analyzes the product ions according to their masses in the second analyzer (Q3) of the tandem mass spectrometer.

The extraction solvent contains a number of internal standards that are stable isotope analogs of the biomarkers. For example, the internal standard for phenylalanine is a d5-phenylalanine with five deuterium atoms. The phenylalanine internal standard has the same chemical behavior as the analyte, but a molecular weight of 5 amu higher than phenylalanine. Use of internal standards is important in mass spectrometry because in the ion source the analytes will be subject to a certain amount of ionization suppression. The environment around the analytes of interest in solution will compete with the analytes for charges, suppressing the response of the analyte of interest in a sample matrix as opposed to the response that may be observed in a pure solvent. Since the DBS samples come from the blood of newborn babies, every environment will be very slightly different and a given concentration of analyte in the sample extract will result in a very slightly different amount of signal. Since the internal standard will experience the same amount of suppression as the target analyte, the concentration of the analyte may be calculated from the response observed for a known concentration of the internal standard in the sample. An example of the calculation of marker concentration is given in Eq. (6.1).

$$\text{Conc of marker} - \text{M} = \frac{\text{Resp of marker} - \text{M} \times \text{Conc IS} \times \text{RRF}}{\text{Resp of IS}} \qquad (6.1)$$

where, Conc of IS is the calculated concentration of the internal standard (IS) in the volume of blood contained in the DBS sample.

RRF is a relative response factor that may be used for correction of extraction efficiency or other variables.

The concentration of a marker in the sample is dependent on the ratio of the response of the marker to the response of a known quantity of the internal standard.

In some laboratories the sample extract is derivatized, to improve the sensitivity and specificity, most often by conversion of amino acids and acylcarnitine to butyl esters. In other laboratories the sample extracts are analyzed directly without derivatization. In the mass spectrometer, amino acid and acylcarnitine markers may be analyzed using either scanning methods or multiple-reaction monitoring (MRM) methods, or a combination of both. A number of detailed reviews of sample preparation and methods of analysis are available.[4–8]

The precision and accuracy of the MS/MS method are dependent on a number of factors including the precision of the instrumentation, the extraction efficiency of the analytes, and the degree of suppression of the analytes. The precision and accuracy of NBS are also dependent on the nature of the DBS sample. The calculation of the concentration of marker in the blood is dependent on the volume of blood in the paper punch sample. This of course may vary slightly from punch-to-punch, spot-to-spot, or sample-to-sample, especially when different hospitals and different health care professionals collect the sample from newborn babies. The Center for Disease Control and Prevention (CDC) has reported the variability of DBS specimens from fortified samples. The volume of blood contained in a punch may vary from 5% to 10% under controlled conditions with fortified specimens. Depending on the analyte, intrarun precision of the method may vary from 15% to 25% and the interrun precision may vary from 20% to 35%. The accuracy of the method, recovery of a known amount of analyte added to a blood sample, may vary from 40% to 140%. If the lab is consistent in its methods, and therefore consistent in its precision and accuracy, these levels are acceptable.

In the MS/MS analysis used in NBS, there is no chromatographic separation of analytes in the sample extract. All analytes in a sample are analyzed together in the mass spectrometer in a single run of two minutes or less. For each sample there may be 50 or more results including analyte concentrations, internal standard responses, and ratios or other mathematical combinations of analyte results that may be informative. Unlike other techniques where a single run for a single sample will provide a single response, analysis of IMDs by MS/MS results in a pattern of analyte concentrations in the sample. The goal of the NBS laboratory is to not miss any truly positive sample, while at the same time minimizing the number of false-positive results. The rules of pattern recognition for reporting positives should be as simple as possible for use in the laboratory and for consistency, but no simpler than necessary to ensure that no true positives are missed and false positives are minimized. Interpretation of the results of the analysis should be based on a set of rules set up with the advice of a consortium of specialists and approved by the laboratory directorship. Programs need to identify those analytes and markers that are critical for a condition and assign cut-off values, a concentration where the analyte results for a particular sample are outside the range of normal results. The evaluation may include several markers and ratios of markers, demographic data such as birth weight or gestation age, and possibly algorithms that will assign a single score based on the evaluation of a pattern of markers. The rest of this chapter will focus on the interpretation of results for IMDs. A list of the markers discussed, their abbreviations, and MRM transitions is presented in Table 6.1.

Table 6.1 Amino Acid and Acylcarnitine Markers Along With Suggested Mass Spectrometry Transitions

Name	Abbrev	Underivatized Ions [M+H]+		Butyl Ester Ions [M+H]+	
		Precursor Ion	Product Ion	Precursor Ion	Product Ion
Amino acids					
Arginine	Arg	175	70	231	70
Citrulline	Cit	176	113	232	113 (130)
Leucine, Isoleucine, Hydroxyproline	Leu, (ile/leu, xle)	132	86	188	86
Methionine	Met	150	104	206	104
Ornithine	Orn	133	70	189	70
Phenylalanine	Phe	166	120	222	120
Tyrosine	Tyr	182	136	238	136
Valine	Val	118	72	174	72
Acylcarnitines					
Free Carnitine	C0	162	85	218	85 (103)
Acetylcarnitine	C2	204	85	260	85
Propionylcarnitine	C3	218	85	274	85
Malonylcarnitine	C3DC	248	85	360	85
Butyryl/Isobutyrylcarnitine	C4	232	85	288	85
Hydroxybutyrylcarnitine	C4OH	248	85	304	85
Tiglylcarnitine	C5:1	244	85	300	85
Isovaleryl/2-Methylbutyryl-carnitine	C5	246	85	302	85
Hydroxyisovalerylcarnitine	C5OH	262	85	318	85
Glutarylcarnitine	C5DC	276	85	388	85
Hexanoylcarnitine	C6	260	85	316	85
Octanoylcarnitine	C8	288	85	344	85
Decadienoylcarnitine	C10:2	312	85	368	85
Decanoylcarnitine	C10	316	85	372	85
Dodecadienoylcarnitine	C12:2	340	85	396	85
Dodecenoylcarnitine	C12:1	342	85	398	85
Dodecanoylcarnitine	C12	344	85	400	85
Tetradecadienoylcarnitine	C14:2	368	85	424	85
Tetradecenoylcarnitine	C14:1	370	85	426	85
Tetradecanoylcarnitine	C14	372	85	428	85
Hexadecanoylcarnitine	C16	400	85	456	85
Hydroxyhexadecanoylcarnitine	C16OH	416	85	472	85
Octadecenoylcarnitine	C18:1	426	85	482	85
Octadecanoylcarnitine	C18	428	85	484	85
Hydroxyoctadecenoylcarnitine	C18:1OH	442	85	498	85

6.2 AMINO ACID DISORDERS

The aminoacidopathies, are those IMDs that inhibit the degradation of amino acids. They are caused by a defect in an enzyme in the degradative pathway and are characterized by an accumulation of the enzyme reactants and a depletion of the enzyme products. The primary markers are the amino acids that accumulate due to the enzyme block. Good primary markers are the reactants closest to the enzyme block. As an example the pathway for the metabolism of phenylalanine is shown in Fig. 6.1. Classical phenylketonuria (PKU) is caused by a mutation in the gene encoding the enzyme phenylalanine hydroxylase (PAH). This enzyme converts phenylalanine (Phe) to tyrosine (Tyr). If there is a defect in the enzyme, Phe will accumulate in the blood and may be detected by NBS.

Secondary markers are usually ratios of two or more analytes. Secondary markers may be useful for the elimination of false positives or to find true positives that are close to the borderline results for the primary markers. In some cases, the secondary marker may be related to the enzyme pathway. Since the PAH enzyme is deficient, the concentration of Tyr in the blood is expected to be depleted since phenylalanine is not being converted to tyrosine (Fig. 6.1). There are other sources, including dietary tyrosine, for tyrosine in the blood, so the concentration of tyrosine is expected to be in the low to low-normal range rather than very low. The ratio of Phe/Tyr is a useful secondary marker[9] since in classic PKU, the ratio should be elevated while in other cases of hyperphenylalaninemia (HPHE), the ratio may approach a normal.

Secondary markers may not be related to the pathway of the deficient enzyme, but instead may be a surrogate internal standard in the blood sample, e.g., the ratio Phe/Leu. These ratios are a useful method for relating the level of an abnormal amino acid observed in the blood to other amino acid levels for the same patient. Total parenteral

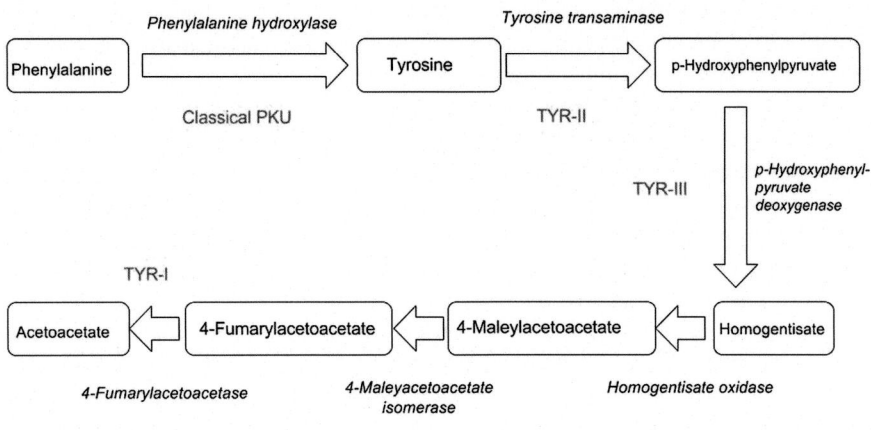

FIGURE 6.1

Schematic diagram of the conversion of phenylalanine to tyrosine and tyrosine to acetoacetate.

nutrition (TPN) or intravenous hyperalimentation, is administered as a nutritional source to infants who are premature or in neonatal intensive care unit (NICU). A patient receiving TPN may have one or several amino acids that show elevated concentrations, but the ratios of the amino acids may likely be in the normal range.

The core conditions and secondary target conditions for aminoacidopathies along with primary markers and secondary markers are listed in Table 6.2.

Phenylalanine and the Phe/Tyr ratio are the primary and secondary markers for the identification of PKU. Other markers, which may also be useful, are listed in Table 6.2. As discussed, PKU is a deficiency of the PAH enzyme, which converts Phe to Tyr. A deficiency of the enzyme leads to an accumulation of Phe and a depletion of Tyr. Left untreated PKU will result in significant mental impairment, seizures, and other complications. If detected, and treated with a phenylalanine restricted diet, normal mental development is possible. With early detection and treatment, the effects of PKU can be minimized or eliminated.

Secondary target conditions, such as HPHE or biopterin (BIOPT) deficiency, also result in elevated Phe and Phe/Tyr ratios, although in the latter conditions the ratio may approach a normal, since both Phe and Tyr catabolism require tetrahydrobiopterin as a cofactor. While there may be some relationship between the magnitude of the results and the condition, there is also a good deal of overlap. The purpose of screening is to identify children at risk. The exact disorder should be determined by confirmatory testing.

Maple syrup urine disease (MSUD), also known as branched-chain ketoaciduria, is an IMD affecting the metabolism of the branched-chain amino acids (leucine, isoleucine, and valine). The common name comes from the presence of sweet-smelling urine similar to maple syrup in affected patients. Newborns with this condition will usually not show symptoms at birth, but will quickly deteriorate. If untreated, MSUD can lead to seizures, coma, and death. MSUD is caused by a deficiency of the branched-chain α-keto acid dehydrogenase complex (BCKDC), which consists of four subunits. A mutation in any one of the four subunits may cause the disease. There are several variations of MSUD; classical, intermediate, thiamine-responsive, and E3-deficient MSUD with lactic acidosis. Only the classical form is reliably detected by NBS. In the other forms the leucine levels may be close to normal and only elevated in times of fasting, stress, or illness.

In screening for MSUD, the tandem mass spectrometer cannot distinguish between leucine and isoleucine. These compounds are structural isomers with the same molecular weight. In practice, the leucine concentrations reported by NBS are the sum of the leucine and isoleucine concentrations. In true cases of MSUD, the increase in leucine/isoleucine is significant enough that this is not a difficulty. Because of the severity of this condition, significantly high concentrations of leucine/isoleucine should be reported to the appropriate care providers without delay. The use of a secondary marker such as Leu/Phe helps to eliminate some false positives for this condition. The leucine concentrations in DBS samples tend to increase slightly with the age of the baby. Age-related cut-off values for Leu help to eliminate false-positive results from samples collected from babies more than 2 weeks old. MSUD is confirmed by the determination of leucine, isoleucine, and allo-isoleucine using

Table 6.2 Newborn Screening Primary and Secondary Markers for Aminoacidopathies

Condition (Abbreviation)	RUSP Status	Enzyme	Primary Marker(s)	Secondary Marker(s)
Classical phenylketonuria (PKU)	Core Condition	Phenylalanine hydroxylase	Phe	Phe/Tyr
Hyperphenylalaninemia (HPHE)	Secondary Target	Phenylalanine hydroxylase	Phe	Phe/Tyr
Disorders of biopterin biosynthesis (BIOPT)	Secondary Target	6-pyruvoyltetrahydropterin synthase	Phe	Phe/Tyr
Maple syrup urine disease (MSUD)	Core Condition	Branched-chain α-keto acid dehydrogenase	Leu, Val	Leu/Phe, Val/Phe
Homocystinuria (HCY)	Core Condition	Cystathionine beta-synthase	Met	Met/Phe, Met/Leu, Met/Tyr
Hypermethioninemia (HMET)	Secondary Target	Methionine adenosyltransferase	Met	Met/Phe, Met/Leu, Met/Tyr
Tyrosinemia type I (TYR-I)	Core Condition	Fumarylacetoacetate hydrolase	SUAC	
Tyrosinemia type II (TYR-II)	Secondary Target	Tyrosine transaminase	Tyr	Tyr/Cit
Tyrosinemia type III (TYR-III)	Secondary Target	4-hydroxyphenylpyruvate acid oxidase	Tyr	Tyr/Cit
Argininemia (ARG)	Secondary Target	Arginase	Arg	Arg/Orn
Citrullinemia type I (CIT-I)	Core Condition	Argininosuccinate synthetase	Cit	Cit/Arg, Cit/Phe, Cit/Met
Argininosuccinic acidemia (ASA)	Core Condition	Argininosuccinate lyase	Cit, ASA	Cit/Arg
Citrullinemia type II (CIT-II)	Secondary Target	Aspartate glutamate carrier [citrin]	Cit	Cit/Arg

Nomenclature for Conditions based upon "Naming and Counting Disorders (Conditions) Included in Newborn Screening Panels." Pediatrics. 2006; 117 (5) Suppl: S308–S314.

high-performance liquid chromatography (HPLC) linked to ultraviolet (UV) detector or a mass spectrometer.[10]

Classical homocystinuria (HCY) is caused by a defect of cystathionine β-synthase (CBS). The condition is also called CBS deficiency. The enzyme deficiency blocks the metabolic conversion of homocysteine to cystathionine. Methionine (Met) is the primary marker for the detection of HCY due to CBS deficiency. Secondary markers are the ratios of Met to other amino acids such as Met/Phe, Met/Leu, and Met/Tyr. These same markers also detect hypermethioninemia (HMET). In the newborn period, methionine concentrations may be low, even in disease cases, making the detection of HCY and HMET challenging.[11] Cases of CBS deficiency have been documented in newborns with normal blood methionine concentrations.[12] In addition, high concentrations of Met may have other causes such as administration of TPN, prematurity, or impaired liver function. The use of the secondary markers can reduce false positives due to TPN administration because the baseline level of the other amino acids will be raised along with Met. In the case of liver prematurity or dysfunction, Tyr will often also be increased, so the ratio Met/Tyr will be within the reference range.

Tyrosinemia is the inability of the body to break down tyrosine. There are three different forms of the disease of which two can be reliably detected as elevated tyrosine levels. Tyrosinemia type II (TYR-II) is caused by a deficiency of tyrosine transaminase. Tyrosinemia type III (TYR-III) is caused by a deficiency of 4-hydroxyphenylpyruvate acid oxidase. Both these conditions may be detected by elevations of tyrosine.

Tyrosinemia type I (TYR-I) is a deficiency of the enzyme fumarylacetoacetase that catalyzes the breakdown of 4-fumarylacetoacetate to acetoacetate (Fig. 6.1). TYR-I is usually asymptomatic in newborns. However, if left untreated, it affects liver, kidney, bone, and peripheral nerves. Infants with the most severe presentations may die from liver failure in the first months of life.[13] The majority of TYR-I patients can be treated with 2-(2-nitro-4-trifluoromethylbenzoyl)-1,3-cyclohexanedione (NTBC) with promising outcomes.[14,15] Since the enzyme deficiency is several steps removed from the tyrosine reactant, tyrosine levels may not rise above the laboratory cut-off in the first few days of life when most NBS samples are collected. Confirmed cases of TYR-I with an NBS result for tyrosine that was only mildly elevated have been reported;[16] however, succinylacetone, a reactant much closer to the enzyme block, is a better marker. Succinylacetone may be analyzed as a separate marker from other amino acids and acylcarnitines, extracted separately and then combined with analysis of the amino acids and acylcarnitines, or extracted and analyzed together with amino acids and acylcarnitines.[17–19]

Urea cycle disorders result from a deficiency of any one of the enzymes that catalyze the removal of ammonia from the bloodstream. The urea cycle is illustrated in Fig. 6.2.[20] An enzyme deficiency in the urea cycle will result in the accumulation of toxic ammonia. Children with severe urea cycle disorders often show symptoms after the first 24 hours of life. Early symptoms may include irritability, followed by vomiting and lethargy. Soon after, seizures, hypotonia (poor muscle tone), respiratory distress, and coma may occur. If untreated, the child will die.

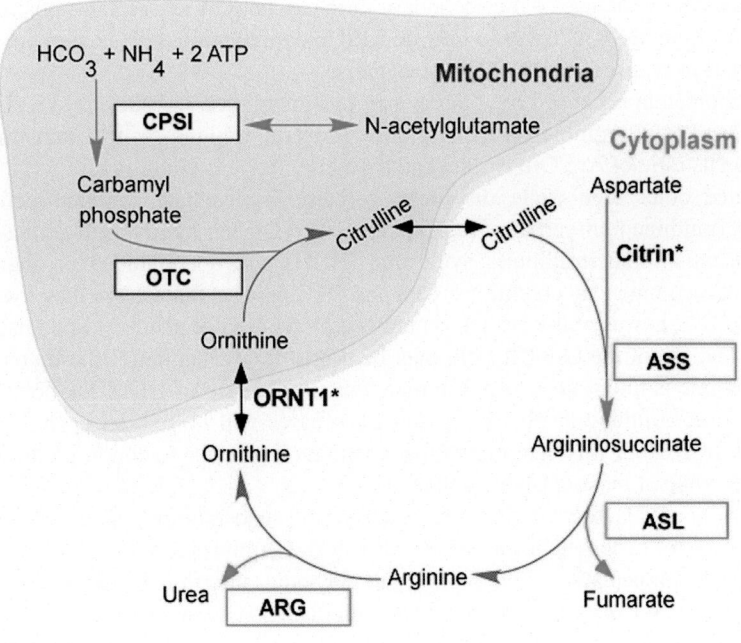

FIGURE 6.2

Schematic diagram of urea cycle disorder.

Re-used with permission from Mew NA, Lanpher BC, Gropman A, Chapman KA, Simpson KL, Urea Cycle Disorders Consortium, et al. Urea Cycle Disorders Overview. GeneReviews® [Internet]. Seattle, WA: Copyright University of Washington. Initial Posting: April 29, 2003; Last Revision: April 9, 2015. <http://www.ncbi. nlm.nih.gov/books/NBK1217/>; 1993–2016 (accessed 19.11.15).

Citrullinemia type I (CIT-I) is a deficiency of the enzyme argininosuccinate synthetase (ASS). ASS catalyzes the formation of argininosuccinate from citrulline and aspartate. In the absence of an active ASS enzyme, citrulline accumulates and is the primary marker for CIT-I. The next step in the urea cycle is the conversion of argininosuccinate to arginine so the CIT-I disorder is also characterized by a deficiency of arginine. A highly elevated Cit/Arg ratio is a useful marker for assessing the disease. Children with significant citrulline elevations should be reported to the appropriate health care professionals as soon as possible. The analysis of citrulline may also detect citrullinemia type II (CIT-II; citrin deficiency), a secondary target.

Argininosuccinic aciduria (ASA) is caused by a deficiency of the enzyme argininosuccinate lyase (ASL). This enzyme cleaves argininosuccinate to arginine and fumarate. A defect in the ASL enzyme leads to an accumulation of citrulline and argininosuccinic acid. Both are reported as primary markers for the evaluation of ASA. In ASA, citrulline levels may be more moderately elevated than CIT-I. As with CIT, the Cit/Arg ratio may be used to eliminate false positives and lower the cut-off used for ASA. The use of the secondary ratio can help to reduce false positives. At the same time, the Cit/Arg ratio may be used in combination with a lower cut-off for Cit levels to reduce the risk of a false negative.

Argininemia is caused by a deficiency of the arginase (ARG) enzyme. The primary marker is arginine (Arg). Arginase converts arginine to urea and ornithine (Orn). The ratio of Arg/Orn is a secondary marker for this condition.

Three other urea cycle disorders, carbamoyl-phosphate synthase deficiency (CPS), ornithine transcarbamylase deficiency (OTC), and hyperornithinemia-hyper-ammonemia-homocitrullinuria syndrome (HHH), are not included on the RUSP panel of recommended conditions. CPS and OTC may be characterized by low levels of citrulline; however, the evaluation may be prone to false positives and false negatives. The use of the Orn/Cit ratio may be useful for evaluation of these conditions as ornithine is the product of these reactions. In the case of HHH, the delay in the increase in ornithine levels means that most cases will be missed in the newborn period. In 2010, it was determined that ornithine levels rise to abnormal levels well after the time of most newborn screens.[21]

A number of factors mimic the high amino acid concentrations that are observed in actual cases of metabolic disorders. The first is the administration of TPN, sometimes called hyperalimentation. TPN supplies all the body's nutritional needs intravenously and bypasses the usual process of eating and digestion. It provides all the necessary nutrients needed for building tissue and expending energy including water, electrolytes, proteins, and lipids. TPN is often administered to premature and very low birth weight babies because they are unable to absorb nutrients through the intestinal tract. While many hospital NICUs will use a standard TPN, the composition may be customized to the individual patient, so the exact composition and concentrations cannot be predicted. Administration of TPN prior to collection of the NBS sample can make the levels of amino acids (and acylcarnitines) appear abnormally high. In certain cases, it may contaminate the NBS sample causing very high amino acid concentrations. TPN is characterized by high concentrations of several amino acids in the same sample, or an elevated amino acid result without a correspondingly elevated secondary ratio.

Immaturity of the liver may result in transient elevated amino acids, particularly tyrosine and methionine.

A number of the amino acids increase in concentration as the age of the baby at collection increases, in particular leucine and citrulline. This may be a problem for programs that obtain a repeat specimen for borderline results. It can also cause difficulties for second samples sent in response to an initial unsuitable specimen. Age-related cut-off values or the use of secondary markers might help reduce the number of false-positive results.

Samples collected before 24 hours of age are not considered reliable for the screening of amino acid disorders. When the sample is collected from a baby less than 24 hours old, it is possible that there has not been adequate time for accumulation of the biomarker. Samples collected before 24 hours of age should be regarded as unsuitable for amino acid screening and a repeat sample should be obtained. However, since the issue is inadequate marker accumulation, those samples that are collected at less than 24 hours and show obviously elevated primary and secondary markers should be considered as positive results. An NBS sample with a high phenylalanine result should be handled according to the laboratories protocols for positive samples, not as an unsuitable sample.

Low extraction efficiency of the basic amino acids, such as Cit, Arg, and Orn, can make these compounds more difficult to accurately quantitate by MS/MS. Extraction methods that use purely organic solvents, such as acetonitrile or methanol, may show a low recovery of these compounds. Extraction solvents that have some water mixed with an organic solvent may show better recovery. The basic amino acids also have lower ionization efficiencies in the mass spectrometer. For the same concentration of marker in the sample, the basic amino acids will have less response than the other amino acids. This lower signal in the mass spectrometer can make the results for Cit, Arg, and Orn more erratic and prone to false positives. The deuterated analogs used as internal standards for these compounds will show the same low-ionization efficiency. Use of repeat analysis or ratios will help mitigate some of these issues.

6.3 ORGANIC ACIDEMIAS

Organic acidemias, screened through NBS, are a group of disorders of the metabolism of the branched-chain amino acids, including, but not limited to, isoleucine, leucine, and valine. Each organic acid disorder is associated with a specific enzyme deficiency. The deficient enzymes in the metabolic pathways result in the build-up of organic acids, which are toxic. Disorders, enzyme deficiencies, and primary and secondary markers are listed in Table 6.3.

The typical presentation of these conditions is a healthy newborn who rapidly becomes ill after the first few days of life. Clinical signs and symptoms may include ketoacidosis, poor feeding, vomiting, dehydration, hypotonia, lethargy, seizures, coma, and possibly death. Organic acidemias are detected in NBS using the acylcarnitine biomarkers. As with the amino acid disorders, the best markers are those closest to the enzyme block. Secondary markers or ratios may be reaction products that will be deficient in the case of an enzyme block, or compounds that represent a surrogate internal standard in the patient's blood and provide a reference point.

Propionylcarnitine (C3) is an important biomarker for the detection of propionic acidemia (PA), methylmalonic acidemia (MUT), and the cobalamin disorders (Cbl A,B, and Cbl C,D). C3 may also be elevated in cases of multiple carboxylase deficiency (MCD). PA and severe cases of MUT may be life-threatening in the first few days of life. In general, C3 elevations are higher for cases of PA and more moderate for cases of MUT or the cobalamin defects; however, there is a good deal of overlap of the NBS C3 results for these conditions and confirmatory tests are required to accurately diagnose the correct disorder.

Secondary ratios are important in the evaluation of elevated C3. The ratios most commonly used are C3/C2 (acetylcarnitine) and C3/C16. These ratios help to relate the C3 concentration to the overall concentration of acylcarnitines in the

Table 6.3 Newborn Screening Primary and Secondary Markers for Organic Acidemias

Condition (Abbreviation)	RUSP Status	Enzyme	Primary Marker(s)	Secondary Marker(s)
Propionic acidemia (PROP)	Core Condition	Propionyl-CoA carboxylase	C3	C3/C2, C3/C16
Methylmalonic acidemia (MUT)	Core Condition	Methylmalonyl-CoA mutase	C3	C3/C2, C3/C16
Methylmalonic acidemia, Cobalamin disorders (Cbl A,B)	Core Condition	Cobalamin disorders	C3	C3/C2, C3/C16
Methylmalonic acidemia with homocystinuria (Cbl C,D)	Secondary Target	Methylmalonyl-CoA mutase and homocysteine	C3, Met (low)	C3/C2, C3/C16, C3/Met
Malonic acidemia (MAL)	Secondary Target	Malonyl-CoA decarboxylase	C3-DC	C5-DC/C3-DC (low)
Isobutyrylglycinuria (IBG)	Secondary Target	Isobutyryl-CoA dehydrogenase	C4	C4/C2, C4/C3, C4/C8
β-Ketothiolase deficiency (βKT)	Core Condition	β-Ketothiolase	C5:1, (C5-OH)	
Isovaleric acidemia (IVA)	Core Condition	Isovaleryl-CoA dehydrogenase	C5	C5/C0, C5/C2, C5/C3
2-Methylbutyrylglycinuria (2MBG)	Secondary Target	2-Methylbutyryl-CoA dehydrogenase	C5	C5/C0, C5/C2, C5/C3
3-Methylcrotonyl-CoA carboxylase (3MCC) deficiency	Core Condition	3-Methylcrotonyl-CoA carboxylase	C5-OH	C5-OH/C8, C5-OH/C0
3-Hydroxy-3-methylglutaric aciduria (HMG)	Core Condition	3-Hydroxy-3-methylglutaryl-CoA lyase	C5-OH	C5-OH/C8, C5-OH/C0
Multiple carboxylase deficiency (MCD)	Core Condition	Holocarboxylase synthetase	C5-OH, C3	C5-OH/C8, C5-OH/C0
3-Methylglutaconic acidemia type I (3MGA)	Secondary Target	3-Methylglutaconyl-CoA hydratase	C5-OH	C5-OH/C8, C5-OH/C0
2-Methyl-3-hydroxybutyric acidemia (2M3HBA)	Secondary Target	2-Methyl-3-hydroxybutyryl-CoA dehydrogenase	C5-OH, (C5:1)	C5-OH/C8, C5-OH/C0
Glutaric acidemia type I (GA I)	Core Condition	Glutaryl-CoA dehydrogenase	C5-DC	C5-DC/C8

Nomenclature for Conditions based upon "Naming and Counting Disorders (Conditions) Included in Newborn Screening Panels." Pediatrics. 2006; 117 (5) Suppl: S308–S314.

blood sample. The C3/C2 ratio may be the best marker for evaluation of true positive cases.[22] Certain methylmalonic acidemia disorders may not produce significant concentrations of C3 and will not be detected.[22]

In the case of methylmalonic acidemia with HCY (Cbl C,D deficiency), elevated C3 and C3/C2 values may be accompanied by abnormally low concentrations of the amino acid methionine for cases of Cbl, C deficiency. One can use low methione as a marker in combination with the C3 and C3/C2. If one only used a lowered C3 as a marker it would greatly increase the number of false positives. By including low Met and a lower cut-off value for C3 it is possible to capture the true positives and minimize the false positives. By using the lowered cut-off value for C3 in combination with a high C3/C2 ratio and low Met concentration, false-positive cases can be minimized and borderline true positive cases identified. In the retrospective evaluation of approximately 250,000 samples from 2008, the New York State NBS program showed a lowered C3 cut-off value would result in three additional referrals, two of which were confirmed cases of Cbl, C deficiency.[23]

Malonic acidemia (MAL), a secondary target, is indicated by a high concentration of malonylcarnitine (C3DC). The ratio of malonylcarnitine to octanoylcarnitine (C3DC/C8) is recommended as a secondary marker for evaluation of this disorder in NBS. C3DC may be elevated in some cases of medium-chain acyl-coenzyme A dehydrogenase (MCAD) deficiency. If the NBS laboratory is using an underivatized method for the determination of amino acids and acylcarnitines, C3DC, and hydroxyisobutyryl-carnitine (C4OH), the marker for medium/short-chain L-3-hydroxy acyl-coenzyme A dehydrogenase deficiency (M/SCHAD), are isobars and cannot be distinguished in the MS/MS analysis.[4] Confirmatory testing will be necessary to determine the true condition.

Isobutyrylglycinuria (IBG) is due to deficiency of the isobutyryl-CoA dehydrogenase enzyme. It is a secondary target characterized by elevations of isobutyrylcarnitine (C4). C4 and butyrylcarnitine (the primary marker for the fatty acid oxidation disorder short-chain acyl-coenzyme A dehydrogenase (SCAD) deficiency, which is also abbreviated as C4) are structural isomers that cannot be distinguished in the mass spectrometer. Therefore elevations in C4 may be indicative of two different disorders. The inability of NBS to separate these two conditions is acceptable since the purpose of screening is to identify those children who are at risk and require further evaluation. The use of ratios of the C4 marker to other short-chain acylcarnitines such as C2 or C3 can help to reduce the number of false positives. C4 may be elevated due to other conditions such as multiple acyl-CoA dehydrogenase deficiency (MADD) or carnitine supplementation. Patterns in the acylcarnitine profile may help distinguish these cases. An elevation in C4 and/or the secondary markers C4/C2, C4/C3, C4/C8 is most likely indicative of IBG or SCAD. MADD will, in general, be characterized by moderate elevations of acylcarnitines ranging from C4 to C16. Carnitine supplementation will often be characterized by significant elevations of free carnitine (C0) and more moderate elevations of short-chain acylcarnitines such as C2, C3, and C4.

β-Ketothiolase deficiency (βKT) is a core condition characterized by the elevation of tiglylcarnitine (C5:1). In some cases of βKT, hydroxyisovalerylcarnitine (C5OH) may also be elevated. In instances where C5:1 or C5OH are elevated, the concentrations of both markers should be reviewed.

Isovaleric acidemia (IVA) is a deficiency of isovaleryl-CoA dehydrogenase, an enzyme important in leucine metabolism. The primary marker for IVA is isovaleryl-carnitine (C5). Babies who have IVA may have a characteristic "sweaty feet" odor. 2-Methylbutyrylcarnitine (also abbreviated as C5) is the primary marker for 2-meth-ylbutyrylglycinuria (2MBG), a secondary target. These structural isomers both pro-duce a signal for the same reactant ion to parent ion transition in the mass spectrometer. Therefore, IVA and 2MBG cannot be differentiated by NBS and confirmatory testing is necessary. Secondary markers such as the ratios of C5/C0, C5/C2, C5/C3 are use-ful in evaluating both of these conditions. C5 may also be increased in newborns with MADD, although the acylcarnitine profile for MADD will likely include elevations of other acylcarnitine markers C4 through C16. Pivalic acid, a compound present in pharmaceutical preparations and topical creams may result in false-positive results for the C5 acylcarnitine marker.[24,25] False-positive results for this marker are more likely in babies who have very low birth weight or are premature.

3-Methylcrotonyl-CoA carboxylase (3MCC) deficiency and 3-hydroxy-3-meth-ylglutaric aciduria (HMG) are core conditions that are indicated by the elevations of C5OH. C5OH is also the primary marker for the secondary target conditions of MCD, 3-methylglutaconic acidemia type I (3MGA), and 2-methyl-3-hydroxybutyric acidemia (2M3HBA). In cases of MCD, the C3 marker may also be moderately ele-vated. The C3 marker result should be reviewed in cases of high C5OH. In cases of 2M3HBA, it is the 2-methyl-3-hydroxybutyrylcarnitine, a structural isomer of C5OH that is, in fact, increased.[26] The C5OH marker may be elevated in cases of maternal 3MCC as number of mothers have been diagnosed with 3MCC after NBS reported a high concentration of C5OH in the baby's sample. The detection of a number of asymptomatic cases of maternal 3MCC raises questions regarding the pathogenicity of this condition. However, cases of decompensation, similar to other organic aci-demias, have been reported.[27] Secondary marker ratios of C5OH/C8 and C5OH/C0 may be useful in reducing false positives.

Glutaric acidemia type I (GA-I) is a core condition resulting from a deficiency of the glutaryl-CoA dehydrogenase. GA-I is relatively rare, but more frequent in Amish popu-lations. Glutarylcarnitine (C5DC) may also be elevated in cases of MADD and occasion-ally in cases of MCAD. There is a possibility of increased C5DC in the cases of MCAD carriers. The use of the C5DC/C8 ratio as a secondary marker may help eliminate any false positives due to MCAD carriers since the C8 levels will also be slightly elevated.

6.4 FATTY ACID OXIDATION DISORDERS

Fatty acid oxidation disorders are genetic disorders that result in the inability to produce or utilize fats as an energy source in the liver or muscles. In a healthy body the usual source of energy is glucose. However, in times of fasting or stress, when all glucose in the body has been used, the body's metabolism will change to catabolism of fats as the primary source of energy. The fatty acid oxidation process involves several different enzymes that break down long-chain fats to medium-chain fats, medium-chain fats to short-chain fats, and short-chain fats to ketone bodies and acetyl-CoA. Individuals with a defect in any one of the enzymes necessary to metabolize fats are unable to use fats as an energy source with subsequent accumulation of toxic metabolites. Left untreated, symptoms may include lethargy, poor feeding, vomiting, an enlarged heart, muscle weakness, heart failure, and coma and death. The primary markers for fatty acid oxidation disorders are the acylcarnitines that accumulate, or, in the case of transport defects, may be deficient. Secondary markers are usually ratios of the accumulated acylcarnitine precursors to the deficient acylcarnitine products. A listing of conditions, enzyme defects, and markers is presented in Table 6.4.

Carnitine uptake defect (CUD) is a defect in the organic carnitine transporter 2 (OCTN2) protein that transports carnitine into the cells. When carnitine cannot be transported into the tissues, fatty acid oxidation is impeded leading to the symptoms of fatty acid oxidation disorders. CUD is detected in NBS as a low level of free carnitine or acylcarnitines. The primary marker is a low value for free carnitine (C0). Secondary markers are low values for other acylcarnitines such as C2, C3, C16, and C18. Detection of CUD can be difficult since some true cases will have carnitine values that are not dramatically low but are close to the laboratory cut-off. Many TPN formulations do not contain carnitine. Therefore, prolonged administration of TPN can deplete free carnitine in the baby. Repeat specimens from low birth weight or premature babies very often show low levels of free carnitine. In addition, values of the long-chain acylcarnitines decrease with age, making the evaluation of premature babies on TPN that are much more difficult.[28]

SCAD is a defect in the short-chain acyl-CoA dehydrogenase enzyme. The deficiency of this enzyme leads to an inability to metabolize the short-chain fatty acids causing an accumulation of butyrylcarnitine (C4). The primary marker is butyrylcarnitine, which in the mass spectrometer cannot be differentiated from its structural isomer isobutyrylcarnitine. Secondary markers ratios include the ratios C4/C2, C4/C3, C4/C8. The use of the ratios C4/C2 and C4/C3 can help eliminate false positives due to an increase in short-chain acylcarnitines caused by carnitine supplements. Since most infants with SCAD, identified through NBS programs, have been well at the time of diagnosis and asymptomatic relatives who meet the diagnostic criteria are reported, the evidence suggests that SCAD as diagnosed by NBS presents as a largely benign condition.[29–31] The clinical significance of this disorder remains a subject of considerable controversy.

MCAD deficiency is a defect in the MCAD enzyme. This enzyme deficiency leads to an inability to metabolize medium-chain fatty acids causing an accumulation medium-chain acylcarnitines (C6 to C10). MCAD is the most commonly occurring inborn error of fatty acid oxidation.[32] In the United States the incidence is estimated to be approximately 1:16,000 live births.[33] The symptoms of MCAD may appear in early infancy and include vomiting, lethargy, and hypoglycemia. In times of stress or fasting, babies with MCAD are at risk of seizures, brain damage, coma, and sudden death.

The primary markers for MCAD include C6, C8, C10, and C10:1. There is some overlap of activity with the short-chain and long-chain acyl-CoA dehydrogenases so that C6 and C10 may be metabolized to some extent. In most cases, the C8 acylcarnitine will show the most accumulation. However, the severity of the disease may

Table 6.4 Newborn Screening Primary and Secondary Markers for Fatty Acid Oxidation (FAO) Disorders

Condition (Abbreviation)	RUSP Status	Enzyme	Primary Marker(s)	Secondary Marker(s)
Carnitine uptake defect/carnitine transport defect (CUD)	Core Condition	Plasma membrane carnitine transporter	C0 (low)	C2 (low), C3 (low), C16 (low), C18 (low), C18:1 (low)
Carnitine palmitoyltransferase type I deficiency (CPT IA)	Secondary Target	Carnitine palmitoyltransferase IA	C0, C16 (low), C18 (low), C18:1 (low)	C0/(C16+C18)
Short-chain acyl-CoA dehydrogenase (SCAD) deficiency	Secondary Target	Short-chain acyl-CoA dehydrogenase	C4	C4/C2, C4/C3, C4/C8
Medium/Short-chain 3-hydroxy acyl-CoA dehydrogenase (M/SCHAD) deficiency	Secondary Target	Medium/short-chain L-3-hydroxy acyl-CoA dehydrogenase	C4-OH, C6-OH	C4-OH/C16, C4-OH/C8, C4-OH/C4
Multiple acyl-CoA dehydrogenase deficiency (MADD, GA-II)	Secondary Target	Electron transfer flavoprotein [ETF; α, β subunit]	C4-C18	All ratios applicable to the primary markers
Medium-chain acyl-CoA dehydrogenase (MCAD) deficiency	Core Condition	Medium-chain acyl-CoA dehydrogenase	C8, C6, C10	C8/C2, C8/C10
Medium-chain ketoacyl-CoA thiolase (MCAT) deficiency	Secondary Target	Medium-chain ketoacyl-CoA thiolase	C8, C10	
2,4-Dienoyl-CoA reductase (DE RED) deficiency	Secondary Target	2,4-Dienoyl-CoA reductase	C10:2	
Very long-chain acyl-CoA dehydrogenase (VLCAD) deficiency	Core Condition	Very long-chain acyl-CoA dehydrogenase	C14:1, C14, C14:2, C12:1, C12	C14:1/C2, C14:1/C16, C14:1/C12:1
Carnitine palmitoyltransferase type II (CPT II) deficiency	Secondary Target	Carnitine palmitoyltransferase II	C14, C16, C18, C16:1, C18:2, C18:1	(C16+C18:1)/C2, C0/(C16+C18) (low), C3/C16 (low)
Carnitine-acylcarnitine translocase (CACT) deficiency	Secondary Target	Carnitine-acylcarnitine translocase	C14, C16, C18, C16:1, C18:2, C18:1	(C16+C18:1)/C2, C0/(C16+C18) (low), C3/C16 (low)
Long-chain L-3-hydroxy acyl-CoA dehydrogenase (LCHAD) deficiency	Core Condition	Long-chain L-3-hydroxy acyl-CoA dehydrogenase	C16-OH, C18:1-OH,	C16-OH/C16, C16-OH/C14
Trifunctional protein (TFP) deficiency	Core Condition	Trifunctional protein [α, β subunit]	C16-OH, C18:1-OH,	C16-OH/C16, C16-OH/C14

Nomenclature for Conditions based upon "Naming and Counting Disorders (Conditions) Included in Newborn Screening Panels." Pediatrics. 2006; 117 (5) Suppl: S308–S314.

not correlate with the concentration of C8 in the NBS sample. Secondary markers include the ratios C8/C2 and C8/C10. Two additional analytes, C3DC and C5DC, are elevated in cases of MCAD deficiency. The presence or absence of C3DC and C5DC does not rule out the risk of MCAD for a sample that has a high C8 value.

Medium-chain triglyceride (MCT) oil is a nutritional supplement used for treating food absorption disorders or added to TPN as a source of fat. The administration of MCT oil to a baby as a nutritional supplement may raise the concentrations of the MCTs and lead to false positives.[6] Certain drugs such as valproate may also interfere. The MCT oil and valproate interferences may be distinguished by the C8/C10 ratio.[34] In true cases of MCAD the C8/C10 ratio is significantly increased, but this same ratio is not significantly increased in patients receiving valproate or MCT oil.

There is the possibility of interfering substances in the blood at high concentration that have a minor fragmentation pathway that will mimic the analyte of interest.[6] This may not be recognized as an interferant if the lab is using a selective reaction monitoring rather than a scanning mode for analysis.[4] An unknown substance has been reported with a mass-to-charge ratio (m/z) of 343. The isotope of this ion, at m/z 344, will interfere with the detection of C8. If this interferant is present, and if the laboratory is using a scanning mode, the result will be a false positive for C8.[6]

A false negative may result, if the newborn suffers from a deficiency of free carnitine (C0). This is due to the fact that there may not be sufficient free carnitine available to complex with the medium-chain C8 fatty acid and form octanoylcarnitine. In this case, the C8 levels may be within the laboratory's reference range even for a true case of MCAD. The use of the secondary ratio C8/C2 should help mitigate this problem and should flag any such samples for additional review. Any samples with a high C8/C2 ratio, low C0, and a borderline or slightly high C8 level should be reviewed carefully.

The age of the baby when the NBS sample is collected may also affect the C8 concentration. The concentrations of acylcarnitines in the blood decrease rapidly with age.[28] Age-related cut-off values should be used for the evaluation of MCAD and the other fatty acid oxidation disorders.

Secondary targets MADD (also called GA-II) and MCKAT will be also detected by elevations of the medium-chain acylcarnitines including C8. Screening will not be able to differentiate/diagnose these different conditions. Confirmatory testing is required.

MADD, also called GA-II, is a deficiency of the electron transfer flavoprotein-dehydrogenase. This enzyme transfers electrons from electron-transferring flavoprotein in the mitochondrial matrix, to the ubiquinone pool in the inner mitochondrial membrane. A defect in this enzyme will result in a wider range of elevated acylcarnitines than MCAD. In cases of MADD, acylcarnitines from C4 to C16 may appear elevated and, in general, the levels will not be as high as might be expected with an MCAD. The name, GA-II, is somewhat misleading since C5DC may or may not be elevated in true cases. In the most severe cases of MADD, affected individuals may also be born with physical abnormalities including brain malformations, an enlarged liver (hepatomegaly), a weakened and enlarged heart (dilated cardiomyopathy), and unusual facial features.

M/SCHAD is a deficiency of the medium/short-chain L-3-hydroxy acyl-CoA dehydrogenase enzyme. The primary markers are hydroxybutyrylcarnitine (C4OH) and hydroxyhexanoylcarnitine (C6OH).

2,4-Dienoyl-CoA reductase deficiency is a very rare condition as only two cases have been reported. The first case was reported in 1990.[35] The second case was reported in 2014.[36] The disease is caused by a defect in the 2,4 dienoyl-CoA reductase enzyme. The primary marker is decadienoylcarnitine (C10:2). Elevated concentrations of this marker may also be detected in newborns to whom MCT oil has been administered as a dietary supplement.

Very long-chain acyl-CoA dehydrogenase (VLCAD) deficiency is a deficiency of the very long-chain Acyl-CoA dehydrogenase enzyme required to break down very long-chain fatty acids. The primary markers for this condition are the acylcarnitines C14:1 (tetradecenoylcarnitine), and C14 (tetradecanoylcarnitine). Other useful markers include C12:1, C12, C14:2. Secondary markers include the ratios C14:1/C2, C14:1/C12:1, and C14:1/C16. There is a good deal of overlap among the markers and conditions for the long-chain fatty acid oxidation disorders. Other long-chain acylcarnitines that may be increased in cases of VLCAD include C16, C18:1, C18. The C14 and C14:1 markers may be elevated in other fatty acid oxidation disorders such as MADD, carnitine palmitoyltransferase II (CPT-II), carnitine-acylcarnitine translocase (CACT), or LCHAD/TPP. Levels of C14 and C14:1 decrease rapidly with age (after 7 days). Collection of a repeat specimen for borderline results therefore is not recommended. All positive results for VLCAD and the other long-chain fatty acid oxidation disorders should be referred for confirmatory testing.

The enzymes CPT-II and CACT are part of the carnitine shuttle system. CACT aids in the transport of long-chain acylcarnitines into the mitochondria. In the mitochondria, CPT-II dissociates the acylcarnitine complex and the fatty acid is bound to CoA. Free carnitine is transported back across the mitochondrial membrane. In CPT-II deficiency and CACT deficiency, there is a failure of the transport mechanism of the long-chain fatty acids into the mitochondria for metabolism. The result is an accumulation of long-chain fatty acids and long-chain acylcarnitines and a depletion of free carnitine. Useful markers for the NBS for these two conditions are elevations of the long-chain acylcarnitines C14, C16, C18, C16:1, C18:2, C18:1. and low C2. The most useful secondary markers are the ratios of short chain or free carnitine to long-chain acylcarnitines. Secondary ratios that have been reported include high (C16+C18:1)/C2 ratios, low C0/(C16+C18) ratios, and low C3/C16 ratios. As with VLCAD there is a significant overlap with other long-chain fatty acid oxidation disorders. And, as with VLCAD, levels of long chain fatty acids may decrease very rapidly with age (after 7 days). Collection of a repeat specimen for borderline results is not recommended. All positive results should be referred for confirmatory testing. False negatives may be seen in cases of secondary carnitine deficiency. If there is a deficiency of free carnitine, there may not be sufficient free carnitine available to complex with the long-chain fatty acids to form the long-chain acylcarnitines. The use of the secondary ratios should help mitigate this problem.

The enzyme carnitine palmitoyltransferase I (CPT-I) catalyzes the transfer of the acyl group of a long-chain fatty acyl-CoA from coenzyme A to free carnitine. A defect in this enzyme will therefore lead to an accumulation of free carnitine, because there will be no formation of the long-chain acylcarnitines, and a subsequent deficit of the long-chain acylcarnitines. CPT-I deficiency is a rare disorder that may be more common in Inuit populations. The NBS profile for CPT-I deficiency will therefore appear as an excess of free carnitine (C0) and a deficiency of the long-chain acylcarnitines (C16, C18:1, C18). Specificity for the detection of CPT-I deficiency may be improved by use of the ratio C0/(C16+C18) as the primary marker.[37] It should be kept in mind that C16 and C18 will decrease rapidly with age while C0 remains relatively constant. Age-related cut-offs are recommended.

Long-chain 3-hydroxyacyl CoA dehydrogenase/trifunctional protein deficiency (LCHAD/TFP) is a defect in the mitochondrial trifunctional protein, which catalyzes three of the four steps in β-oxidation. The primary markers for LCHAD/TFP are C16OH and C18:1OH. Other hydroxylated long-chain acylcarnitine markers including C14OH, C16:1OH, C18OH, and C18:2OH may also be elevated. In cases of LCHAD, there may be increases in C14, C16, C18, or C18:1. NBS cannot differentiate between LCHAD and TFP deficiency.

6.5 REGION 4 STORK

The Region 4 Stork (R4S) consortium is a collaboration of 47 US states and Puerto Rico and 80 programs in 45 countries.[38] The Region 4 Genetics Collaborative was funded by the Health Resources and Services Administration from 2003 to 2012 and since 2012 by the Newborn Screening Translational Research Network, funded by the Eunice Kennedy Shriver National Institute of Child Health and Human Development. The consortium collects amino acid and acylcarnitine profiles data from patients affected with metabolic disorders as well as profiles for other disorders. The Mayo Clinic of Rochester, MN, has been instrumental in developing, organizing, and maintaining software for the evaluation of data contained in this database. As of December 15, 2011, the MS/MS profiles of 12,077 patients affected with 60 metabolic disorders, along with 644 heterozygote carriers for 12 conditions has been collected in the database.[39] True positive cases are defined by the participants according to the established local protocols and/or professional guidelines.[38] Normal profiles are based on cumulative percentiles of amino acids and acylcarnitines in DBSs of approximately 25–30 million normal newborns.[38] The cumulative results collected by the project have generated 91 high and 23 low cut-off target ranges and related ratios for amino acids, acylcarnitines for 64 conditions. Since so much data is collected for confirmed cases, analyte ranges may be calculated for both normal patients and those affected with an inborn error of metabolism. The effectiveness of markers and ratios may be evaluated on the basis of the degree of separation or overlap between the normal and disease ranges. Better markers show more separation between the disease and normal ranges. As an example, the useful acylcarnitine markers for the evaluation of β-ketothiolase (BKT) are shown in Fig. 6.3.[38] What develops from this analysis is a pattern of results rather than a single cut-off value of a single marker.

The key element of this project, which is now integrated into the Newborn Screening Translational Research Network, is freely available, on-demand access to the R4S website (http://www.clir-r4s.org). This website contains a number of tools and applications. Once logged in, users have access to profiles unique to their screening program for data submission and to comparison tools, as well as to common

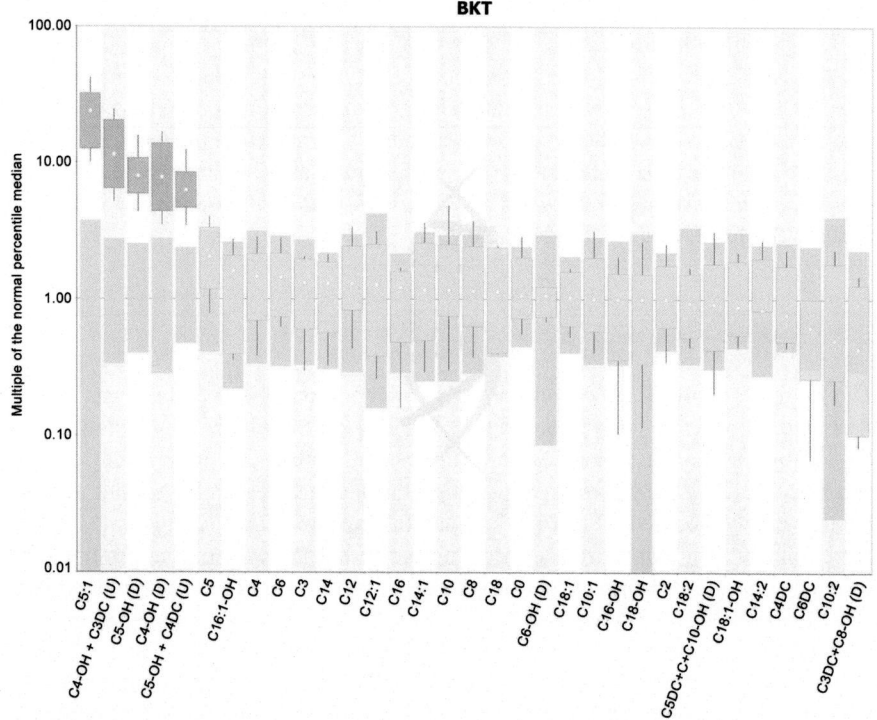

FIGURE 6.3

R4S plot by condition for β-ketothiolase (BKT) deficiency. This plot converts each case value to the corresponding multiple of the cumulative median (MoM). Each box represents the interval between the 10 and 90 percentile, the upper and lower lines extend to the 99 percentile and 1 percentile, respectively. The median is shown as a white circle in the body of the box. Color-coding: red: disorder ranges of informative markers; gray: disorder range of uninformative markers; and green: range of normal population. Abbreviations are listed in the legend of Table 6.1.

Re-used with permission from McHugh DMS, Cameron CA, Abdenu JE, Abdulrahman M, Adair O, Al Nuaimi SA, et al. Clinical validation of cutoff target ranges in newborn screening of metabolic disorders by tandem mass spectrometry: a worldwide collaborative project. Genet Med 2011;13(3):230–54.

folders inclusive of more than 30 project tools and reports. Users may access the website to assess their cut-off values (compare cut-off values to disease ranges), compare their normal percentiles to other labs, compare their cut-off values to other labs, and evaluate the effectiveness of markers for particular conditions. As an illustration, the analyte comparison tool is shown in Fig. 6.4 for the Phe analyte.[38] The analyte comparison tool shows the cumulative normal percentiles for Phe, the percentiles for each program submitting normal results, cut-off values for Phe used by

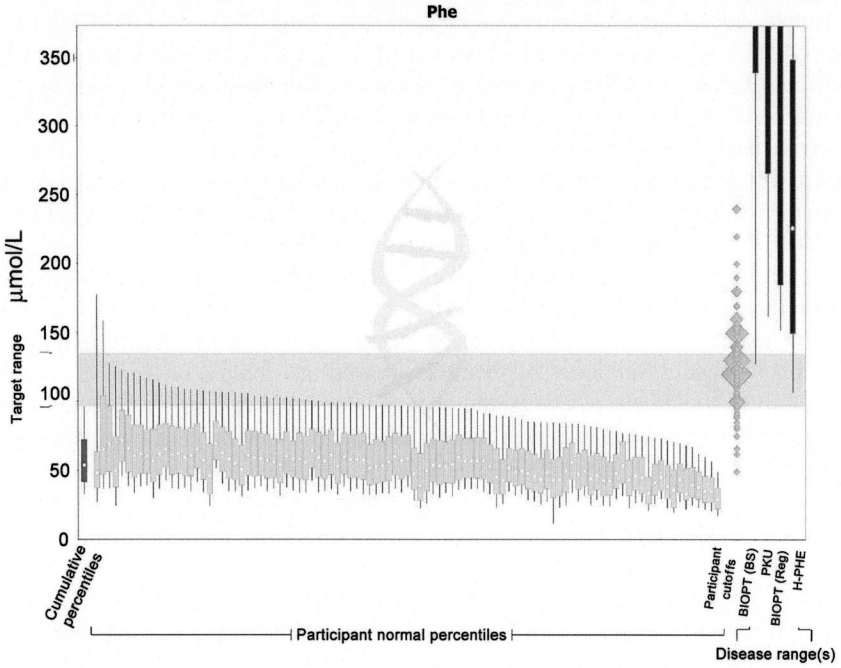

FIGURE 6.4

R4S analyte comparison tool for the amino acid phenylalanine in neonatal dried blood spots. Each box represents the interval between the 10 and 90 percentile, the upper and lower lines extend to the 99 percentile and 1 percentile, respectively. The median is shown as a white circle in the body of the box. Color coding: dark green: cumulative percentiles; light green: percentiles of individual participants, sorted in descending order of the 99 percentile value; orange: cut-off target range (see text for details); light blue diamonds: actual cut-off values of participants; the marker size is proportional to the number of laboratories using the same value; and bright red bars: disorder ranges (partially hidden by *Y*-axis reduction to allow the normal percentiles to be visible). Abbreviations are listed in the legend of Table 6.2.

*Re-used with permission from McHugh DMS, Cameron CA, Abdenu JE, Abdulrahman M, Adair O, Al Nuaimi SA, et al. Clinical validation of cutoff target ranges in newborn screening of metabolic disorders by tandem mass spectrometry: a worldwide collaborative project. Genet Med 2011;**13**(3):230–54.*

programs submitting data, the recommended range for Phe cut-off values based on the project data, and the range of results for confirmed cases of PKU, HPHE, and Biopterin deficiency. Using this tool, a program can assess how their cut-offs and normal values compare to other programs in the R4S collaboration.

Other tools available include condition-specific, postanalytical tools designed to interpret analyte profiles of a single case.[39] These tools generate a composite score driven by the degree of overlap between a normal population and a disease range. Site-specific customization of these tools is available to correct for differences in analyte panels and sample preparation (derivatized vs underivatized method). For example, eight different amino acids are considered informative for OTC/CPS. Users can build custom tools based on analytes available in their profile, but fewer analytes will result in a loss of sensitivity and specificity. Condition-specific tools may be set up by each program to account for analyte profiles (missing analytes) or method (derivatized or underivatized). The user may change between cumulative normal values and program-specific normal values to account for program differences in normal value. An example of the postanalytical tool for the evaluation of ASA is shown in Fig. 6.5.[39] The result provided shows the degree of penetration into the disease range for each informative analyte and marker, and the degree of overlap between each marker and the normal range.

An examination of VLCAD screen positive cases from the Western States Regional Genetics Services Collaborative showed that the use of the R4S postanalytical tools could help reduce the number of false-positive samples.[40] Other postanalytical tools are available such as a two-condition tool to generate a score and suggest interpretation guidelines for a specific condition and a direct comparison with a second related condition. A multiple conditions tool generates a score and suggests interpretation guidelines for a specific condition and a direct comparison with multiple other conditions.

R4S has developed additional tools (tool runner), which may be used to upload and process large numbers of samples and calculate composite scores for all available tools for each case within the batch in real time.[39] A retrospective review of 176,186 subjects born in California between January 1 and June 30, 2012 showed that the utilization of the R4S tools could reduce the false-positive rate and improve the positive predictive value.[41]

6.6 GALACTOSEMIA

Galactosemia is a metabolic disorder that affects an individual's ability to metabolize the sugar galactose. Galactose-1-phosphate (Gal-1-P), the activated metabolite of galactose is highly toxic. Newborn babies affected with galactosemia are typically symptomatic in the first few days of life. Symptoms include lethargy, vomiting, failure to thrive, and jaundice. If left untreated, the disease will rapidly progress to liver and kidney failure. Death may occur within two weeks generally from septicemia, although some affected babies may survive 2–3 years before developing

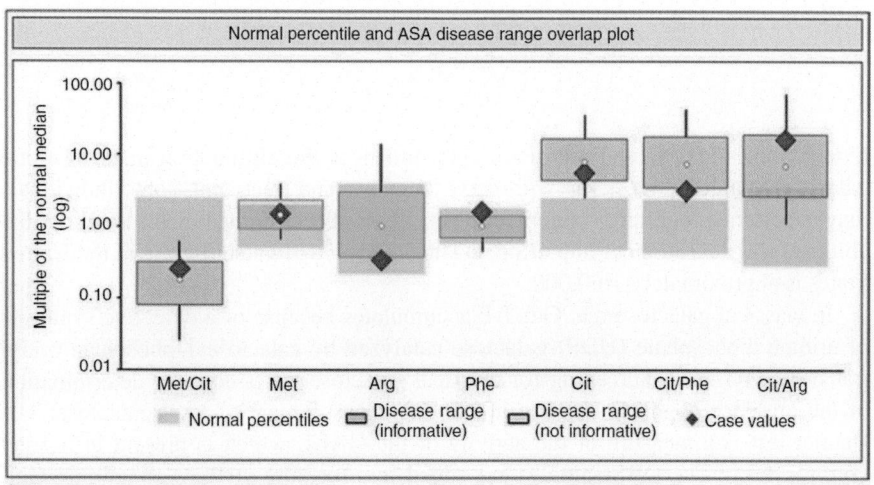

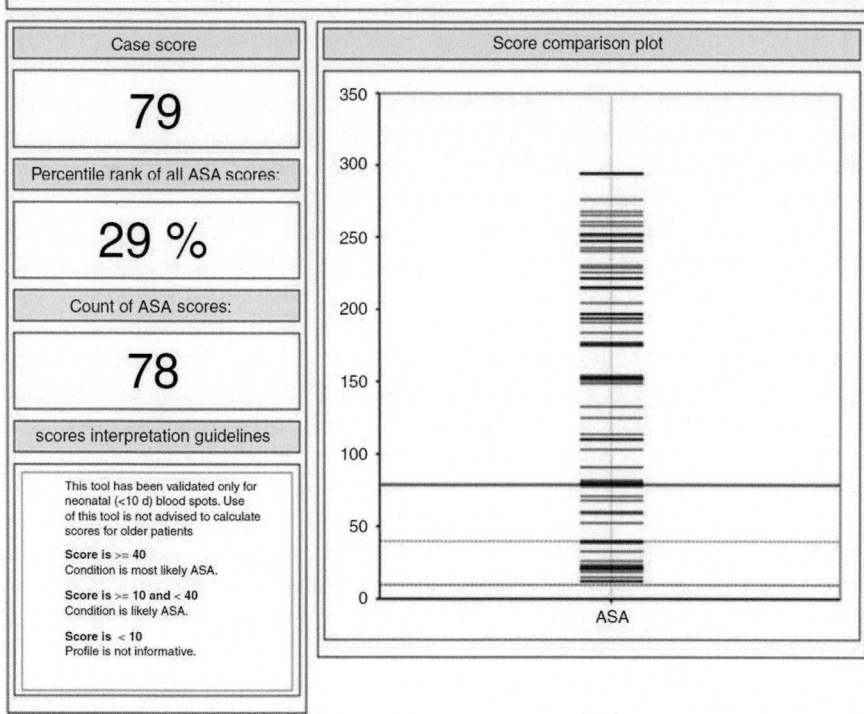

FIGURE 6.5

Partial display of the tool for argininosuccinic acid (ASA) lyase deficiency (two of the three panels). This case was considered not informative on the basis of a cut-off for citrulline set inappropriately high. The top panel is an overlay graph of normal population, disease range, and the values entered to calculate a score. All values are expressed as µmol/L and converted to multiples of the normal median on a log scale. The bottom panel shows the calculated score, the percentile rank comparison to all available scores and the case count along with a graphic display of all available scores for the chosen condition, and a summary of interpretation guidelines.

liver cirrhosis and mental retardation. Treatment is the elimination of lactose and galactose from the diet. Even with early diagnosis and treatment, some individuals may experience long-term complications such as speech impediment, learning disabilities, and neurological impairment. This incidence of galactosemia in the United States is approximately 1:60,000.

In classical galactosemia, Gal-1-P accumulates because of a defective synthesis of uridine diphosphate (UDP)-galactose catalyzed by galactose-1-phosphate uridyl transferase (GALT). Screening for classical galactosemia is done by determination of the presence of the GALT enzyme and/or measurement of total galactose. The Beutler test is a measure of the activity of the GALT, which is present in normal erythrocytes.[42] The DBS samples are added to a reaction mixture containing Gal-1-P, UDPG (uridine-5-diphosphoglucose), NADP (nicotinamide adenine dinucleotide phosphate, also called TP, not to be confused with TPN), buffer, and a reagent to hemolyze the red cells. If GALT is present, UDPG and Gal-1-P react to form glucose-1-phosphate. This is transformed by phosphoglucomutase, which is present in the sample, to α-glucose-6-phosphate. α-Glucose-6-phosphate mutorotates completely spontaneously and with the help of phosphohexose isomerase to β-glucose-6-phosphate. Glucose-6-phosphate dehydrogenase, present in the samples, oxidizes β-glucose-6-phosphate to 6-phosphogluconate, which is, in turn, oxidized to ribulose-5-phosphate. Both these steps result in the reduction of TPN. Reduced TPN fluoresces brightly when activated with long-wavelength UV light. This test may be readily adapted to the high sample volumes required for NBS. The materials for the method are commercially available. In-house methods may be set up and validated by the screening programs. In-house methods often treat the results as qualitative, reporting the enzyme as either present or absent. Commercial kits that automate the method and quantitate the amount of enzyme activity present are also available.

A large number of mutations have been reported for the GALT gene. One particular mutation is known as the Duarte variant. This variant is associated with an approximately 50% reduction in enzyme activity; individuals who carry this mutation are usually not symptomatic. Even compound heterozygotes with a second more severe mutation on the second allele may have sufficient enzyme activity so that dietary intervention is not necessary. Those NBS programs that use qualitative methods to determine the presence or absence of the GALT enzyme may miss individuals who have the Duarte variant and therefore have enough GALT enzyme activity to test negative for galactosemia.

Several factors in testing may lead to false-negative results. Newborns who may have received transfusions cannot be reliably screened by this method as enough enzyme to test negative for galactosemia may be transferred from the donor blood. If a transfusion is known or suspected, samples should be tested for total galactose. Although active enzyme contributed by donor blood may cause a false-negative result for the Beutler test, it will likely not be enough to achieve a normal level of total galactose. Results for total galactose will be elevated even though there is apparently active enzyme present.

False-positive results may be caused by mishandling of the samples, such as exposure to heat, or organic solvents (possibly in preparing the site of the heel stick to obtain the sample) that will denature the GALT enzyme.

Two other enzyme deficiencies in the conversion of galactose to glucose are not detected by the Beutler test and can lead to galactosemia. Galactokinase (GALK) deficiency is the mildest form, the chief symptom being cataract formation as elevated galactose is reduced to galactitol in the lens. Galactose-4-epimerase (GALE) deficiency, the rarest form, is in most cases a biochemical abnormality with no clinical symptoms. However, a more severe form of this disorder has been reported presenting with symptoms similar to those of classical galactosemia. GALE and GALK are both secondary targets on the RUSP.

Detection of all three recommended enzyme deficiencies can be accomplished by screening all samples for total galactose. Commercial kits that automate the method and quantitate the amount of total galactose present are available from several vendors. While the determination of total galactose is not prone to the false negatives that may be caused by transfusion or to the false positives that may be caused by mishandling of the samples, there are some difficulties. A false-negative result may be observed if the baby has not fed sufficiently for total galactose to accumulate or if the baby is fed a lactose-free product such as soy milk. A number of NBS programs measure both GALT enzyme and total galactose for all samples.

6.7 BIOTINIDASE DEFICIENCY

The biotinidase enzyme catalyzes the release of biotin from dietary and endogenous protein. A defect in the biotinidase enzyme causes a deficiency of free biotinidase. Symptoms of profound biotinidase deficiency, the most severe form of the condition, usually appear in the first few months of life and may include seizures, developmental delay, weak muscle tone, hearing and vision loss, uncoordinated movement, skin rash, and hair loss. Profound biotinidase deficiency is generally characterized by an enzyme activity of less than 10% of normal. Partial biotinidase deficiency, a milder form of the condition, may only cause these symptoms in times of stress or illness. Profound biotinidase deficiency affects about 1 in 130,000 births (worldwide). The overall incidence of profound biotinidase deficiency together with partial biotinidase deficiency is approximately 1 in 60,000 births (worldwide). Treatment is oral supplementation with biotin. If treated prior to the onset of symptoms, most people with biotinidase deficiency are asymptomatic.

A semiquantitative colorimetric screening test for biotinidase activity was developed by Heard and Wolf.[43] An aqueous solution of biotin-4-amidobenzoic acid is added to DBS samples as a substrate. The biotinidase enzyme is extracted from the DBS by the substrate solution and reacts with the substrate to produce a reaction product containing a free primary aromatic amino group. After an incubation period the enzyme reaction is stopped. A colorimetric reaction then detects the presence of any free primary aromatic amino groups in the sample. Samples containing

Table 6.5 Newborn Screening Primary and Secondary Markers for Other Inherited Metabolic Disorders

Condition (Abbreviation)	RUSP Status	Enzyme	Primary Marker(s)	Secondary Marker(s)
Biotinidase Deficiency	Core Condition	Biotinidase	Biotinidase enzyme	
Galactosemia, Classical	Core Condition	Galactose-1-phosphate uridyl transferase	GALT enzyme, Total Galactose	
Galactokinase Deficiency (GALK)	Secondary Target	Galactokinase	Total Galactose	
Galactoepimerase Deficiency (GALE)	Secondary Target	Galactose-4-epimerase	Total Galactose	

a free primary aromatic amino group, indicating the presence of the biotinidase enzyme, will turn purple. Samples with no free primary aromatic amino groups (enzyme reaction products) will remain brown or straw-colored. The materials for the method are commercially available and the analysis lends itself to the high volumes necessary for NBS (up to 2000 samples per day can be processed by a single analyst). As with GALT testing for galactosemia, in-house methods often treat the results as qualitative, reporting the enzyme as either present or absent. Cases of partial biotinidase deficiency may be missed by qualitative methods. Commercial kits that automate the method and quantitate the amount of enzyme activity present are also available.

False-positive results may be caused by mishandling of the samples such as exposure to heat, or organic solvents (possibly in preparing the site of the heel stick to obtain the sample) that will denature the biotinidase enzyme. False-negative results may be caused by blood transfusion or the administration of drugs containing a free primary aromatic amine group (Table 6.5).

6.8 CONCLUSION

NBS for IMDs includes over 45 different core and secondary conditions. The primary purpose of NBS is to identify those babies who may be at risk for a metabolic disorder receive treatment or further testing. A number of the IMDs are immediately life-threatening; therefore, there is an emphasis on time analysis and reporting. While some of the condition such as biotinidase deficiency or galactosemia are based on a single test for a single biomarker, the use of MS/MS for most of the metabolic disorders has significantly changed the scope of NBS. MS/MS is a true multiplex method capable of quantitating over 50 analytes from a single analysis of a single sample. Evaluation of the results has become a matter of pattern recognition rather than a single out-of-range analyte.

REFERENCES

1. Watson AS, Mann MY, Lloyd-Puryear MA, Rinaldo P, Howell RR. Newborn screening: toward a uniform panel and system. *Genet Med* 2006;**8**(Suppl 1):1S–11S.
2. Advisory Committee on Heritable Disorders in Newborns and Children. Recommended Uniform Screening Panel (as of March 2015). US Department of Health and Human Services. <http://www.hrsa.gov/advisorycommittees/mchbadvisory/heritabledisorders/recommendedpanel> (accessed 25.11.15).
3. CLSI. Blood Collection on Filter Paper for Newborn Screening Programs; Approved Standard - Sixth Edition. CLSI document NBS01-A6, vol 29, No. 25, Wayne, PA. Clinical and Laboratory Standards Institute, 2013.
4. CLSI. Newborn Screening by Tandem Mass Spectrometry; Approved Guideline. CLSI document NBS04-A, vol 29, No. 25, Wayne, PA. Clinical and Laboratory Standards Institute, 2010.
5. Zytkovicz TH, Fitzgerald EF, Marsden D, Larson CA, Shih VE, Johnson DM, et al. Tandem mass spectrometric analysis for amino, organic, and fatty acid disorders in newborn dried blood spots: a two-year summary from the New England Newborn Screening Program. *Clin Chem* 2001;**47**:1945–55.
6. Chace DH, Theodore A, Kalas TA, Naylor EW. Use of tandem mass spectrometry for multianalyte screening of dried blood specimens from newborns. *Clin Chem* 2003;**49**(11):1797–817.
7. Frazier DM, Millington DS, McCandless SE, Koeberl DD, Weavil SD, Chaing SH, et al. The tandem mass spectrometry newborn screening experience in North Carolina: 1997–2005. *J Inherit Metab Dis* 2006;**29**:76–85.
8. Rashed MS, Ozand PT, Bucknall MP, Little D. Diagnosis of inborn errors of metabolism from blood spots by acylcarnitines and amino acids profiling using automated electrospray tandem mass spectrometry. *Pediatr Res* 1995;**38**(3):324–31.
9. Chace DH, Sherwin JE, Hillman SL, Lorey F, Cunningham GC. Use of phenylalanine-to-tyrosine ratio determined by tandem mass spectrometry to improve newborn screening for phenylketonuria. *Clin Chem* 2003;**49**(11):1813–4.
10. Oglesbee D, Sanders KA, Lacey JM, Magera MJ, Casetta B, Strauss KA, et al. Second-tier test for quantification of alloisoleucine and branched-chain amino acids in dried blood spots to improve newborn screening for maple syrup urine disease (MSUD). *Clin Chem* 2008;**54**(3):542–9.
11. Chace DH, Hillman SL, Millington DS, Kahler SG, Adam BW, Levy HL. Rapid diagnosis of homocystinuria and other hypermethioninemias from newborns' blood spots by tandem mass spectrometry. *Clin Chem* 1996;**42**(3):349–55.
12. Peterschmitt MJ, Simmons JR, Levy HL. Reduction of false negative results in screening of newborns for homocystinuria. *N Engl J Med* 1999;**341**(21):1572–6.
13. Mitchell GM, Grompe M, Lambert M. Tanguay RM. Hypertyrosinemia 8th ed. Scriver C.R.Beaudet AL, Sly WS, Valle D, editors. *The metabolic and molecular bases of inherited disease*, **Vol. 2**. New York: McGraw-Hill; 2001. p. 1777–805.
14. Holme E, Lindstedt S. Diagnosis and management of tyrosinemia type I. *Curr Opin Pediatr* 1995;**7**:726–32.
15. Kvittingen EA. Tyrosinemia type I: an update. *J Inherit Metab Dis* 1991;**14**:554–62.
16. Schulze A, Frommhold D, Hoffmann GF, Mayatepek E. Spectrophotometric microassay for delta-aminolevulinate dehydratase in dried-blood spots as confirmation for hereditary tyrosinemia type I. *Clin Chem* 2001;**47**:1424–9.

17. Morrissey MA, Sunny S, Fahim A, Lubowski C, Caggana M. Newborn screening for Tyr-I: Two years' experience of the New York State program. *Mol Genet Metab* 2011;**103**:191–2.

18. Turgeon C, Magera MJ, Allard P, Tortorelli S, Gavrilov D, Oglesbee D, et al. Combined determination of succinylacetone, amino acids and acylcarnitines in dried blood spots for newborn screening. *Clin Chem* 2008;**4**:657–64.

19. Dhillon K, Bhandal A, Aznar CP, Lorey F, Neogi P. Improved tandem mass spectrometry (MS/MS) derivatized method for the detection of tyrosinemia type I, amino acids and acylcarnitine disorders using a single extraction process. *Clinica Chimica Acta* 2011;**412**(11–12):873–9.

20. Mew NA, Lanpher BC, Gropman A, Chapman KA, Simpson KL, Urea Cycle Disorders Consortium, et al. Urea Cycle Disorders Overview. *GeneReviews®* [Internet]. Seattle, WA: Copyright University of Washington. Initial Posting: April 29, 2003; Last Revision: April 9, 2015. <http://www.ncbi.nlm.nih.gov/books/NBK1217/>; 1993–2016 (accessed 19.11.15).

21. Sokoro AA, Lepage J, Antonishyn N, McDonald R, Rockman-Greenberg C, Irvine J, et al. Diagnosis and high incidence of hyperornithinemia-hyperammonemia-homocitrullinemia (HHH) syndrome in northern Saskatchewan. *J Inherit Metab Dis* 2010;**33**(S3): S275–81. http://dx.doi.org/10.1007/s10545-010-9148-9.

22. Chace DH, DiPerna JC, Kalas TA, Johnson RW, Naylor EW. Rapid diagnosis of methylmalonic and propionic acidemias: quantitative tandem mass spectrometric analysis of propionylcarnitine in filter-paper blood specimens obtained from newborns. *Clin Chem* 2001;**47**:2040–4.

23. Weisfeld-Adams JD, Morrissey MA, Kirmse BM, Salveson BR, Wasserstein MP, McGuire PJ, et al. Newborn screening and early biochemical follow-up in combined methylmalonic aciduria and homocystinuria, cblC type, and utility of methionine as a secondary screening analyte. *Mol Genet Metab* 2010;**99**(2):116–23. http://dx.doi. org/10.1016/j.ymgme.2009.09.008.

24. Abdenur JE, Chamoles NA, Guinle AE, Schenone AB, Fuertes AN. Diagnosis of isovaleric acidaemia by tandem mass spectrometry: false positive result due to pivaloylcarnitine in a newborn screening programme. *J Inherit Metab Dis* 1998;**21**:624–30.

25. Boemer F, Schoos R, de Halleux V, Kalenga M, Debray FG. Surprising causes of C5-carnitine false positive results in newborn screening. *Mol Genet Metab* 2014;**111**(1):52–4. http://dx.doi.org/10.1016/j.ymgme.2013.11.005. Epub 2013 Nov 19.

26. Zschocke J, Ruiter JP, Brand J, Lindner M, Hoffmann GF, Wanders RJ, et al. Progressive infantile neurodegeneration caused by 2-methyl-3-hydroxybutyryl-CoA dehydrogenase deficiency: a novel inborn error of branched-chain fatty acid and isoleucine metabolism. *Pediatr Res* 2000;**48**:852–5.

27. Grünert SC, Stucki M, Morscher RJ, Suormala T, Bürer C, Burda P, et al. 3-methylcrotonyl-CoA carboxylase deficiency: Clinical, biochemical, enzymatic and molecular studies in 88 individuals. *Orphanet J Rare Dis* 2012;**7**(31):1–24.

28. Cavedon CT, Bourdoux P, Mertens K. Hong Vien Van Thi, Herremans N, de Laet C, and Goyens P. Age-related variations in acylcarnitine and free carnitine concentrations measured by tandem mass spectrometry. *Clin Chem* 2005;**51**(4):745–52.

29. Waisbren SE, Levy HL, Noble M, Matern D, Gregersen N, Pasley K, et al. Short-chain acyl-CoA dehydrogenase (SCAD) deficiency: An examination of the medical and neurodevelopmental characteristics of 14 cases identified through newborn screening or clinical symptoms. *Mol Genet Metab* 2008;**95**:39–45.

30. Gallant NM, Leydiker K, Tang H, Feuchtbaum L, Lorey F, Puckett R, et al. Biochemical, molecular, and clinical characteristics of children with short chain acyl-CoA dehydrogenase deficiency detected by newborn screening in California. *Mol Genet Metab* 2012;**106**:55–61.

31. Wolfe L, Jethva R, Oglesbee D, Vockley J. Short-Chain Acyl-CoA Dehydrogenase Deficiency. *GeneReviews®* [Internet]. Initial Posting: September 22, 2011; Last Update: August 7, 2014. <http://www.ncbi.nlm.nih.gov/books/NBK63582/> (accessed 11.04.16).

32. Banta-Wright SA, Steiner RD. Tandem mass spectrometry in newborn screening A primer for neonatal and perinatal nurses. *J Perinat Neonat Nurs* 2004;**18**(1):41–58.

33. Chace DH, Kalas TA, Naylor EW. The application of tandem mass spectrometry to neonatal screening for inherited disorders of intermediary metabolism. *Annu Rev Genomics Hum Genet* 2002;**3**:17–45.

34. Van Hove JL, Zhang W, Kahler SG, Roe CR, Chen YT, Terada N, et al. Medium-chain acyl-CoA dehydrogenase (MCAD) deficiency: diagnosis by acylcarnitine analysis in blood. *Am J Hum Genet* 1993;**52**:958–66.

35. Roe CR, Millington DS, Norwood DL, Kodo N, Sprecher H, Mohammed BS, et al. 2,4-Dienoyl-coenzyme A reductase deficiency: a possible new disorder of fatty acid oxidation. *J Clin Invest* 1990;**85**:1703–7.

36. Houten SM, Denis S, te Brinke H, Jongejan A, van Kampen AHC, Bradley EJ, et al. Mitochondrial NADP(H) deficiency due to a mutation in *NADK2* causes dienoyl-CoA reductase deficiency with hyperlysinemia. *Hum Mol Genet* 2014;**23**(18):5009–16. http://dx.doi.org/10.1093/hmg/ddu218.

37. Fingerhut R, Roeschinger W, Muntau AC, Dame T, Kreischer J, Arnecke R, et al. Hepatic carnitine palmitoyltransferase I deficiency: acylcarnitine profiles in blood spots are highly specific. *Clin Chem* 2001;**47**(10):1763–8.

38. McHugh DMS, Cameron CA, Abdenu JE, Abdulrahman M, Adair O, Al Nuaimi SA, et al. Clinical validation of cutoff target ranges in newborn screening of metabolic disorders by tandem mass spectrometry: a worldwide collaborative project. *Genet Med* 2011;**13**(3):230–54.

39. Marquardt G, Robert Currier R, McHugh DMS, Gavrilov D, Magera MJ, Matern D, et al. Enhanced interpretation of newborn screening results without analyte cutoff values. *Genet Med* 2012;**14**(7):648–55.

40. Merritt JL, Vedal S, Abdenur JE, Au SM, Barshop BA, Feuchtbaum L, et al. Infants suspected to have very-long chain acyl-CoA dehydrogenase deficiency from newborn screening. *Mol Genet Metab* 2014;**111**:484–92.

41. Hall PL, Marquardt G, McHugh DMS, Currier RJ, Tang H, Stoway. Postanalytical tools improve performance of newborn screening by tandem mass spectrometry. *Genet Med* 2014;**16**(12):889–95.

42. Beutler E, Balude ME. A simple spot screening test for galactosemia. *J Lab Clin Med* 1966;**68**:137–41.

43. Heard G, McVoy JRS, Wolf B. A screening method for biotinidase deficiency in newborns. *Clin Chem* 1984;**3**(1):125–7.

CHAPTER

Carbohydrate disorders

7

A.M. Ferguson

University of Missouri School of Medicine, Kansas City, MO, United States;
Children's Mercy Hospitals and Clinics, Kansas City, MO, United States

7.1 INTRODUCTION

Carbohydrates play both a structural role in the cell, as elements of nucleic acids and glycoproteins, and a metabolic role, as a major energy source. There are several key clues to the diagnosis of an inherited disorder of carbohydrate metabolism, but in most cases, the differential diagnosis is quite broad. Glucose is the primary carbohydrate energy source, and hypoglycemia is a common presenting symptom among the various disorders. When not being used by the body, glucose is stored in the muscles and liver as glycogen, and thus hepatomegaly or hypotonia and muscle weakness may also be seen. As with other biochemical pathways, the biomarker of choice to measure for either diagnosis or follow up for disorders of carbohydrate metabolism depends on which pathway has the blockade. In most cases, this involves determining the enzymatic activity of the dysfunctional enzyme or measuring the concentration of metabolites that accumulate due to the obstruction. This chapter describes the clinical picture, biomarkers for diagnosis, and treatment for disorders of carbohydrate metabolism including galactosemia, glycogen storage diseases (GSDs), and disorders of fructose metabolism.

7.2 GALACTOSEMIA

Galactosemia is a family of autosomal recessive disorders in which the metabolism of the sugar galactose is disrupted. There are three forms of galactosemia, depending on which enzyme in the Leloir pathway of galactose metabolism is nonfunctional (Fig. 7.1). Classic galactosemia is the most common of the three disorders, and it is caused by mutation in the gene for the galactose-1-phosphate uridylyltransferase (GALT) enzyme.[1–4] Defects in this enzyme result in the accumulation of galactitol and galactose-1-phosphate metabolites.[1] Galactokinase (GALK) deficiency is a much rarer form of galactosemia, and it is caused by mutation in the gene that encodes the enzyme GALK, causing an accumulation of galactose in the blood and tissues.[2] The

Biomarkers in Inborn Errors of Metabolism. DOI: http://dx.doi.org/10.1016/B978-0-12-802896-4.00013-4

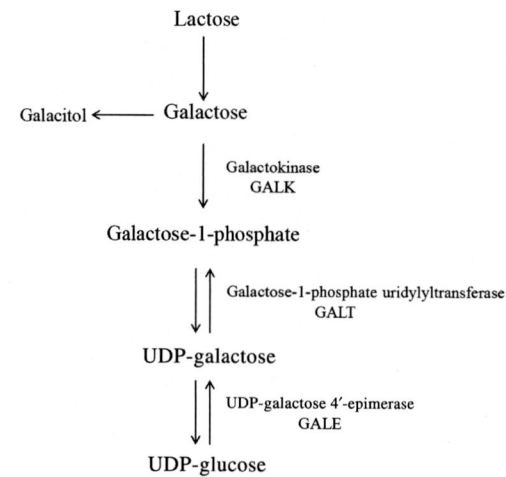

FIGURE 7.1

The Leloir pathway of galactose metabolism.

third type of galactosemia is termed epimerase deficiency galactosemia and is caused by mutation in the gene for the enzyme UDP-galactose-4′-epimerase (GALE). These patients also accumulate galactose and galactose-1-phosphate in erythrocytes as well as high levels of UDP-galactose.[2]

7.2.1 CLINICAL PRESENTATION

Patients with classic galactosemia are asymptomatic at birth, but develop life-threatening complications after exposure to milk. Symptoms include feeding difficulties, hypoglycemia, renal tubular dysfunction, vomiting, diarrhea, hepatomegaly, *Escherichia coli* sepsis, and cataracts.[1,2] Long-term complications can include speech and cognitive disabilities, decreased bone mass and hypergonadotrophic hypogonadism in the majority of females.[1,2] In contrast to patients with classic galactosemia, patients with GALK deficiency do not have the same issue with consuming milk-based products. They do have high levels of galactose and galactitol in their blood and tissues and can develop cataracts, and rarely, central nervous system abnormalities including mental retardation and pseudotumor cerebri, but these conditions can resolve after eliminating galactose from their diet early in life.[2,5] Patients experience no long-term complications as long as the dietary restriction is followed. Epimerase deficiency results in a lack of phenotype in most patients, as the enzyme deficiency is usually restricted to red and white blood cells, but there is a very rare manifestation of the disease that has a symptom profile similar to that of classic galactosemia.[2]

7.2.2 TREATMENT

Treatment for all forms of galactosemia is immediate dietary restriction of galactose-containing foods. Infants can be given soy milk or formula containing other carbohydrate sources, or amino acid–based elemental formulas.[1,6] When the patients reach childhood and beyond, galactose restriction is still recommended, but it is increasingly difficult to remove all galactose from the diet, as trace amounts are found in fruits, vegetables, bread, and legumes.[1] A study that compared treatment variation and outcomes in different countries around the world found that in spite of widely disparate manners of monitoring patients, timing of treatment initiation, and levels of dietary restriction, negative outcomes still occurred in the majority of cases.[3] It has been hypothesized that increased concentrations of galactose-1-phosphate is the cause of the pathogenesis in classic galactosemia, and that small inhibitors of GALK could decrease the buildup of this metabolite. Identification of inhibitors of GALK is in the early stages of scientific discovery, and use of these molecules is far from being implemented clinically.[7,8]

7.2.3 BIOMARKERS FOR DIFFERENTIAL DIAGNOSIS

Testing for galactosemia is included in the newborn screening panels in all states in the United States and is also included in the newborn screening panels in many countries around the world. The analytes tested vary from state to state, however. Most laboratories measure the activity of the GALT enzyme in dried blood spots, and while this will identify newborns with classic galactosemia, it could miss patients with a milder form of classic galactosemia referred to as the Duarte variant and patients with defects in the GALK and GALE enzymes.[9,10] In addition to testing for GALT activity, some laboratories also measure the concentration of total galactose (galactose plus galactose-1-phosphate), which can identify the other forms of galactosemia.[10] Owing to increased false-positive rate, many newborn screening laboratories have discontinued testing for total galactose. Presence of reducing substances in the urine can also be a clue toward the diagnosis of galactosemia, but this must be confirmed with a more specific test measuring enzyme activity or molecular testing, as this can be a nonspecific finding.[4]

7.2.4 BIOMARKERS FOLLOWED FOR TREATMENT EFFICACY

Dietary compliance in patients with galactosemia is monitored by measuring either galactose-1-phosphate in red blood cells or galactitol levels in the urine.[11] However, levels do not correlate with either the clinical condition or potential complications that can occur in patients, and the levels never decrease to that found in unaffected subjects even when compliance with the diet is very good.[11] Because of the limitations of galactose-1-phosphate and urinary galactitol as biomarkers for treatment efficacy, many groups have searched for biomarkers with less intraindividual variation and better correlation with patient outcomes. A study led by Coss looked at the differences in N-glycosylation patterns of immunoglobulin G (IgG) molecules to see if they could be used as a more informative clinical marker.[11] When compared to red blood cell galactose-1-phosphate and urinary galactitol levels, IgG N-glycan profiles showed alterations when patients ingested galactose and were more informative than the traditional markers.[11] Ovarian function is monitored in female patients as they reach puberty by measurement of follicle stimulating hormone (FSH), luteinizing hormone (LH), and estradiol.[3]

7.2.5 CONFOUNDING CONDITIONS

Disorders of galactose metabolism can be mistaken for several other conditions. Presenting symptoms can mimic liver disease or liver failure due to jaundice, hepatomegaly, and elevated liver enzymes. Secondary galactosemia can result from liver dysfunction that is found with congenital infectious hepatitis, hepatic arteriovenous malformations, patent ductus venosus, or tyrosinemia.[12] Untreated patients can present with *E. coli* sepsis, and in the newborn population, galactosemia as a contributing factor to the infection should be included in the differential diagnosis.

7.3 INBORN ERRORS IN FRUCTOSE METABOLISM

Fructose is found in high concentrations in fruits and in an increasing number of processed foods in the form of high fructose corn syrup (HFCS). There are three recognized inherited disorders of fructose metabolism, which vary quite a bit in severity. Essential fructosuria results from a deficiency of fructokinase and leads to benign elevations of fructose in the blood and urine.[13] As this disorder is asymptomatic and usually diagnosed incidentally, it will not be discussed further. Hereditary fructose intolerance (HFI) is an autosomal recessive disorder caused by a mutation in the gene encoding the enzyme aldolase B. This gives rise to an accumulation of fructose-1-phosphate that inhibits glycogenolysis and gluconeogenesis.[13] Fructose-1,6-bisphosphate (FBP) deficiency is also an autosomal recessive disorder due to mutation in the gene that encodes the FBP enzyme that causes impaired formation of glucose from all precursors.[13]

7.3.1 CLINICAL PRESENTATION

Patients with HFI are usually healthy in the neonatal period and only manifest symptoms once they are weaned and exposed to fructose, sucrose, or sorbitol in fruits and vegetables.[13] Presenting symptoms include bloating, nausea and vomiting, hypoglycemia, restlessness, lethargy, and often with progression to coma.[13,14] If ingestion of fructose is continued, patients exhibit chronic conditions such as failure to thrive, liver disease, and kidney dysfunction.[13] In contrast to infants with HFI, infants with

FBP can present as neonates with hypoglycemia and severe lactic acidosis due to reduced glycogen stores.[13] As the patient ages and the tolerance to fasting improves, the symptoms decrease in both frequency and severity. These symptoms can include irritability, hepatomegaly, coma, and somnolence.[13] In both conditions, exposure to intravenous solutions containing fructose can be fatal, so it is prudent to determine the sugar used in the solution prior to administration.

7.3.2 CONFOUNDING CONDITIONS

Disorders of fructose metabolism can be confused with and misdiagnosed as several illnesses including fructose malabsorption, GLUT5 transporter deficiency, food allergy, acute viral gastroenteritis, liver disease, or sepsis. Symptoms that are shared include nausea, vomiting, abdominal pain, and hypoglycemia. Fructose malabsorption and food allergies can present in a similar time frame, after weaning and the introduction of fruit to the diet, but may present earlier, as most commercial formulas contain sucrose. A case report by Wenzel et al.[15] described a 5-year-old patient who presented with recurrent watery diarrhea, abdominal pain, and food refusal, particularly avoiding sweets and fruit. The patient's initial symptoms began at the age of 1, after she had been weaned. After ingesting fructose as a part of a fructose breath hydrogen test to confirm or exclude the diagnosis of fructose malabsorption, the patient exhibited a severe reaction including seizures, severe hypoglycemia, and coma, but she recovered quickly after receiving an infusion of glucose. This case exemplifies why a detailed history, including nutritional information, should be obtained before provocative diagnostic testing is undertaken, and why this type of testing is not recommended.

7.3.3 BIOMARKERS FOR DIFFERENTIAL DIAGNOSIS

Patients with HFI have elevated levels of fructose-1-phosphate, but there is not a clinical test available for this biomarker. Discovery of fructose in the urine can suggest a disorder of fructose metabolism, but the absence of fructosuria does not rule out these conditions due to variation in the timing of the fructose ingestion. After collecting an extensive dietary and nutritional history of the patient, the least invasive and most common method of diagnosis for both HFI and FBP is DNA analysis. If no mutations are found, then determination of enzymatic activity from liver biopsy can be performed. Provocative testing such as a fructose loading test is not recommended, as mentioned previously.

7.3.4 TREATMENT

The treatment for HFI is the elimination of fructose from the diet. Once the patient no longer ingests fructose, sucrose, or sorbitol, clinical symptoms resolve and the prognosis is quite good. As the patient ages, tolerance for fructose increases slightly.[13] For patients with FBP, restriction of fructose is only recommended in small children. The most critical feature to control is an avoidance of fasting, especially during a febrile illness, and the ability to fast improves with age.[13] Treatment for an acute episode is oral or intravenous glucose and long-term treatment includes frequent feeding or use of uncooked cornstarch or other slowly absorbed carbohydrates.[13]

7.3.5 BIOMARKERS FOLLOWED FOR TREATMENT EFFICACY

There is no current biomarker that is followed in patients with HFI or FBP. Research studies have shown that patients with untreated HFI have defective glycoprotein glycosylation due to the inhibition of enzyme activity by accumulated fructose-1-phosphate.[16] This defect disappears after fructose restriction and can be detected by analyzing plasma transferrin isoelectric focusing (TfIEF) patterns. Such analysis could be useful for monitoring compliance to dietary treatment as well as diagnosing indolent cases.

7.4 GLYCOGEN STORAGE DISEASES

GSDs comprise a number of disorders that affect the metabolism of glycogen (Table 7.1). Glycogen serves as a reservoir of glucose, and mutations are found in the genes encoding the enzymes that regulate its processing, leading to abnormal concentrations or structures. Glycogenolysis, gluconeogenesis, and the production of lactate and ketone bodies can be affected, depending on the disorder.[17]

7.4.1 CLINICAL PRESENTATION

The liver and the muscles are the main organs that are affected in GSD, as those organs are the primary sites for storage or utilization of glycogen. Presenting symptoms can

Table 7.1 Glycogen Storage Diseases

Type	Name	Enzyme Defect
0		Glycogen synthase
I	von Gierke	Glucose 6-phosphatase
II	Pompe	Acid-α-glucosidase
III	Cori	Glycogen debrancher enzyme
IV	Anderson	Glycogen branching enzyme
V	McArdle	Muscle phosphorylase
VI	Hers	Liver phosphorylase
VII	Tarui	Muscle fructokinase
IX		Liver phosphorylase kinase

include hepatomegaly with recurrent hypoglycemia, intermittent myalgia and muscle weakness, and rhabdomyolysis, with slight variations depending on the specific disorder.[18]

GSD type 0 is due to mutations in the glycogen synthase gene, *GYS2*, which lead to a decrease in liver glycogen content.[19] Patients have hypoglycemia and ketosis after short fasts and hyperlipidemia, as excess glucose cannot be converted to glycogen.[18]

Patients with GSD type I (von Gierke disease) are unable to generate glucose through gluconeogenesis or by the breakdown of glycogen due to a mutation in the *G6PC* gene, resulting in glucose 6-phosphatase deficiency.[19] Instead, patients form glucose-6-phosphate, which when utilized in the cell, results in increased lactate, lipids, and uric acid.[18–21] Patients present in either the newborn period with hypoglycemic seizures or later in infancy, as the time between feedings is increased. By 6 months of age, hepatomegaly and doll-like facies are apparent. Platelet dysfunction and renal tubular acidosis can be added complications.[18,21] GSD type Ib is caused by mutations in the glucose-6-phosphate translocase gene, *SLC37A4*, and also includes neutropenia and neutrophil dysfunction, leading to recurrent infections and poor wound healing.[18,19]

GSD type II (Pompe disease) is caused by mutation in the *GAA* gene and deficiency of lysosomal acid-α-glucosidase enzyme (GAA). Pompe disease is the only GSD that is also classified as a lysosomal storage disease.[22] Patients can present at a variety of different ages, with variable age of onset, severity, and progression of the disease. Despite these differences, all patients show an accumulation of glycogen in skeletal, cardiac, and smooth muscle, which leads to weakness, hypotonia, respiratory distress, and poor linear growth and weight gain.[22,23] The infantile form tends to be rapidly progressing and lethal, with death due to cardiorespiratory failure by the age of 1 year, while the late-onset form proceeds more slowly and lacks cardiac involvement, with the age of death dependent on the rate of disease progression.[22,23]

GSD type III (Cori disease) results from a mutation in the *AGL* gene. This causes a defect in the glycogen debranching enzyme, resulting in a phenotype that includes hypoglycemia with ketosis, hyperlipidemia, hepatosplenomegaly, and myopathy.[24] This disorder is further stratified by the involvement of skeletal muscle (GSD type IIIa) or nonskeletal muscle (GSD type IIIb).[18,19] As patients reach adolescence, their hypoglycemia becomes more stable, but myopathy, including cardiomyopathy and exercise intolerance, worsens.[18,19]

GSD type IV (Anderson disease) is caused by a mutation in the *GBE1* gene encoding the glycogen branching enzyme and has a variable presentation, depending on where the deficiency is located.[25] Patients can have severe or mild liver forms, severe or mild neuromuscular forms, or a generalized severe form that is fatal. As expected with numerous forms, the presenting symptoms are quite variable and can include hepatosplenomegaly and hepatic fibrosis, hypotonia, muscular atrophy, myopathy, cardiomyopathy, hydrops fetalis, exercise intolerance, and central and peripheral nervous system dysfunction.[25]

GSD type V (McArdle disease) is due to mutation in the *PYGM* gene and deficiency of muscle phosphorylase activity, and muscles are not able to utilize muscle glycogen in the initial phase of physical activity.[26] After the blood supply increases and supplies the muscles with energy, patients are able to function normally, in what is referred to as the "second wind" phenomenon.[26] Symptoms don't present until the second or third decade of life and include exercise-induced muscle pain, fatigue, and, in some cases, rhabdomyolysis.[26]

GSD type VI (Hers disease) is caused by mutation in the *PGYL* gene and deficiency of the hepatic glycogen phosphorylase and is the rarest of the GSDs. Unlike the other GSDs, it is not associated with hypoglycemia as the presenting symptom, but instead with hepatomegaly, mild liver dysfunction, short stature, and hyperlipidemia.[18,19] The clinical course for this disorder is quite benign, and most adults are asymptomatic.[19,27]

GSD type VII (Tarui disease) results from a mutation in the *PFKM* gene, leading to deficiency of muscle fructokinase.[26] It is clinically very similar to GSD type V, not only with exercise-induced pain, muscle cramps, and fatigue, but also includes nausea and vomiting, hemolytic anemia, and hyperuricemia.[26]

GSD type IX is subdivided into types IXa, IXb, and IXc, depending on which of the genes encoding the subunits of phosphorylase kinase contains the defect, *PHKA2, PHKB*, or *PHKG2*, respectively. Most patients have a mild course, with isolated hepatomegaly and fasting ketosis.[18,27]

7.4.2 CONFOUNDING CONDITIONS

Patients who present in the newborn period with hypoglycemia and seizures can be confused for multiple different diagnoses, especially if the secondary symptoms of acidosis and hepatomegaly have yet to manifest.[18,20] Persistent hypoglycemic hyperinsulinemia of infancy, galactosemia, or fatty oxidation disorders are other diagnoses that should be considered along with one of the GSDs.[20] Hyperglycemia after meals and glucosuria can be confused for diabetes.[19] When Pompe disease is suspected, the differential diagnosis could also include spinal muscular atrophy I, hypothyroidism, myocarditis, mitochondrial/respiratory chain disorders, Danon disease, peroxisomal disorders, muscular dystrophy, myasthenia gravis, and rheumatoid arthritis.[22]

7.4.3 BIOMARKERS FOR DIFFERENTIAL DIAGNOSIS

Laboratory testing for GSDs should include glucose, electrolytes, liver function tests, complete blood count, creatine kinase, uric acid, cholesterol, triglycerides, ammonia, and lactate, preferably after the patient has fasted.[18–20] In most cases, genetic testing has replaced enzyme assays as the diagnostic method of choice since enzyme assays are difficult to perform and must be done by an experienced laboratory. Liver biopsy shows hepatocytes bulging with glycogen and a vacuolated appearance, but this is now rarely performed since genetic testing is readily available and less invasive.[18,20] To help in the diagnosis of GSDs involving the muscles, the lactate-ischemia test can be performed.[26] Compared to healthy controls, the ammonia level is similarly elevated but the lactate response is attenuated after vigorous forearm exercise. For Pompe disease, a chest X-ray and electrocardiogram (ECG) are useful to arrive at the correct diagnosis and will show cardiomegaly and an abnormal, pathognomic ECG.[22] A diagnosis of Pompe disease can be confirmed by measuring GAA enzymatic activity from cultured fibroblasts, muscle biopsy, or dried blood spot, elevation of glucose tetrasaccharide (GLc$_4$) in urine, or molecular testing.[22,23,28] In 2013, the Discretionary Advisory Committee on Heritable Disorders in Newborns and Children (DACHDNC) voted to add Pompe disease to the recommended uniform screening panel. The recommendation was confirmed by the US Secretary of Health and Human Services in 2015.[29] In 2016, several states have implemented screening for Pompe disease as part of their newborn screening panel, with several other states pursuing implementation. The question remains, however, of how to determine the treatment for the patients diagnosed via newborn screening. Mutation analysis is not predictive of the patient's phenotype, and patients with infantile-onset cannot be distinguished from those with late-onset or mild disease.[30]

7.4.4 TREATMENT

The main treatment for most GSDs is dietary, with the goal to maintain a normal blood glucose concentration via carbohydrates in the diet. Uncooked cornstarch is commonly used, with continuous feeding overnight to prevent fasting and frequent feeding during the day.[19,31,32] Continuous glucose monitoring can be utilized to minimize peaks and troughs in glucose levels.[18,20] Enzyme replacement therapy (ERT) with recombinant human GAA (rhGAA) has emerged as a viable treatment for patients with Pompe disease who also have cross-reactive immunologic material (CRIM-positive).[33] An assessment of a cohort of 10 patients with infantile-onset Pompe disease who were identified at birth via newborn screening results and treated with rhGAA for a median time period of 63 months showed the benefits of ERT. The patients showed long-term survival when compared to untreated cases, and all the patients could walk independently and did not require mechanical ventilation. Muscle weakness did appear after 2 years of age, as well as ptosis and speech disorders.[33] CRIM-negative patients, as well as CRIM-positive patients with high-sustained anti-rhGAA IgG antibody titers (HSAT) have been successfully treated with ERT in combination with immunosuppressive regimens including rituximab, methotrexate, intravenous immunoglobulin, and bortezomib.[34]

Treatment of patients with adult-onset Pompe disease appears to be less effective in halting disease progression. A 5-year retrospective study found that pulmonary function was stabilized but muscle endurance was not significantly enhanced as seen in previous studies.[35] A separate study that focused on quality of life in patients with adult-onset Pompe disease reported that ERT had a positive effect on patients' physical health status and participation in daily life, as well as not only halting the decline of their health status, but improving it in the first 2 years of treatment.[36]

7.4.5 BIOMARKERS FOLLOWED FOR TREATMENT EFFICACY

Patients should be monitored for growth and other markers of glycemic control, including glucose, uric acid, triglycerides, liver function tests, lactate, or ketones, depending on the disorder being managed. Monitoring of the size of the liver by ultrasound is also recommended. Patients with GSD type I should have measured glomerular filtration rates (GFR) performed to screen for developing end-stage renal disease.[18–20] Patients with Pompe should be monitored for cardiomyopathy, respiratory function, muscle weakness, and neurological sequelae.[22]

7.5 CONCLUSIONS

Disorders of carbohydrate metabolism include galactosemia, GSDs, and disorders of fructose metabolism. The prognosis of these disorders runs the spectrum from life-threatening to completely benign. The majority of these disorders can be managed by restricting the diet of the patient and avoiding the specific carbohydrate involved. Emerging treatment for Pompe disease, the only GSD that is also a lysosomal storage disease, includes enzyme replacement therapy. Traditional diagnosis of these disorders is accomplished by assessing enzyme activity, but this is being replaced by noninvasive molecular testing on an increasing basis. The biomarker of choice for monitoring treatment compliance is dependent on the disorder in question, but patients with all disorders require routine laboratory testing for long-term patient management.

REFERENCES

1. Bosch AM. Classic galactosemia: dietary dilemmas. *J Inherit Metab Dis* 2011;**34**(2):257–60.
2. Fridovich-Keil JL. Galactosemia: the good, the bad, and the unknown. *J Cell Physiol* 2006;**209**(3):701–5.
3. Jumbo-Lucioni PP, Garber K, Kiel J, et al. Diversity of approaches to classic galactosemia around the world: a comparison of diagnosis, intervention, and outcomes. *J Inherit Metab Dis* 2012;**35**(6):1037–49.
4. Karadag N, Zenciroglu A, Eminoglu FT, et al. Literature review and outcome of classic galactosemia diagnosed in the neonatal period. *Clin Lab* 2013;**59**(9-10):1139–46.
5. Bosch AM, Bakker HD, van Gennip AH, van Kempen JV, Wanders RJ, Wijburg FA. Clinical features of galactokinase deficiency: a review of the literature. *J Inherit Metab Dis* 2002;**25**(8):629–34.
6. Van Calcar SC, Bernstein LE, Rohr FJ, Scaman CH, Yannicelli S, Berry GT. A re-evaluation of life-long severe galactose restriction for the nutrition management of classic galactosemia. *Mol Genet Metab* 2014;**112**(3):191–7.
7. Boxer MB, Shen M, Tanega C, Tang M, Lai K, Auld DS. Toward improved therapy for classic galactosemia. Probe reports from the NIH molecular libraries program. Bethesda (MD); 2010.

8. Tang M, Odejinmi SI, Vankayalapati H, Wierenga KJ, Lai K. Innovative therapy for Classic Galactosemia – tale of two HTS. *Mol Genet Metab* 2012;**105**(1):44–55.
9. Lehotay DC, Hall P, Lepage J, Eichhorst JC, Etter ML, Greenberg CR. LC–MS/MS progress in newborn screening. *Clin Biochem* 2011;**44**(1):21–31.
10. Pyhtila BM, Shaw KA, Neumann SE, Fridovich-Keil JL. Newborn screening for galactosemia in the United States: looking back, looking around, and looking ahead. *JIMD Rep* 2015;**15**:79–93.
11. Coss KP, Byrne JC, Coman DJ, et al. IgG N-glycans as potential biomarkers for determining galactose tolerance in Classical Galactosaemia. *Mol Genet Metab* 2012;**105**(2):212–20.
12. Berry GT. Galactosemia: when is it a newborn screening emergency? *Mol Genet Metab* 2012;**106**(1):7–11.
13. Mayatepek E, Hoffmann B, Meissner T. Inborn errors of carbohydrate metabolism. *Best Pract Res Clin Gastroenterol* 2010;**24**(5):607–18.
14. Bouteldja N, Timson DJ. The biochemical basis of hereditary fructose intolerance. *J Inherit Metab Dis* 2010;**33**(2):105–12.
15. Wenzel JJ, Rossmann H, Kullmer U, et al. Chronic diarrhea in a 5-year-old girl: pitfall in routine laboratory testing with potentially severe consequences. *Clin Chem* 2009;**55**(5):1026–30. discussion 1030-1.
16. Moraitou M, Dimitriou E, Mavridou I, et al. Transferrin isoelectric focusing and plasma lysosomal enzyme activities in the diagnosis and follow-up of hereditary fructose intolerance. *Clin Chim Acta* 2012;**413**(19–20):1714–5.
17. Haack KAaB MJ. Genetic metabolic disorders. In: Dietzen DJ, Bennett MJ, Wong ECC, editors. *Biochemical and molecular basis of pediatric disease* 4th ed. Washington, DC: AACC Press; 2010. p. 235–60.
18. Bhattacharya K. Investigation and management of the hepatic glycogen storage diseases. *Transl Pediatr* 2015;**4**(3):240–8.
19. Wolfsdorf JI, Weinstein DA. Glycogen storage diseases. *Rev Endocr Metab Disord* 2003;**4**(1):95–102.
20. Kishnani PS, Austin SL, Abdenur JE, et al. Diagnosis and management of glycogen storage disease type I: a practice guideline of the American College of Medical Genetics and Genomics. *Genet Med* 2014;**16**(11):e1.
21. Santos BL, Souza CF, Schuler-Faccini L, et al. Glycogen storage disease type I: clinical and laboratory profile. *J Pediatr (Rio J)* 2014;**90**(6):572–9.
22. Kishnani PS, Steiner RD, Bali D, et al. Pompe disease diagnosis and management guideline. *Genet Med* 2006;**8**(5):267–88.
23. Dasouki M, Jawdat O, Almadhoun O, et al. Pompe disease: literature review and case series. *Neurol Clin* 2014;**32**(3):751–76. ix.
24. Kishnani PS, Austin SL, Arn P, et al. Glycogen storage disease type III diagnosis and management guidelines. *Genet Med* 2010;**12**(7):446–63.
25. Shin YS. Glycogen storage disease: clinical, biochemical, and molecular heterogeneity. *Semin Pediatr Neurol* 2006;**13**(2):115–20.
26. Das AM, Steuerwald U, Illsinger S. Inborn errors of energy metabolism associated with myopathies. *J Biomed Biotechnol* 2010;**2010**:340849.
27. Roscher A, Patel J, Hewson S, et al. The natural history of glycogen storage disease types VI and IX: long-term outcome from the largest metabolic center in Canada. *Mol Genet Metab* 2014;**113**(3):171–6.
28. Kishnani PS, Amartino HM, Lindberg C, Miller TM, Wilson A, Keutzer J. Methods of diagnosis of patients with Pompe disease: data from the Pompe Registry. *Mol Genet Metab* 2014;**113**(1–2):84–91.

29. www.newsteps.org/pompe.
30. Andersson HC. Newborn screening+ enzyme replacement therapy= improved lysosomal storage disorder: outcomes in infantile-onset Pompe disease. *J Pediatr* 2015;**166**(4):800–1.
31. El-Shabrawi MH, Kamal NM. Medical management of chronic liver diseases in children (part I): focus on curable or potentially curable diseases. *Paediatr Drugs* 2011;**13**(6):357–70.
32. Heller S, Worona L, Consuelo A. Nutritional therapy for glycogen storage diseases. *J Pediatr Gastroenterol Nutr* 2008;**47**(Suppl. 1):S15–21.
33. Chien YH, Lee NC, Chen CA, et al. Long-term prognosis of patients with infantile-onset Pompe disease diagnosed by newborn screening and treated since birth. *J Pediatr* 2015;**166**(4):985–91. e1-2.
34. Stenger EO, Kazi Z, Lisi E, Gambello MJ, Kishnani P. Immune tolerance strategies in siblings with infantile Pompe disease-advantages for a preemptive approach to high-sustained antibody titers. *Mol Genet Metab Rep* 2015;**4**:30–4.
35. Stepien KM, Hendriksz CJ, Roberts M, Sharma R. Observational clinical study of 22 adult-onset Pompe disease patients undergoing enzyme replacement therapy over 5 years. *Mol Genet Metab* 2016;**117**(4):413–8.
36. Gungor D, Kruijshaar ME, Plug I, et al. Quality of life and participation in daily life of adults with Pompe disease receiving enzyme replacement therapy: 10 years of international follow-up. *J Inherit Metab Dis* 2016;**39**(2):253–60.

Mitochondrial disorders

8

N. Couser and M. Gucsavas-Calikoglu

University of North Carolina, Chapel Hill, NC, United States

8.1 INTRODUCTION

The mitochondrion is a complex cellular organelle involved in key metabolic pathways such as fatty acid oxidation, amino acid metabolism, and oxidative phosphorylation (OXPHOS). Most human nucleated cells have 500–2000 mitochondria. Their function is to produce energy from oxygen consumption as well as to detoxify intermediary metabolites. Mitochondria are unique in having both their own genome, mitochondrial DNA (mtDNA) and requiring nuclear encoded gene products for pyruvate utilization, Krebs cycle function, and mitochondrial genome maintenance.

Mitochondrial disease often results from defects in respiratory chain complexes as well as defects in numerous pathways that require mitochondrial function such as replication, translation, transcription, transport, fusion and fission, ribosome structure or assembly. Organ systems that have high energy demands, such as the heart, skeletal muscle, central nervous system, kidneys, pancreas, liver, and eyes, are often affected. The disease process can be progressive and even fatal.

The mitochondrion is composed of an inner and outer membrane enclosing an intermembrane space (Fig. 8.1). Cristae are folds in the inner membrane that extend into the matrix, increasing the functional surface area of the inner membrane—the physical location of the electron transport chain protein complexes required for OXPHOS. The interior organelle matrix contains enzymes necessary for pyruvate, amino acid, and fatty acid oxidation, as well as those enzymes that comprise the tricarboxylic acid cycle (Krebs cycle). Urea, glucose, and heme biosynthesis have steps that occur in the mitochondrial matrix. Furthermore, the matrix contains both nicotinamide adenine dinucleotide (NAD^+) and flavin adenine dinucleotide (FAD), the coenzymes required as hydrogen acceptors in the electron transport chain (ETC), as well as adenosine diphosphate (ADP) and Pi, which is necessary for the final step of adenosine triphosphate (ATP) production, that help to carry out the key function of OXPHOS.[1] The OXPHOS is comprised of five functional enzyme complexes each with multiple subunits: Complex I (NADH–CoQ reductase), Complex II (succinate:CoQ reductase), Complex III (ubiquinol:cytochrome *c* oxidoreductase),

Biomarkers in Inborn Errors of Metabolism. DOI: http://dx.doi.org/10.1016/B978-0-12-802896-4.00008-0

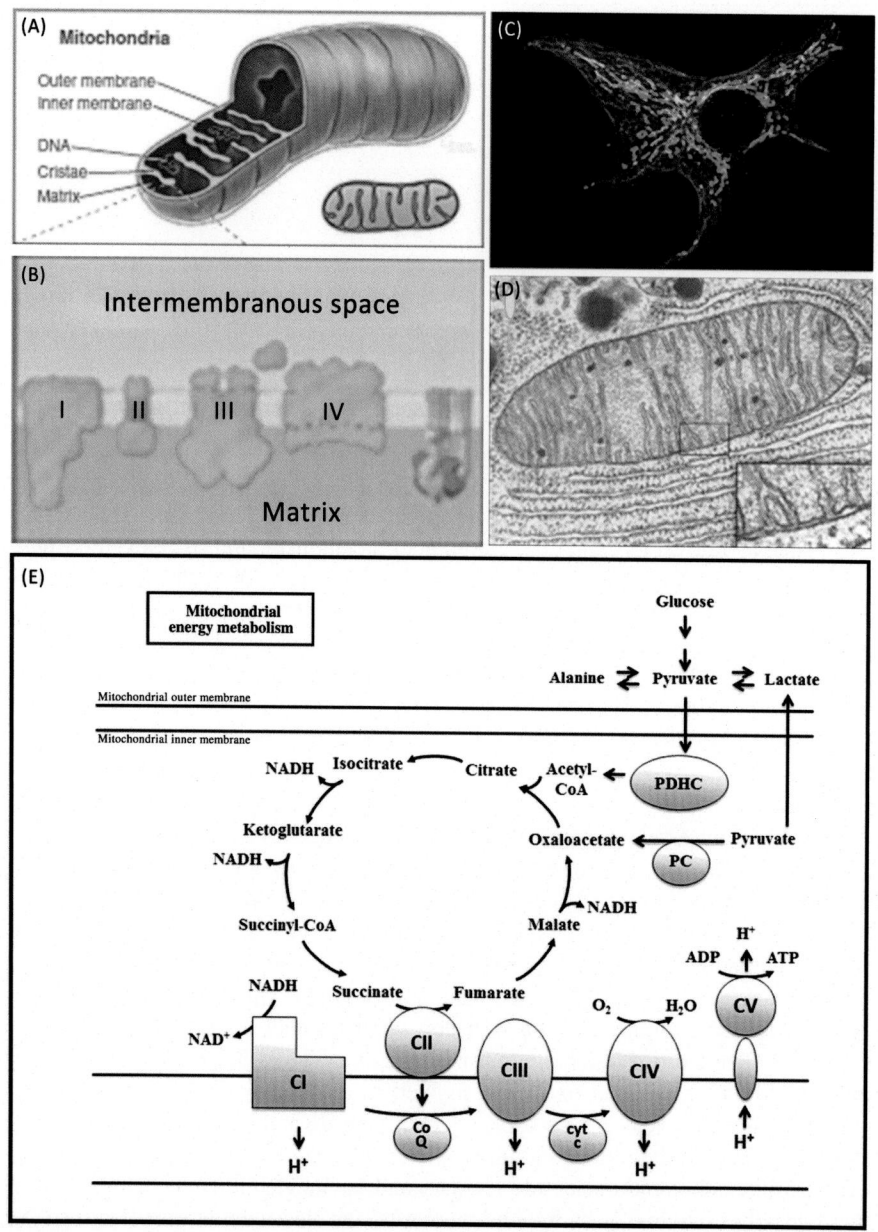

FIGURE 8.1

Basic structure of mammalian mitochondrion. (A, B) Mitochondrial compartments and organization of the electron transport chain. (C) Fluorescence light micrograph of cell with mitochondria labeled with a green-fluorescent antibody (*Cell Biology*. 2nd ed., courtesy of Michael Yaffee, University of San Diego).[62] (D) Thin-section electron micrograph of a mitochondrion (*Cell Biology*. 2nd ed., courtesy of Don Fawcett, Harvard Medical School, Boston, Massachusetts).[62] (E) Biochemical energy metabolism within the mitochondrion.

Complex IV (cytochrome c oxidase) and Complex V (ATP synthetase). Oxidation of substrates from multiple biochemical pathways results in reduced electrons that are transferred from one unit to the other, generating a proton gradient and ultimately, forming ATP from ADP, which provides energy for critical cellular functions. Defects in any of the enzymes forming these complexes result in mitochondrial dysfunction in affected organs.

8.2 CLINICAL PRESENTATION

The prevalence of mitochondrial diseases is estimated to be about 1 in 5000 across all ages.[2] The clinical presentation tends to be complex and may involve all organ systems. Those organs with high energy demands, such as brain, nerves, heart, gut, ears, and the eye, are particularly at risk. Disease may appear at any age, from a newborn with hypotonia, cardiomyopathy, and lactic acidosis, to a child with hearing loss and seizures, to an adolescent or adult with migraines or isolated vision loss secondary to retinal degeneration. Phenotypic expression is highly variable in affected members within or between families and across the same disease spectrum. For example, a family affected with MELAS (mitochondrial encephalopathy with lactic acidosis and stroke-like episodes) may present with a healthy carrier mother, a son with cardiomyopathy needing heart transplant, and a daughter with recurrent strokes and hearing loss.

Although certain patterns of organ involvement such as MELAS, MERRF (mitochondrial encephalopathy with ragged red fibers), NARP (neuropathy, ataxia, retinitis pigmentosa, and ptosis) or Leigh syndrome (LS) have been well described in the literature (see below), in reality there can be considerable overlap between these entities and providers must be adept at keeping an open mind when confronted with unexplained or puzzling disease symptomatology.

The more severe defects present earlier, often with intrauterine fetal involvement, while symptoms in adults may be milder. Intrauterine growth retardation in the fetus may be associated with poly- or oligohydramnios and structural anomalies such as arthrogryposis, limb defects, or cardiac defects. A neonate may have severe lactic acidosis, recurrent apnea, seizures, or cardiomyopathy with hepatic failure. Infants may present with chronic watery diarrhea and villous atrophy or sideroblastic anemia. Progressive neurological deterioration with intractable seizures is often observed.

Although most textbooks and articles emphasize that a suspicion for mitochondrial disease should be considered when symptoms occur in more than three organ systems, one must also be aware of certain red flags or symptoms that may be more specific (Tables 8.1 and 8.2). Depending on the specificity of the underlying symptom, consideration of and testing for mitochondrial disorders may be initiated earlier rather awaiting for further organ involvement.

A hallmark of mitochondrial disease is the variability of the disease process within the same family or individuals despite similar mutations, which may complicate the diagnosis.[3] Also the disease process may evolve over time with intermittent stabilization in one organ system with decline in another.

Table 8.1 Common Red Flags in Mitochondrial Disorders

Examples of Red Flag Symptoms	Disorder
Myoclonus	MERRF
Stroke in nonvascular distribution	MELAS
Epilepsy partialis continua	POLG
Encephalopathy-hepatopathy with valproic acid	POLG
Bilateral basal ganglia lesions	Leigh syndrome
Sensorineural hearing loss in multisystem disorder	Mitochondrial depletion syndrome
Sudden central vision loss	LHON
Progressive external ophthalmoplegia	KSS
Concentric hypertrophic cardiomyopathy, neutropenia, 3-methylglutaconic acid in boys	Barth syndrome
Exocrine pancreatic dysfunction with sideroblastic anemia	Pearson marrow–pancreas syndrome

The neurological system is commonly affected. Some neurological symptoms are more specific than others and should be considered red flags such as myoclonus (suggestive of MERRF), strokes in a nonvascular pattern (suggestive of MELAS), or epilepsy partialis continua, recurrent focal motor epileptic seizures that can recur every few seconds or minutes for extended periods (suggestive of polymerase gamma (POLG) disorders).

Other neurological symptoms include hypotonia or hypertonia. Global developmental delays are common. Seizures (generalized, partial, focal, myoclonic, drop attacks, or astatic) may be present at birth or start at any age and may be difficult to treat and intractable. Myopathy is often seen and may be progressive. Apnea may be recurrent, suggestive of brain stem dysfunction. Axonal neuropathy may be confused with other neurological diseases such as several subtypes of Charcot–Marie–Tooth syndrome. Encephalopathy is a general feature with varying degrees of intellectual disability, recurrent coma, or global delays. Regression of skills is a major concern. Cerebellar involvement may result in ataxia and autonomic dysfunction may also be present. Basal ganglia involvement may result in persistent choreoathetoid movements or other movement disorders. Migraines may represent mild stroke-like episodes. Leukodystrophy may be present and identifiable on magnetic resonance imaging (MRI). Peripheral neuropathy may also be present. Some elderly patients may have dementia.

Although this symptom list is extensive, providers must remember that the above neurological symptoms wax and wane and may progress over time. It is also important to note that symptom severity can be exacerbated at times of illness or stress. Also the association of other major organs as further described below indicates the need for further diagnostic work-up. Particularly, the development of sensorineural hearing loss over time with associated neurological symptoms is concerning. Decline

Table 8.2 Clinical Features of Selected Mitochondrial Disorders

Disorder	Inheritance	Prominent Clinical Features
Alpers–Huttenlocher disease (AHS)	Autosomal recessive	Seizures, developmental regression, liver dysfunction
Kearns–Sayre syndrome (KSS)	Mitochondrial	Ophthalmoplegia, ptosis, pigmentary retinopathy, cardiac conduction defects
Leber hereditary optic neuropathy (LHON)	Mitochondrial	Acute or subacute painless loss of central vision
Leigh syndrome (LS)	Autosomal recessive Mitochondrial	Hypotonia, spasticity, chorea or other movement disorders, cerebellar ataxia and/or a peripheral neuropathy, hypertrophic cardiomyopathy
Maternally inherited diabetes-deafness syndrome (MIDD)	Mitochondrial	Insulin-dependent diabetes mellitus, hearing loss
Mitochondrial encephalopathy, lactic acidosis, stroke-like episodes (MELAS)	Mitochondrial	Seizures, stroke, hearing loss, gastric dysmotility
Mitochondrial neurogastrointestinal encephalopathy syndrome (MNGIE)	Autosomal recessive	Gastrointestinal dysmotility, ophthalmoplegia, ptosis, peripheral neuropathy, cachexia, leukoencephalopathy
Myoclonic epilepsy with ragged red fibers syndrome (MERRF)	Mitochondrial	Myoclonus, myopathy, progressive spasticity, epilepsy, ataxia, peripheral neuropathy, dementia
Neuropathy, ataxia, retinitis pigmentosa syndrome (NARP)	Mitochondrial	Proximal neurogenic muscle weakness, sensory neuropathy, ataxia, pigmentary retinopathy
Pearson marrow–pancreas syndrome (PMPS)	Mitochondrial	Anemia, pancreatic insufficiency, liver steatosis, malabsorption, growth failure
Progressive external opthalmoplegia (PEO)	Autosomal dominant Autosomal recessive	Ophthalmoplegia, ptosis

in hearing, particularly after exposure to aminoglycosides, is also highly specific. Cochlear implants may be used to improve hearing but aminoglycoside antibiotics should be avoided in confirmed mitochondrial patients.

Intellectual disability may be present but often may be a consequence of strokes or seizures and isolated intellectual disability is not sufficient to make a diagnosis of a mitochondrial disorder. Similarly autistic behaviors have been reported, but autism spectrum disorders in mitochondrial disorders are often accompanied by other organ system involvement. The presence of psychiatric disease is also increasingly appreciated, and depression, anxiety, and even obsessive behaviors may be noted. Certain diseases such as Alzheimer or Parkinson disease may also present with secondary mitochondrial dysfunction as the destruction of healthy nerve cells and accumulation of plaques may impede OXPHOS.[2,4]

Other clinical features often seen in mitochondrial disease, although nonspecific, include developmental delays including speech delay, fatigue, and exercise intolerance. Although chronic fatigue is often reported in affected adults, there is often objective evidence of exercise intolerance as determined by exercise stress testing.

Varying degrees of cardiomyopathy (hypertrophic and dilated as well as concentric) and arrhythmias are also seen in mitochondrial disorders. Suspected patients need to have a cardiac echo for evaluation for cardiomyopathy (dilated or hypertrophic—concentric) and electrocardiogram (EKG) for identification of varying types of cardiac block or dysrhythmias. Cardiac function and arrhythmias may worsen during illness and may sometimes improve but pacemaker placement may be needed.

Ophthalmological findings are also extensive and usually develop over time. Initially, optic atrophy, ptosis, or progressive external ophthalmoplegia may be present. Over time, retinal degeneration, pigmentary retinopathy, and cataracts may develop. A comprehensive ophthalmological evaluation is needed including retinal evaluation in suspected cases. Sudden onset central vision loss is also typical for Leber hereditary optic neuropathy (LHON).

The kidneys have high energy requirement: renal concentration defects and generalized aminoaciduria are commonly seen. Proximal tubulopathy and tubule-interstitial nephritis may progress to renal failure. Nephrotic syndrome can be present. Kidney disease may worsen during illness but may also intermittently improve.

The liver and gut are consistently involved. Some patients will present with recurrent vomiting, failure to gain weight, malnutrition, and even chronic diarrhea with villous atrophy unresponsive to typical interventions. Chronic intestinal pseudo-obstruction and gastric dysmotility are often present. Exocrine pancreatic dysfunction may also be present and a warning sign for Pearson syndrome. Liver failure may be severe in infants. Valproate-induced liver failure is typical for POLG disorders and testing should be immediately initiated. It is prudent to avoid valproate in patients with suspected mitochondrial disorders.

The endocrine system is often involved with symptoms varying from recurrent hypoglycemia to diabetes mellitus. Thyroid and parathyroid deficiencies may develop over time. There may be insufficient adrenocorticotropic hormone (ACTH) secretion, particularly during illness, and stress dose steroids may be needed in some patients. Hypothalamic dysfunction may also result in diabetes insipidus or growth hormone deficiency. Periodic evaluation of the endocrine system function is needed in known patients.

Regression after minor illness or exposure to medications is often reported and increased susceptibility to infections is seen although specific immune deficiencies have not been identified.

The pulmonary system may also be involved as a consequence of neuromuscular myopathy. Continuous positive airway pressure (CPAP) or ventilator support may be necessary in patients with respiratory failure. Low-dose oxygen therapy may be beneficial in some patients, particularly those with sleep apnea.

A list of medications to avoid in mitochondrial is present at the United Mitochondrial Disease Foundation (www.umdf.org) website, Mito101 section.

8.3 GENETICS

The mitochondrion is the only organelle in humans whose structure and function is under dual genetic control. It contains its own genome but many structures and functions are also under nuclear genetic control. The human mitochondrial genome is composed of 16,569 base pairs arranged as circular DNA, similar to the bacterial genome, and contains genes for 22 transfer RNAs, 12S and 16S ribosomal RNAs, and 13 protein coding sequences that encode components of respiratory complexes I (NADH–CoQ reductase), Complex III (ubiquinone:cytochrome c oxidoreductase), IV (cytochrome c oxidase), or V (ATP synthetase). Complex II (succinate dehydrogenase) is the only respiratory chain complex whose subunits are encoded solely by nuclear DNA sequences. Defects within mtDNA are maternally inherited, in contrast to nuclear DNA (nDNA) defects that may be inherited from either parent; mutations in genes encoded by either may lead to mitochondrial dysfunction.

The mode of inheritance in mitochondrial diseases is quite complex, since the structure of mitochondria and the respiratory chain proteins are a consequence of both the mitochondrial and nuclear genomes. Mitochondrial DNA has a high mutation rate with mutations encompassing point mutations or deletions/duplications. The reported frequency of pathogenic mutations in mitochondrial DNA is about 1 in 200 births.[5]

Mitochondrial DNA mutations can either be de novo or inherited from the mother. If inherited from the mother, and the mother is homoplasmic (i.e., all of her mitochondria carry the mutation), all of her children will be affected. If the mother is heteroplasmic (heteroplasmy: the presence of more than one type of organellar genome within a cell or individual), clinical severity may be variable depending on the number of normal and affected mitochondria that are present in the offspring (Fig. 8.2). Generally speaking, the limit of detection of heteroplasmy is ≥15% in blood by Sanger sequencing,[6] while newer techniques have the potential to improve this to identifying heteroplasmy of ≤1.33%.[7,8] Defects in genes of nuclear origin may result in autosomal recessive, dominant inheritance or X-linked inheritance. A common misperception among providers is that mitochondrial diseases are always of maternal origin but, in reality, most mitochondrial disease is secondary to nuclear gene defects and exhibit autosomal recessive inheritance. Determining the precise inheritance pattern of mitochondrial diseases is crucial for accurate reproductive counseling.

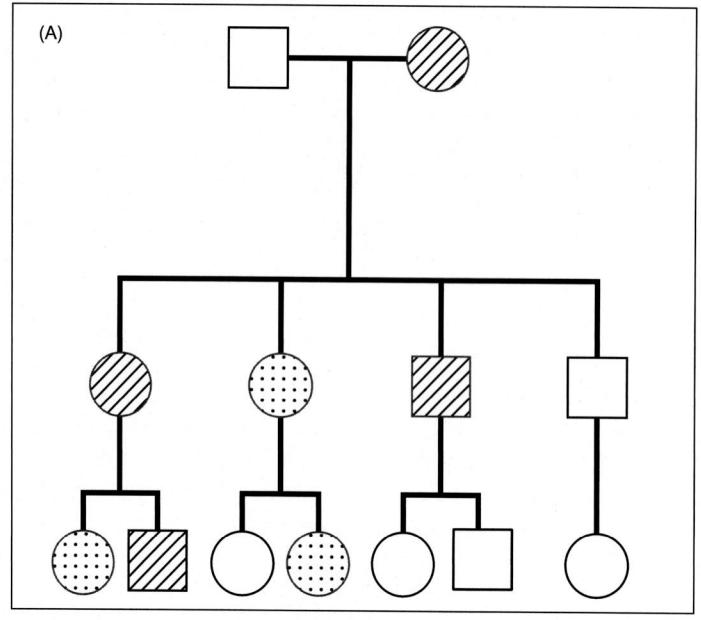

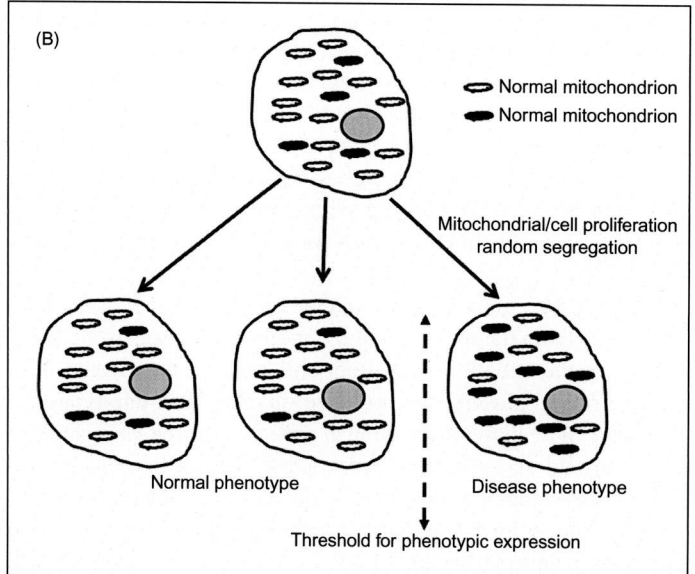

FIGURE 8.2

(A) Mitochondrial (maternal) inheritance. Both males and females may be affected to varying degrees, but only females will pass on the trait to subsequent generations. (B) Heteroplasmy and the bottleneck affect. Variations in the number of normal and mutated mitochondria exist within the same cell. Phenotypic expression of a pathogenic trait occurs only after a threshold is reached or surpassed.

8.4 DIAGNOSIS

Owing to the vast array of clinical phenotypes and age of onset, establishing a diagnosis is often challenging. Along with obtaining a detailed personal and family history, and comprehensive physical exam, an evaluation in suspected cases should include a cardiology evaluation, ophthalmic assessment, neuroimaging including both MRI and magnetic resonance spectroscopy (MRS), and lactate level measurement in blood and/or cerebrospinal fluid (CSF). Muscle biopsy or fibroblast skin biopsy to assess for abnormal mitochondrial respiratory chain function has been considered the gold standard for diagnosis but results may be negative, even if disease is present. It is important to note that lactic acidosis may be seen in other conditions. An ischemic cerebrovascular event may cause an elevated lactate concentration in the CSF after the episode, and seizures unrelated to mitochondrial disease may cause elevated lactate levels in plasma and CSF, for example. With the advent of newer testing modalities, the need for more invasive studies is decreasing. For example, molecular genetic testing panels are now more readily available and able to identify mtDNA or nDNA mutations and can be used for confirmation of the diagnosis.

8.5 DIAGNOSTIC STUDIES

8.5.1 BIOCHEMICAL TESTING

8.5.1.1 Metabolic panel and creatine kinase

When evaluating a patient with suspected mitochondrial disease, it is important to develop an understanding of the body's acid–base system, kidney and liver function, as well as nutrition parameters. Therefore a metabolic panel including sodium (Na), potassium (K), chloride (Cl), carbondioxide (CO_2), BUN (blood urea nitrogen), creatinine (Cr), glucose, liver function tests (AST, ALT, bilirubin), total protein (TP), albumin (Alb), and creatine kinase (CK) should be requested. Anion gap should be calculated. Metabolic acidosis can be present and anion gap can be increased. Liver dysfunction can be present.

8.5.1.2 Lactate and pyruvate levels

Lactate levels should be obtained in blood gas collection syringes and placed on ice. Results are often available quickly as most blood gas machines also simultaneously measure lactate. There is often a misconception among providers that elevated blood lactate levels (>2.1 mM) are diagnostic for mitochondrial disease. However, lactate levels are nonspecific and may be elevated from prolonged tourniquet use or poor specimen handling, in addition to medical causes of lactic acidemia. Ideally, samples should be obtained from a free-flowing arterial sample, although this is often not practical or possible in most outpatient clinics. Also many patients with mitochondrial disease may have normal lactate levels when well but have distinct elevations only with intense exercise or significant illness. A nonischemic forearm test, as compared to the traditional ischemic forearm exercise test, has been proven to be a safe and useful tool in the detection of some individuals with either glycogenolysis defects or mitochondrial disorders.[9,10]

CSF lactate elevations may also be secondary to infection, seizures, or stroke. Therefore, elevations in blood or CSF lactate should be evaluated in the context of other biochemical parameters.

Pyruvate levels require special processing and special collection tubes containing perchlorate and placement on ice. Most pyruvate samples will be sent out to specialty laboratories and therefore results may take several days, making immediate clinical interpretation difficult. Blood lactate/pyruvate ratios reflect $NAD^+/NADH$ redox states. While pyruvate elevations are seen in pyruvate decarboxylase and dehydrogenase deficiencies, the ratio of lactic acid to pyruvic acid may be more helpful in generating a differential diagnosis. A normal lactic:pyruvate ratio is <25. If a ratio of greater than 25 is found, this is highly suggestive of a mitochondrial disorder. The only caveat to this interpretation is that deficiency of pyruvate dehydrogenase complex activity maintains a normal lactate:pyruvate ratio in the face of lactatemia and lactic acidemia.

8.5.1.3 Plasma amino acid profile

Samples should be obtained in a green top tube (heparin or EDTA (ethylenediamine-tetraacetic acid)) and placed on ice for proper handling and be analyzed by quantitative methods. Although alanine elevations >450 mM are suggestive of mitochondrial dysfunction, this is nonspecific and not diagnostic.

8.5.1.4 Urine organic acid profile

Since organic acids are by-products of amino acid catabolism and the Krebs cycle, qualitative urine organic acid analysis is often diagnostic for the organic acidemias. However, it is not specific for identification of mitochondrial disorders. Often there will be general markers of global mitochondrial dysfunction such as elevations in lactate, and presence of ethylmalonic acid, dicarboxylic aciduria, Krebs cycle intermediates, and methylglutaconic acid. Although these are suggestive, they are neither pathognomonic nor definitive for diagnosis.

8.5.1.5 Carnitine

There is no acylcarnitine profile that is diagnostic for any of the mitochondrial disorders. Carnitine deficiency is frequently seen in mitochondrial and respiratory chain disorders[11] and is thought to be related to compromised energy-dependent carnitine transport at the membrane.[12]

8.5.1.6 Magnetic resonance spectroscopy

Magnetic resonance spectroscopy (MRS) is a relatively new radiologic modality that can be used to identify and quantitate intracranial cellular metabolites. It is a non-invasive method that does not use ionizing radiation with excellent signal-to-noise ratio and contrast resolution, along with multiplanar imaging capabilities. Its role in the evaluation of congenital and developmental brain abnormalities, as well as evaluation of inborn errors of metabolism has been expanding.[13–15] A recent study by Lunsing et al. evaluated 88 children with neurometabolic disease and subdivided into groups that had a definite, probable, possible, or unlikely diagnosis of a mitochondrial disorder. Of these 88 children, CSF lactate levels were available for 61. There was a statistical difference between the MRS lactate level and the lactate-to-creatinine ratio between the definite and the unlikely group ($p = 0.015$ and $p = 0.001$, respectively). There was a difference between the lactate-to-creatinine ratio between those with a probable diagnosis and an MRS reference subgroup ($p = 0.03$). Interestingly, there were no significant differences between measured CSF lactate levels. The authors conclude that MRS-quantified brain tissue lactate levels can be a diagnostic marker for mitochondrial disease in children and that brain tissue lactate levels are quantifiable, that the MRS lactate and L/Cr ratios are increased in children with mitochondrial disease and that CSF lactate biochemical quantification may be a less accurate measure than that obtained by MRS.[14] Thus, it may be that in the future, MRS as a diagnostic modality for mitochondrial disorders may become the standard of care.

8.5.1.7 Whole exome sequencing

Recent advances in next-generation sequencing technology have allowed for improved diagnosis of mitochondrial disorders.[16–18] Several studies have shown improved diagnostic rates up to 47% in suspected cases.[2,4,19–21]

Currently available next-generation sequencing panels such as "MitoExome" have led to the identification of a molecular etiology in up to 47% of individuals with OXPHOS deficiencies. Also low-level mtDNA heteroplasmy can be reliably identified. With technical improvements and addition of new genes to existing panels, the above technologies are likely to replace invasive tissue studies except in select cases.

8.6 TREATMENT

The treatment of mitochondrial disorders is supportive. Often, management includes a multidisciplinary approach while utilizing a combination of vitamins and cofactors, optimizing health status including nutrition and exercise, and treating illnesses and other physiologic stresses appropriately.[22]

Patients with mitochondrial disease may be malnourished from difficulties with feeding secondary to neurological involvement to malabsorption from the gut or liver dysfunction. Therefore, a metabolic nutritionist should be involved in management to determine caloric intake, protein status, and vitamin and mineral deficiencies. A determination of resting metabolic rate is often available at major medical centers. Caloric intake can be tailored accordingly with frequent, small meals, and prevention of prolonged fasting. The goal is to prevent catabolic states.

If needed, gastric tubes or jejunostomy tubes may be considered. Some patients will do better on restriction of fat or protein and some will restrict carbohydrates. In some patients, total parenteral nutrition may be indicated although it should be used judiciously in some patients with mitochondrial neurogastrointestinal encephalopathy (MNGIE) as it may precipitate liver dysfunction. Feeding therapies for swallowing difficulties, medical management of gut motility, and gastroesophageal reflux disease (GERD) is also indicated.

Illness management is paramount and patients should be treated early during illness or febrile episodes. Patients have inappropriate stress responses and may decompensate quickly even with minor illness. Admission to the hospital should be earlier rather than later, with the initiation of intravenous (IV) fluids to prevent catabolism and treat dehydration. Unstable patients should be in the intensive care unit and general principles of airway and circulatory management should be applied. Fluids should contain 10% dextrose solution with electrolytes and provided at a rate of 1.5 times maintenance. However, in patients with existing cardiomyopathy or the elderly, caution should be exercised in order to prevent fluid overload and pulmonary edema.

Lactated ringer is contraindicated as lactic acidosis may be present and worsen. Acute and persistent acidosis can be treated with sodium bicarbonate at 1 mEq/kg as a slow infusion. Higher rates of glucose infusion or parental nutrition may require a central line and even insulin infusion (0.005–0.1 U/kg) for anabolic effects.

Additionally, tailoring a treatment strategy for the early diagnosis and intervention for treatable complications due to the underlying mitochondrial disease should be done, such as cochlear implants for sensorineural hearing loss, low vision services for visual impairments, optimal blood glucose control for diabetes mellitus, and internal cardiac defibrillators for cardiac rhythm management.

Although there are no absolute medical contraindications, mitochondrial toxins should be also be avoided if possible; pharmacologic agents with reported mitochondrial toxicity include acetaminophen, aminoglycoside antibiotics, aminoglycoside and platinum chemotherapeutics, antiretrovirals, aspirin, beta-blockers, erythromycin, metformin, statins, and particularly valproic acid.[22–32]

Doses of certain anesthetic agents such as volatile compounds may need to be reduced and sevoflurane may be better tolerated. The use of propofol is controversial and is not recommended for procedures lasting longer than 30–60 minutes.

Although there is a lack of consensus as to clear evidence for any particular intervention, agents commonly used in the medical management include alpha-lipoic acid, coenzyme Q10, arginine, folinic acid, L-carnitine, creatine, riboflavin, thiamine, vitamins C and E.[22,33]

Vitamins and supplements may act as cofactors to critical enzymatic reactions in mitochondria; these include riboflavin and thiamine, vitamin C, vitamin E, alpha-lipoic acid, and creatine. See Table 8.3 for currently accepted doses.

Coenzyme Q10 (ubiquinone) is a cofactor in complex I and II and is present in all cells where it works in redox shuttling. Ubiquinol is a more effective reduced version and is preferred, although can be difficult to obtain and relatively costly. Several clinical trials are currently underway for new derivatives of CoQ. Ubiquinol doses are 2–8 mg/kg with 50–600 mg daily in adults. Ubiquinone is 5–30 mg/kg per day with

Table 8.3 Currently Accepted Doses of Vitamins and Supplements

Vitamin or Supplement	Accepted Dose
Alpha-lipoic acid	50–200 mg/kg daily
Creatine	0.1 g/kg daily, 5 g po in adults
Riboflavin	50–400 mg daily
Thiamine	B-complex vitamins as 50–100 mg daily
Vitamin C	5 mg/kg daily
Vitamin E	1–2 IU/kg po daily

300–2400 mg daily in adults. Both forms may be given in two divided doses with meals for improved absorbtion. CoQ10 levels decrease with age, and some providers advocate supplementation in healthy adults for its antioxidant properties.

Levo-carnitine has been a mainstay of the metabolic physicians' medical management regimen. L-carnitine is a quaternary ammonium compound that binds-carboxylic acids at its -hydroxyl position. It is needed for long-chain fatty acid transport into the mitochondrion as well as modulating coenzyme A homeostasis. It has been used in the treatment of respiratory chain defects and mtDNA encephalopathies to prevent secondary carnitine deficiency and coenzyme A depletion by the transesterification of toxic acyl-CoA intermediates to acyl-L-carnitines and releasing CoA.[34] While its use in fatty acid oxidation disorders is somewhat controversial, carnitine deficiency is frequently seen in mitochondrial and respiratory chain disorders[11] and is thought to be related to compromised energy-dependent carnitine transport at the membrane.[12] While no clinical trials have been performed demonstrating benefits of isolated carnitine use, a report by Campos et al. demonstrated improvement in muscle weakness, growth failure, encephalopathic symptoms, and cardiomyopathy in patients with documented carnitine deficiency.[11] While there is little evidence for efficacy, there is also little evidence for associated harm, although recent concern about trimethylamines generated by metabolism by gut bacteria and atherothrombosis has been raised.[35] If used, it tends to be given in doses between 50 and 200 mg/kg per day. The main side effects of treatment include a fishy body odor (from the aforementioned trimethylamines), nausea, vomiting, loose stools, and stomach upset.

While there is a theoretic risk for cardiac rhythm disturbances in the longer chain fatty acid oxidation disorders, it is unclear if a similar risk is present for those with other mitochondrial disorders.

Folinic acid, the reduced form of folic acid, is more efficiently transported across the blood brain barrier. It is available as leucovorin (D and L isomers), Deplin (5-MTHF (5-methyl tetrahydrofolate)) and isovorin (D isomer). Cerebral folate deficiency is present in certain mitochondrial disorders such as Kearns–Sayre syndrome (KSS) and supplementation is suggested on a case-by-case basis.

L-arginine is an amino acid that has recently been shown to be effective in MELAS patients. Arginine produces nitric oxide and has vasodilatory effects, which is useful in stroke-like episodes. IV administration during the acute phase of the episode as well as chronic oral administration has been shown to reduce severity and frequency of strokes and reduce tissue injury and improve circulation. The recommended dose is 500 mg/kg IV for several days during the acute episode. Maintenance dose is 150–300 mg/g orally or IV daily in two to three divided doses. Hypotension and hyperchloremic acidosis may occur with high IV arginine doses as the IV form is bound to HCl.

Most specialists advocate for immunizations to prevent potential infectious diseases that could be uniquely life-threatening for an individual with mitochondrial disease.[22] Further specific management issues may include ptosis correction and intraocular lens replacement for cataracts.

It is known that exercise can have a positive effect as a treatment for mitochondrial disorders.[36] Exercise is important in mitochondrial diseases as it may improve mitochondrial function as well as affecting overall mitochondrial biogenesis.[37] Several recent studies have shown improved well-being and muscle strength with endurance exercise. A rehabilitation specialist should monitor the exercise regimen.

8.7 CONFOUNDING CONDITIONS

While lactic acidemia is often considered a hallmark of mitochondrial disorders, lactic acidemia has many other causes. Thus, if one is presented with a patient with lactic acidemia, more common causes in an age-dependent fashion, such as poor perfusion of any etiology, sepsis, HIV, neoplasm, renal failure, or other inborn errors of metabolism (such as the organic acidemias or fatty acid oxidation disorders) should be considered. Other causes of lactic acidemia include cardiopulmonary disease, severe anemia, diabetes mellitus, and seizures. Since there is no specific biochemical test that is pathognomonic for a mitochondrial disorder, consideration of the diagnosis should be made in any patient with multisystem involvement and/or little response to usually effective interventions.

8.8 SELECTED DISORDERS

8.8.1 ALPERS–HUTTENLOCHER SYNDROME[38,39] (OMIM #203700)

Alpers–Huttenlocher syndrome (AHS) is an autosomal recessive disorder caused by mutations in the *POLG* gene. This gene encodes DNA polymerase gamma, which is essential for mitochondrial DNA replication. Over 60 mutations are currently known that result in this phenotype. Deficiency of this function results in a mitochondrial DNA depletion syndrome. While mutations in *POLG* can result in other phenotypes, Alpers–Huttenlocher disease is the most severe. Hallmark features of this disorder, with typical onset between the ages of 2 and 4 years of age, include intractable seizures, developmental regression, and liver dysfunction. While lactic acid levels may be within reference ranges, liver dysfunction is always present. There is a bimodal age of onset, with a second peak of onset between the ages of 17 and 24 years of age. Symptoms are progressive and ultimately fatal. Exposure to valproic acid is often implicated as a trigger and CSF pleocytosis is often present.

8.8.2 LEBER HEREDITARY OPTIC NEUROPATHY[40,41] (OMIM #535000)

Leber hereditary optic neuropathy (LHON) is a mitochondrially inherited form of vision loss. Onset of symptoms, which includes acute or subacute painless loss of central vision, is usually in the teens to twenties, although early childhood and later adult onset has been reported. Onset usually involves blurred and clouded vision, either unilaterally or bilaterally. If unilateral, bilateral involvement tends to occur rapidly (weeks–months). In a few, central vision will gradually improve; however, most cases progress to profound and permanent vision loss. Symptoms are related to optic disc atrophy. Ophthalmologic findings, including the aforementioned vision loss include disk hyperemia, edema of the peripapillary retinal nerve fiber layer, retinal telangecteses, and increased vascular tortuosity, although up to 20% of affected individuals will have no abnormalities of the fundi. Optic disk atrophy and electroretinogram abnormalities (pattern and visual evoked potentials) will be consistent with optic nerve dysfunction rather than retinal disease. Extraocular manifestations may include tremors, unusual movements, a peripheral neuropathy, and a multiple-sclerosis-like illness. Cardiac dysrhythmias have also been identified. MRI may be normal but may also demonstrate white matter abnormalities or a high signal within the optic nerves.[42]

Despite maternal inheritance, males tend to be more affected than females, although, interestingly approximately 50% of male and 85% of female carriers of the mutation manifest no symptoms. Mutations in the mitochondrial genes MT-ND1, MT-ND4, MT-ND4L, and MT-ND6 are all known to cause this phenotype. All of the encoded proteins are involved in electron transport chain and OXPHOS. Environmental factors such as smoking and alcohol use have been implicated in symptom development; hence, these activities should be particularly discouraged. There are no specific biochemical markers for this condition, rather, it must be suspected on symptom development.

8.8.3 LEIGH SYNDROME[43] (OMIM #256000) AND NEUROPATHY, ATAXIA, RETINITIS PIGMENTOSA SYNDROME [44,45] (OMIM #551500)

Leigh syndrome (LS) and Neuropathy, Ataxia, Retinitis Pigmentosa Syndrome (NARP) are both progressive neurodegenerative mitochondrial diseases. They are both on the continuum of disorders related to inadequate mitochondrial energy production. While LS can be caused by mutations in *MT-ATP6, MT-TL1, MT-TK, MT-TW, MT-TV, MT-ND1, MT-ND2, MT-ND3, MT-ND4, MT-ND5, MT-ND6,* and *MT-CO3*, NARP is exclusively caused by mutations in *MT-ATP6*.

LS, also known as subacute necrotizing encephalophyelopathy, typically has symptom onset between 3 and 12 months of age, often following an acute viral infection. Biochemically, blood and/or CSF lactate levels are elevated during illness and are associated with psychomotor retardation or regression. Features that may suggest the diagnosis include hypotonia, spasticity, chorea, or other movement disorders, cerebellar ataxia and/or a peripheral neuropathy. Infants may also present with hypertrophic cardiomyopathy. Diagnosis can be made by clinical criteria and molecular genetic testing. Diagnostic criteria include progressive neurologic disease with motor and intellectual developmental delay, signs and symptoms of brain stem and/or basal ganglia disease, and elevated blood and/or CSF lactate. One or more of the following must also be present to meet strict diagnostic criteria: characteristic features of LS on neuroimaging (bilateral symmetric hypodensities in the basal ganglia on computed tomography (CT) or bilateral symmetric hyperintense signal in brain stem and/or basal ganglia on T2-weighted MRI), typical neuropathologic changes (multiple focal symmetric necrotic lesions in the basal ganglia, thalamus, brain stem, dentate nuclei, and optic nerves representative of demyelination, gliosis, and vascular proliferation with a spongiform appearance to the lesions), or typical neuropathology in a similarly affected sibling.[46] Muscle biopsy is less commonly used in the diagnosis. Molecular genetic testing confirms the diagnosis. Treatment is supportive with the use of sodium bicarbonate or sodium citrate for acute acidotic episodes, antiepileptic medications (avoiding valproic acid and barbiturates because of their inhibitory effect on the electron transport chain), medications to treat dystonia (benzhexol, baclofen, tetrabenazine, gabapentin, or botulinum toxin injection), and management of cardiomyopathy under the care of a cardiologist. Prognosis is poor, with about 50% of affected individuals dying by the age of three years, secondary to cardiac or respiratory failure.

On the less severe end of the spectrum, individuals with NARP tend to have proximal neurogenic muscle weakness complicated by a sensory neuropathy, ataxia, and a pigmentary retinopathy. Unlike LS, onset of symptoms tends to be later, usually in early childhood, with ataxia and learning difficulties. Episodic deteriorations in association with viral illness may be interspersed in an otherwise relatively stable disease state. While diagnostic criteria exist for LS, this is not the case for NARP. The diagnosis tends to be established after identifications of neurogenic muscle weakness, which may have an accompanying peripheral neuropathy identified on electromyography and nerve conduction studies, ataxia with cerebral and cerebellar atrophy identified on MRI and retinitis pigmentosa, ranging from a mild salt-and-pepper retinopathy to bone spicule formation to bull's-eye maculopathy.[47,48]

As noted earlier, while LS can be caused by mutations in several genes, NARP is caused by mutations in *MT-ATP6*. While there is little strong genotype–phenotype correlation due to the effects of heteroplasmy, and hence, mutation copy number, the m.8993 T > G and the m.8993 T > C pathogenic variants do show some correlation. There is very little tissue-dependent or age-dependent variation in mutation load along with a strong correlation between mutation load and disease severity.[49,50] Individuals who have a mutation load of <60% of the m.8993 T > G pathogenic variant may be asymptomatic or suffer from a mild pigmentary retinopathy or migraine headaches, while those with mutations loads between 70% and 90% will have NARP and those with mutations loads of greater than 90% will have LS, although there may be overlap between asymptomatic individual and affected individual mutation load. In general, the m.8993 T > C mutation results in a less severe presentation, requiring more than a 90% mutation load for symptoms to be present.[51]

No specific treatments exist for NARP. Again, it is prudent to avoid sodium valproate and barbiturates, as well as to exert care during procedures that require anesthesia as this has the potential to lead to worsening of respiratory symptoms with resultant respiratory failure.[52]

8.8.4 MATERNALLY INHERITED DIABETES-DEAFNESS SYNDROME[53,54] (OMIM #520000)

It has long been recognized that hearing loss and insulin-dependent diabetes mellitus often represented mitochondrial dysfunction. It is now known that maternally inherited diabetes-deafness syndrome (MIDD) is caused by pathogenic variants in *MT-TL1*, *MT-TE*, and *MT-TK* genes. Affected individuals typically have symptom onset in mid-adulthood, although age of onset can range from childhood through late adulthood. Hearing loss tends to occur before insulin deficiency. Macular retinal dystrophy may also develop in affected individuals, although vision impairment is rare. Other possible manifestations include muscle cramping and weakness, cardiomyopathy, renal disease, gastrointestinal tract involvement (particularly constipation), or seizures.

8.8.5 MITOCHONDRIAL ENCEPHALOPATHY, LACTIC ACIDOSIS, STROKE-LIKE EPISODES[55,56] (OMIM #540000)

Mitochondrial encephalopathy, lactic acidosis, stroke-like episodes (MELAS) is a severe multisystem disease with initial presentation in early childhood. Often failure to gain weight and developmental delays are reported and sometimes initial soft neurological signs may be mistakenly interpreted as cerebral palsy. The disease process evolves over time with development of seizures and strokes. In infants and toddlers, stroke-like episodes may present initially as limb weakness or speech delays. Seizures may be generalized or focal and may present with recurrent hemiparesis or cortical blindness. Recurrent headaches may be interpreted as migraines but may be the prodrome of new stroke-like episodes. Although lactic acidosis is often elevated during episodes, it may be normal between episodes. Recurrent episodes, if untreated, result in motor, cognitive, and visual deficits. Sensorineural hearing loss is common and gastric dysmotility is present. Renal complications such as renal tubular acidosis may occur. Although cognition is initially normal, recurrent episodes may also affect the intellect. Anxiety and depression have been reported.

The incidence of MELAS not precisely known but is estimated to occur in about 1 in 4000 individuals. In the past, the gold standard of diagnosis was demonstration of ragged red fibers on muscle biopsy; however, inherent difficulties led to inconclusive biopsy results. Since diagnosis can now be easily confirmed by sequencing of DNA from either lymphocytes or cells from urine sediment, the need for muscle biopsy had declined but has not been completely eliminated (PIMD 15199381; 15372523).

MELAS is caused by mutations in several mitochondrially encoded genes (*MT-CO1, MT-CO2, MT-CO3, MT-CYB, MT-ND1, MT-ND5, MT-ND6, MT-TC, MT-TF, MT-TH, MT-TK, MT-TL1, MT-TQ, MT-TS1, MT-TS2, MT-TV, MT-TW*) and thus exhibits maternal inheritance.

The most common mutation is m.3243 A > G in *MT-TL1*, coding a mitochondrial tRNA leucine. Other more frequently occurring mitochondrial mutations seen in *MT-TL1* are the m.3271 T > C and m.3252 A > G pathogenic variants. These three mutations account for over 80% of the cases of MELAS.

8.8.6 MITOCHONDRIAL NEUROGASTROINTESTINAL ENCEPHALOPATHY SYNDROME[57] (OMIM #603041)

Mitochondrial neurogastrointestinal encephalopathy (MNGIE) syndrome is characterized by a progressive external ophthalmoplegia, ptosis, gastrointestinal dysmotility, peripheral neuropathy, cachexia, and leukoencephalopathy. The age of onset is usually between the second and fifth decades of life. Gastrointestinal dysmotility is the hallmark symptom of the disease. The prevalence of the condition is not known. The disorder results from pathogenic mutations in the *TYMP* gene. This nuclear gene encodes the enzyme thymidine phosphorylase, which breaks down thymidine and is critical for the regulation of intracellular nucleoside concentrations. Disruption of the intramitochondrial nucleoside pool with accumulation of thymidine and deoxyuridine is felt to be the underlying pathologic mechanism since nucleoside imbalance is postulated to disrupt mitochondrial DNA synthesis and repair (15571233, 20561600). This ultimately results in DNA depletion and mitochondrial dysfunction. Since *TYMP* is a nuclear gene, inheritance of MNGIE is in an autosomal recessive fashion, rather than maternally inherited.

Diagnosis requires a level of suspicion, with DNA analysis confirmation. Management is supportive with surveillance for swallowing difficulties and aspiration pneumonia, dromperidone for nausea and vomiting, parenteral nutrition support, and antibiotics for bacterial overgrowth. Neuropathic symptoms have been successfully managed with amitryptiine, nortryptyline, and gabapentin. Diverticulitis can occur and there should be a high suspicion for diverticular rupture in the presence of acute-onset abdominal pain.

8.8.7 MYOCLONIC EPILEPSY WITH RAGGED RED FIBERS SYNDROME[58] (OMIM #545000)

Myoclonic epilepsy with ragged red fibers (MERRF) is another multisystemic mitochondrial disorder, so named because of the "canonical features" of myoclonus, epilepsy, ataxia, and ragged red fibers on muscle biopsy. Signs and symptoms tend to present in childhood or adolescence, with wide variation among affected individuals, even within the same family. Features include myoclonus, myopathy, and progressive spasticity. Epilepsy is also common, as are ataxia, peripheral neuropathy, and dementia. Hearing loss and optic atrophy may also occur. Cardiomyopathy, along with Wolff–Parkinson–White rhythm disturbance, may also develop. Affected individuals may develop lipomas and may have short stature.

It is estimated to affect about 1 in 5000 people worldwide. While several mutations in several mitochondrial genes can lead to the MERRF phenotype (*MT-TH, MT-TK, MT-TL1, MT-TP, MT-TS1, MT-TS2, MT-TT*), mutations in *MT-TK*, which encodes a mitochondrial tRNA(Lys), are the most commonly identified mutations, present in greater than 80% of affected individuals. In fact, the most common change is m.8344 A > G. Pathogenic mutations tend to be identifiable in all tissue types, including leukocytes, fibroblasts, urine sediment, buccal cells, hair follicles, and skeletal muscle.

As with other mitochondrial disorders, treatment is supportive. Conventional antiepileptic medications are helpful with seizure control. Valproic acid and barbiturates should be avoided.

8.8.8 PEARSON MARROW–PANCREAS SYNDROME[59,60] (OMIM #557000)

Pearson marrow–pancreas syndrome (PMPS) is a very severe condition that typically begins in infancy. Infants with PMPS exhibit a refractory, transfusion-dependent sideroblastic anemia with vacuolization of hematopoietic precursors, along with exocrine pancreatic insufficiency. This results in severe anemia. Pancytopenia may also occur. Liver steatosis is common, as is malabsorption that leads to growth failure. Hyperglycemia, secondary to pancreatic damage and insulin deficiency has been seen. This condition is often fatal early in life, with mortality associated with kidney or liver failure. Lactic acidosis occurs, which can also be life-threatening. This condition is quite rare. For those children who survive, in addition to pancreatic insufficiency and insulin dependence, there can be progression to KSS: progressive external ophthalmoplegia, pigmentary retinitis, deafness, cerebellar ataxia, and/or cardiac conduction defects.

PMPS is caused by heteroplasmic deletions of mitochondrial DNA, ranging from 1000 to 10,000 bp in length. These deletions result in loss of coding sequences for proteins involved in OXPHOS. It is thought that lack of cellular energy plays a role in overall pathogenesis, although the mechanism is not completely clear. The most common deletion is a 4977-bp mt-DNA deletion, which is found in about 20% of affected individuals. In addition to deletions, duplications that functionally act like deletions can also cause this phenotype.

Complete blood count consistent with refractory anemia and paucity of white blood cells and platelets suggest the diagnosis but must be differentiated from other causes of anemia. Bone marrow biopsy will show a decrease in cellular precursors with an abnormal vacuolar appearance. Ringed sideroblasts biochemical parameters include lactic acidosis, hypoglycemia, elevated alanine levels on plasma amino acid profile and lactic acidosis, and Krebs cycle intermediates in urine organic acids.

Diagnosis is made through mtDNA deletion testing and identification of the common deletion. Fibroblast testing or muscle biopsy is not useful since the primary defect is in the bone marrow.

The disease is often fatal in early childhood. There is no treatment for this condition and efficacy of supplements is limited. Pancreatic enzyme replacement may provide some symptomatic relief for pancreatic dysfunction. Infection risk is increased, given bone marrow involvement. Early involvement of hospice providers may provide support to families. Longer term survival is associated with progression to KSS.

8.8.9 PROGRESSIVE EXTERNAL OPTHALMOPLEGIA AND KEARNS–SAYRE SYNDROME[61] (OMIM #530000)

Progressive external opthalmoplegia (PEO) and Kearns–Sayre Syndrome (KSS) represents two ends of the spectrum of the same disease. PEO presents with onset of eye muscle weakness, usually between the ages of 18 and 40. The initial presentation is typically ptosis that worsens over time. Ophthalmoplegia (weakness or paralysis of the extraocular muscles) also develops over time. The condition may further progress to a more generalized myopathy involving the neck, arms, or legs, along with dysphagia. Exercise intolerance is common. PEO can progress to KSS.

KSS tends to be more generalized than PEO. Ocular involvement, including progressive ophthalmoplegia along with ptosis, tends to be the cardinal symptom, occurring before the age of 20. In addition, individuals with KSS develop a pigmentary retinopathy, characterized by a speckled and streaked appearance, which may result in vision loss. Other symptoms associated with KSS include cardiac conduction defects, ataxia, generalized muscle weakness, deafness, and renal problems. Dementia is also a complication of KSS.

If muscle biopsy is performed, ragged red fibers are often apparent. Ragged red fibers represent mitochondrial proliferation in the cell and are pathognomonic for mitochondrial dysfunction. DNA sequencing is becoming the diagnostic modality of choice. Both conditions are caused by mutations in one of several genes, including *POLG, C10orf2, RRM2B, SLC25A4,* or *MT-TL1*. All but *MT-TL1* are nuclearly encoded genes, while *MT-TL1* is a mitochondrially encoded gene.

8.9 CONCLUSION

Providing the cell with energy in the form of ATP is the critical job of the mitochondrial respiratory chain. Mutations in genes encoded by mitochondrial or nuclear DNA can cause mitochondrial dysfunction, which may result in a disruption in the coordinated process of ATP synthesis that can lead to mitochondrial disease, thus, diagnosis of a specific mitochondrial disorder can be difficult. Dysfunction in the mitochondrial respiratory chain may manifest in a variety of clinical symptoms at any age with a variable mode of inheritance. Establishing the diagnosis often involves some combination of a careful personal and family history account, detailed physical examination, cardiology evaluation, ophthalmologic assessment, neuroimaging, obtaining lactate levels in blood and/or CSF, molecular genetic testing, or muscle biopsy. Management is supportive; specialized vitamin and cofactor therapy may provide some symptomatic improvement.

REFERENCES

1. Cooper GM, Hausman RE. The cell: a molecular approach. Sunderland, MA: Sinauer Associates; 2013.
2. Falk MJ, Sondheimer N. Mitochondrial genetic diseases. Curr Opin Pediatr 2010;**22**:711–6.
3. Haas RH, Parikh S, Falk MJ, Saneto RP, Wolf NI, Darin N, et al. Mitochondrial disease: a practical approach for primary care physicians. Pediatrics 2007;**120**:1326–33.
4. Falk MJ. Neurodevelopmental manifestations of mitochondrial disease. J Dev Behav Pediatr 2010;**31**:610–21.
5. Elliott HR, Samuels DC, Eden JA, Relton CL, Chinnery PF. Pathogenic mitochondrial DNA mutations are common in the general population. Am J Hum Genet 2008;**83**:254–60.
6. Rohlin A, Wernersson J, Engwall Y, Wiklund L, Bjork J, Nordling M. Parallel sequencing used in detection of mosaic mutations: comparison with four diagnostic DNA screening techniques. Hum Mutat 2009;**30**:1012–20.
7. Zhang W, Cui H, Wong LJ. Comprehensive one-step molecular analyses of mitochondrial genome by massively parallel sequencing. Clin Chem 2012;**58**:1322–31.
8. Cui H, Li F, Chen D, Wang G, Truong CK, Enns GM, et al. Comprehensive next-generation sequence analyses of the entire mitochondrial genome reveal new insights into the molecular diagnosis of mitochondrial DNA disorders. Genet Med 2013;**15**:388–94.
9. Kazemi-Esfarjani P, Skomorowska E, Jensen TD, Haller RG, Vissing J. A nonischemic forearm exercise test for McArdle disease. Ann Neurol 2002;**52**:153–9.
10. Hanisch F, Eger K, Bork S, Lehnich H, Deschauer M, Zierz S. Lactate production upon short-term non-ischemic forearm exercise in mitochondrial disorders and other myopathies. J Neurol 2006;**253**:735–40.
11. Campos Y, Huertas R, Lorenzo G, Bautista J, Gutierrez E, Aparicio M, et al. Plasma carnitine insufficiency and effectiveness of L-carnitine therapy in patients with mitochondrial myopathy. Muscle Nerve 1993;**16**:150–3.
12. Pons R, De Vivo DC. Primary and secondary carnitine deficiency syndromes. J Child Neurol 1995;**10**(Suppl 2) S8-24.
13. Shekdar K, Wang DJ. Role of magnetic resonance spectroscopy in evaluation of congenital/developmental brain abnormalities. Semin Ultrasound CT MR 2011;**32**:510–38.
14. Lunsing RJ, Strating K, de Koning TJ, Sijens PE. Diagnostic value of MRS-quantified brain tissue lactate level in identifying children with mitochondrial disorders. Eur Radiol 2016.
15. Haas RH, Parikh S, Falk MJ, Saneto RP, Wolf NI, Darin N, et al. The in-depth evaluation of suspected mitochondrial disease and Diagnosis, M.M.S.s.C.o. Mol Genet Metab 2008;**94**:16–37.
16. Dinwiddie DL, Smith LD, Miller NA, Atherton AM, Farrow EG, Strenk ME, et al. Diagnosis of mitochondrial disorders by concomitant next-generation sequencing of the exome and mitochondrial genome. Genomics 2013;**102**:148–56.

17. McCormick E, Place E, Falk MJ. Molecular genetic testing for mitochondrial disease: from one generation to the next. Neurotherapeutics 2013;**10**:251–61.

18. Wortmann SB, Koolen DA, Smeitink JA, van den Heuvel L, Rodenburg RJ. Whole exome sequencing of suspected mitochondrial patients in clinical practice. J Inherit Metab Dis 2015;**38**:437–43.

19. Lieber DS, Calvo SE, Shanahan K, Slate NG, Liu S, Hershman SG, et al. Targeted exome sequencing of suspected mitochondrial disorders. Neurology 2013;**80**:1762–70.

20. Falk MJ, Pierce EA, Consugar M, Xie MH, Guadalupe M, Hardy O, et al. Mitochondrial disease genetic diagnostics: optimized whole-exome analysis for all MitoCarta nuclear genes and the mitochondrial genome. Discov Med 2012;**14**:389–99.

21. Falk MJ, Shen L, Gonzalez M, Leipzig J, Lott MT, Stassen AP, et al. Mitochondrial Disease Sequence Data Resource (MSeqDR): a global grass-roots consortium to facilitate deposition, curation, annotation, and integrated analysis of genomic data for the mitochondrial disease clinical and research communities. Mol Genet Metab 2015;**114**:388–96.

22. Parikh S, Saneto R, Falk MJ, Anselm I, Cohen BH, Haas R. A modern approach to the treatment of mitochondrial disease Medicine Society, T.M. Curr Treat Options Neurol 2009;**11**:414–30.

23. Silva MF, Aires CC, Luis PB, Ruiter JP, IJlst L, Duran M, et al. Valproic acid metabolism and its effects on mitochondrial fatty acid oxidation: a review. J Inherit Metab Dis 2008;**31**:205–16.

24. Dalakas MC. Peripheral neuropathy and antiretroviral drugs. J Peripher Nerv Syst 2001;**6**:14–20.

25. Scruggs ER, Dirks Naylor AJ. Mechanisms of zidovudine-induced mitochondrial toxicity and myopathy. Pharmacology 2008;**82**:83–8.

26. Pinti M, Salomoni P, Cossarizza A. Anti-HIV drugs and the mitochondria. Biochim Biophys Acta 2006;**1757**:700–7.

27. Littarru GP, Langsjoen P. Coenzyme Q10 and statins: biochemical and clinical implications. Mitochondrion 2007;**7**(Suppl):S168–74.

28. Sirvent P, Mercier J, Lacampagne A. New insights into mechanisms of statin-associated myotoxicity. Curr Opin Pharmacol 2008;**8**:333–8.

29. Wagner BK, Kitami T, Gilbert TJ, Peck D, Ramanathan A, Schreiber SL, et al. Large-scale chemical dissection of mitochondrial function. Nat Biotechnol 2008;**26**:343–51.

30. Bindu LH, Reddy PP. Genetics of aminoglycoside-induced and prelingual non-syndromic mitochondrial hearing impairment: a review. Int J Audiol 2008;**47**:702–7.

31. Kovacic P, Pozos RS, Somanathan R, Shangari N, O'Brien PJ. Mechanism of mitochondrial uncouplers, inhibitors, and toxins: focus on electron transfer, free radicals, and structure-activity relationships. Curr Med Chem 2005;**12**:2601–23.

32. Spiller HA, Sawyer TS. Toxicology of oral antidiabetic medications. Am J Health Syst Pharm 2006;**63**:929–38.

33. Pfeffer G, Majamaa K, Turnbull DM, Thorburn D, Chinnery PF. Treatment for mitochondrial disorders. Cochrane Database Syst Rev 2012;**4** CD004426.

34. Pons R, De Vivo DC. Mitochondrial Disease. Curr Treat Options Neurol 2001;**3**:271–88.

35. Chhibber-Goel J, Gaur A, Singhal V, Parakh N, Bhargava B, Sharma A. The complex metabolism of trimethylamine in humans: endogenous and exogenous sources. Expert Rev Mol Med 2016;**18**:e8.

36. Mahoney DJ, Parise G, Tarnopolsky MA. Nutritional and exercise-based therapies in the treatment of mitochondrial disease. Curr Opin Clin Nutr Metab Care 2002;**5**:619–29.

37. Menshikova EV, Ritov VB, Fairfull L, Ferrell RE, Kelley DE, Goodpaster BH. Effects of exercise on mitochondrial content and function in aging human skeletal muscle. J Gerontol A Biol Sci Med Sci 2006;**61**:534–40.
38. Saneto RP, Cohen BH, Copeland WC, Naviaux RK. Alpers-Huttenlocher syndrome. Pediatr Neurol 2013;**48**:167–78.
39. Harding BN. Progressive neuronal degeneration of childhood with liver disease (Alpers-Huttenlocher syndrome): a personal review. J Child Neurol 1990;**5**:273–87.
40. Newman NJ. Leber's hereditary optic neuropathy. New genetic considerations. Arch Neurol 1993;**50**:540–8.
41. Newman NJ, Wallace DC. Mitochondria and Leber's hereditary optic neuropathy. Am J Ophthalmol 1990;**109**:726–30.
42. Yu-Wai-Man P, Chinnery PF. Leber hereditary optic neuropathy. In: Pagon RA, Adam MP, Ardinger HH, Wallace SE, Amemiya A, Bean LJH, Bird TD, Fong CT, Mefford HC, Smith RJH, et al., editors. *GeneReviews*®. Seattle, WA: University of Washington; 1993.
43. Van Maldergem L, Trijbels F, DiMauro S, Sindelar PJ, Musumeci O, Janssen A, et al. Coenzyme Q-responsive Leigh's encephalopathy in two sisters. Ann Neurol 2002;**52**:750–4.
44. Kerrison JB, Biousse V, Newman NJ. Retinopathy of NARP syndrome. Arch Ophthalmol 2000;**118**:298–9.
45. López-Gallardo E, Solano A, Herrero-Martín MD, Martínez-Romero I, Castaño-Pérez MD, Andreu AL, et al. NARP syndrome in a patient harbouring an insertion in the MT-ATP6 gene that results in a truncated protein. J Med Genet 2009;**46**:64–7.
46. Rahman S, Blok RB, Dahl HH, Danks DM, Kirby DM, Chow CW, et al. Leigh syndrome: clinical features and biochemical and DNA abnormalities. Ann Neurol 1996;**39**:343–51.
47. Ortiz RG, Newman NJ, Shoffner JM, Kaufman AE, Koontz DA, Wallace DC. Variable retinal and neurologic manifestations in patients harboring the mitochondrial DNA 8993 mutation. Arch Ophthalmol 1993;**111**:1525–30.
48. Chowers I, Lerman-Sagie T, Elpeleg ON, Shaag A, Merin S. Cone and rod dysfunction in the NARP syndrome. Br J Ophthalmol 1999;**83**:190–3.
49. White SL, Shanske S, McGill JJ, Mountain H, Geraghty MT, DiMauro S, et al. Mitochondrial DNA mutations at nucleotide 8993 show a lack of tissue- or age-related variation. J Inherit Metab Dis 1999;**22**:899–914.
50. White SL, Collins VR, Wolfe R, Cleary MA, Shanske S, DiMauro S, et al. Genetic counseling and prenatal diagnosis for the mitochondrial DNA mutations at nucleotide 8993. Am J Hum Genet 1999;**65**:474–82.
51. Thorburn DR, Rahman S. Mitochondrial DNA-associated leigh syndrome and NARP. In: Pagon RA, Adam MP, Ardinger HH, Wallace SE, Amemiya A, Bean LJH, Bird TD, Fong CT, Mefford HC, Smith RJH, et al., editors. *GeneReviews*®. Seattle, WA: University of Washington; 1993.
52. Niezgoda J, Morgan PG. Anesthetic considerations in patients with mitochondrial defects. Paediatr Anaesth 2013;**23**:785–93.
53. Ballinger SW, Shoffner JM, Hedaya EV, Trounce I, Polak MA, Koontz DA, et al. Maternally transmitted diabetes and deafness associated with a 10.4 kb mitochondrial DNA deletion. Nat Genet 1992;**1**:11–15.
54. Guillausseau PJ, Massin P, Dubois-LaForgue D, Timsit J, Virally M, Gin H, et al. Maternally inherited diabetes and deafness: a multicenter study. Ann Intern Med 2001;**134**:721–8.

55. Malfatti E, Laforêt P, Jardel C, Stojkovic T, Behin A, Eymard B, et al. High risk of severe cardiac adverse events in patients with mitochondrial m.3243A> G mutation. Neurology 2013;**80**:100–5.

56. Parsons T, Weimer L, Engelstad K, Linker A, Battista V, Wei Y, et al. Autonomic symptoms in carriers of the m.3243A> G mitochondrial DNA mutation. Arch Neurol 2010;**67**:976–9.

57. Taanman JW, Daras M, Albrecht J, Davie CA, Mallam EA, Muddle JR, et al. Characterization of a novel TYMP splice site mutation associated with mitochondrial neurogastrointestinal encephalomyopathy (MNGIE). Neuromuscul Disord 2009;**19**:151–4.

58. Blakely EL, Trip SA, Swalwell H, He L, Wren DR, Rich P, et al. A new mitochondrial transfer RNAPro gene mutation associated with myoclonic epilepsy with ragged-red fibers and other neurological features. Arch Neurol 2009;**66**:399–402.

59. Pearson HA, Lobel JS, Kocoshis SA, Naiman JL, Windmiller J, Lammi AT, et al. A new syndrome of refractory sideroblastic anemia with vacuolization of marrow precursors and exocrine pancreatic dysfunction. J Pediatr 1979;**95**:976–84.

60. Blaw ME, Mize CE. Juvenile Pearson syndrome. J Child Neurol 1990;**5**:187–90.

61. Barshop BA, Nyhan WL, Naviaux RK, McGowan KA, Friedlander M, Haas RH. Kearns-Sayre syndrome presenting as 2-oxoadipic aciduria. Mol Genet Metab 2000;**69**:64–8.

62. Pollard TD, Earnshaw WC, Lippincott-Schwartz J. Cell biology. Philadelphia, PA: Saunders/Elsevier; 2008.

Lysosomal storage disorders: mucopolysaccharidoses

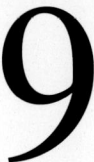

9

C. Yu

Icahn School of Medicine at Mount Sinai, New York, NY, United States

9.1 INTRODUCTION

Mucopolysaccharidoses (MPS) are a group of lysosomal storage disorders with defects in enzymes needed for degradation of mucopolysaccharides or glycosaminoglycans (GAGs). Eleven enzymes are involved in the catabolic pathways of chondroitin sulfate, dermatan sulfate, heparan sulfate, keratan sulfate, or hyaluronan. Deficiencies of these enzymes result in specific GAG accumulations in lysosomes and cellular dysfunction ultimately leading to clinical manifestations in various tissues and organs. Seven types of MPS disorders have been identified to date depending on the enzymatic defects and storage material (Table 9.1). MPS disorders are typically multisystemic, with progressive involvements of brain, visceral organs, and bones. Nondegraded or partially degraded fragments of GAGs are excreted in the urine, which can be used for screening and diagnosis of MPS disorders. Various enzyme replacement therapies (ERTs) have been developed or are under investigation for treatment of MPS. There are also analytical developments that enable newborn screening for several conditions, with the hope that early identification and treatment may reduce the morbidity and mortality of these rare diseases.

9.2 BRIEF DESCRIPTION OF CLINCIAL PRESENTATIONS

MPS disorders are heterogeneous and progressive disorders involving multiple systems. Most infants with an MPS disorder appear normal at birth, but develop characteristics of the disorder over time. MPS disorders share many common clinical features to variable degrees. These include coarse facial features, short stature, skeletal dysplasia (dysostosis multiplex), joint stiffness, organomegaly, cardiac valve disease, corneal clouding, hearing loss, airway obstruction, and respiratory infections.[1,2] These clinical features are strong indications for MPS. There are also characteristic clinical manifestations that are specific to certain MPS disorders and can be useful for differential diagnosis. Corneal clouding, while a feature of the majority of MPS disorders is not considered a primary characteristic of either MPS II (Hunter syndrome)

Biomarkers in Inborn Errors of Metabolism. DOI: http://dx.doi.org/10.1016/B978-0-12-802896-4.00006-7

191

Table 9.1 Summary of Mucopolysaccharidoses (MPS)

MPS Subtype	Eponym	Enzyme Deficiency	Gene Symbols	Accumulating Substrates	Key Clinical Features
MPS I	Hurler/Hurler-Scheie/Scheie	α-L-Iduronidase	IDUA	Dermatan sulfate Heparan sulfate	Characteristic coarse facies, organomegaly, dysostosis multiplex, joint stiffness, cardiac disease, cognitive impairment.
MPS II	Hunter	Iduronate 2-sulfatase	IDS	Dermatan sulfate Heparan sulfate	Similar to MPS I. X-linked. Corneal clouding is not present.
MPS III A	Sanfilippo A	Heparan-N-sulfatase (Heparan sulfamidase)	SGSH	Heparan sulfate	Progressive behavioral deterioration, hyperactivity, aggression, sleep disturbances, mild dysmorphisms with hirsutism. Mild somatic changes.
MPS III B	Sanfilippo B	α-N-Acetylglucosaminidase	NAGLU		
MPS III C	Sanfilippo C	AcetylCoA-glucosaminide acetyltransferase	HGSNAT		
MPS III D	Sanfilippo D	N-Acetylglucosamine 6-sulfatase	GNS		
MPS IV A	Morquio A	N-Acetylgalactosamine 6-sulfatase	GALNS	Keratan sulfate Chondroitin-6-sulfate	Characteristic skeletal dysplasia with short trunk dwarfism, kyphosis and genu valgum. Odontoid hypoplasia is common. Normal intelligence.
MPS IV B	Morquio B	β-Galactosidase	GLB1	Keratan sulfate	
MPS VI	Maroteaux-Lamy	N-Acetylgalactosamine-4-sulfatase (Arylsulfatase B)	ARSB	Dermatan sulfate	Hurler-like phenotype with normal cognitive function.
MPS VII	Sly	β-Glucuronidase	GUSB	Dermatan sulfate Heparan sulfate Chondroitin sulfates	Similar to MPS I. Variable presentations. Severe form presents in utero with fetalis hydrops or neonatal period.
MPS IX	Natowitz	Hyaluronidase	HYAL1	Hyaluronan	Soft tissue masses. Only a few case reports.

or MPS III (Sanfilippo syndrome).[3] Profound intellectual disability is characteristic of severe forms of MPS I (Hurler syndrome), MPS II, and all subtypes of MPS III, but intelligence may be preserved in MPS IV (Morquio syndrome) and MPS VI (Maroteaux–Lamy syndrome) where heparan sulfate is not elevated. Distinctive skeletal abnormalities are specific to MPS IV as keratan sulfate accumulates selectively in bones. For each of the MPS disorders, there is a wide range of phenotypic variability among affected individuals. When an MPS is clinically suspected, urine GAG analysis should be performed. Detection of an abnormal GAG pattern can narrow down the abnormalities to the catabolic pathways of dermatan sulfate, heparan sulfate, keratan sulfate, or chondroitin sulfate. A definitive diagnosis can be made after measurement of specific enzyme activities and identification of disease-causing mutations in the encoding gene.

9.3 MUCOPOLYSACCHARIDOSES

9.3.1 MPS I (HURLER, HURLER-SCHEIE, AND SCHEIE SYNDROMES)

MPS I is an autosomal recessive disorder caused by mutations of the *IDUA* gene leading to a deficiency of lysosomal α-L-iduronidase. The estimated incidence is approximately 1:100,000 live births. This enzyme cleaves the L-iduronic acid from the nonreducing terminus of dermatan sulfate and heparan sulfate (Fig. 9.1). The excess storage of dermatan sulfate primarily causes somatic symptoms of bones, cartilage, and visceral organs while the accumulation of heparan sulfate affects the central nervous system (CNS).

Historically, MPS I has been classified into three clinical syndromes—Hurler, Hurler-Scheie, and Scheie, with disease severity ranging from severe (Hurler) to mild (Scheie). The current recommended nomenclature is to use severe MPS I for patients with cognitive deficits and attenuated MPS I for those without. Approximately 60% of patients with MPS I have the Hurler phenotype.[4] Patients with Hurler present early with classic features of MPS, including hepatosplenomegaly, coarse facial features, dysostosis multiplex, joint stiffness, and contractures. Hurler syndrome is often suspected by the characteristic coarse facies and an enlarged tongue, with developmental delay apparent during the first year of life. The somatic changes and cognitive impairment progress rapidly in Hurler syndrome. Without ERT or bone marrow transplantation, most patients with Hurler die within the first decade of life from airway disease, respiratory infection, and heart disease. Individuals with attenuated MPS I have milder symptoms and slower disease progression and may live well into adulthood.[1,2,4,5]

9.3.2 MPS II (HUNTER SYNDROME)

MPS II, also known as Hunter syndrome, is an X-linked recessive disorder that primarily affects males, although a few females with milder phenotype have been identified due to skewed X-inactivation patterns or inheritance of another sex chromosome

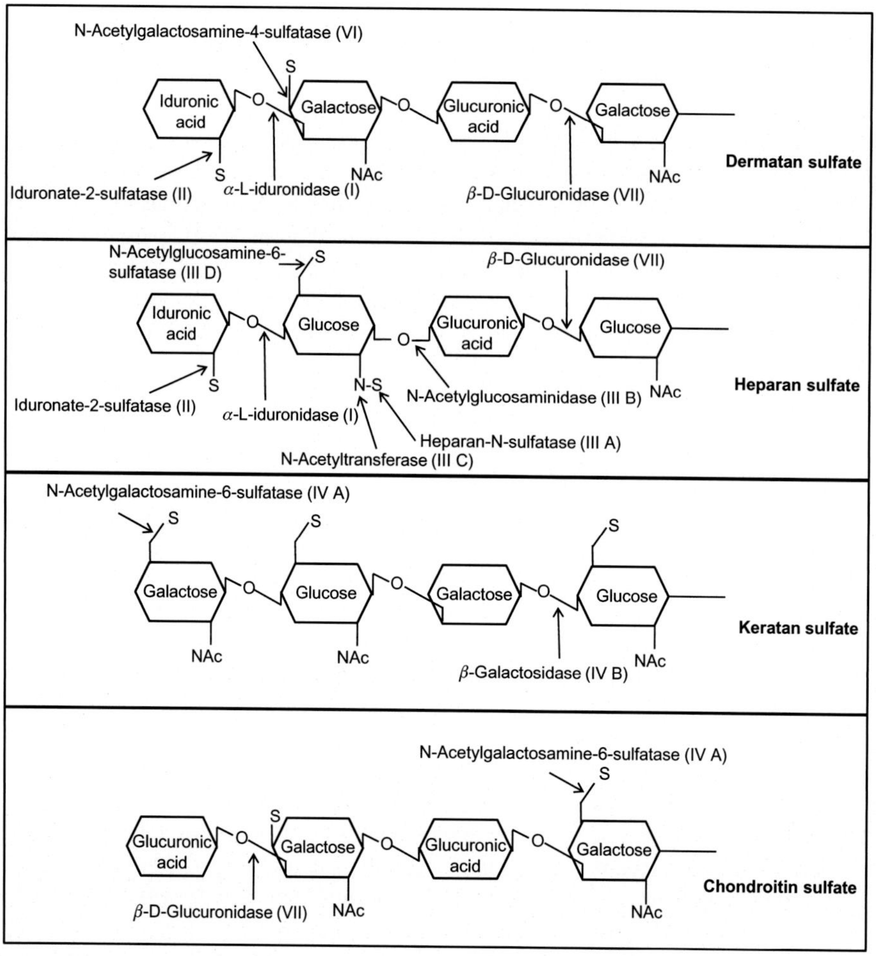

FIGURE 9.1

The catabolism of GAGs. The catabolism starts from the nonreducing (left) end of GAGs. Enzyme deficiencies in different MPS types are shown in parentheses.

abnormality.[6] The incidence of MPS II is estimated between 1:100,000 and 1:170,000 male births.[7,8] Mutations in the *IDS* gene on the X-chromosome lead to a deficiency of iduronate-2-sulfatase, which cleaves the C2 sulfate from L-iduronic acid residues at the nonreducing ends (NREs) of heparin, heparan sulfate, and dermatan sulfate (Fig. 9.1). More than 500 mutations have been identified to date, approximately 40% of which are deletions, duplications, insertions, indels, or complex rearrangements mechanisms (Human Gene Mutation Database (HGMD)). Affected individuals, similarly to those with MPS I, excrete high levels of urinary dermatan and heparan sulfate.

Similar to MPS I, MPS II is also a chronic and progressive lysosomal storage disorder affecting multiple organ systems with variable age of onset, presentation of symptoms, and rate of progression. Patients with MPS II are often classified as severe MPS II or a more mild attenuated form (attenuated MPS II). The more severe form of MPS II is characterized by progressive cognitive impairment, progressive airway disease, and heart disease. Death usually occurs in the first, second, or third decades of life. Those with an attenuated form of MPS II typically have no-to-minimal cognitive involvement, living well into adulthood. Pebbly, cream/white-colored skin lesions (peau d'orange) are seen in some individuals with MPS II that are not seen in any other MPS disorder and can aid in the diagnosis of MPS II. Corneal clouding is not typically seen in MPS II.[1,2,9,10]

9.3.3 MPS III A, B, C, AND D (SANFILIPPO SYNDROME, TYPE A, B, C, AND D)

MPS III, also known as Sanfilippo syndrome, is a group of four lysosomal storage disorders that share similar clinical features but are caused by four distinct enzyme deficiencies (Table 9.1). The combined incidence is 0.28–4.1 per 100,000 live births, making MPS III the most common type of MPS.[11] All four enzymes are required for the removal of N-sulfated or N-acetylated glucosamine residues during the degradation of heparan sulfate: heparan-N-sulfatase (type A), α-N-acetylglucosaminidase (type B), glucosamine-N-acetyltransferase (type C), and N-acetylglucosamine-6-sulfatase (type D) (Fig. 9.1). MPS III A and B are the most common forms accounted for 60% and 30% of Sanfilippo syndromes, respectively. All types of MPS III are associated with abnormal storage of heparan sulfate, predominantly affecting the CNS. Urinary heparan sulfate is also highly elevated. Somatic changes are relatively mild, unlike MPS I and II. Features of MPS III are not typically apparent until after the first year of life with most symptoms developing between the ages of 2 and 6 years. The hallmark of MPS III is progressive behavioral problems including hyperactivity and aggression. Sleep disturbances are also very common among MPS III patients. Other signs and symptoms include cognitive impairment with regression, mild coarse facial features with full lips, thick eyebrows with synophrys, diarrhea, hearing impairment, vision loss (retinopathy), and seizures.[2,11]

9.3.4 MPS IV (MORQUIO SYNDROME)

MPS IV, also known as Morquio syndrome, is caused by a deficiency in one of two enzymes: N-acetylgalactosamine-6-sulfatase (MPS IVA) or β-galactosidase (MPS IVB). N-acetylgalactosamine-6-sulfatase (*GALNS*) cleaves the C6 sulfate group from the N-acetylgalactosamine-6-sulfate residue of chondroitin-6-sulfate and the galactose-6-sulfate residue of keratan sulfate. β-galactosidase further hydrolyzes β-linked galactose from keratan sulfate (Fig. 9.1). It needs to be pointed out that G_{M1} gangliosidosis is also caused by a deficiency of β-galactosidase due to different mutations in the *GLB1* gene. Mutations that are associated with total absence of

β-galactosidase activity result in G_{M1} gangliosidosis, while mutations that selectively impair catalytic activity toward keratan sulfate cause MPS IVB.

Type A and type B Morquio syndromes are clinically and biochemically indistinguishable. Abnormal lysosomal storage of keratan sulfate selectively affects the skeletal system and connective tissues. Both types are characterized by short-trunk dwarfism with kyphosis and scoliosis, genu valgum, corneal opacity, and severe skeletal dysplasia that is distinct from other MPS disorders. Intelligence is intact. Affected individuals appear normal at birth like other MPS patients. Skeletal signs become apparent between 1 and 4 years of age and worsen over time. Neurological symptoms may develop secondary to severe skeletal involvement and spinal cord compression. Odontoid hypoplasia is common in Morquio syndrome and can result in life-threatening atlantoaxial subluxation. Surgical intervention may be needed to stabilize the upper cervical spine.

9.3.5 MPS VI (MAROTEAUX–LAMY SYNDROME)

Maroteaux–Lamy syndrome is an autosomal recessive disorder caused by mutations in the *ARSB* gene, which encodes N-Acetylgalactosamine-4-sulfatase (arylsulfatase B). The enzyme removes C4 sulfate from the nonreducing terminus of chondroitin-4-sulfate and dermatan sulfate. Deficiency leads to lysosomal storage of dermatan sulfate and elevated dermatan sulfate excretion without elevated heparan sulfate. The somatic involvement in the severe form of Maroteaux–Lamy is similar to that seen in Hurler syndrome with the exception that the CNS is spared as heparan sulfate is not elevated. In severe MPS VI patients, cardiac failure leads to death in the second or third decade.

9.3.6 MPS VII (SLY SYNDROME)

MPS VII is an autosomal recessive genetic disorder caused by mutations in the *GUSB* gene, leading to a deficiency of the enzyme β-glucuronidase. The enzyme cleaves the glucuronide residue from dermatan sulfate, heparan sulfate, and chondroitin sulfate. Deficiency of β-glucuronidase leads to the accumulation of these abnormal GAGs and their elevated urinary excretion. MPS VII is very rare, occurring at a frequency of less than 1:250,000 births.

MPS VII is a highly variable lysosomal storage disorder with a range of presentation from severe hydrops fetalis *in utero* to a milder form with an intermediate phenotype consisting of hepatomegaly, coarse facial features, skeletal abnormalities, cardiac valve disease, and varying degrees of cognitive impairment. Many features are similar to MPS I and MPS II. This is one of the few lysosomal disorders that has a neonatal form with clinical manifestations *in utero* or at birth.

9.3.7 MPS IX

This extremely rare MPS is caused by a deficiency of hyaluronidase and abnormal storage of hyaluronan, which is abundant in the extracellular matrix of connective tissue. Only a few cases have been reported. The first-described patient was a 14-year-old girl with multiple soft tissue masses surrounding the joints of her ankles, knees, and fingers.[12]

9.4 OTHER DISEASES WITH MPS-LIKE PHENOTYPES

9.4.1 MULTIPLE SULFATASE DEFICIENCY

Multiple sulfatase deficiency (MSD) is a rare autosomal recessive disorder of a single gene that affects 17 sulfatases in the body. Mutations in the *SUMF1* gene result in functional defects of the formylglycine-generating enzyme (FGE), a critical protein localized in the endoplasmic reticulum and involved in the posttranslational modification of a specific cysteine residue located at the catalytic site of all sulfatases to C_α-formylglycine (FGly).[13,14] Six of the seventeen sulfatases are implicated in lysosomal disorders including iduronate-2-sulfatase (MPS II), sulfamidase (MPS III A), glucosamine-6-sulfatase (MPS III D), N-actylgalactosamine-6-sulfatase (MPS IV A), arylsulfatase B (MPS VI), and arylsulfatase A (metachromatic leukodystrophy, or MLD). Other sulfatases are located in the microsome and golgi apparatus and at the cell surface. Microsomal arylsulfatase C is associated with X-linked ichthyosis, a skin disorder due to steroid sulfatase deficiency. Another nonlysosomal sulfatase causes chondrodysplasia punctata, a disorder affecting bone and cartilage due to arylsulfatase E deficiency. Deficiencies in all these enzymes lead to complex substrate accumulations including mucopolysaccharides, oligosaccharides, and glycoproteins.[13–15]

Patients with MSD present with combined clinical and biochemical features of MPS and MLD. Specific clinical findings include psychomotor retardation and neurological deterioration as well as dysostosis multiplex, organomegaly, cardiac valve disease, corneal clouding, retinopathy with vision loss, hearing loss, recurrent infections, gingival hypertrophy, joint stiffness, carpal tunnel syndrome, and neuropathy. Ichthyosis is also a common finding in MSD due to steroid sulfatase deficiency. Urinary excretions of GAGs, oligosaccharides, and sulfatides are elevated in MSD. Most individuals with MSD die before the age of 10 although several individuals have been reported to have lived into the second and third decades of life.[15,16] Approximately 50 mutations of *SUMF1* have been reported. Impacts of these mutations on individual sulfatases are heterogeneous. Mean residual sulfatase activity seems to correlate with disease severity. The onset of nonneurological symptoms before 2 years and psychomotor regression are the clinical prognostic markers for a rapid disease progression.[15]

MSD should be considered on the differential diagnosis when there is clinical suspicion of a lysosomal storage disease, particularly when a specific sulfatase is deficient and mutation analysis is negative. Diagnosis of MSD can be established by identifying deficiencies of multiple sulfatase activities and two mutations in the *SUMF1* gene.

9.4.2 SIALIDOSIS OR MUCOLIPIDOSES I (ML I)

Mucolipidoses (ML I) is a severe condition caused a deficiency of lysosomal α-neuraminidase due to mutations of the *NEU1* gene.[17] Neuraminidase catalyzes sialic acid removal from sialylated glycoproteins and oligosaccharides. Deficiency of neuraminidase results in lysosomal storage of sialylated glycopeptides and sialo-oligosaccharides and their urinary excretion.[18] Recently, neuraminidase has been found to play important role in desialylation of LAMP1 (lysosomal associated membrane protein). In turn, abnormally desialylated LAMP1 leads to increased lysosomal enzyme exocytosis and relevant clinical symptoms.[19]

The variability of patients encompasses two ends of a clinical spectrum. Type I, the milder form, presents later in life with macular cherry red spots, seizures, and generalized myoclonus. Prolonged survival is common with preserved cognitive function and fewer somatic changes. Type II is the more severe disease form, which presents prenatally with hydrops fetalis or soon after birth with dysmorphic facial features, hepatosplenomegaly, skeletal dysplasia, and many other clinical features similar to Hurler syndrome. Clinical outcome is poor and patients with type II ML I usually die in very early childhood.[5,17]

Abnormal urinary oligosaccharides and sialic acid (bound form) and deficiency of neuraminidase activity in leukocytes or fibroblasts are diagnostic for ML I. The disorder can be further confirmed with identification of disease causing mutations of the *NEU1* gene.

9.4.3 MUCOLIPIDOSIS II (ML II OR I-CELL DISEASE) AND MUCOLIPIDOSIS III (ML III OR PSEUDO-HURLER POLYDYSTROPHY)

ML II and ML III are allelic disorders of deficiencies of UDP-N-actyloglucosamine:lysosomal hydrolase N-acetyl-1-phophotransferase, or UDP-GlcNAc-1-phosphate transferase (GNPT) with ML II being the most severe end of the clinical spectrum. This enzyme catalyzes the synthesis of the mannose-6-phosphate (M6P) recognition marker on lysosomal hydrolases or other glycoproteins. Without this recognition marker, receptor-mediated targeting of hydrolytic enzymes to the lysosomes from the Golgi apparatus does not occur and the hydrolases are secreted into plasma and other body fluids. This defect impacts multiple lysosomal enzyme functions and therefore leads to lysosomal storage of mucopolysaccharides, oligosaccharides, and sphingolipids. The GNPT enzyme is a hexameric protein consisted of α, β, and γ subunits ($\alpha2\beta2\gamma2$). α and β subunits are encoded by the *GNPTAB* gene on chromosome 12q23.3. Mutations in the *GNPTAB* gene result in either ML II or ML III. The γ subunit is encoded by the *GNPTG* gene on chromosome 16p13.3. Mutations in the *GNPTG* gene is only associated with ML III phenotypes.[20,21]

Patients with ML II present in the newborn period with many clinical features resembling MPS I. Notably, there is no or minimal elevation of urine mucopolysaccharides. Poor feeding and respiratory difficulties are common during infancy. All patients invariably show severe psychomotor retardation. The majority of ML II patients die in the first decade of life. ML III is an attenuated form of ML II. Patients with ML III have a later onset and a milder and slower disease progression. Clinical manifestations include mild learning disability, short stature, cardiac valve lesions, and skeletal abnormalities. The skeletal involvement is prominent in ML III, primarily affecting the hip joints and shoulders. Claw-hand deformities have also been observed.[22]

Inclusion bodies are found in fibroblasts of ML II patients. Significant increases of serum or plasma lysosomal enzyme activities and severe deficiencies of multiple lysosomal enzymes in cultured fibroblasts are indicative of ML II or III. Deficiency of GNPT activity in leukocytes and identification of *GNPTAB* or *GNPTG* mutations establishes the specific diagnosis of ML II, ML III, or ML IIIγ.[20]

9.4.4 MUCOLIPIDOSIS IV (ML IV)

TRPML1 (also known as mucolipin 1 or MCOLN1) is a lysosomal ion channel protein belonging to the mucolipin subfamily of Transient Receptor Potential (TRP) proteins.[23] Mutations in the *TRPML1* gene result in mucolipidosis type IV (ML IV). ML IV is a progressive neurological disease that presents in early infancy with psychomotor delay, severe mental retardation, retinal degeneration, corneal clouding, iron-deficiency anemia, and achlorhydria with elevated blood gastrin levels. The accumulated substrates include sphingolipids, phospholipids, and mucopolysaccharides. Although the disease pathogenesis is not fully understood, some studies indicate that ML IV is caused by defective ion transport[23] and chaperone-mediated autophagy.[24]

9.5 GLYCOSAMINOGLYCANS AND GAGS ANALYSIS

GAGs are negatively charged, sulfated polysaccharides made of repeating disaccharides, which consist of hexosamines and uronic acid (or galactose in keratan sulfate). Hyaluronan is the only GAG that is not sulfated. GAGs covalently bind to the core protein to form proteoglycans for diverse physiological functions (Table 9.2).

Table 9.2 Classifications of GAGs and their Biological Distributions

GAGs	Disaccharide Repeat Unit	Distributions
Chondroitin 4- and 6-sulfates	N-Acetyl-D-galactosamine-4 or 6-sulfate and glucuronic acid	Cartilage, tendon, ligament, bone, cardiac valves
Dermatan sulfate	N-Acetyl-D-galactosamine-4-sulfate and iduronic acid	Skin, blood vessels, cardiac valves
Heparan sulfate	N-Sulfo-D-glucosamine-6-sulfate and iduronate-2-sulfate	Mainly in central nervous system involving extracellular component of basement membrane, and components of cell surfaces
Keratan sulfate	N-Acetyl-D-glucosamine-6-sulfate and galactose	Cornea, bone, cartilage aggregated with chondroitin sulfates

GAGs were previously called mucopolysaccharides because of their viscous and elastic properties due to highly sulfated residues. Proteoglycans and associated GAGs are primarily localized at cell surfaces and in extracellular matrices and are also found in basement membranes and cytoplasmic secretory granules. GAGs play an important role in maintaining structural integrity of most tissues, particularly connective tissues by forming hydrated matrices and interacting with collagen. Proteoglycan and GAGs can also bind to cytokines, chemokines, growth factors, and morphogens to regulate cell adhesion, differentiation, and migration during development.

Quantitative and qualitative fractioning of GAGs have been widely used in screening for MPS disorders for many years. Chemical or enzymatic digestion of GAG species yields disaccharide biomarkers that are disease-specific. Recently, liquid chromatography tandem mass spectrometry (LC-MS/MS) analysis of these disaccharide biomarkers has been applied in clinical biochemical genetics laboratories for diagnostic and disease monitoring purposes of MPS disorders.

9.5.1 TOTAL GAGS ANALYSIS BY DIMETHYLENE BLUE BINDING ASSAY

Total urinary GAGs excretion is commonly performed by a dye-binding assay with dimethylene blue (DMB) followed by spectrophotometric analysis. The total GAG measurement is normalized to creatinine concentration and is interpreted based on age-specific reference intervals. Urinary GAG excretion is high in infants and young children, decreases with age, then remains constant through adulthood.[25,26] This measurement has been widely used in diagnosis and has also been applied to monitor the therapeutic responses in clinical trials for MPS I, II, and VI.[27–29] However, this assay can be falsely negative in some MPS cases when the total GAG excretion is not elevated, particularly MPS IV and some attenuated forms of MPS. For this reason, simultaneous testing of qualitative fractionation with total GAG quantitation is strongly recommended when an MPS disorder is clinically suspected.[30,31]

9.5.2 QUALITATIVE FRACTIONATION OF GAGS

Qualitative fractionation of GAG species can be achieved by thin-layer chromatography (TLC) or gel electrophoresis. Both assays require purification of GAGs from a urine sample via cetylpyridinium chloride (CPC) precipitation. Purified GAGs are then separated by either TLC with a solvent gradient or gel electrophoresis based on charge and molecular weight.[32,33] Separated GAGs can be visualized by staining with dye and destaining (e.g., alcian blue and acetic acid). Bands of chondroitin sulfate, dermatan sulfate, heparan sulfate, and keratan sulfate are visually interpreted. There are subtle differences in the banding pattern of these two methods. Two bands for dermatan sulfate can be observed upon gel electrophoresis, while TLC gives only one band. In contrast, chondroitin-4-sulfate and chondroitin-6-sulfate can be

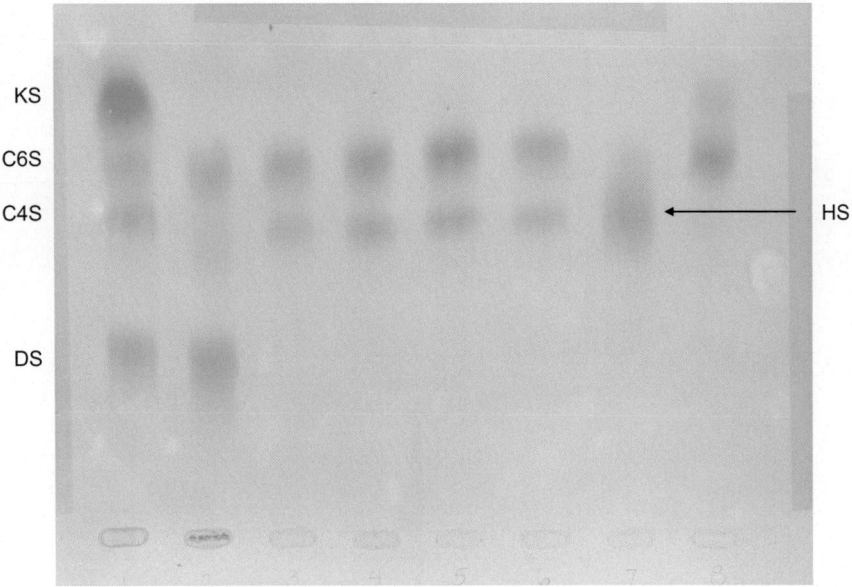

FIGURE 9.2

Thin-layer chromatography of GAGs. *C4S*, chondroitin-4-sulfate; *C6S*, chondroitin-6-sulfate; *DS*, dermatan sulfate; *KS*, keratan sulfate. Lane 1—GAG standards; Lane 2—MPS I; Lane 3, 4, 5, 6—Normal samples; Lane 7—MPS III; Lane 8—MPS IV.

separated on TLC plate but not by gel electrophoresis. Heparan sulfate shows as a smear rather than a band in both methods. A representative TLC plate with standards and patterns of various MPS disorders is shown in Fig. 9.2.

Fractionation of GAGs provides clues for the diagnosis of MPS. However, these assays are still considered screening tests and cannot be used for monitoring of disease progression. The sensitivity and specificity are both limited. Interpretation can be challenging and subjective when the banding is faint. This is particularly true for the interpretation of heparan sulfate and keratan sulfate. Thus enzymatic and/or genetic testing is needed for definitive diagnosis. Another limitation of these methods is that high-throughput screening is not possible.

9.5.3 LC-MS/MS ANALYSES

Recently quantitative LC-MS/MS analysis of specific GAGs has become possible after enzymatic or chemical digestion of GAGs into disaccharide fragments. These disaccharide products represent and correlate with the levels of the precursor GAGs and can be used as new biomarkers for the different MPS disorders. The enzymes keratanase II, heparitinase, and chondroitinase B have been used to produce disaccharides

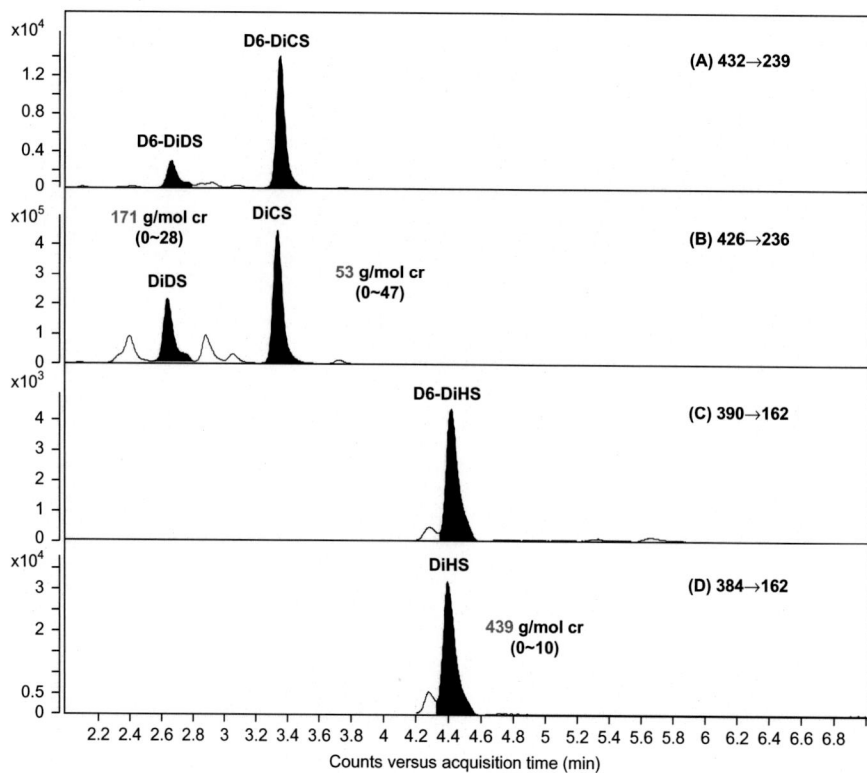

FIGURE 9.3

Extracted ion chromatograms of methanolyzed disaccharides of dermatan, heparan, and chondroitin sulfates from a patient with MPS I. (A) *m/z* of 432 → 239: Internal standards derived from deuteriomethanolysis products of dermatan and chondroitin sulfates; (B) *m/z* of 426 → 236: Disaccharide derived from dermatan and chondroitin sulfates; (C) *m/z* of 390 → 162: Internal standard derived from deuteriomethanolysis products of heparan sulfate; (D) *m/z* of 384 → 162: Disaccharide derived from heparan sulfate. *DiDS*, disaccharide from dermatan sulfate; *DiHS*, disaccharide from heparan sulfate; *DiCS*, disaccharide from chondroitin sulfate; *D6-DiDS*, *D6-DiHS*, and *D6-DiCS*, deuterated disaccharide internal standards.

of keratan sulfate, heparan sulfate, and dermatan sulfate, which are then measured by LC-MS/MS analysis.[34–36] Methanolysis of GAGs using methanolic HCl generates GAG specific disaccharides for heparan, dermatan, and chondroitin sulfates, which can be readily quantitated by LC-MS/MS. The deuterated disaccharide internal standards used for the assay are derived from methanolysis of GAG standards using deuterated methanolic HCl.[37,38] A limitation of this approach is that it cannot measure keratan sulfate. Both enzyme digestion and methanolysis LC-MS/MS methods are highly sensitive for measurement of GAGs from plasma (or serum), CSF, and even tissues, in addition to urine samples.[35,36,39,40] Urine, however, seems to be the best matrix for GAG analysis given the abundance of GAGs. In a large study of an MPS IV patient cohort, urinary keratan sulfate measured by LC-MS/MS analysis demonstrated better discrimination between MPS IV and normal controls when compared to classic methodologies.[34] Some overlap between patients and controls was observed for plasma samples. Urine and plasma keratan sulfates concentrations showed an increase from 0 to 6 years and peak at 7 to 10 years and decline from 11 to 15 years.[34] High sensitivity and specificity of these assays permit accurate measurement of the specific GAGs for the attenuated forms of disease. These new LC-MS/MS methods will likely replace measurement of total urinary GAGs for screening as well as monitoring disease progression and therapeutic responses in patients with MPS. A representative extracted ion chromatogram of GAGs from a MPS I patient using the methanolysis method is illustrated in Fig. 9.3. The structures and MS/MS parameters for the disaccharides derived from GAGs after methanolysis are shown in Table 9.3.

9.6 LABORATORY DIAGNOSIS OF MPS DISORDERS

Urinary GAG analysis is an effective screening test in patients suspected to have MPS. Elevated excretions of dermatan, heparan or keratan sulfate indicate a specific enzyme activity assay to diagnose the disorder, which can be further confirmed by mutation analysis of the encoding gene. The clinical diagnosis of MPS, however, will soon transition to diagnosis by newborn screening. As of 2016, MPS I has been added to the Recommended Uniform Screening Panel for newborn screening. To confirm a diagnosis in babies with positive screens prior to symptom manifestations can be challenging and involves a combination of GAG quantitation, enzyme activity, and mutation analysis.

9.7 BRIEF DESCRIPTION OF TREATMENT

Historically, supportive care with a multidisciplinary clinical team was the only treatment option for MPS. Surgical repairs are often needed for patients with severe somatic involvement. Currently, enzyme replacement therapy (ERT) has become the mainstay treatment option for several MPS disorders. Over the years, ERT with recombinant human enzyme has been approved by the Food and Drug Administration (FDA) for the treatment of MPS I, II, and VI. Recently, ERT has also been approved by the FDA for the treatment of MPS IVA.[41,42] ERT is generally well tolerated. Patients treated with ERT demonstrated some improvements in walking

Table 9.3 MS/MS Parameters for the Disaccharide Products of Methanolysis

Compound	Structure	SRM Transition (m/z)	Collision Energy (V)	High-Pressure RF (V)	Low-Pressure RF (V)
D$_6$-DiCS		432/239	6	70	40
DiCS		426/236	4	70	40
D$_6$-DiDS		432/239	6	70	40
DiDS		426/236	4	70	40
D$_6$-DiHS		390/162	11	70	40
DiHS		384/162	13	70	40

ability, joint mobility, pulmonary functions, reduced liver and spleen volumes, and decreased urinary GAG excretion. However, there is no benefit for the neurological symptoms as the recombinant enzymes via intravenous infusion do not cross the blood-brain barrier, a limitation that may be improved by intrathecal infusions. ERT also has limited benefits toward cardiac valve disease and skeletal deformities if the pathological changes are already present when ERT is started.[41–43]

Hematopoietic stem cell transplantation (HSCT) is another available therapy for MPS. HSCT has been shown to prevent many of the clinical features in MPS I, VI, and VII.[44–47] If performed before the mental deterioration, HSCT can preserve the cognitive function in these children. HSCT has not proven effective in treating MPS II, III, or IV.[48–50] Again, HSCT cannot reverse corneal clouding, cardiac valve deformities, and skeletal abnormalities if already present.[50] Unfortunately, HSCT is associated with significant morbidity and mortality.

Many novel therapeutic options are on the horizons to treat MPS. ERT for MPS VII has been developed and is currently in a phase III clinical trial (https://clinical-trials.gov). Intrathecal ERT is currently under investigation for treatment of MPS I, MPS II, MPS III A, and MPS III B.[42] Several gene therapy approaches are under pre-clinical studies for MPS I, II, III A, III B, VI, and VII.[42] Substrate reduction therapy (SRT) with small molecules that inhibit the GAG synthesis has been proposed for MPS, particularly MPS III.[51,52]

9.8 CONCLUSION

MPS disorders are a group of heterogenous lysosomal disorders with primary defects in the GAGs catabolic pathways. Accumulations of dermatan, heparan, keratan sulfate, or hyaluronan determine the pathophysiology and clinical phenotypes of MPS. Other secondary defects of GAG degradation due to primary defects of other enzyme or proteins can also have MPS-like phenotypes. Urinary GAGs analysis, particularly the new LC-MS/MS analysis of disaccharide biomarkers, provides useful information for the diagnosis and monitoring of MPS. Other biomarkers such as cytokines and short saccharides from the NRE are also used for clinical testing or under investigation. With more and better therapeutic options becoming available, there is a parallel development to include MPS in newborn screening because early identification and intervention may reduce the morbidity and mortality of these diseases.

ACKNOWLEDGMENT

The author would like to thank Mei Lu, PhD for her assistance with the preparations of Fig. 9.3 and Table 9.3. The author would also like to thank Dr. Sander Houten for the critical review of the manuscript.

REFERENCES

1. Muenzer J. Overview of the mucopolysaccharidoses. *Rheumatology (Oxford)* 2011; **50**(Suppl 5):v4–12.
2. Neufeld E, Muenzer J. *The Mucopolysaccharidoses*. New York, NY: McGraw-Hill; 2014.
3. Ashworth JL, Biswas S, Wraith E, Lloyd IC. Mucopolysaccharidoses and the eye. *Surv Ophthalmol* 2006;**51**(1):1–17.
4. Beck M, Arn P, Giugliani R, Muenzer J, Okuyama T, Taylor J, et al. The natural history of MPS I: global perspectives from the MPS I Registry. *Genet Med* 2014;**16**(10):759–65.
5. Wraith JE. Mucopolysaccharidoses and mucolipidoses. *Handb Clin Neurol* 2013;**113**:1723–9.
6. Tuschl K, Gal A, Paschke E, Kircher S, Bodamer OA. Mucopolysaccharidosis type II in females: case report and review of literature. *Pediatr Neurol* 2005;**32**(4):270–2.
7. Baehner F, Schmiedeskamp C, Krummenauer F, Miebach E, Bajbouj M, Whybra C, et al. Cumulative incidence rates of the mucopolysaccharidoses in Germany. *J Inherit Metab Dis* 2005;**28**(6):1011–7.
8. Nelson J, Crowhurst J, Carey B, Greed L. Incidence of the mucopolysaccharidoses in Western Australia. *Am J Med Genet A* 2003;**123A**(3):310–3.
9. Wraith JE, Beck M, Giugliani R, Clarke J, Martin R, Muenzer J, et al. Initial report from the Hunter Outcome Survey. *Genet Med* 2008;**10**(7):508–16.
10. Wraith JE, Scarpa M, Beck M, Bodamer OA, De Meirleir L, Guffon N, et al. Mucopolysaccharidosis type II (Hunter syndrome): a clinical review and recommendations for treatment in the era of enzyme replacement therapy. *Eur J Pediatr* 2008;**167**(3):267–77.
11. Valstar MJ, Ruijter GJ, van Diggelen OP, Poorthuis BJ, Wijburg FA. Sanfilippo syndrome: a mini-review. *J Inherit Metab Dis* 2008;**31**(2):240–52.
12. Natowicz MR, Short MP, Wang Y, Dickersin GR, Gebhardt MC, Rosenthal DI, et al. Clinical and biochemical manifestations of hyaluronidase deficiency. *N Engl J Med* 1996;**335**(14):1029–33.
13. Cosma MP, Pepe S, Annunziata I, Newbold RF, Grompe M, Parenti G, et al. The multiple sulfatase deficiency gene encodes an essential and limiting factor for the activity of sulfatases. *Cell* 2003;**113**(4):445–56.
14. Dierks T, Schmidt B, Borissenko LV, Peng J, Preusser A, Mariappan M, et al. Multiple sulfatase deficiency is caused by mutations in the gene encoding the human C(alpha)-formylglycine generating enzyme. *Cell* 2003;**113**(4):435–44.
15. Sabourdy F, Mourey L, Le Trionnaire E, Bednarek N, Caillaud C, Chaix Y, et al. Natural disease history and characterisation of SUMF1 molecular defects in ten unrelated patients with multiple sulfatase deficiency. *Orphanet J Rare Dis* 2015;**10**:31.
16. Eto Y, Gomibuchi I, Umezawa F, Tsuda T. Pathochemistry, pathogenesis and enzyme replacement in multiple-sulfatase deficiency. *Enzyme* 1987;**38**(1–4):273–9.
17. Lowden JA, O'Brien JS. Sialidosis: a review of human neuraminidase deficiency. *Am J Hum Genet* 1979;**31**(1):1–18.
18. Seyrantepe V, Poupetova H, Froissart R, Zabot MT, Maire I, Pshezhetsky AV. Molecular pathology of NEU1 gene in sialidosis. *Hum Mutat* 2003;**22**(5):343–52.
19. Yogalingam G, Bonten EJ, van de Vlekkert D, Hu H, Moshiach S, Connell SA, et al. Neuraminidase 1 is a negative regulator of lysosomal exocytosis. *Dev Cell* 2008;**15**(1):74–86.

20. Cathey SS, Leroy JG, Wood T, Eaves K, Simensen RJ, Kudo M, et al. Phenotype and genotype in mucolipidoses II and III alpha/beta: a study of 61 probands. *J Med Genet* 2010;**47**(1):38–48.

21. Cathey SS, Kudo M, Tiede S, Raas-Rothschild A, Braulke T, Beck M, et al. Molecular order in mucolipidosis II and III nomenclature. *Am J Med Genet A* 2008;**146A**(4):512–3.

22. Robinson C, Baker N, Noble J, King A, David G, Sillence D, et al. The osteodystrophy of mucolipidosis type III and the effects of intravenous pamidronate treatment. *J Inherit Metab Dis* 2002;**25**(8):681–93.

23. Dong XP, Cheng X, Mills E, Delling M, Wang F, Kurz T, et al. The type IV mucolipidosis-associated protein TRPML1 is an endolysosomal iron release channel. *Nature* 2008;**455**(7215):992–6.

24. Venugopal B, Mesires NT, Kennedy JC, Curcio-Morelli C, Laplante JM, Dice JF, et al. Chaperone-mediated autophagy is defective in mucolipidosis type IV. *J Cell Physiol* 2009;**219**(2):344–53.

25. de Jong JG, Wevers RA, Laarakkers C, Poorthuis BJ. Dimethylmethylene blue-based spectrophotometry of glycosaminoglycans in untreated urine: a rapid screening procedure for mucopolysaccharidoses. *Clin Chem* 1989;**35**(7):1472–7.

26. Whitley CB, Ridnour MD, Draper KA, Dutton CM, Neglia JP. Diagnostic test for mucopolysaccharidosis. I. Direct method for quantifying excessive urinary glycosaminoglycan excretion. *Clin Chem* 1989;**35**(3):374–9.

27. Clarke LA, Wraith JE, Beck M, Kolodny EH, Pastores GM, Muenzer J, et al. Long-term efficacy and safety of laronidase in the treatment of mucopolysaccharidosis I. *Pediatrics* 2009;**123**(1):229–40.

28. Muenzer J, Wraith JE, Beck M, Giugliani R, Harmatz P, Eng CM, et al. A phase II/III clinical study of enzyme replacement therapy with idursulfase in mucopolysaccharidosis II (Hunter syndrome). *Genet Med* 2006;**8**(8):465–73.

29. Harmatz P, Giugliani R, Schwartz I, Guffon N, Teles EL, Miranda MC, et al. Enzyme replacement therapy for mucopolysaccharidosis VI: a phase 3, randomized, double-blind, placebo-controlled, multinational study of recombinant human N-acetylgalactosamine 4-sulfatase (recombinant human arylsulfatase B or rhASB) and follow-on, open-label extension study. *J Pediatr* 2006;**148**(4):533–9.

30. Gray G, Claridge P, Jenkinson L, Green A. Quantitation of urinary glycosaminoglycans using dimethylene blue as a screening technique for the diagnosis of mucopolysaccharidoses: an evaluation. *Ann Clin Biochem* 2007;**44**(Pt 4):360–3.

31. Piraud M, Boyer S, Mathieu M, Maire I. Diagnosis of mucopolysaccharidoses in a clinically selected population by urinary glycosaminoglycan analysis: a study of 2,000 urine samples. *Clin Chim Acta* 1993;**221**(1–2):171–81.

32. Hopwood JJ, Harrison JR. High-resolution electrophoresis of urinary glycosaminoglycans: an improved screening test for the mucopolysaccharidoses. *Anal Biochem* 1982;**119**(1):120–7.

33. Dembure PP, roesel RA. Screening for mucopolysaccharidoses by analysis of urinary glycosaminoglycans. In: Hommes FA, editor. *Techniques in diagnostic human biochemical genetics A laboratory manual*. : Wiley-Liss; 1991. p. 77–86.

34. Martell LA, Cunico RL, Ohh J, Fulkerson W, Furneaux R, Foehr ED. Validation of an LC-MS/MS assay for detecting relevant disaccharides from keratan sulfate as a biomarker for Morquio A syndrome. *Bioanalysis* 2011;**3**(16):1855–66.

35. Tomatsu S, Montano AM, Oguma T, Dung VC, Oikawa H, Gutierrez ML, et al. Validation of disaccharide compositions derived from dermatan sulfate and heparan sulfate in

mucopolysaccharidoses and mucolipidoses II and III by tandem mass spectrometry. *Mol Genet Metab* 2010;**99**(2):124–31.

36. Oguma T, Tomatsu S, Montano AM, Okazaki O. Analytical method for the determination of disaccharides derived from keratan, heparan, and dermatan sulfates in human serum and plasma by high-performance liquid chromatography/turbo ionspray ionization tandem mass spectrometry. *Anal Biochem* 2007;**368**(1):79–86.

37. Zhang H, Wood T, Young SP, Millington DS. A straightforward, quantitative ultra-performance liquid chromatography-tandem mass spectrometric method for heparan sulfate, dermatan sulfate and chondroitin sulfate in urine: an improved clinical screening test for the mucopolysaccharidoses. *Mol Genet Metab* 2015;**114**(2):123–8.

38. Zhang H, Young SP, Millington DS. Quantification of glycosaminoglycans in urine by isotope-dilution liquid chromatography-electrospray ionization tandem mass spectrometry. *Curr Protoc Hum Genet* 2013 Chapter 17:Unit 17 2.

39. Oguma T, Toyoda H, Toida T, Imanari T. Analytical method of chondroitin/dermatan sulfates using high performance liquid chromatography/turbo ionspray ionization mass spectrometry: application to analyses of the tumor tissue sections on glass slides. *Biomed Chromatogr* 2001;**15**(5):356–62.

40. Zhang H, Young SP, Auray-Blais C, Orchard PJ, Tolar J, Millington DS. Analysis of glycosaminoglycans in cerebrospinal fluid from patients with mucopolysaccharidoses by isotope-dilution ultra-performance liquid chromatography-tandem mass spectrometry. *Clin Chem* 2011;**57**(7):1005–12.

41. Muenzer J, Fisher A. Advances in the treatment of mucopolysaccharidosis type I. *N Engl J Med* 2004;**350**(19):1932–4.

42. Giugliani R, Federhen A, Vairo F, Vanzella C, Pasqualim G, da Silva LM, et al. Emerging drugs for the treatment of mucopolysaccharidoses. *Expert Opin Emerg Drugs* 2016; **21**(1):9–26.

43. Muenzer J. Early initiation of enzyme replacement therapy for the mucopolysaccharidoses. *Mol Genet Metab* 2014;**111**(2):63–72.

44. Hobbs JR, Hugh-Jones K, Barrett AJ, Byrom N, Chambers D, Henry K, et al. Reversal of clinical features of Hurler's disease and biochemical improvement after treatment by bone-marrow transplantation. *Lancet* 1981;**2**(8249):709–12.

45. Herskhovitz E, Young E, Rainer J, Hall CM, Lidchi V, Chong K, et al. Bone marrow transplantation for Maroteaux–Lamy syndrome (MPS VI): long-term follow-up. *J Inherit Metab Dis* 1999;**22**(1):50–62.

46. Souillet G, Guffon N, Maire I, Pujol M, Taylor P, Sevin F, et al. Outcome of 27 patients with Hurler's syndrome transplanted from either related or unrelated haematopoietic stem cell sources. *Bone Marrow Transplant* 2003;**31**(12):1105–17.

47. Weisstein JS, Delgado E, Steinbach LS, Hart K, Packman S. Musculoskeletal manifestations of Hurler syndrome: long-term follow-up after bone marrow transplantation. *J Pediatr Orthop* 2004;**24**(1):97–101.

48. Sivakumur P, Wraith JE. Bone marrow transplantation in mucopolysaccharidosis type IIIA: a comparison of an early treated patient with his untreated sibling. *J Inherit Metab Dis* 1999;**22**(7):849–50.

49. Peters C, Krivit W. Hematopoietic cell transplantation for mucopolysaccharidosis IIB (Hunter syndrome). *Bone Marrow Transplant* 2000;**25**(10):1097–9.

50. Prasad VK, Kurtzberg J. Transplant outcomes in mucopolysaccharidoses. *Semin Hematol* 2010;**47**(1):59–69.

51. Malinowska M, Wilkinson FL, Langford-Smith KJ, Langford-Smith A, Brown JR, Crawford BE, et al. Genistein improves neuropathology and corrects behaviour in a mouse model of neurodegenerative metabolic disease. *PLoS One* 2010;**5**(12):e14192.
52. Piotrowska E, Jakobkiewicz-Banecka J, Maryniak A, Tylki-Szymanska A, Puk E, Liberek A, et al. Two-year follow-up of Sanfilippo Disease patients treated with a genistein-rich isoflavone extract: assessment of effects on cognitive functions and general status of patients. *Med Sci Monit* 2011;**17**(4):CR196–202.

Lysosomal storage disorders: sphingolipidoses 10

C. Yu

Icahn School of Medicine at Mount Sinai, New York, NY, United States

10.1 INTRODUCTION

Sphingolipidoses are a group of lysosomal storage diseases with defects in enzymes or activator proteins needed for the degradation of sphingolipids. Accumulation of sphingolipids in one or several organs leads to visceral, neurovisceral, or purely neurological manifestations. Niemann–Pick C disease, a primary disorder of impaired cellular lipid trafficking, is also included in this group due to secondary accumulation of sphingolipids. The defects of enzymes, accumulated substrates, and key clinical features of these diseases are summarized in Table 10.1.

10.2 OVERVIEW OF SPHINGOLIPIDS METABOLISM

Sphingolipids refer to a class of complex phospholipids with a core hydrophobic structure of ceremide, which is composed of a sphingosine head and a long-chain fatty acid chain. They are essential components of plasma membranes. De novo synthesis of sphingolipids begins in the endoplasmic reticulum (ER) and ends in the Golgi apparatus by adding carbohydrates and other modifications onto the backbone of ceremide. Sphingolipids are also constantly being recycled. Deficiencies of the lysosomal enzymes that are required for the degradation of these lipid compounds result in the sphinolipidoses. Depending on the modifying structures, sphingolipids are classified into sphingomyelins and glycosphingolipids. Sphingomyelins consist of phosphocholine or phosphoethanolmine and ceremide. Deficiency of acid sphingomyelinase results in Niemann–Pick disease type A or type B (NPD-A or NPD-B). Sphingomyelins can also secondarily accumulate in Niemann–Pick disease type C (NPD-C) due to abnormal cellular lipid trafficking. Glycosphingolipids include cerebrosides, sulfatides, globosides, and gangliosides with carbohydrate groups attached to the 1-OH position of sphingosine. Cerebrosides contain a mono sugar group (galactose or glucose) and ceremide. Galactocerebroside is primarily present in neuronal cell membranes. Galactocerebrosidase deficency, associated with Krabbe disease, is

Table 10.1 Summary of Sphingolipidoses

Diseases	Enzyme Deficiency	Gene Symbols	Accumulating Substrates (Site of Storage)	Key Clinical Features
G$_{M1}$ gangliosidosis	β-Galatosidase	GLB1	• G$_{M1}$ gangliosides (CNS) • Oligosaccharides (CNS and visceral organs) • Keratan sulfate (Skeleton)	60% patients present during early infancy with coarse features, hepatosplenomegaly, dysostosis multiplex, macular cherry-red spots, rapid neurological deterioration, and death by 2 years. Juvenile and adult forms have slower rate of regression.
G$_{M2}$ gangliosidoses • Tay–Sachs disease • Sandhoff disease • G$_{M2}$ activator deficiency	• β-Hexosaminidase A • β-Hexosaminidase A&B • G$_{M2}$ activator	• HEXA • HEXB • GM2A	G$_{M2}$ gangliosides (CNS)	Infantile Tay–Sachs presents at 3–6 months with rapid and progressive cerebral and retinal degeneration, death usually by 4 years. An exaggerated startle response and macular cherry-red spots are typical signs. Juvenile and adult forms exist. Sandhoff and G$_{M2}$ activator deficiency are clinically indistinguishable from Tay–Sachs.
Fabry disease	α-Galatosidase A	GLA	• Globotriaosylceramide • Galabiosylceramide • Globotriaosylsphingosine (vascular system, kidney, heart, autonomic nervous system)	Pain and acroparesthesia in the extremities, angiokeratoma and hypohidrosis in childhood. Renal failure in adulthood. Whorl-like corneal dystrophy is common in both males and females. Attenuated forms exist. Female heterozygotes may be symptomatic.
Gaucher disease	Acid β-glucosidase	GBA	• Glucosylceramide • Glucosylsphingosine (monocytes/macrophage system affecting liver, spleen, bone marrow, and CNS)	Type 1: Hepatosplenomegaly, hypersplenism, avascular necrosis of the hip. Childhood or adult onset. Some patients may be asymptomatic. Type 2: Hepatosplenomegaly and rapid neurodegeneration in infancy. Type 3: Intermediate between type 1 and 2.
Niemann–Pick disease type A and type B	Acid sphingomyelinase	SMPD1	Sphingomyelin (liver, spleen, bone marrow, lung, and CNS)	Type A: Hepatosplenomegaly and rapid neurodegeneration in infancy. Tye B: Hepatosplenomegaly in children or adults. Pulmonary involvement may occur. Hyperlipidemia is common.
Metachromatic leukodystrophy	Arylsulfatase A	ARSA	Sulfatides (myelins of CNS and peripheral nerves)	Progressive neurodegeneration and psychomotor regression. No organomegaly. Late-infantile, juvenile, or adult onset.
Krabbe disease	Galactosylceramidase	GALC	Galactosylceramide (CNS)	Extremely sensitive to sounds, light, or touch with screaming and rigidity. Progressive neurodegeneration. No organomegaly.
Farber disease	Acid ceramidase	ASAH	Ceramide (subtaneous tissues, joints, liver, spleen, lung, larynx, and CNS)	Painful swelling of joints, subcutaneous nodules (lipogranulomatosis) and progressive hoarseness.
Niemann–Pick disease type C	• NPC1 (95%) • NPC2 (5%)	• NPC1 • NPC2	Free cholesterol (CNS and visceral organs)	Liver disease in infants. Supranuclear gaze palsy, developmental regression, ataxia, seizures in childhood. Psychotic episodes in adults.

characterized by demyelination of the central nervous system (CNS) and peripheral nervous system. Glucocerebroside or glucosylceramide is widedly distributed in different tissues and not limited to the CNS. Glucocerebrosidase or β-glucosidase deficiency is associated with Gaucher disease and has heterogenous clinical phenotypes. Sulfatides are sulfated galactosylceramides that are abundant in the myelin sheath of the central and peripheral nervous system. Excess accumulation of sulfatides is the hallmark of metachromatic leukodystrophy (MLD) due to a deficiency of arylsulfatase A or its cofactor. Globosides have more than one carbohydrate grouplinked to ceramide. Globotetraosylceramide (Gb4) is the substrate for β-hexosaminidase A and B (Sandhoff). Globotriaosylceramide (Gb3) and galabiosylceramide (Gb2) are degraded by α-galactosidase A (Fabry). Gangliosides are structurally similar to globosides with an additional sialic acid attached to a galactose residue. Defects in β-galactosidase (G_{M1} gangliosidosis) and β-hexosaminidase A and B (Tay–Sachs and Sandhoff, or G_{M2} gangliosidoses) lead to accumultion of gangliosides and neurodegeneration. As sphingolipids are mostly hydrophobic, several enzymatic reactions in the degration pathways require small nonenzymatic glycoprotein cofactors to bind to their lipid substrates to facilitate catalytic reaction. These proteins are called sphinolipid activator proteins (SAPs), including saposins and the G_{M2} activator protein. Genetic defects of these activator proteins also lead to the same clinical manifestations. The degradation pathways of sphingolipids and associated enzymes and sphingolipidoses are illustrated in Fig. 10.1.

10.3 SPHINGOLIPIDOSES

10.3.1 G_{M1} GANGLIOSIDOSIS

G_{M1} gangliosidosis (GM1) is an autosomal recessive lysosomal disorder caused by mutations in the *GLB1* gene and subsequent deficiency of β-galactosidase enzyme. This lysosomal enzyme hydrolyzes the terminal β-linked galactose residue from G_{M1} gangliosides, glycoproteins, and glycosaminoglycans. Massive storage of G_{M1} gangliosides, and less elevated asialo ganglioside derivatives are found primarily in brain in patients with GM1. Other abnormal storage materials include galactose-containing oligosaccharides derived from various sources and keratan sulfate are found in both neuronal and somatic tissues and visceral organs and excreted in the urine. Therefore, G_{M1} gangliosidosis shows combined features of a sphingolipidosis, an oligosaccharidosis, and a mucopolysaccharidosis.

More than 60% of GM1 patients present with an infantile form (type I).[1] A late infantile/juvenile form (type II) and an adult/chronic form (type III) also exist. In typical type I cases, affected infants initially present with hypotonia and then develop spasticity as the disease progresses. An exaggerated startle reflex may be present as seen in Tay–Sachs and Sandhoff diseases. Developmental delay or arrest is observed at 3–6 months of age followed by a rapid neurologic and psychomotor deterioration. A macular "cherry red" spot is found in 50% of the cases. Other symptoms include

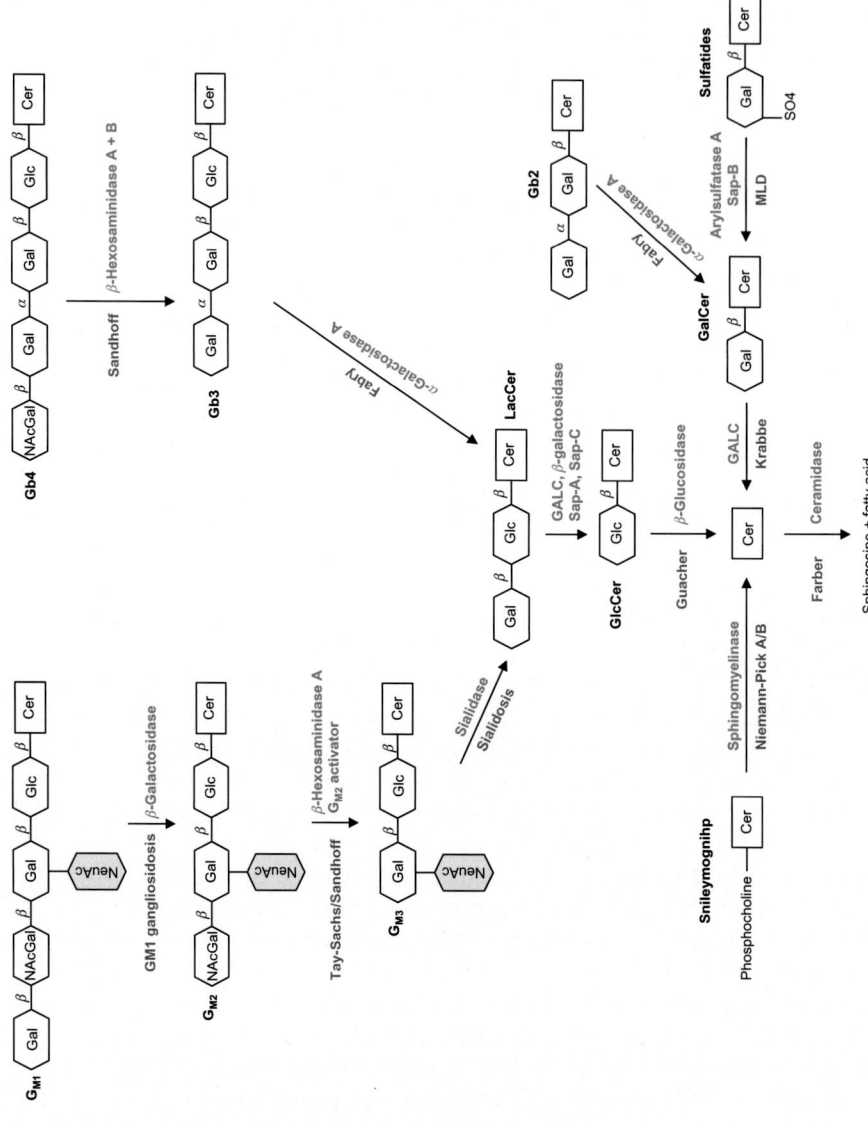

FIGURE 10.1

The degradation pathway of sphingolipids. The sphingolipids are shown in black, the enzymes are in *green*, and the diseases are in *red*. *Cer*, ceramide; *Gal*, galactose; *GALC*, galactocerebrosidase; *GalCer*, galactosylceramide; *NacGal*, N-acetylgalactosamine; *Gb2*, galabiosylceramide; *Gb3*, globotriaosylceramide; *Gb4*, globotetraosylceramide; *Glc*, glucose; *GlcCer*, glucosylceramide; *G*$_{M1}$, G$_{M1}$ ganglioside; *G*$_{M2}$, G$_{M2}$ ganglioside; *G*$_{M3}$, G$_{M3}$ ganglioside; *LacCer*, lactosylceramide; *MLD*, metachromatic leukodystrophy; *NeuAc*, N-acetylneuraminic acid or sialic acid; *Sap*, saposin.

dysmorphic facial features, hepatosplenomegaly, and skeletal involvement (dysostosis multiplex). Death usually occurs by 2 years of age. Type II disease usually presents between 7 months and 3 years of life with neurocognitive and psychomotor regression. The disease progression is slower and hepatic and splenic involvement and cherry-red macular changes are less common than in type I. Type III is characterized by onset between the second and third decades of life with extrapyramidal signs (dystonia, ataxia, or speech disturbances) due to local deposition of gangliosides in the caudate nucleus. Hepatosplenomegaly and cherry-red spots are not generally present in type III.[1,2]

Urinary oligosaccharide (OS) analysis shows elevated galactose-containing OS either by qualitative visualization by thin-layer chromatography (TLC)[3] or mass profile by MALDI TOF with details of structural information.[4] Keratan sulfate excretion can also be elevated in patients with GM1; however, the amount is much lower than that seen in patients with Morquio syndrome (MPS Type IV). Demonstration of deficient β-galactosidase activity in leukocytes or cultured fibroblasts can establish a diagnosis of G_{M1} gangliosidosis. The residual enzyme activity correlates inversely with disease severity.[5] β-Galactosidase activity in leukocytes or cultured fibroblasts are severely deficient in infantile and junvenile forms (<5% of normal), and higher residual activity (5–10% of normal) is seen in patients with adult form G_{M1} gangliosidosis and Morquio B syndrome. β-Galactosidase activity is also deficient in galactosialidosis, where combined deficiencies of β-galactosidase and neuraminidase are present due to primary defects in the protective protein/cathepsin A (PPCA) that is shared by both enzymes. For this reason, it is recommended that neuraminidase activity be measured in the patients with β-galactosidase deficiency to rule out galactosialidosis.

Currently treatment is limited to supportive and symptomatic management.

10.3.2 G_{M2} GANGLIOSIDOSES (TAY–SACHS DISEASE, SANDHOFF DISEASE, AND GM2 ACTIVATOR PROTEIN DEFICIENCY)

The G_{M2} gangliosidoses are a group of lysosomal storage disorders that are characterized by deficiency of β-hexoaminidase A and accumulations of G_{M2} gangliosides and other glycolipids in the lysosomes, mainly in the neurons. Two lysosomal β-hexosaminidase isoenzymes exist, Hex A ($\alpha\beta$) and Hex B ($\beta\beta$). The α- and β-subunits of these two isozymes are encoded by two different genes, *HEXA* and *HEXB*, respectively. Both Hex A and Hex B hydrolyze the β-linked terminal nonreducing sugars *N*-acetylgalactosamine (GalNAc) and *N*-acetylglucosamine (GlcNAc) from glycolipids, glycoproteins, oligosaccharides, and glycosaminoglycans. However, the pathologic substrate G_{M2} gangliosides are almost exclusively cleaved by the Hex A enzyme in the presence of G_{M2} activator. Tay–Sachs disease is caused by a deficiency of the Hex A enzyme due to mutations in the *HEXA* gene. Sandhoff disease is caused by deficiencies of both Hex A and Hex B due to mutations in the *HEXB* gene. G_{M2} activator deficiency is caused by mutations in the *GM2A* gene and functional Hex A deficiency with similar clinical features to Tay–Sachs disease but normal Hex A activity in blood.

Infantile Tay–Sachs disease is the prototype of GM2 gangliosidosis. Patients with infantile Tay–Sachs disease present with progressive cerebral and retinal degeneration that initially becomes clinically apparent around 3–6 months of age. The symptoms include weakness, loss of motor skills, decreased attentiveness and increased startle response, and cherry-red spots on the macula. The disease is rapidly progressing with blindness, rigidity, and decerebrate posturing by 12–18 months followed by death, usually from aspiration and pneumonia, by the age of 4 years. Infantile Sandhoff disease is clinically indistinguishable from Tay–Sachs disease, although the deficiency of Hex B results in additional substrate storage of globosides and oligosaccharides. Hepatosplenomegaly, skeletal abnormalities, and other somatic changes may occur in Sandhoff disease, which are not commonly seen in Tay–Sachs disease. G_{M2} activator deficiency is also almost clinically identical to Tay-Sachs disease in its presentation and course.

The subacute or juvenile form of G_{M2} gangliosidosis presents between 2 and 10 years of age with development of ataxia, lack of coordination, dystonia, dementia, progressive seizures, and spasticity. Death usually occurs in the second decade of life. The chronic or adult form of G_{M2} gangliosidosis can have its onset from childhood to adulthood with slower rate of disease progression. Intelligence is normally intact. Neurological symptoms include dystonia, ataxia, and psychosis.

Enzyme analyses are crucial for the diagnosis of Tay–Sachs and Sandhoff diseases. The enzyme assay can be performed using serum (or plasma), white blood cells, chorionic villi, amniotic fluid, amniocytes, and other tissues. 4-Methylumbelliferyl-2-acetamido-2-deoxy-β-D-glucopyranoside (4-MUG) is the most commonly used artificial substrate that measures total β-hexosaminidase activity (Hex A and Hex B) and percentage of Hex A (Hex A%) after a two- to three-hour heat inactivation of the thermolabile Hex A. Synthetic sulfated substrate 4-methylumbelliferyl-6-sulfo-2-acetamido-2-deoxy-β-D-glucopyranoside (4-MUGS) is used to measure the specific Hex A activity. Tay–Sachs disease is characterized by absent or extremely low specific Hex A activity and a very low Hex A% (<10%) with normal or even elevated Hex B activity. Sandhoff disease has absent or extremely low total β-hexosaminidase activity with a very high Hex A% (90–100%). The heat inactivation enzyme analysis with 4MUG substrate has been the primary method for carrier testing of Tay–Sachs disease in non-Jewish populations with a detection rate of >98%. Carriers of Tay–Sachs disease have an intermediate Hex A% (20–50%) that can be discriminated from non-carriers (60–65% ± 5%). When screening for Tay–Sachs carriers, Sandhoff carriers can also be identified by a characteristic high Hex A% activity (≥75–80%) and relatively low total activity.[6]

Molecular analysis of the *HEXA* gene also plays important role in the diagnosis of Tay–Sachs disease. Three mutations c.1274_1277dupTATC (1278+ TATC), c.1421+ 1G> C (IVS12+ 1G> C), and c.805G> A (p.G269S) account for more than 98% disease causing alleles in Ashkenizi Jewish individuals.[7,8] Other founder mutations include c.1073+ 1G> A (IVS9+ 1G> A) in the Irish[9] and g.2644_10588del (del7.6kb) in French Canadians.[10] More than 180 mutations in the *HEXA* gene have been reported to date in Human Gene Mutation Database (http://www.hgmd.cf.ac.uk/).

Most of the mutations are associated with infantile Tay–Sachs disease. The residual Hex A activity correlates inversely with the severity of the disease. Individuals with acute infantile Tay–Sachs usually have two null alleles. Individuals with juvenile or chronic and adult-onset Tay–Sachs are usually compound heterozygotes for a null allele and an allele that results in low residual Hex A activity, or compound heterozygotes of two alleles that result in low residual Hex A activity.[6,11,12] Missense mutations at two codons (178 and 258), c.532C> T (p.R178C), c.533G> A (p.R178H), c.533G> T (p.R178L), and c.772G> C (p.D258H), are associated with B1 variant of Tay–Sachs disease, presenting with juvenile or adult disease.[13] The B1 variants could have normal enzyme activities toward the 4-MUG substrate, however, are inactive toward natural substrates or the 4-MUGS substrate.[14] Carriers of the B1 variants may be falsely negative by the routine heat inactivation assay with the 4-MUG substrate. Two pseudo-deficiency variants c.739C> T (p.R247W) and c.745C> T (p.R249W) cause false-positive enzyme results resembling a Tay–Sachs carrier but are not associated with Tay–Sachs disease.[15] It has been reported about 35% of non-Jewish and 2% of Jewish individuals who are carriers by enzyme analysis are carriers for one of these two pseudo-deficiency alleles.[15] Therefore, combined enzyme and molecular testing are recommended by American College of Obstetrics and Gynecology (ACOG) for the accurate detection of Tay–Sachs carriers.

Sandhoff disease is a panethnic disorder, with a population carrier frequency of 1:300. The majority of the *HEXB* mutations are private mutations. A 16 kb deletion spanning the promoter region and exons 1–5 is the only common mutation and accounts for 27% of alleles in Sandhoff patients. Therefore, sequencing analysis is the best option for molecular diagnosis.

G_{M2} activator deficiency is suspected in patients who clinically appear to have Tay–Sachs but have normal Hex A and Hex B activities. G_{M2} activator deficiency is often diagnosed by demonstration of disease causing mutations in the *GM2A* gene.

Treatment of the G_{M2} gangliosidoses is limited to supportive care. Recently, pyrimethamine (PMT) has been tested as a potential pharmacological chaperone (PC) to treat late-onset G_{M2} gangliosidosis.[16] The enhancement of β-hexosaminidase activity has been demonstrated; however, the clinical safety and efficacy are still under investigation.[17,18]

10.3.3 FABRY DISEASE

Fabry disease is an X-linked recessive disorder caused by a deficiency of α-galactosidase A due to mutations in the *GLA* gene. This enzyme removes the α-galactose residue from globotriaosylceramide (Gb3) and to a lesser degree, from galabiosylceramide (Gb2). The isoenzyme α-galactosidase B or α-N-acetylgalactosaminidase also hydrolyzes the terminal galactose moiety toward artificial substrate; however, it is encoded by a separate but evolutionarily related gene (*NAGA*), the mutation of which causes a neuroaxonal dystrophy known as Schindler disease.[19] Deficiency of α-galactosidase A results in the accumulation of Gb3 in the lysosomes of endothelial, perithelial, and smooth muscle cells of the vascular system, as well as cells in the kidney, heart, eyes, and ganglion cells of the autonomic nervous system. However, there is a missing link between the Gb3 storage and disease pathogenesis and disease progression. The deacylated substrate globotriaosylsphingosine or lyso-Gb3 has recently been recognized as a better biochemical marker of severity and progression for Fabry disease.[20]

The prevalence of Fabry disease is about 1 in 40,000–60,000 males. Males with classic Fabry disease have almost no detectable α-galactosidase A activity with disease onset in childhood or adolescence. The typical symptoms include pain and acroparesthesia in the extremities, angiokeratomas in the skin and mucous membranes, and hypohidrosis. The whorl-like corneal dystrophy (corneal verticillata) is also characteristic for Fabry disease (Fig. 10.2). Progressive deposition of glycosphingolipids in kidney results in proteinuria initially and progresses to end-stage renal disease. Pulmonary and cardiac involvements, along with cerebral vascular disease, are also known complications that often lead to premature death. Psychiatric illness (depression, bipolar disorder) and GI symptoms can also occur. Without ERT, death in males usually occurs in the third or fourth decade from renal or heart disease. Males with attenuated forms of Fabry disease have partial residual α-galactosidase A activity and later onset. These patients lack many classic features of the disease. The clinical findings are often limited to mild proteinuria and cardiac abnormalities. The c.936+ 919G> A (IVS4+ 919G> A) variant associated with late onset cardiac variant form is highly prevalent in the Taiwan Chinese population as identified through a pilot newborn screening study.[21]

Female heterozygotes have intermediate enzyme activity levels and variable presentations ranging from asymptomatic to classic Fabry disease due to random X-inactivation. The whorl-like corneal opacity is the most common feature which can be observed in approximately 70% of female carriers.[22]

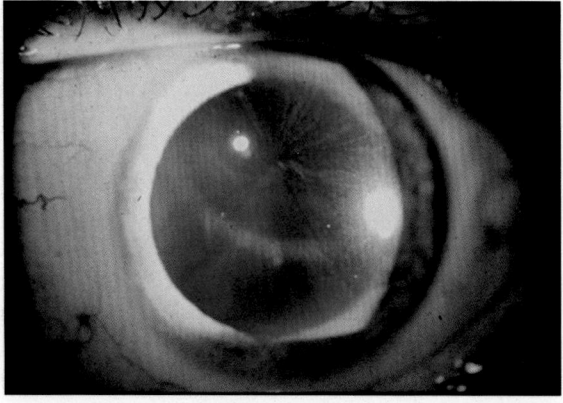

FIGURE 10.2

Corneal verticillata of Fabry disease.

Courtesy of Dr. Robert J. Desnick.

Diagnosis of classic Fabry disease is straight forward by demonstration of near absent α-galactosidase Activity in plasma, leukocytes or cultured cells and a mutation in the *GLA* gene. However, diagnosis of the attenuated form of disease and female Fabry patients can be challenging. Patients with an attenuated form of disease may have substantial residual enzyme activity and approximately 30% female carriers may have normal enzyme activity. Since these patients can potentially be missed by enzyme analysis, both enzymatic and molecular testing should be performed for diagnostic accuracy when the diagnosis is suspected. Measurement of plasma lyso-Gb3 is now considered a diagnostic test for Fabry disease, particularly for the interpretation of variants of unknown significance (VOUS) and unequivocal enzyme testing results. The α-galactosidase A activity can be measured using a flurogenic 4-methylumbelliferyl-α-D-galactopyranoside substrate or synthetic lipid substrate using tandem mass spectrometry.[23] Inhibitor of isoenzyme α-galactosidase B or α-N-acetylgalactosaminidase is usually needed for the accurate measurement of α-galactosidase A activity.

Enzyme replacement therapy (ERT) with agalsidase beta (Fabrazyme) is available for the treatment of Fabry disease. The agalsidase alfa (Replagal) is available in Europe for treating Fabry disease. ERT is of proven benefit in slowing the progression of the renal and cardiac disease associated with Fabry disease.[24] Other therapeutic options include pharmacological chaperones and substrate reduction treatment. Pain management and supportive treatment for cardiac and renal disease are also needed.

10.3.4 GAUCHER DISEASE

Gaucher disease is one of the most common lysosomal storage diseases with a prevalence of 1:40,000 to 1:50,000 in the general population and much more frequent (as high as 1:850) in the Ashkenazi Jewish individuals due to the founder mutations. This autosomal recessive disorder is caused by mutations in the *GBA* gene and subsequent deficient activity of glucocerebrosidase (acid β-glucosidase). As a result, glycosylceramide (GL1) and deacylated substrate glycosylsphingosine (Lyso-GL1) accumulate in cells of the monocytes/macrophage system. The lipid-laden "Gaucher cells" have unique wrinkled tissue paper or crumpled silk appearance in the cytoplasm and are characteristic for Gaucher disease. Gaucher cells are especially prominent in the liver and spleen, leading to hepatosplenomegaly. Progressive accumulation of Gaucher cells in the bone marrow results in bone disease including osteopenia, osteosclerosis, and osteonecrosis. In neuropathic forms of Gaucher disease, significant amounts of GL1 and Lyso-GL1 are present in the CNS.[25,26] Similar to Lyso-GB3 in Fabry disease, Lyso-GL1 appears to be correlated with disease progression and seems to be a better biomarker for the diagnosis and monitoring of Gaucher disease.[27] In addition, macrophage activation also plays a role in the pathophysiology of Gaucher disease. Several protein markers including angiotensin converting enzyme (ACE), chitotriosidase, tartrate-resistant acid phosphatase (TRAP), and the chemokine PARC/CCL18 are considered surrogate markers for lipid burden and macrophage activation and are used in monitoring progression of the disease and treatment efficacy in Gaucher disease.[25]

There are three clinical subtypes of Gaucher disease based on the involvement of CNS and rate of disease progression. Type 1 is nonneuronopathic and the most common form. Type 2 is a fatal neurodegenerative disorder of infancy in addition to the visceral involvements. Type 3 has a severity intermediate between type 1 and type 2.

Type 1 has a variable clinical phenotype, ranging from asymptomatic to severe. The classic presentations in childhood include massive hepatosplenomegaly, pancytopenia, and severe skeletal abnormalities. Some patients were initially misdiagnosed as hematologic malignancies because of pancytopenia. Despite massive hepatomegaly, liver failure is rare. Patients may also present with chronic fatigue, epistaxis, and easy bruising. The bony problems and episodic painful bone crises usually occur later than the development of visceral enlargements. Erlenmeyer flask deformity of the distal femur is a characteristic radiological finding of Gaucher bone disease. Type 2 is a more severe and fast progressing disorder with infantile onset. In addition to massive hepatosplenomegaly, neurologic abnormalities include oculomotor apraxia, cognitive impairment, psychomotor impairment, and seizures. Death usually occurs between 2 and 4 years of age. Type 3 is a more slowly progressive neuropathic form of Gaucher disease with onset in childhood or adolescence.

Recently, the association of mutations in the *GBA* gene and Parkinson disease has been studied extensively. Patients with Gaucher disease, asymptomatic patients and Gaucher carriers have a significantly increased risk for developing Parkinson disease compared to the general population.[28]

Diagnosis of Gaucher disease can be established by demonstration of reduced acid β-glucosidase activity in leukocytes or cultured fibroblasts (<15% of normal). The β-glucosidase activity can also be readily measured in dried blood spot sample for newborn screening of Gaucher disease. Molecular testing involving targeted mutational or sequence analysis of the *GBA* gene is available. Although more than 400 *GBA* mutations have been identified, four mutations, p.N409S (N370S), p.L483P (L444P), c.84dupG (84GG), and c.115+ 1G> A (IVS2+ 1), account for approximately 95% of the disease-causing alleles in the Ashkenazi Jewish population and approximately 50–60% in other populations.[26] Molecular testing of the *GBA* gene can not only confirm and diagnose Gaucher disease but can also detect Gaucher carriers for reproductive counseling. There is some genotype–phenotype correlation toward prediction of a phenotype. The p.N409S (N370S) mutation is predicative of non-neuronopathic (type 1) Gaucher disease. The p.L483P (L444P) mutation is strongly associated with the development of neuronopathic Gaucher disease: homozygosity for this mutation is associated with type 3 Gaucher disease. The p.L483P (L444P) in combination with a more severe mutation results in type 2 Gaucher disease. Measurements of biomarkers including lyso-GL1, chitotriosidase, ACE, TRAP, and CCL18 can also facilitate diagnosis.

ERT has been the standard of care for the treatment of Gaucher disease since 1992. Three enzyme preparations are available worldwide: imiglucerase (Cerezyme), velalglucerasealfa (VPRIV), and taligucerase (Elelyso). Regular ERT infusions leads to decreased plasma levels of the biochemical markers and improvement and stabilization of hematologic and visceral (liver/spleen) involvement. There has been also improvement in frequency of bone crises and bone disease with prolonged treatment with ERT. Miglustat (Zavesca) and eliglustat are inhibitors of glucosylceramide synthase and have been approved by the US Food and Drug Administration (FDA) to treat type 1 Gaucher disease. Substrate reduction therapy (SRT) can be used alone or in combination with ERT. Pharmacological chaperones are under investigation and clinical trials for the treatment of Gaucher disease. Both SRT and pharmacological chaperones can be taken orally and may have potential to cross the blood–brain barrier for possible treatment of neuronopathic Gaucher disease. Bisphosphonates can be used as a supportive treatment for osteopenia.

10.3.5 NIEMANN–PICK A/B (NPD-A AND NPD-B)

NPD-A and NPD-B are autosomal recessive conditions caused by deficient activity of lysosomal acid sphingomyelinase (ASM), which breakdowns sphingomyelin to ceramide. As a result, sphingomyelin accumulates in the lysosomes. In addition, cholesterol and bis (monoacylglycero) phosphate and some other sphingolipids are also highly elevated. These sphingolipids play important roles in cellular signal transduction and may contribute to the disease pathophysiology in NPD-A&B. For example, sphingosine is a potent inhibitor of protein kinase C, which mediates multiple cell-signaling pathways.[29] Ceramide is a second messenger in diverse pathways involving apoptosis.[30] The deacylated sphingomyelin or sphingosylphosphorylcholine is elevated in NPD-A&B and may contribute to cell dysfunctions and apoptosis. The foam cells or Niemann–Pick cells are lipid laden macrophages found primarily in the bone marrow, liver, spleen, and lungs of all NPD-A&B patients, as well as the brains of NPD-A patients. Although Niemann–Pick cells are the histologic hallmark of NPD-A&B, histologically similarly appearing cells may be also found in GM1 gangliosidosis, Wolman disease, and cholesterol ester storage disease, and lipoprotein lipase deficiency.[31]

NPD-A and NPD-B are examples of allelic heterogeneity where different mutations in the same gene locus, *SMPD1* gene on chromosome 11p15, result in different clinical phenotypes. NPD-A is a progressive neurodegenerative disorder of infancy with less than 5% ASM activity, whereas NPD-B is a nonneuronopathic disorder with a broad range of phenotypic severity and higher residual ASM activity. Both types of NPD are panethnic; however, NPD-A is more common in the Ashkenazi Jewish population. Three founder mutations p.L304P (L302P), p.R498L (R496L), and c996delC (fsp330) account for approximately 90% of pathogenic alleles in NPD-A in this population. The other mutation, p.R610del (delR608), is found in 15–20% NPD-B patients in Western Europe and North America and is predicted to have a neuroprotective effect.

NPD-A presents within the first few months of life with massive hepatosplenomegaly, feeding difficulties, recurrent vomiting, constipation and failure to thrive. Psychomotor retardation becomes apparent after 6 months of age with hypotonia, weakness and regression in developmental milestones and at later stages, is superseded with spasticity and rigidity. Cherry-red maculae are observed in ~50% of patients. Interstitial lung disease can result in recurrent infection and respiratory failure and death. The neurological deterioration is debilitating and most NPD-A patients die before 3 years of age.

NPD-B has more variable presentation with childhood, adolescent, or adult onset of symptoms. The clinical presentations and course are more variable. Most patients develop liver and spleen enlargement in childhood with progressive hypersplenism. Liver dysfunction is stable but, in some cases, liver disease can be severe with progression to cirrhosis. Hyperlipidemia is common with elevations of total cholesterol (elevated LDL), triglycerides, and low HDL levels. By the time of diagnosis, pulmonary infiltrations are usually present with progression to restrictive lung disease. Despite absence of neurological symptoms, cherry-red maculae are detected in 20% of NPD-B patients.[32,33]

Diagnosis of NPD-A and NPD-B is made by demonstrating deficient ASM activity (<10% of normal) in leukocytes or cultured fibroblasts. Although ASM activity is relatively higher in NPD-B, the residual ASM activity is not accurate in predicting the disease phenotype. The ASM activity can be measured in DBS specimens and there have been pilot newborn screening studies for this condition. It is important to note that individuals with the *SMPD1* mutation p.Gln294Lys may have apparently normal enzymatic activity when using artificial fluorogenic substrates.

Molecular testing involving targeted mutational or sequence analysis of the *SMPD1* gene is available. Targeted mutational analysis of common NPD-A mutations are useful in testing Ashkenazi Jewish individuals for NPD-A or their carrier status for NPD-A. Targeted mutation analysis is also effective for testing family members and for prenatal diagnosis. Analysis of other disease causing mutations can be achieved by sequence analysis of the *SMPD1* gene.

Treatment for both NPD-A and NPD-B is generally supportive. ERT with human recombinant acid sphingomyelinase (olipudase alfa) has been developed and is in clinical trial for NPD-B.[34,35]

10.3.6 METACHROMATIC LEUKODYSTROPHY

MLD is an autosomal recessive genetic condition with defective desulfation of 3-O-sulfogalactosyl containing glycolipids, particularly sulfatides. Sulfatides are mainly present in myelin sheaths of the central and peripheral nervous tissues. Degradation requires both arylsulfatase A enzyme and its activator protein saposin B. MLD is caused by the deficient activity of arylsulfatase A, which is encoded by the *ARSA* gene located on chromosome 22q13.31-qter. Sulfatides accumulate in the lysosomes and plasma membrane of myelin resulting in demyelination and characteristic deposition of metachromatic staining granules. A characteristic leukodystrophy is seen on magnetic resonance imaging (MRI) with bilateral symmetrical confluent areas of periventricular deep white matter signal change in the region of the atria and frontal horns with sparing of the subcortical U fibers (Fig. 10.3). This is described as a "butterfly" pattern. With progression, cortical and subcortical atrophy develop.[36] Excess sulfatides in non-neuronal tissues are excreted in the urine.

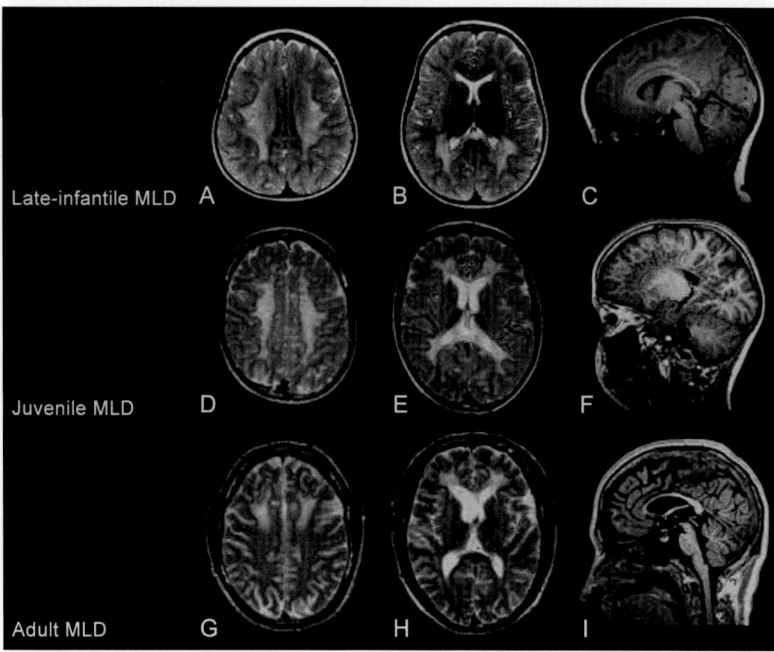

FIGURE 10.3

Axial T2-weighted (A, B, D, E, G, H) and sagittal T1-weighted (C, F, I) MR images of three patients with MLD. (A–C): 2-year-old patient with late-infantile MLD. Involvement of the periventricular white matter and centrum semiovale with parietooccipital predominance and involvement of the splenium. U fibers are spared. (D–F): 7-year-old patient with juvenile MLD. (F) Shows the typical pattern of radiating stripes with bands of normal signal intensity in between. U fibers are spared. (G–I): 28-year-old patient with adult MLD. In addition to the white matter signal abnormalities with frontal predominance, there is mild supratentorial atrophy (G, H).[36]

Saposin B deficiency and multiple sulfatase deficiency, which both have deficient function of arylsulfatase A, are different diseases with different enzymatic defects.

Late-infantile, juvenile, and adult forms have been described based on the age at disease onset. The late-infantile form accounts for 50–60% of MLD with onset between the ages of 1 to 2 years. Presenting symptoms include hypotonia, weakness, clumsiness, toe walking, and slurred speech. Regression of neurocognitive and psychomotor skills ensues (rigidity, hypertonia, hearing and vision loss, pain, peripheral neuropathy, seizures). Affected individuals eventually progress to posturing, tonic spasms, and loss of awareness with death by the age of 5 years. The juvenile form accounts for 20–30% of MLD and presents with behavioral problems, decline in school performance, gait disturbances, clumsiness, slurred speech, and incontinence before 6 years of age. Onset in adolescence may occur as well. Progression and features of juvenile MLD are similar to but slower than late-infantile with death usually occurring before the age of 20 years. Adult-onset MLD is the least common form of MLD presenting much later in life with personality changes, decline in the ability to function in a professional setting, emotional issues, progressing to loss of coordination, peripheral neuropathy, and seizures. Disease progression is highly variable. Death, resulting from pneumonia or another related illness, usually occurs about 20 years after the onset of symptoms.

Reduced nerve conduction velocity and white matter demyelination by MRI are the major clinical findings pointed to the diagnosis of MLD. Biochemical diagnosis of MLD is based on the demonstration of deficiency of the enzyme arylsulfatase A in leukocytes or cultured fibroblasts. However, interpretation of enzyme findings could be complicated by the presence of pseudodeficiency alleles. Between 0.2% and 0.5% of normal individuals can have a considerable degree of deficiency of arylsulfatase A activity (5–15%) due to the high prevalence of the pseudodeficiency allele.[37] Therefore sequence analysis of the *ARSA* gene and urinary sulfatides analysis are needed for accurate diagnosis. In patients where there is a high clinical suspicion of disease but normal arylsulfatase A activity, saposin B deficiency should be ruled out. Diagnosis of multiple sulfatase deficiency requires testing additional sulfatases.

Treatment for MLD is palliative. Bone marrow transplantation (BMT) is used to primarily treat the CNS manifestations of the disease and may slow disease progression. BMT option remains controversial because of the high morbidity and mortality rate associated with the procedure. Long-term outcome study indicates that BMT benefits presymptomatic children with late-infantile MLD or minimally symptomatic juvenile MLD.[38] ERT has been developed and is undergoing clinical trials (rhARSA; metazyme). Hematopoietic stem cell gene therapy is another treatment modality for this devastating demyelination disorder. Preliminary outcome studies show evidence of safety and efficacy in early-onset MLD patients who received gene therapy in the presymptomatic or very early symptomatic stage.[39]

10.3.7 KRABBE DISEASE (GLOBOID CELL LEUKODYSTROPHY)

Krabbe disease is an autosomal recessive condition caused by a deficiency of lysosomal galactosylceramidase (GALC), which is encoded by the *GALC* gene on chromosome 14q31. The deficiency of GALC enzyme results in galactosylceramide storage and formation of multinucleated macrophages (globoid cells) in the CNS and almost total loss of myelin and oligodendroglia and astrocytic gliosis in the white matter. White matter disease with progressive cerebellar atrophy is identified on MRI. The peripheral nervous system is also affected in Krabbe disease. Another compound, galactsylsphingosine (psychosine), is also a substrate for the GALC enzyme and is essentially absent in normal brains but is increased in the CNS of Krabbe patients. It is postulated that psychosine plays important roles in the pathogenesis of Krabbe disease and brain psychosine levels appear to be correlated with disease severity.[40]

The incidence of Krabbe disease was estimated at 1:100,000 live births, with 90% being infantile form and 10% being late-onset form. Infantile Krabbe disease presents with irritability, feeding difficulties, reflux, spasticity, seizures, and hypertonia at 3–6 months of age followed by rapid neurologic deterioration. Infants with Krabbe disease are extremely sensitive to sounds, light, or touch, resulting in screaming and rigidity. Blindness, deafness, and peripheral neuropathy are also common features of Krabbe disease. Organomegaly is not present. Seizures become frequent and death usually occurs before the age of two. Late-onset Krabbe disease presents between the first year of life and the fifth decade of life with a variable onset of vision disturbance/loss, weakness, and cognitive decline.[40]

Diagnosis of Krabbe disease is based on the demonstration of deficiency of the GALC enzyme and identification of the *GALC* mutations. The GALC activity can be measured in leukocytes or cultured fibroblasts by the use of radiolabeled natural substrate galactosylceramide or synthetic florescent substrate 6-hexadecanoylamino-4-methylumbelliferyl-β-D-galactopyranoside. Methods using synthetic lipid substrates and tandem mass spectrometry have recently become available. Several common disease-causing mutations are known. A 30-kb deletion (or 502T/del) is the most common mutation in populations of European ancestry accounting for approximately 40% of infantile Krabbe alleles. Two missense mutations p.T513M and p.Y551S make up for additional 0–15% of the infantile Krabbe alleles.[40,41] Another missense mutation p.G270D is common in patients with late-onset Krabbe disease.[40] Three pseudodeficiency alleles (p.R168C, p.D232N, and p.I546T) are known to cause reduced GALC activity but do not cause Krabbe disease.[40]

New York State has screened almost 2 million infants for Krabbe disease since 2006. Only 5 infants were diagnosed with infantile Krabbe disease and 46 children were identified as having moderate to high risk for later-onset disease. The incidence of infantile Krabbe disease is 1:394,000 in New York population, which is lower than the previous estimate; however, the incidence of later-onset Krabbe disease seems more prevalent than previously thought.[42,43]

At present, the treatment option for Krabbe disease is limited to hematopoietic stem cell transplantation (HSCT). This treatment remains controversial. Earlier literature reported evidence for stabilization and possible improvements in 4 patients with late-onset disease[44] and favorable outcomes in 11 presymptomatic newborns with infantile Krabbe disease[45] indicating the benefits of HSCT. However, high mortality and morbidity were reported in the patients identified by New York State newborn screening. Out of the four infantile Krabbe patients who received HSCT, two patients died from HSCT complications and two patients who survived transplantation had moderate-to-severe disability.[43]

10.3.8 FARBER DISEASE

Farber disease is a rare recessive condition of lipid metabolism associated with a deficiency of lysosomal acid ceramidase and accumulation of ceramide. Abnormal storage of ceramide is confined to the lysosomes of multiple organs and tissues leading to progressive formation of subcutaneous nodules (lipogranulomata) and granulomatous infiltrations in subcutaneous tissues and joints as well as larynx, liver, spleen, lung, heart, and CNS system.

Approximately 50% of patients described to date have classic Farber disease presenting in early infancy with the characteristic triad of painful swelling of joints, subcutaneous nodules (lipogranulomata), and progressive hoarseness. Other symptoms include feeding and breathing difficulties, poor weight gain, and intermittent fever. Neurological symptoms occur in most patients. However, the evaluation of neurological function can be difficult in Farber patients because of the joint pain. Diagnosis can almost be made from the striking appearance with cachexia, flexion contractures along with periarticular swelling and subcutaneous nodules. Demonstration of reduced or absent acid ceramidase in leukocytes or cultured fibroblast samples and two mutations in the *ASAH* gene confirm the diagnosis. Other confirmatory evidence includes the presence of perivascular aggregates of foamy histiocytes and the identification of "Farber bodies" (crescentic-shaped bodies within Schwann cells) by electron microscopy in the biopsy sample and elevated ceramide levels in cultured cells and urine.

The therapy for Farber disease is mainly palliative. BMT in two classic Farber patients resulted in improvements of somatic symptoms but was not helpful for CNS involvement.[46] BMT might be appropriate for patients with mild or no neurological symptoms.

10.3.9 NIEMANN–PICK DISEASE TYPE C

Niemann–Pick disease type C (NPD-C) is an autosomal recessive disorder with dysregulated intracellular lipid trafficking. NPD-C is panethnic with an estimated incidence of 1:100,000 to 1:120,000 live birth. NPD-C is caused by mutations in one of two genes, *NPC1* (in 95% cases) or *NPC2* (in 5% cases). *NPC1* encodes a large protein that resides in the membrane of endosomes and lysosomes and functions to allow appropriate transport of cholesterol and lipids across cell membranes. *NPC2* encodes a protein that binds to cholesterol and transports it out of the luminal space of the late endosome/lysosome into the delimiting membrane. Defects of either protein essentially trap free cholesterol and other lipids, including glycosphingolipids, in the lysosomes and result in cellular dysfunction and apoptosis.[47]

NPD-C is a highly variable neurovisceral condition that can present in infancy, childhood, or adulthood. Classically, NPD-C presents in mid-to-late childhood with vertical supranuclear gaze palsy, ataxia, dementia, and psychiatric disturbances. Seizures, dystonia, dysarthria, loss of learned speech, and dysphagia may also be present. Death occurs in the second or third decade of life, usually from aspiration pneumonia. Infants can present with liver disease, ascites, or lung disease, or may simply present with hypotonia and developmental delay. About half of NPD-C patients have neonatal cholestasis with hepatosplenomegaly and are initially suspected of having a cytomegalovirus (CMV) infection, a peroxisomal disorder or a mitochondrial disorder. Adults typically present with the classical features later in life and are more likely to present with a psychotic episode or dementia.[47,48]

The diagnosis can be suspected with the identification of foamy macrophages in blood smears or other tissue samples (liver, tonsil). Demonstration of impaired cholesterol esterification followed by filipin staining in cultured fibroblasts used to be the key diagnostic biochemical test for NPD-C. However, the sensitivity and specificity of filipin staining test is less ideal and requires an invasive skin biopsy procedure and cell culture. It is particularly insensitive in non-classic NPD-C. The plasma biomarkers chitotriosidase and oxycholesterol can be effective in screening for NPD-C and, if abnormal, molecular genetic testing of the *NPC1* or *NPC2* gene can confirm the diagnosis.

Treatment is generally symptomatic and supportive. Miglustat has been approved in Europe, Japan, and Canada, as a therapy for treatment of progressive neurological manifestations in pediatric and adult patients with NPD-C because of the demonstration of treatment-related stabilization of key neurological manifestations.[49] Cyclodextrin is a small molecule that is designed to bind cholesterol bypassing NPC1 and NPC2 protein. It has been shown effective in treating NPD-C in animal models. Clinical trials of various forms of cyclodextrin are under way.

10.4 BIOMARKERS IN CURRENT USE

10.4.1 PLASMA CHITOTRIOSIDASE

Chitotriosidase is a biomarker of macrophage activation that can be elevated in various lipid storage lysosomal diseases including Gaucher disease, Niemann–Pick disease, galactosialidosis, and cholesteryl ester storage disease. Plasma chitotriosidase is elevated several hundred-fold in the plasma of symptomatic non-neuronopathic Gaucher patients and decreases and stabilizes with adequate ERT or SRT. It is commonly used as a surrogate marker for the assessment of disease severity and monitoring efficacy of treatment.[50,51] Chitotriosidase activity could be moderately increased in Niemann–Pick and other lipid storage diseases. However, a null *CHIT1* allele, 24 bp duplication in exon 10, is highly prevalent. About 5% of individuals are homozygous and 35% individuals are heterozygous for this null allele in the Caucasian population. Therefore, the interpretation of chitotriosidase activity needs to be in the context of the *CHIT1* genotype.[52,53] Hypomorphic alleles (p.G102S) are also reported to affect the activity of chitotriosidase.[53]

Besides chitotriosidase, ACE and TRAP have been used to monitor patients with Gaucher disease. However, these two biomarkers are not as elevated as chitotriosidase and their use for monitoring has fallen out of favor.

10.4.2 PLASMA PARC/CCL18

The high frequency of chitotriosidase deficiency prompted the search for an alternative marker for Gaucher disease treatment and management. The pulmonary and activation-regulated chemokine (PARC/CCL18) is found to be approximately 30-fold elevated in symptomatic Gaucher patients, which is far more pronounced than ACE and TRAP. Plasma PARC/CCL18 level decreases with ERT, comparably to chitotriosidase. Immunohistochemistry studies have demonstrated that Gaucher cells are the prominent source of PARC/CCL18, making it a surrogate marker for monitoring therapeutic intervention, particularly for monitoring chitotriosidase-deficient Gaucher patients. However, PARC/CCL18 is less specific for diagnosing Gaucher disease as the level can be massively elevated in other medical conditions associated with inflammation.[54]

10.4.3 PLASMA GLUCOSYLSPHIGOSINE (LYSO-GL1)

Although glucosylceramide (GL1) is the primary lipid storage in Gaucher disease, plasma GL1 is generally not used as a biomarker for monitoring Gaucher disease. Plasma GL1 is only slightly elevated because most of it is present in lipoproteins. The relation between circulating GL1 with Gaucher cell burden in the tissues is also unclear. The deacylated substrate glucosylsphingosine (lyso-GL1) has been found to be markedly increased to approximately 200-fold in plasma of symptomatic non-neuronopathic Gaucher patients and seems to correlate with the current Gaucher cell markers chitotriosidase and PARC/CCL18. Plasma lyso-GL1 level decreases with ERT and a less pronounced reduction with miglustat. Moreover, in vitro study in the cultured macrophages indicated that the elevated circulating lyso-GL1 was originated from Gaucher cells.[55] These findings have been used to justify the use of lyso-GL1 as a biomarker for type 1 Gaucher disease. In a recent larger clinical study, lyso-GL1 has also shown to be correlated with liver and spleen volume. In patients treated with the new SRT drug eliglustat, more reduction of plasma lyso-GL1 was observed compared to ERT-treated patients.[27]

10.4.4 PLASMA (OR URINE) GLOBOTRIAOSYLSPHINGOSINE (LYSO-G$_B$3)

Similarly to Gaucher disease, globotriaosylceramide (Gb3), also named ceramidetrihexoside (CTH), is the primary lipid storage in Fabry disease. However, recently, the deacylated substrate lyso-Gb3 has proven to be the hallmark biochemical marker for Fabry disease manifestation. In vitro exposure with lyso-Gb3, not Gb3, resulted in marked proliferation of smooth muscle cells in culture, which indicates the vasoactive effects of this metabolite.[20] Plasma lyso-Gb3 concentration is elevated 250-fold in classic male Fabry patients, in contrast to the 3-fold increase of Gb3. Plasma lyso-Gb3 level is also unequivocally highly elevated in classic female patients, in contrast to the normal Gb3 level in female carriers. Therefore the plasma lyso-Gb3 can be used as a diagnostic test for Fabry disease in both males and females.[20,56] Additional analogs of lyso-Gb3 have been reported in urine and can be quite abundant in Fabry patients. The diagnostic and monitoring values of these analogs for Fabry disease have yet to be determined.[57–59]

10.4.5 URINE SULFATIDES

Urine sulfatides are extremely low in normal individuals and highly elevated in patients with MLD. This marker is clinically useful in discriminating MLD patients from individuals with pseudodeficiencies. Traditionally, urine sulfatides were qualitatively visualized by TLC analysis.[60] Quantitative sulfatide analysis using high-performance liquid chromatography (HPLC) revealed a 50-fold increase of urine total sulfatides in MLD patients.[61] Specific and sensitive liquid chromatography and tandem mass spectrometry (LC-MS/MS) analysis have been developed and used for the screening and diagnosis of MLD. A recent study using dried blood spot samples showed 20-fold and 5-fold increases of total sulfatides concentration for early- and late-onset MLD patients, respectively, when compared to normal controls and those with pseudodeficiencies. A corresponding 160-fold and 80-fold increase was found for early- and late-onset MLD in dried urine spot samples suggesting that sulfatides might be a feasible marker for newborn screening for MLD.[62]

10.4.6 OXYSTEROLS

Oxysterols are a group of non-enzymaticoxidative derivatives of cholesterol. Biomarker studies of oxysterols were initiated in patients with NPD-C because of the notion that oxidative stress plays an important role in the pathogenesis of NPD-C disease. Two of the oxysterolscholestane-3β-5α-6β-triol and 7-ketocholesterol were found to be highly elevated in the plasma of NPD-C patients and have been proposed to be the biomarkers for NPD-C.[63,64] These two markers are similarly elevated in patients with NPD-A and NPD-B.[65,66] Moderate elevations of both 3β-5α-6β-triol and 7-ketocholesterol are observed in plasma from patients with cholesteryl ester storage disease. 7-Ketocholesterol is highly elevated in patients with Smith–Lemli–Opitz syndrome. Interestingly, oxysterols are not elevated in patients with familial hypercholesterolemia.[66]

10.5 CONCLUSION

While rare, the sphingolipidoses nonetheless result in significant morbitidy and mortality for those affected individuals. The largest hurdle in recognizing these disorders is considering them on the differential diagnosis. Biomarkers play important roles in screening, diagnosis, and monitoring of sphingolipidoses. Some of these biomarkers are not necessarily the direct substrates of deficient enzymes but may reflect disease pathophysiology. For example, the protein markers chitotriosidase and PARC/CCL18 are not substrates for β-glucosidase but represent the macrophage lipid burden of Gaucher disease. This is also true for oxysterols as biomarkers for NPD-C (as well as NPD-A and NPD-B), which are the results of abnormal cholesterol oxidation that is associated with the pathogenesis of these conditions. These markers are more associated with the disease progression and better for monitoring therapeutic responses. Similarly deacylated disease substrates, lyso-GL1 (Gaucher) and lyso-Gb3 (Fabry) are predicted to be better associated with disease pathology and therefore better biomarkers for Gaucher disease and Fabry disease than their respective disease substrates. These markers are particularly useful in resolving the diagnosis in individuals having pseudodeficiencies or having VOUS or questionable enzyme results.

REFERENCES

1. Brunetti-Pierri N, Scaglia F. GM1 gangliosidosis: review of clinical, molecular, and therapeutic aspects. *Mol Genet Metab* 2008;**94**(4):391–6.
2. Suzuki Y, et al. β-Galactosidase deficiency (β-galactosidosis): GM1 ganagliosidosis and Morquio B disease. In: Valle D, Beaudet AL, Vogelstein B,Kinzler KW, editors. *The online metabolic & molecular bases of inherited disease*. New York, NY: McGraw-Hill; 2014.
3. Sewell AC. Urinary oligosaacharides. In: Hommes FA, editor. *Techniques in diagnostic human biochemical genetics. A laboratory manual*. New York: Wiley-Liss; 1991. p. 219–31.
4. Xia B, et al. Oligosaccharide analysis in urine by maldi-tof mass spectrometry for the diagnosis of lysosomal storage diseases. *Clin Chem* 2013;**59**(9):1357–68.
5. Suzuki Y, Nakamura N, Fukuoka K. GM1-gangliosidosis: accumulation of ganglioside GM1 in cultured skin fibroblasts and correlation with clinical types. *Hum Genet* 1978;**43**(2):127–31.
6. Kaback MM, Desnick RJ. Hexosaminidase A deficiency. In: Pagon RA, editor. *Gene Reviews (R)*. Seattle (WA); 1993.
7. Fernandes MJ, et al. Specificity and sensitivity of hexosaminidase assays and DNA analysis for the detection of Tay-Sachs disease gene carriers among Ashkenazic Jews. *Genet Epidemiol* 1992;**9**(3):169–75.
8. Scott SA, et al. Experience with carrier screening and prenatal diagnosis for 16 Ashkenazi Jewish genetic diseases. *Hum Mutat* 2010;**31**(11):1240–50.
9. van Bael M, et al. Heterozygosity for Tay-Sachs disease in non-Jewish Americans with ancestry from Ireland or Great Britain. *J Med Genet* 1996;**33**(10):829–32.
10. De Braekeleer M, et al. The French Canadian Tay-Sachs disease deletion mutation: identification of probable founders. *Hum Genet* 1992;**89**(1):83–7.
11. Maegawa GH, et al. The natural history of juvenile or subacute GM2 gangliosidosis: 21 new cases and literature review of 134 previously reported. *Pediatrics* 2006;**118**(5):e1550–62.
12. Gravel RA, Clarke JTR, Kaback MM, Mahuran D, Sandhoff K, Suzuki K. The GM2 gangliosidoses. In: Scriver CR, Beaudet AL, Sly WS, editors. *The metabolic and molecular basis of inherited disease* 7th edn. New York: McGraw-Hill; 1995. p. 2839–79.
13. Mahuran DJ. Biochemical consequences of mutations causing the GM2 gangliosidoses. *Biochim Biophys Acta* 1999;**1455**(2-3):105–38.
14. Peleg L, et al. GM2 gangliosidosis B1 variant: biochemical and molecular characterization of hexosaminidase A. *Biochem Mol Med* 1995;**54**(2):126–32.
15. Cao Z, et al. A second mutation associated with apparent beta-hexosaminidase A pseudodeficiency: identification and frequency estimation. *Am J Hum Genet* 1993;**53**(6):1198–205.
16. Maegawa GH, et al. Pyrimethamine as a potential pharmacological chaperone for late-onset forms of GM2 gangliosidosis. *J Biol Chem* 2007;**282**(12):9150–61.
17. Clarke JT, et al. An open-label phase I/II clinical trial of pyrimethamine for the treatment of patients affected with chronic GM2 gangliosidosis (Tay-Sachs or Sandhoff variants). *Mol Genet Metab* 2011;**102**(1):6–12.
18. Osher E, et al. Pyrimethamine increases beta-hexosaminidase A activity in patients with Late Onset Tay Sachs. *Mol Genet Metab* 2011;**102**(3):356–63.
19. Wang AM, Desnick RJ. Structural organization and complete sequence of the human alpha-N-acetylgalactosaminidase gene: homology with the alpha-galactosidase A

gene provides evidence for evolution from a common ancestral gene. *Genomics* 1991;**10**(1):133–42.

20. Aerts JM, et al. Elevated globotriaosylsphingosine is a hallmark of Fabry disease. *Proc Natl Acad Sci U S A* 2008;**105**(8):2812–17.

21. Chien YH, et al. Fabry disease: incidence of the common later-onset alpha-galactosidase A IVS4+ 919G--> A mutation in Taiwanese newborns--superiority of DNA-based to enzyme-based newborn screening for common mutations. *Mol Med* 2012;**18**:780–4.

22. Nguyen TT, et al. Ophthalmological manifestations of Fabry disease: a survey of patients at the Royal Melbourne Fabry Disease Treatment Centre. *Clin Experiment Ophthalmol* 2005;**33**(2):164–8.

23. Li Y, et al. Direct multiplex assay of lysosomal enzymes in dried blood spots for newborn screening. *Clin Chem* 2004;**50**(10):1785–96.

24. Beck M, et al. Long-term effectiveness of agalsidase alfa enzyme replacement in Fabry disease: A Fabry Outcome Survey analysis. *Mol Genet Metab Rep* 2015;**3**:21–7.

25. Grabowski GA. Phenotype, diagnosis, and treatment of Gaucher's disease. *Lancet* 2008;**372**(9645):1263–71.

26. Baris HN, Cohen IJ, Mistry PK. Gaucher disease: the metabolic defect, pathophysiology, phenotypes and natural history. *Pediatr Endocrinol Rev* 2014;**12**(Suppl 1):72–81.

27. Murugesan V, et al. Glucosylsphingosine is a key biomarker of Gaucher disease. *Am J Hematol* 2016;**91**(11):1082–9.

28. Rosenbloom B, et al. The incidence of Parkinsonism in patients with type 1 Gaucher disease: data from the ICGG Gaucher Registry. *Blood Cells Mol Dis* 2011;**46**(1):95–102.

29. Lai MK, et al. Biological effects of naturally occurring sphingolipids, uncommon variants, and their analogs. *Neuromolecular Med* 2016;**18**(3):396–414.

30. Hsieh CT, et al. Ceramide inhibits insulin-stimulated Akt phosphorylation through activation of Rheb/mTORC1/S6K signaling in skeletal muscle. *Cell Signal* 2014;**26**(7):1400–8.

31. Schuchman EH, Wasserstein MP. Types A and B Niemann-Pick disease. *Best Pract Res Clin Endocrinol Metab* 2015;**29**(2):237–47.

32. McGovern MM, et al. Lipid abnormalities in children with types A and B Niemann Pick disease. *J Pediatr* 2004;**145**(1):77–81.

33. Wasserstein MP, et al. The natural history of type B Niemann-Pick disease: results from a 10-year longitudinal study. *Pediatrics* 2004;**114**(6):e672–7.

34. Wasserstein MP, et al. Successful within-patient dose escalation of olipudase alfa in acid sphingomyelinase deficiency. *Mol Genet Metab* 2015;**116**(1-2):88–97.

35. Thurberg BL, et al. Clearance of hepatic sphingomyelin by olipudase alfa is associated with improvement in lipid profiles in acid sphingomyelinase deficiency. *Am J Surg Pathol* 2016;**40**(9):1232–42.

36. van Rappard DF, Boelens JJ, Wolf NI. Metachromatic leukodystrophy: disease spectrum and approaches for treatment. *Best Pract Res Clin Endocrinol Metab* 2015;**29**(2):261–73.

37. Gieselmann V, Krageloh-Mann I. Metachromatic leukodystrophy--an update. *Neuropediatrics* 2010;**41**(1):1–6.

38. Martin HR, et al. Neurodevelopmental outcomes of umbilical cord blood transplantation in metachromatic leukodystrophy. *Biol Blood Marrow Transplant* 2013;**19**(4):616–24.

39. Sessa M, et al. Lentiviral haemopoietic stem-cell gene therapy in early-onset metachromatic leukodystrophy: an ad-hoc analysis of a non-randomised, open-label, phase 1/2 trial. *Lancet* 2016;**388**(10043):476–87.

40. Wenger DA, Escolar ML, Luzi P, Rafi MA. Krabbe disease (Globoid Cell Leukodystrophy). In: Valle D, Beaudet AL, Vogelstein B, Kinzler KW, Antonarakis SE, Ballabio A,

editors. *The online metabolic and molecular bases of inherited disease*. New York, NY: McGraw-Hill; 2014. http://ommbid.mhmedical.com/content.aspx?bookid=971&Sectio nid=62644214.

41. Kleijer WJ, et al. Prevalent mutations in the GALC gene of patients with Krabbe disease of Dutch and other European origin. *J Inherit Metab Dis* 1997;**20**(4):587–94.

42. Orsini JJ, et al. Newborn screening for Krabbe disease in New York State: the first eight years' experience. *Genet Med* 2016;**18**(3):239–48.

43. Wasserstein MP, et al. Clinical outcomes of children with abnormal newborn screening results for Krabbe disease in New York State. *Genet Med* 2016;**18**(12):1235–43.

44. Krivit W, et al. Hematopoietic stem-cell transplantation in globoid-cell leukodystrophy. *N Engl J Med* 1998;**338**(16):1119–26.

45. Escolar ML, et al. Transplantation of umbilical-cord blood in babies with infantile Krabbe's disease. *N Engl J Med* 2005;**352**(20):2069–81.

46. Yeager AM, et al. Bone marrow transplantation for infantile ceramidase deficiency (Farber disease). *Bone Marrow Transplant* 2000;**26**(3):357–63.

47. Patterson MC, et al. Recommendations for the diagnosis and management of Niemann-Pick disease type C: an update. *Mol Genet Metab* 2012;**106**(3):330–44.

48. Vanier MT. Niemann-Pick disease type C. *Orphanet J Rare Dis* 2010;**5**:16.

49. Patterson MC, et al. Miglustat for treatment of Niemann-Pick C disease: a randomised controlled study. *Lancet Neurol* 2007;**6**(9):765–72.

50. Hollak CE, et al. Marked elevation of plasma chitotriosidase activity. A novel hallmark of Gaucher disease. *J Clin Invest* 1994;**93**(3):1288–92.

51. van Dussen L, et al. Value of plasma chitotriosidase to assess non-neuronopathic Gaucher disease severity and progression in the era of enzyme replacement therapy. *J Inherit Metab Dis* 2014;**37**(6):991–1001.

52. Boot RG, et al. The human chitotriosidase gene. Nature of inherited enzyme deficiency. *J Biol Chem* 1998;**273**(40):25680–5.

53. Grace ME, et al. Type 1 Gaucher disease: null and hypomorphic novel chitotriosidase mutations-implications for diagnosis and therapeutic monitoring. *Hum Mutat* 2007;**28**(9):866–73.

54. Boot RG, et al. Marked elevation of the chemokine CCL18/PARC in Gaucher disease: a novel surrogate marker for assessing therapeutic intervention. *Blood* 2004;**103**(1):33–9.

55. Dekker N, et al. Elevated plasma glucosylsphingosine in Gaucher disease: relation to phenotype, storage cell markers, and therapeutic response. *Blood* 2011;**118**(16):e118–27.

56. Smid BE, et al. Plasma globotriaosylsphingosine in relation to phenotypes of Fabry disease. *J Med Genet* 2015;**52**(4):262–8.

57. Boutin M, Auray-Blais C. Multiplex tandem mass spectrometry analysis of novel plasma lyso-Gb(3)-related analogues in Fabry disease. *Anal Chem* 2014;**86**(7):3476–83.

58. Auray-Blais C, et al. Urinary biomarker investigation in children with Fabry disease using tandem mass spectrometry. *Clin Chim Acta* 2015;**438**:195–204.

59. Boutin M, Auray-Blais C. Metabolomic discovery of novel urinary galabiosylceramide analogs as Fabry disease biomarkers. *J Am Soc Mass Spectrom* 2015;**26**(3):499–510.

60. Rafi MA, et al. Disease-causing mutations in cis with the common arylsulfatase A pseudodeficiency allele compound the difficulties in accurately identifying patients and carriers of metachromatic leukodystrophy. *Mol Genet Metab* 2003;**79**(2):83–90.

61. Natowicz MR, et al. Urine sulfatides and the diagnosis of metachromatic leukodystrophy. *Clin Chem* 1996;**42**(2):232–8.

62. Spacil Z, et al. Sulfatide analysis by mass spectrometry for screening of metachromatic leukodystrophy in dried blood and urine samples. *Clin Chem* 2016;**62**(1):279–86.
63. Porter FD, et al. Cholesterol oxidation products are sensitive and specific blood-based biomarkers for Niemann-Pick C1 disease. *Sci Transl Med* 2010;**2**(56):56ra81.
64. Jiang X, et al. A sensitive and specific LC-MS/MS method for rapid diagnosis of Niemann-Pick C1 disease from human plasma. *J Lipid Res* 2011;**52**(7):1435–45.
65. Lin N, et al. Determination of 7-ketocholesterol in plasma by LC-MS for rapid diagnosis of acid SMase-deficient Niemann-Pick disease. *J Lipid Res* 2014;**55**(2):338–43.
66. Boenzi S, et al. Evaluation of plasma cholestane-3beta,5alpha,6beta-triol and 7-keto-cholesterol in inherited disorders related to cholesterol metabolism. *J Lipid Res* 2016;**57**(3):361–7.

Peroxisomal disorders: clinical and biochemical laboratory aspects

M. Dasouki

King Faisal Specialist Hospital and Research Center, Riyadh, Saudi Arabia;
University of Kansas Medical Center, Kansas City, KS, United States

11.1 PEROXISOME STRUCTURE, BIOGENESIS, AND FUNCTION

11.1.1 INTRODUCTION

Peroxisomes are ubiquitous single membrane lined spherical cytoplasmic organelles, 0.1–1.0 μm in diameter, with finely granular matrices. They are primarily concerned with lipid (especially but not limited to very long chain fatty acids, VLCFAs) and redox homeostasis (Fig. 11.1). However, newer roles in innate immunity, aging, neurodegeneration, obesity-related diabetes, and cancer are emerging.[1] They are found in multiple copies (100–1000) in all eukaryotic cells. They were first described morphologically by Rhodin in 1954 who identified them in mouse kidney convoluted tubule cells as microbodies.[2,3] De Duve coined the term *peroxisome* (i.e., cytoplasmic body responsible for peroxidation) and through various biochemical and density gradient studies showed the peroxisomes' combined urate oxidase, D-amino acid oxidase, L-α-hydroxy acid oxidase, and catalase activities.[4–6] In 1973, absent peroxisomes and secondary mitochondrial abnormalities were first linked with the human disease, cerebrohepatorenal (Zellweger) syndrome, by Goldfischer et al.,[7] while the associated biochemical marker (elevated VLCFAs) was first reported in 1984.[8] *PEX2* (PAF: peroxisome assembly factor 1) was the first gene found to be mutated in a peroxisomal disorder (Zellweger syndrome, ZS).[9]

While significant progress has been made in understanding the peroxisome's complex function and mechanisms of biogenesis, there are still gaps in this understanding. Over the last few years, several excellent reviews have been published in the literature describing mammalian peroxisome biogenesis, structure, and function, as well as related human genetic disorders. Several of these reviews will be cited throughout this chapter.

Peroxisomes do not contain nucleic acid of their own, and are thought to be impermeable to small molecules. Therefore they must have their own transporters. It has recently been demonstrated that peroxisomes have one-membrane channel pore

Biomarkers in Inborn Errors of Metabolism. DOI: http://dx.doi.org/10.1016/B978-0-12-802896-4.00007-9

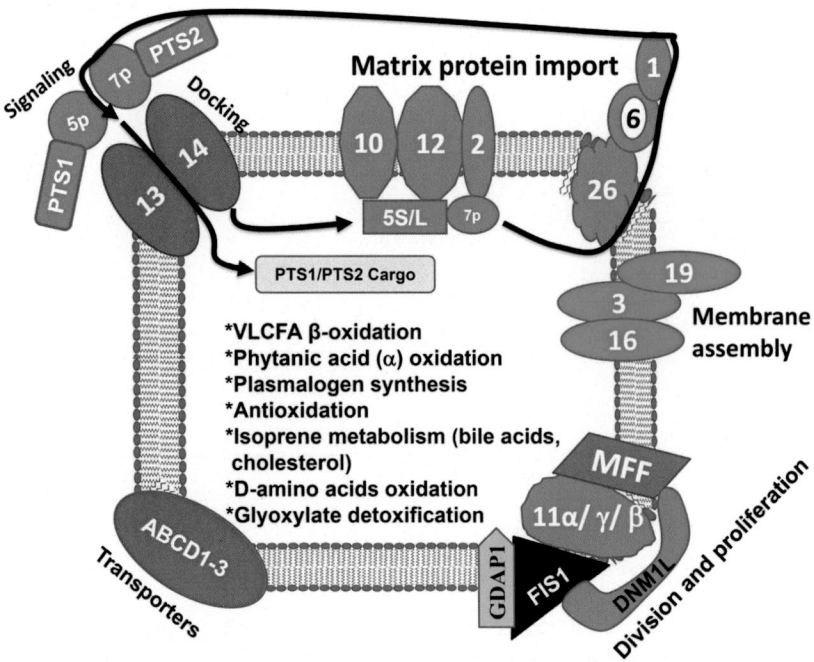

FIGURE 11.1

Peroxisome structure and function. Several peroxisome membrane proteins (VLCFA transporters, membrane assembly, docking, division and proliferation, signaling and importer proteins) and matrix proteins are necessary to ensure normal structure and function of peroxisomes. Peroxisomal matrix proteins are synthesized on free cytoplasmic polyribosomes and then transported using either PTS1 or PTS2 signals recognized by their respective cytosolic receptors "PEX5p and PEX7p." The imported matrix proteins perform diverse biochemical functions as shown.

Adapted from Fujiki Y et al. Front Physiol 2015;5:307.

(PXMP2, peroxisomal membrane protein 2) of unknown function[10] and one transporter (SLC25A17, solute carrier family 25 member 17), which is responsible for the transport of Co-A (coenzyme-A), FAD (flavin adenine dinucleotide), NAD^+ (nicotinamide adenine dinucleotide) in exchange for PAP (phospho-adenosine phosphate), FMN (flavin mononucleotide), and AMP (adenosine monophosphate).[11,12] They have complex machinery involving their membrane and matrix structures that allows them to carry out such diverse metabolic functions (Fig. 11.1) as fatty acid oxidation (VLCFA, phytanic acid), hydrogen peroxide detoxification (catalase), docohexanoic acid (DHA) synthesis, bile acid synthesis, plasmalogen (ether phospholipid) biosynthesis, cholesterol and isoprenes synthesis, glyoxylate detoxification, and lysine catabolism (pipecolic acid).[13–15] To perform these functions, peroxisomes need a large set of peroxisome assembly proteins (peroxins), encoded by several PEX genes, that function both in the peroxisome membrane as well the matrix. Various peroxins required for matrix protein import, peroxisome division, and membrane formation have been identified. More than 30 peroxins necessary for the formation of functional peroxisomes have been identified using genetic screens in several model organisms. Previously, it was thought that new peroxisomes originate from old ones only through growth (elongation, constriction) and fission;[16] however, recent studies support a semiautonomous model of peroxisomal biogenesis. As such, peroxisomal membrane proteins (PMPs) and matrix enzymes first traffic from the endoplasmic reticulum (ER) to the peroxisome by a vesicular budding, targeting, and fusion process while peroxisomal matrix proteins are imported into the organelle through an autonomous, posttranslational mechanism.[17–20] Most peroxisome matrix proteins contain the C-terminal (-S-K-L) peroxisome targeting sequence 1 (PTS1) motif and bind to their soluble cytosolic membrane receptor PEX5p encoded by *PEX5*, while a small number of matrix proteins use the (PTS2) N-terminal (-R/K-L-X5-Q/H-L-) targeting sequence and bind to their receptor PEX7p. However, several exceptions had been reported such as those peroxisomal matrix proteins without a typical PTS1 signal, which are still targeted to peroxisomes via PEX5p.[21]

11.1.2 PEROXISOME BIOGENESIS

Using the *de novo* biogenesis pathway, a selected group of PMPs is inserted into the ER through the translocon and then sequestered into specialized PEX3p-containing ER structures from which vesicles are pinched-off in a PEX19p-dependent manner.[22] These preperoxisome vesicles subsequently develop into mature peroxisomes that are capable of importing matrix proteins, a multistage process that consists of cargo-recognition by a PTS1/2 receptor (PEX5p/PEX7p respectively), docking of the PTS receptor-cargo complexes at the peroxisomal membrane (PEX13, 14), cargo translocation and delivery across the peroxisomal membrane (PEX5, 7, 15), cargo release (PEX14) into the peroxisome matrix, and finally receptor recycling. Recycling involves extraction of the receptor from the peroxisome membrane, followed by ubiquitination (PEX2, 10, 12) by the receptor export module. Peroxisomes also have quality control machinery, which includes Lon protease (LONP1) that removes oxidatively damaged matrix proteins, the proteasome that removes and degrades unneeded PMPs, and pexophagy (p62, Atg30, Atg36), which removes dysfunctional organelles.[23]

11.1.3 PEROXISOME DYNAMICS

Peroxisomes are dynamic cytoplasmic structures whose morphology, size, number, and function adapt to the tissue specificity as well as internal and external stimuli such as experimental focal cerebral ischemia or pharmacological induction.[24] The peroxisome transcriptional control is quite complex and not fully understood yet. For example, in yeast, peroxisomes are able to import folded proteins or peptides, which may also enhance the cell's antioxidant capacity. Successful trafficking of human proteins into the peroxisomes may serve an important therapeutic function in diverse clinical disorders that are associated with production of injurious reactive oxygen species (ROS).[25] Peroxisomes also share machinery and interact with mitochondria in particular, which appear to be secondarily affected in various human peroxisomal disorders.[26–30]

The peroxin 11 (PEX11) family controls peroxisome proliferation and regulates morphology, size, and number by participating in the elongation process. However, regulators of the following constriction stage are still unknown. To undergo fission, peroxisomes need machinery, which includes dynamin-like proteins (DNM1L), a GTPase that is anchored to the peroxisome through FIS1 (fission factor 1) and MFF (mitochondrial fission factor) (Fig. 11.1). While the MFF-DNM1L complex promotes mitochondrial and peroxisomal fission, MIEF1 and MIEF2 (mitochondrial elongation factors 1 and 2, also known as MiD49 and 51) proteins may sequester DNM1L, thus inhibiting its function and promoting mitochondrial fusion.[31]

11.1.4 PEROXISOME INHERITANCE

The subcellular transmission and distribution of peroxisomes from parent to daughter cells (inheritance) is another fascinating biological process, which will likely have an impact on our understanding of the role(s) of peroxisomes in health and disease. It is becoming evident that a number of factors, yet to be fully elucidated, are needed for the peroxisomes to be efficiently and equitably transmitted through successive generations of mitosis. These factors are generally classified into three groups: motors, tethers, and receptors, which the organelles need for transport, retention, and attachment, respectively. Several transport motor, tethers, and connector (receptor) proteins necessary for peroxisome inheritance in yeast have been identified,[32–34] although similar proteins have not, as yet, been identified in mammals. Examples of proteins involved in peroxisome inheritance include Myo2p, Inp1, and Inp2. These proteins play a role in moving the peroxisome along the microtubule cytoskeleton and across the cytoplasm.[35] It is likely that proteins from the dynein and kinesin families are also important in intracellular movement and distribution into daughter cells, therefore regulating their metabolic efficiency.[34,36]

11.1.5 TRANSCRIPTIONAL REGULATION

Peroxisome biogenesis requires the involvement of a regulatory network, some members of which had been identified including the "fatty-acid-mediated" oleate-activated transcription factor 1 and peroxisome induction pathway 2 (Oaf1/Pip2) and peroxisome proliferator-activated receptors/retinoid acid receptors (PPAR/RAR) heterodimers, which function as asymmetric positive feedback loops (upregulation impacts the expression of only one member of the heterodimer pair).[37] The network also includes alcohol dehydrogenase regulator 1 (Adr1), a negative regulator of Oaf1/Pip2 dimer.

In addition, the regulation of peroxisome proliferation and function in response to various stimuli also involves both PPAR-dependent as well as PPAR-independent mechanisms such as protein phosphorylation.[29] PPARs are a three-member (PPARA, PPARB, and PPARG also referred to as PPARα, PPARβ/δ, and PPARγ, respectively) nuclear receptor protein that belong to the nuclear hormone receptor superfamily and have tissue-specific expression pattern and also vary in the responses they mediate. All PPARs heterodimerize with the retinoid X receptor (RXR) and bind to their specific DNA response elements (PPREs/PPAR response elements) that have a consensus sequence (AGGTCAC TGGTCA), a direct repeat of hexamer half-sites interspaced by a single nucleotide, which is generally located in the 5′ region of target genes. PPREs have been identified in various human enzymes of the peroxisomal β-oxidation pathway such as acyl-CoA oxidase 1 (ACOX1), the bifunctional enzymes (D and L-bifunctional enzymes), and 3-ketoacyl-CoA thiolases (SCP2, ACAA1) as well as apolipoprotein A1.[38–40]

PPARα is the best studied among the three PPARs, and in humans, PPARα plays a role in the regulation of lipid and glucose homeostasis and inflammatory responses. It responds to stimulation by fibrates, hypoxia, glucocorticoid (GC) pathway, as well as sterol regulatory element binding protein (SREBP) among others. PPARB and PPARG are less well studied and have been implicated in different biological processes. Stimulation of PPARG by rosiglitazone results in peroxisome proliferation and increases in levels of the antioxidant, catalase. PPARA stimulation is not associated with the same response, suggesting that catalase upregulation is mediated by PPARG specific response elements. In humans, mutations/variants in *PPARG* have been linked to several metabolic disorders including carotid intimal medial thickness 1 (MIM 609338), severe (digenic) insulin resistance (MIM 604367), autosomal dominant type 3 familial partial lipodystrophy (MIM 604367), both autosomal recessive and dominant forms of severe obesity (MIM 601665), and type 2 diabetes mellitus (MIM 125853). In mice, cardiomyocyte-restricted *PPARD* deletion caused lipotoxic hypertrophic cardiomyopathy although a similar phenotype has not yet been described in humans.[41] PPARD has also been implicated in vascular homeostasis[42] suggesting a potential role for PPARD in the treatment of atherosclerosis. More recently, variants in PPARD have been implicated in the pathogenesis and progression of colorectal cancer.[43]

Other PPAR-independent inducers of peroxisome proliferation include PPARγ coactivator-1α (PGC1-α), mechanistic target of rapamycin (mTOR) as well as kinases and phosphatases involved in peroxisome biogenesis and metabolism.[44]

11.1.6 PEROXISOMES AND THE IMMUNE RESPONSE

Peroxisomes are also linked to the immune response. Upon intracellular invasion by a pathogen, an innate immune response is mounted via RIG-I (retinoic acid-inducible gene I)-like receptors (RLRs), which induce the expression of various interferon-stimulated genes (ISGs).[45] Both peroxisomes and mitochondria carry the mitochondrial antiviral signaling protein (MAVS). If targeted only to peroxisomes, a transient innate immune response is produced. Targeting only to the mitochondrion produces a sustained type 1 interferon-like response. Cooperative signaling of peroxisomes and mitochondria results in a maximal immune response.[46] Rotavirus, influenza, and human immune deficiency (HIV1) viruses exploit peroxisomes and their metabolic machinery during intracellular replication in human cells,[47] a process that is mediated by peroxisome-targeting signals demonstrable in several viral proteins.[48,49] Either PTS1 or PTS2 signals have been detected in various viral proteins suggesting that viruses may exploit or modify, at least in part, some of the wide variety of the peroxisome functions ranging from cholesterol or lipid metabolism to toxin degradation.

11.1.7 PEROXISOMES AND CANCER

Based on the observation that cancer cells of various origins had high levels of alkyl ether lipids, aberrant lipid metabolism has become an established hallmark of cancer cells.[50–52] This phenomenon correlates with the somatic overexpression of the critical peroxisomal ether lipid biosynthetic enzyme, alkylglyceronephosphate synthase (AGPS) in various tumors,[53,54] an effect that is probably mediated by generating procarcinogenic structural and signaling lipids.[55–58]

11.2 PEROXISOMAL METABOLISM

VLCFAs (Fig. 11.2) are metabolized primarily in the peroxisomes and require transport into the matrix for activation, followed by α- or β-oxidation (Fig. 11.3). Plasmalogen (Fig. 11.4) and bile acids biosynthesis are the other main peroxisomal biochemical processes.

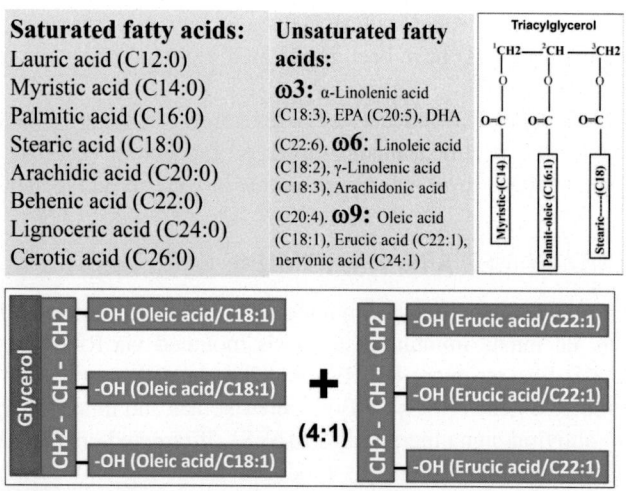

FIGURE 11.2

Common lipids and their structures. In most naturally occurring unsaturated fatty acids, double bonds are cis. Triacylglycerols have a glycerol backbone with either similar fatty acids (simple type) or three different fatty acids (mixed type). Lorenzo's oil is a (4:1) glyceryl trioleate (GTO) and glyceryl trierucate (GTE) mixture.

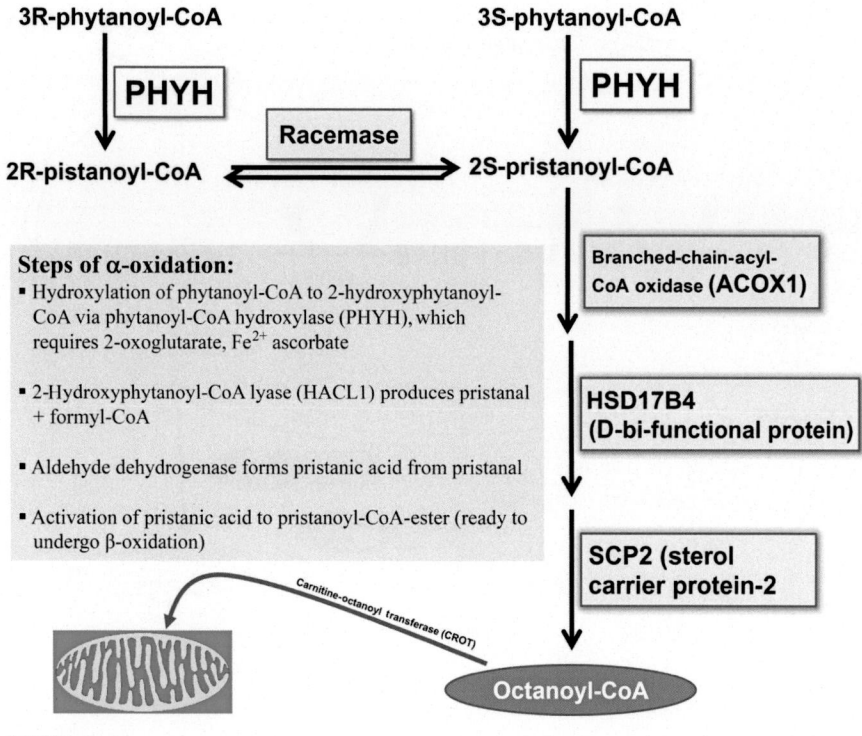

FIGURE 11.3

Peroxisomal branched-chain fatty acids α- and β-oxidation. Phytanic acid, being a 3-methyl-branched (C20) fatty acid first undergoes α-oxidation before entering the β-oxidation pathway. In addition to VLCFAs, peroxisomal fatty acids β-oxidation also handles monounsaturated (MUFA), polyunsaturated fatty acids (PUFA) and their derivatives (eicosanoids and docosanoids), 2-methyl branched-chain fatty acids, and dicarboxylic acids.

11.2.1 ABCD TRANSPORTERS

There are three known peroxisomal ATP-binding cassette (ABC) half-transporters: adrenoleukodystrophy protein (ALDP encoded by *ABCD1*), adrenoleukodystrophy-related protein (ALDRP, encoded by *ABCD2*), and 70-kDa PMP (PMP70, encoded by *ABCD3*) and PMP70-related protein (P70R, encoded by *ABCD4*), that are essential for the transport of various substrates needed for peroxisomal metabolism. Each transporter has a different substrate preference. ALDP preferentially transports straight chain VLCFAs, ALDRP preferentially transports unsaturated VLCFAs and PMP70 preferentially transports branched-chain fatty acids, dicarboxylic acids (DCA), and bile acid precursors.[59–61] Mutations causing human disease have been identified only in *ABCD1* and cause X-linked adrenoleukodystrophy (X-ALD: MIM 300100), the most common peroxisomal disorder and most commonly inherited leukodystrophy. Knockout (KO) mouse models for *Abcd1*,[62–64] *Abcd2*,[65] and *Abcd3*[64–68] had been generated.

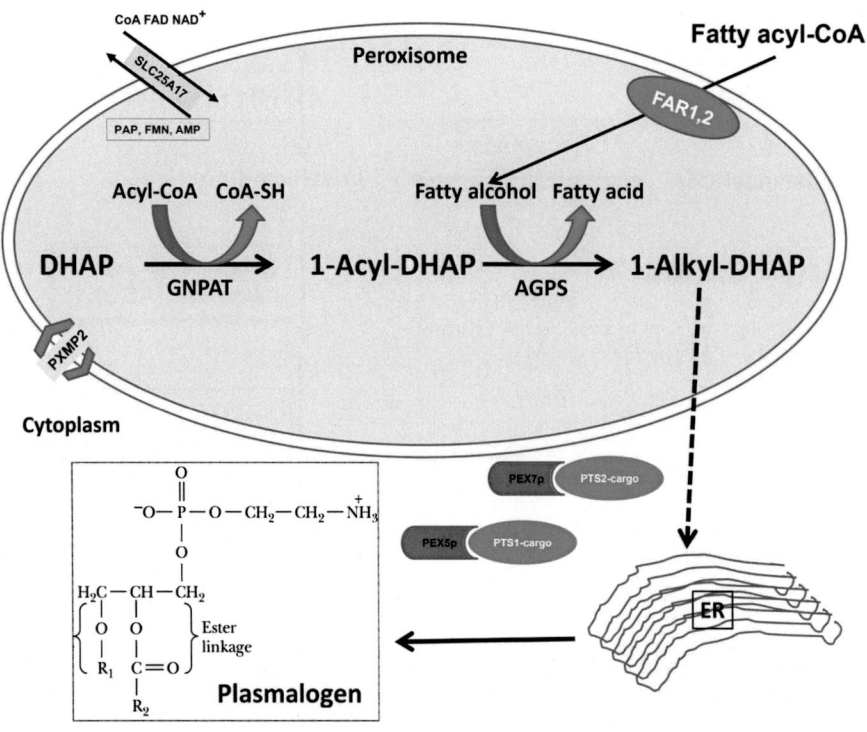

FIGURE 11.4

Peroxisomal plasmalogen biosynthesis. Only the first two steps in plasmalogen synthesis occur in the peroxisome. Fatty acyl-CoAs are converted to corresponding fatty alcohols using the membrane enzymes FAR1 and 2, a process needed to ensure proper synthesis of plasmalogens. Mutations in *GNPAT*, *AGPS*, and *FAR1* are responsible for RCDP types 2, 3, and 4, respectively, with type 4 being the mildest. PXMP2 is the only peroxisome membrane channel (of unknown function) and SLC25A17 is the only transporter described so far.

11.2.2 FATTY ACYL-CoA SYNTHETASES (ACSs), THIOESTERASES (ACOTs), AND ACYLTRANSFERASES

Acyl-CoA synthetases (ACSs) are enzymes required for activation of fatty acids in the peroxisomes in order for α- and β-oxidation to proceed, several of which (ACSL4, SLC27A2, and SLC27A4) reside in the peroxisomes.[69–71] Only two human acyl-CoA thioesterases (ACOT4 and ACOT8 important in α- and β-oxidation of fatty acyl-CoAs, DCA, bile acid-CoAs, and methyl branched-CoAs to free fatty acid + CoA) and one human acyltransferase (peroxisomal bile acid-CoA:amino acid N-acyltransferase, BAAT, necessary for amidation of bile acid-CoAs and acyl-CoAs to amino acids) have been described.[69] Succinyl-CoA, glutaryl-CoA, and long-chain acyl-CoAs are the substrates for human ACOT4 while medium- and long-chain acyl-CoAs are substrates for ACOT8. Control of cellular levels of acyl-CoA:CoA:fatty acid depends on the relative activities of the ACSs and ACOTs.

11.2.3 PEROXISOMAL FATTY ACID α- AND β-OXIDATION

Human peroxisomes contain complex biochemical machinery responsible for the biosynthesis and metabolism of bile acids, docosahexaneoic acids, and ether phospholipids (plasmalogens). Also, through their α- and β-oxidation capabilities (Fig. 11.3), they catabolize a variety of fatty acids such as long chain, very long chain, and 3-methyl-branched fatty acids, as well as eicosanoids including prostaglandins, thromboxanes, and leukotrienes. They also detoxify hydrogen peroxide, glyoxylate, and certain xenobiotics. Since phytanic acid is a 3-methyl branched chain fatty acid that cannot be processed via peroxisomal β-oxidation, it is first oxidized to a 2-methyl compound via peroxisomal α-oxidation, which allows its entry into the β-oxidation pathway.[72–75] Peroxisomal enzyme activities are altered during pathophysiological conditions through various endogenously produced biomolecules such as nitric oxide (NO) that is produced by cytokines or NO-donors. NO modulates peroxisomal functions through cyclic guanosine monophosphate (cGMP); however, L-carnitine prevents these effects in skin fibroblasts.[76]

Similar to the mitochondrial β-oxidation, the four steps of the cyclical peroxisomal fatty acid oxidation (oxidation, hydration, dehydrogenation, and thiolytic cleavage) start with the activation of VLCFAs, bile acids, and DCA to their corresponding acyl-CoA followed by transport into the peroxisome via ALDP. ACOX1 (acyl-CoA oxidase 1) is the first and rate-limiting enzyme in the peroxisomal fatty acid beta-oxidation that produces hydrogen peroxide. HSD17B4, also known as D-bifunctional protein (DBP), or multifunctional protein-2 (MFP2), uses very long chain acyl-CoAs, branched-chain acyl-CoAs including pristanoyl-CoA, and bile acid precursors as substrates and has both hydratase and dehydrogenase activities (D-3-hydroxyacyl-CoA dehydratase/D-3-hydroxyacyl-CoA dehydrogenase bifunctional protein), which it needs for the next two steps, respectively.[77–79] In fibroblasts, the DBP (HSD17B4) is more abundant and more active than L-bifunctional protein (EHHADH, **E**noyl-CoA **H**ydratase/3-**H**ydroxy**A**cyl-CoA **DH**ydrogenase).[80] ACAA (acetyl-coenzyme A acyltransferase) and SCP2 (sterol carrier protein-2) are two peroxisomal thiolases that cause the release of acetyl-CoA. After multiple rounds of β-oxidation, fatty acids are reduced to octanoyl-CoA, which is then transported into the mitochondria via carnitine octanoyl transferase (CROT) for complete oxidation. While no humans with mutations in *CROT* had been described so far, leukoencephalopathy with dystonia and motor neuropathy had been demonstrated in a patient with a homozygous mutation in *SCP2* (see disorders of peroxisomal β-oxidation below). Accumulation of branched-chain pristanic acid in plasma and abnormal bile urinary alcohol glucuronides were demonstrated.

The *EHHADH* gene encodes the peroxisomal L-bifunctional protein and is expressed in the proximal renal tubule. Some of the earlier patients thought to have

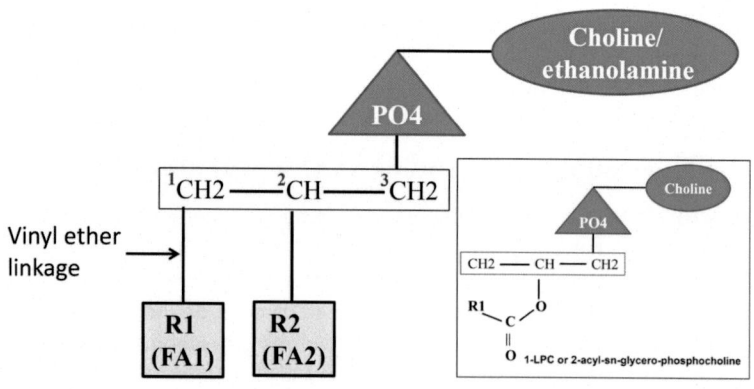

FIGURE 11.5

Plasmalogen structure. Ether glycerophospholipids (also known as plasmalogens) have ether (platelet activating factors, PAF) or vinyl-ether (plasmalogens) bond at the sn-1 position of glycerol linking it with an aliphatic group (R1/FA1) such as C16:0 (palmitic acid), C18:0 (stearic acid), or C18:1 (oleic acid). The sn-2 position is occupied by polyunsaturated fatty acids (PUFAs) while the head group is usually of the ethanolamine or choline type. 1-LPC (inset) also known as 1-lysophosphatidylcholine, also known as 2-acyl-sn-glycero-3-phosphocholine.

deficient EHHADH were reclassified as DBP-deficient individuals.[81] EHHADH deficiency has been recently linked with Fanconi renal tubular syndrome type 3 (see below).

11.2.4 PEROXISOMAL FATTY ACYL-CoA REDUCTASES 1, 2 (FAR1, 2)

The conversion of fatty acids to fatty alcohols is required for the synthesis of ether lipids (plasmalogens) and wax monoesters. In 2004, Cheng and Russell isolated and characterized two mammalian peroxisomal fatty acyl-CoA reductases (FAR1 and 2), which reduce fatty acids to fatty alcohols (Fig. 11.4). The two FARs have different fatty acid substrate preferences and differential tissue expression profiles. As these two enzymes lack transmembrane domains and lack any recognizable PTS motif, it is still not clear whether they are integral membrane proteins or just tightly bound to the phospholipid bilayer of the peroxisome.[82]

11.2.5 BIOSYNTHESIS OF PLASMALOGENS (ETHER PHOSPHOLIPIDS)

Ether phospholipids represent a special class of phospholipids in which the glycerol backbone has an ether or vinyl-ether bond at the sn-1 position (Fig. 11.5), of which the vinyl-ethers constitute a class of ether phospholipids called plasmalogens. Found in major organs (brain, heart, kidney), brain myelin has a high content of phosphatidylethanolamine while myocardium contains phosphatidylcholine. Biosynthesis of plasmalogens starts with dihydroxyacetone phosphate (DHAP), a product of glycolysis, which is used to form the glycerol backbone of the plasmalogen (Fig. 11.4). This biosynthetic pathway starts in the peroxisome utilizing the first two peroxisomal enzymes, "Dihydroxyacetone phosphate acyltransferase/*GNPAT*; Alkyl dihydroxyacetone phosphate synthase/*AGPS* then Acyl/alkyl dihydroxyacetone reductase," and ends in the ER with the formation of 1-alkenyl-2-acyl-glycerophosphocholine.[83–85] The flavoenzyme alkyl dihydroxyacetone phosphate synthase (ADHAPS) carries out the critical step of formation of the vinyl ether bond through an intermediate imino compound.[86] While the exact function of plasmalogens is still not fully understood, they are considered to be essential for membrane fluidity and their function(s) may vary in different tissues and organs, and in various metabolic processes and developmental stages. They are essential for the normal development of major organs (heart, kidney, brain, lung, liver) and their deficiency causes major malformations of these organs as exemplified by the patients with peroxisomal biogenesis disorders (PBDs) and rhizomelic chondrodysplasia punctate (RCDP).[87] In addition, they appear to be important in postnatal life as their secondary deficiency is linked to various age-related diseases.

11.2.6 BILE ACIDS BIOSYNTHESIS

Di- and tri-hydroxycholestanoic (DHC/THC) acids are C27-bile acid intermediates synthesized from cholesterol in the liver but undergo β-oxidation in the peroxisome mainly via HSD17B4, which results in the production of chenodeoxycholic and cholic acid CoA-esters, respectively, which are then conjugated by BAAT with either taurine or glycine within peroxisomes. DHCA and THCA conjugated taurine- and glycine-esters are then transported out of the peroxisome into the hepatocyte cytosol followed by secretion into bile via ABCB11, the canalicular membrane bile salt export pump.[88]

11.3 PEROXISOMAL DISORDERS PHENOTYPES AND ASSOCIATED BIOCHEMICAL ABNORMALITIES

Given the wide variety of biological and biochemical processes in which peroxisomes are involved and associated severe clinical phenotypes resulting from major peroxisomal disorders such as ZS, it is clear that having normal peroxisomal function is essential for normal cell physiology and overall health of the organism (Fig. 11.6). Over the last few decades, the essential role of peroxisomes in health and increasing number of clinical disorders resulting from peroxisomal dysfunction had been elucidated. In Table 11.1, all currently known peroxisomal genes and associated genetic disorders are listed.

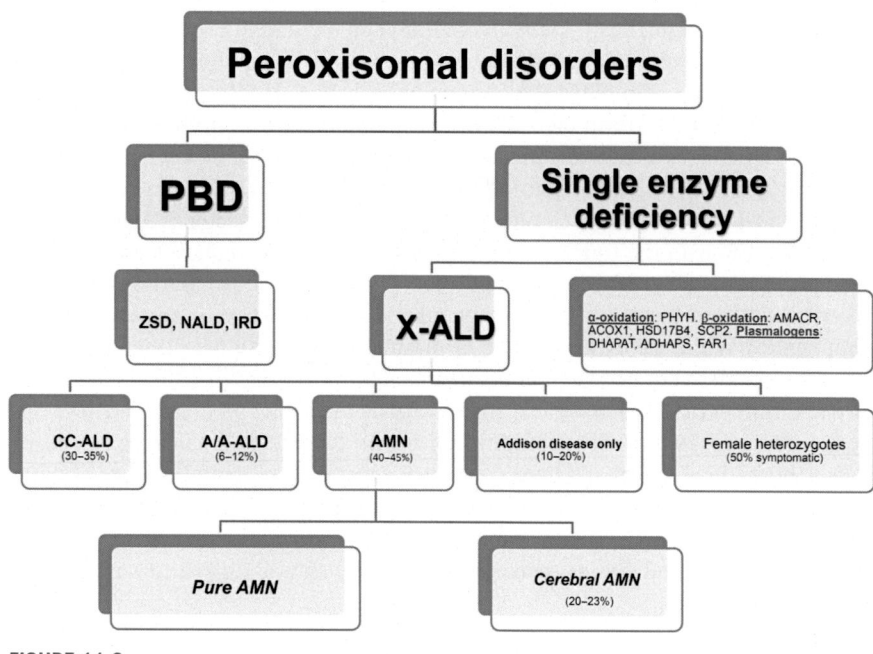

FIGURE 11.6

Clinical classification of peroxisomal disorders. Peroxisomal biogenesis disorders (PBDs) and single enzyme deficiencies represent the two main groups of peroxisomal disorders. Abbreviations: *PBD*, Peroxisome biogenesis disorder; *ZSD*, Zellweger spectrum disorder; *NALD*, Neonatal adrenoleukodystrophy; *IRD*, Infantile Refsum disease; *cc-ALD*, Childhood cerebral adrenoleukodystrophy; *A-ALD*, Adult adrenoleukodystrophy; *AMN*, Adrenomyeloneuropathy.

11.3.1 PEROXISOME BIOGENESIS DISORDERS

Peroxisomal disorders are generally divided into (1) peroxisome biogenesis disorders (PBDs) and (2) peroxisomal single enzyme deficiencies. ZS, the prototype of PBDs, was first described in 1964.[89] Typically, affected children present with multiple major health problems including severe neurological abnormalities (hypotonia, developmental delay, typical facial dysmorphism, epilepsy), skeletal abnormalities (rhizomelia, abnormal calcification), and hepatic dysfunction (hepatomegaly, abnormal liver function). In addition to classical ZS, milder forms of ZS are collectively referred to as Zellweger spectrum disorders (ZSD) and include neonatal adrenoleukodystrophy (NALD), and infantile Refsum disease (IRD). In such patients, peroxisome function is disrupted due to mutations in one of the many peroxins (*PEX*) whose proper expression is required for normal peroxisome biogenesis. ZSD results from mutations in any of the currently known 15 different PEX genes. The early studies of Moser and coworkers in 1982 delineated the important role of peroxisomes in fatty

Table 11.1 Human Peroxisomal Genes and Related Peroxisomal Disorders

Peroxisome Function	Peroxin (%)*	Genome Position (GRCh38/hg38)	Disorder Phenotype and Complementation Group
Peroxisome biogenesis disorders			
Peroxisomal membrane proteins (PMP)	PEX3 (<1%)	chr6q24.2:143450781-143490614 (NM_003630)	ZS (PBD 10A), (MIM 614882)
	PEX16 (<1)	chr11p11.2:45,909,669-45,918,123 (isoform 1: NM_004813; isoform 2: NM_057174)	ZS (PBD 8A & 8B), (MIM 614876 & 614877)
	PEX19 (<1)	chr1q23.2:160276809-160285151 (NR_036493), 3 isoforms	ZS (PBD 12A), (MIM 614886)
Docking peroxins	PEX13 (<1)	chr2p15:61017677-61051990 (NM_002618)	ZS, NALD* (PBD 11A & 11B), (MIM 614883, 614885)
	PEX14	chr1p36.22:10474946-10630761 (NM_004565)	ZS (PBD 13A), (MIM 614887)
Peroxisome importome	PEX2 (3)	chr8q21.13:76980258-77000288 (NM_000318)	ZS, IRD* (PBD 5A & 5B), (MIM 614866, 614867)
	PEX10 (3)	chr1p36.32:2404802-2412571 (NM_153818), isoforms 1,2	ZS, NALD (PBD 6A & 6B), (MIM 614870, 614871)
	PEX12 (5)	chr17:35574795-35578637 (NM_000286)	ZS, NALD, IRD (PBD 3A & 3B), (MIM 614859, 266510)
RING peroxins	PEX1 (70)	chr7q21.2:92487023-92528531 (NM_000466), isoforms 1,2,3	ZS (PBD 1A, MIM# 214100), NALD/ IRD (PBD 1B, MIM 601539); Heimler syndrome 1 (MIM 234580)
	PEX6 (10)	chr6p21.1:42963873-42979243 (NR_133009), isoforms 1,2	ZS (PBD 4A, (MIM 614862), NALD (PBD 4B, (MIM 614863), Heimler syndrome 2 (HMLR2, MIM 616617)
	PEX26 (26)	chr22q11.21:18077920-18091031 (NM_017929), isoforms a,b	ZS (PBD 7A, (MIM 614872), NALD/IRD (PBD 7B, MIM 614873)

(Continued)

Table 11.1 Human Peroxisomal Genes and Related Peroxisomal Disorders (Continued)

Peroxisome Function	Peroxin (%)[◆]	Genome Position (GRCh38/hg38)	Disorder Phenotype and Complementation Group
Proliferation and fission peroxins	PEX11A/α	chr15q26.1:89681531-89690784 (NM_003847), isoforms 1,2,3	None
	PEX11B/β	chr1q21.1:145911348-145918458 (NR_073493), isoforms 1,2	ZS (PBD 14B, (MIM 614920)
	PEX11G/γ	chr19p13.2:7476870-7489038 (NM_080662), isoforms 1,2,3	None
	FIS1	chr7q22.1:101239612-101245090 (NM_016068)	None
	MFF	chr2q36.3:227325151-227357836 (NR_102266), isoforms a–g	Mitochondrial encephalomyopathy (MIM 614785)
	DNM1L (Dlp1)	chr12p11.21:32679200-32745650 (NM_012062), isoforms 1–7	Lethal encephalopahty, lethal, due to defective mitochondrial peroxisomal fission/EMPF (MIM 614388)
	GDAP1	chr8q21.11:74350383-74367100 (NR_046346), isoforms a,b	CMT4A (MIM 214400), CMTIA (MIM 608340), CMT2K (MIM 607831), CMT + vocal cord paresis (MIM 607706)
Peroxisomal targeting			
PTS1-linked signaling	PEX5 (<2)	chr12p13.31:7189686-7211483 (NM_001131023), isoforms a–e	ZS (PBD 2A, MIM 214110), NALD (PBD 2B, MIM 202370), RCDP5 (MIM 202370)
	PEX5L	chr3q26.33:179899537-179921899 (NR_110061), isoforms 1–8	None
PTS2-linked signaling	PEX7	chr6q23.3:136822564-136913934 (NM_000288)	RCDP1 (PBD 9, MIM 215100)

Peroxisome VLCFA transporters

VLCFA transporters	ABCD1	chrXq28:153724868-153744762 (NM_000033)	X-ALD, X-AMN (ALDP, MIM 300100)
	ABCD2	chr12q12:39551220-39620041 (NM_005164)	None (ALDRP)
	ABCD3	chr1p21.3:94418377-94518663 (NM_002858), isoforms a,b	Bile acid synthesis defect, congenital, 5 (PMP70, MIM 616278)
	ABCD4	chr14q24.3:74285277-74303064 (NM_005050)	Methylmalonic aciduria and homocystinuria, cblJ type (P70R, MIM 614857)

Peroxisome matrix proteins

Peroxisomal α-oxidation	PHYH	chr10p13:13277796-13300130 (NM_006214), isoforms: a,b	Refsum disease (MIM 266500)
	HACL1	chr3p25.1:15560704-15601852 (NR_104315), isoforms a-d	None
	AMACR	chr5p13.2:33986986-34008115 (NM_014324), isoforms 1,2,3	Alpha-methylacyl-CoA racemase deficiency (MIM 614307); Bile acid synthesis defect, congenital, 4 (MIM 214950)
Peroxisomal β-oxidation	ACOX1	chr17q25.1:75941511-75979434 (NM_004035), isoforms a,b,c	Peroxisomal acyl-CoA oxidase deficiency (MIM 264470)
	HSD17B4	chr5q23.1:119452497-119542335 (NM_001199291), isoforms 1-5	D-Bifunctional protein deficiency (MIM 261515); Perrault syndrome 1 (MIM 233400)
	EHHADH	chr3q27.2:185190624-185254098 (NM_001966), isoforms 1,2	"Autosomal dominant" Fanconi renotubular syndrome 3 (L-Bifunctional protein deficiency, MIM 615605)
	ACAA1	chr3p22.2:38122710-38137242 (NR_024024), isoforms a,b	None (Peroxisomal 3-oxoacyl-CoA thiolase, Acetyl-CoA Acyl transferase)

(Continued)

Table 11.1 Human Peroxisomal Genes and Related Peroxisomal Disorders (Continued)

Peroxisome Function	Peroxin (%)[a]	Genome Position (GRCh38/hg38)	Disorder Phenotype and Complementation Group
Peroxisomal glyoxalate cycle	AGXT	chr2q37.3:240868745-240879119 (NM_000030)	Hyperoxaluria, primary, type 1 (MIM 259900)
D-amino acid oxidation	DOA	chr12q24.11:108,880,030-108,901,043 (NM_001917)	Schizophrenia
	DDO	chr6q21:110392180-110415550 (NM_003649), isoforms a,b	None
	HAO1	chr20p12.3:7882984-7940446 (NM_017545)	None
	HAO2	chr1p12:119368776-119394130 (NM_016527)	None
Antioxidants	EPHX2	chr8p21.2:27491002-27544922 (NM_001979), isoforms a,b,c	Hypercholesterolemia, familial, due to LDLR defect, modifier of (MIM 132811)
	GSTK1	chr7q34:143263429-143269129 (NM_015917)	None
	CAT	chr11p13:34,439,014-34,471,433 (NM_001752)	Acatalasemia (MIM 614097)
	PRDX1	chr1p34.1:45511035-45522890 (NM_001202431)	None
	PRDX5	chr11q13.1:64318088-64321823 (NM_012094)	None
	SOD1	chr21q22.11:31659622-31668930 (NM_000454)	Amyotrophic lateral sclerosis 1 /ALS1 (MIM 105400)
	SOD2	chr6q25.3:159679116-159693321 (NM_001024465)	Microvascular complications of diabetes 6 (MIM 612634)
L-lysine metabolism	PIPOX	chr17q11.2:29042900-29057218 (NM_016518)	None

Purine metabolism	XDH	chr2p23.1:31334322-31414745 (NM_000379)	Xanthinuria, type I (MIM 278300)
Polyamine metabolism	PAOX	chr10q26.3:133379237-133391696 (NM_152911)	None
Retinoid metabolism	DHRS4	chr14q11.2:23953735-23969281 (NM_021004), isoforms 1–6	None
Proteases	LONP2	chr16q12.1:48244167-48353979 (NM_031490), isoforms 1,2	None
	IDE	chr10q23.33:92451684-92574095 (NM_004969), isoforms 1,2	None

Plasmalogen deficiency-related defects

Plasmalogens synthesis	PEX7	chr6q23.3:136822564-136913934 (NM_000288)	RCDP1 (PBD9, MIM 215100)
	GNPAT	chr1q42.2:231241173-231277973 (NM_014236), isoforms a,b	RCDP2 (MIM 222765)
	AGPS	chr2q31.2:177392743-177543836 (NM_003659)	RCDP3 (MIM 600121)
	FAR1	chr11p15.3:13,668,670-13,732,346 (NM_032228)	RCDP4 (MIM 616107)
	PEX5	chr12p13.31:7189686-7211483 (NM_001131023), isoforms a–e	RCDP5 (MIM 202370)
	FAR2	chr12p11.22:29149003-29335616 (NM_001271783), isoforms 1,2	None

(Continued)

Table 11.1 Human Peroxisomal Genes and Related Peroxisomal Disorders (Continued)

Peroxisome Function	Peroxin (%)♠	Genome Position (GRCh38/hg38)	Disorder Phenotype and Complementation Group
Peroxisomal acyl-CoA thioesterases (ACOTs)			
Acyl-CoA thioesterases	ACOT4	chr14q24.3:73591706-73595766 (NM_152331)	Substrates: succinyl-CoA, glutaryl-CoA, long-chain acyl-CoAs
	ACOT6	chr14q24.3:73616844-73619888, (uc001xop.3)	Substrates: phytanoyl-CoA, pristanoyl-CoA
	ACOT8	chr20q13.12:45841721-45857409 (NM_005469)	Substrates: medium- and long-chain acyl-CoAs
	ACOT12	chr5q14.1:81330128-81394169 - (NM_130767)	Substrates: short-chain acyl-CoAs
Peroxisomal acyl-CoA acyltransfearses			
	BAAT	chr9q31.1:101360417-101385005 (NM_001701)	Substrates: bile acid-CoAs, long- and very long-chain acyl-CoAs
Peroxisomal acyl-CoA synthetases (fatty acid+ ATP→fatty acyl-AMP+ PPi)			
Peroxisomal acyl-CoA synthetases	ACSL4	chrXq23:109641335-109733392 (NM_004458), isoforms 1,2	Mental retardation, X-linked 63 (MIM 300387)
	ACSS1	chr20p11.21:25006230-25058182 (NM_032501), isoforms 1–4	None
	ACSS2	chr20q11.22:34876525-34927966 (NM_018677), isoforms 1–3	None
	SLC27A1	chr19p13.11:17470444-17506168 (NM_198580)	None (long-chain fatty acid transport protein 1)
	SLC27A2	chr15:50182196-50236392 (NM_003645), isoforms 1,2	None (very long chain fatty acyl-CoA ligase/transporter 2)

	Gene	Location	Disease/Function
	SLC27A3	chr1q21.3:153775292-153780157 (NM_024330), isoforms 1,2	None (very long chain fatty acyl-CoA ligase/transporter 3)
	SLC27A4	chr9q34.11:128340560-128361470 (NM_005094)	Ichthyosis prematurity syndrome; Insulin resistance syndrome (MIM# 604194)
	SLC27A5	chr19q13.43:58498333-58512065 (NM_012254)	None (bile acyl-CoA synthetase; very long chain fatty acyl-CoA ligase/ transporter 5)
	SLC27A6	chr5q23.3:128965517-129033642 (NM_014031)	None (very long chain fatty acyl-CoA ligase/transporter 6)
	ACSF2	chr17q21.33:50468329-50474845 (NR_110232), isoforms 1-5	None
	ACSF3	chr16q24.3:89136548-89155846 (NR_045667), isoforms 1,2	Combined malonic and methylmalonic aciduria, (MIM 614265)
	AASDH	chr4q12:56338285-56387508 (NM_181806), isofroms 1-6	none
Peroxisomal membrane transporters, channels	MPV17L	chr16p13.11:15,395,779-15,408,439 (NM_001128423)	Murine nephrotic syndrome
	PXMP2	chr12q24.33:132687606-132704991 (NM_018663)	None (membrane channel)
	SLC25A17	chr22q13.2:40789630-40819399 (NR_104235), isoforms 1-3	None (Co-A and adenine nucleotide transporter)
	PXMP4	chr20q11.22:33702744-33720330 (NM_007238), isoforms a,b	None (prostate carcinogenesis via silencing by hypermethylation)
	TRIM37	chr17q22:58998200-59106905 (NM_015294) E3 ubiquitin-protein ligase	Mulibrey nanism (autosomal recessive)
	MLYCD	chr16q23.3:83899125-83916182 (NM_012213)	Malonic aciduria

(Continued)

Table 11.1 Human Peroxisomal Genes and Related Peroxisomal Disorders   (Continued)

Peroxisome Function		Peroxin (%)♣	Genome Position (GRCh38/hg38)	Disorder Phenotype and Complementation Group
Peroxisome quality check systems	Ubiquitination	UBE2D1 (UbcH5)	chr10q21.1:58334979-58370753 (NM_003338), isoforms 1,2	None; ubiquitin-conjugating enzymes: E2(Pex4,22); E3(Pex2,10,12)
	Dislocation	ZFAND6	chr15q25.1:80059568-80138393 (NM_019006), isoforms a-d	none
	Deubiquitination	USP9X	chrX:41085635-41236579 (NM_001039590), isoforms 3,4 ??	None
		Ubp15p		
	Lon protease	LONP1 (Lon)	chr19p13.3:5691834-5720165 (NR_076392), isoforms1-3	CODAS syndrome (MIM 600373)
	Pexophagy	SQSTM1 (P62)	chr5q35.3:179820842-179838077 (NM_003900), isoform 1,2	Autosomal dominant frontotemporal dementia and/or amyotrophic lateral sclerosis 3 (MIM 616437), and Paget disease of bone 3 (MIM 167250)
		Atg30	Unknown	
		Atg36	Unknown	

Abbreviations: AASDH, Aminoadipate-semialdehyde dehydrogenase; ABCD1, ATP-binding cassette, subfamily D, member 1; ACAA1, Acetyl-CoA acyltransferase 1; ACOT1, Acyl-CoA thioesterase 1; ACOTs, Acyl-CoA thioesterases; ACOX1, Acyl-CoA oxidase 1, Palmitoyl; ACSBG1, Acyl-CoA synthetase bubblegum family member 1; ACSF2, Acyl-CoA synthetase family member 2; ACSF3, Acyl-CoA synthetase family member 3; ACSL1, Acyl-CoA synthetase long-chain family, member 1; ACSS1, Acyl-CoA synthetase short-chain family, member 1; AGPS, Alkyldihydroxyacetonephosphate synthase; AGXT, Alanine-glyoxylate aminotransferase; AMACR, Alpha-methyl-acyl-CoA racemase; CPP, Cell penetrating peptide; CROT: Carnitine octanoyltransferase; CODAS, Cerebral, ocular, dental, auricular, and skeletal; DHAP-AT, Dihydroxyacetonephosphate acyltransferase; DLP1, Dynamin1-like; EH-HADH, Enoyl-CoA hydratase/3-Hydroxyacyl-CoA dehydrogenase; FAR1, Fatty acyl-CoA reductase 1; GNPAT, Glyceronephosphate O-acyltransferase; HACL1, 2-Hydroxyacyl-CoA lyase 1; HSD17B4, 17-Betahydroxysteroid dehydrogenase IV; IDH1: Isocitrate dehydrogenase 1; IRD, Infantile Refsum disease; KANL, Lysine-alanine-asparagine-leucine; MFF, Mitochondrial fusion factor; MIEF1& MIEF2, Mitochondrial elongation factor 1 & 2; Mulibrey nanism, Autosomal recessive muscle-liver-brain-eye nanism, severe growth failure of perinatal onset, dysmorphism, pericardial constriction, and hepatomegaly; NALD, Neonatal adrenoleukodystrophy; NLS, Nuclear localization signal; PBD, Peroxisomal biogenesis disorder, PEX, Peroxin; PH1: Primary hyperoxaluria type 1; PHYH, Phytanoyl-CoA hydroxylase; PMP, Peroxisome membrane protein; PTS1 (or 2), Peroxisomal targeting signal type 1 (or 2); RCDP, Rhizomelic chondrodysplasia punctata; RING, Really interesting new gene; ROS, Reactive oxygen species; SCP2, Sterol carrier protein 2; SKL, Serine-lysine-leucine; SLC27A2, Solute carrier family 27 (fatty acid transporter), member 2; ZS, Zellweger syndrome.

#Human peroxisomes contain at least two ACOTs (ACOT4 and ACOT8) and one bile acid-CoA:amino acid N-acyltransferase (BAAT). *ACOTs (acyl-CoA thioesterase enzymes) catalyze the hydrolysis of acyl-CoAs (short-, medium-, long-, and very long-chain), bile acid-CoAs, and methyl branched-CoAs, to the free fatty acid and coenzyme A. **Acyltransferase enzymes, which are structurally and functionally related to ACOTs, conjugate (or amidate) bile acid-CoAs and acyl-CoAs to amino acids, resulting in the production of amidated bile acids and fatty acids. ♣ Frequency of peroxin mutations were taken from Steinberg et al. (2006).

ABCD2 encodes ALD-related protein (ALDRP), ABCD3 (PMP70), and ABCD4 (PMP70-related protein, which is located in the endoplasmic reticulum). Zellweger spectrum disorder include: ZS (related peroxins: PEX1, 2, 3, 5, 6, 10, 12, 13, 14, 16, 19, 26), NALD (related peroxins: PEX1, 3, 5, 6, 10, 12, 13), and IRD (related peroxins: PEX1, 2, 5, 6, 10, 12).

acid β-oxidation[90,91] and the discovery that plasmalogens deficiency in patients with ZS by Heymans et al.[92] in 1983 identified the critical roles of peroxisomes in plasmalogen (etherphospholipid) biosynthesis. Also, the essential role of peroxisomes in fatty acid α-oxidation was confirmed by the identification of significantly elevated phytanic acid levels in patients with ZS.[93]

Tissues of patients with PBDs usually show morphologically aberrant peroxisomes called peroxisomal ghosts. In addition, large peroxisomes as well as different horseshoe-shaped membrane structures were also demonstrated in fibroblasts from patients with peroxisomal β-oxidation defects.[94] Accumulation of VLCFAs and phytanic acid and deficient plasmalogens are the biochemical hallmark of PBD.

11.3.2 X-LINKED ADRENOLEUKODYSTROPHY

Both X-linked adrenoleukodystrophy (X-ALD, MIM 300100) and X-linked adrenomyeloneuropathy (X-AMN) are clinically, radiographically, and biochemically well-recognized neurometabolic syndromes, which are caused by mutations in the X-linked VLCFA transporter (*ABCD1*) gene that encodes ALDP protein.[95] Probably as many as 19% of boys affected with X-ALD have de novo mutations in the *ABCD1* gene,[96] which maps to human chromosome Xq28 and has many intragenic mutations in addition to very few microdeletions (see below) involving neighboring genes. A 9.7 kb segment encompassing exons 7–10 of the *ABCD1* gene has duplicated to specific locations near the pericentromeric regions of human chromosomes 2p11, 10p11, 16p11, and 22q11 creating multiple copies of pseudogenes, which may complicate mutation detection by DNA-sequencing methods.[97]

Both X-ALD and X-AMN phenotype can coexist in the same family, a phenomenon known as variable expressivity. The biochemical hallmarks of X-ALD and X-AMN are the significant elevation of saturated VLCFA (C22:0, C24:0, C26:0) in various body fluids and tissues in association with varying degrees of malfunction of the adrenal cortex and nervous system myelin, which distiguish these clinical phenotypes. Unlike the (infantile) autosomal recessive form of adrenoleukodystrophy that phenotypically and biochemically overlaps with ZS, patients with X-ALD have normal physical appearance, as well as growth and development for the first few years of life until the onset of symptoms between four and eight years of age. Also, they have normal phytanic acid and plasmalogen levels.

X-ALD is the most common peroxisomal disorder and inherited leukodystrophy with an estimated panethnic incidence of 1:20,000 and 1:30,000 males.[95] There are several distinct clinical phenotypes (Fig. 11.6). The progressive neurodegenerative acute childhood cerebral demyelinating inflammatory form (ccX-ALD) is the most severe with onset between four and eight years of age. Early in the course of the disease, affected boys present with nonspecific health concerns including learning problems, attention deficit that then progress to loss of speech, cognitive decline, ataxia, seizures, hearing and vision loss, and ultimately to a vegetative state within a few years. The majority (90%) of these boys develop adrenal insufficiency (Addison disease) as well. ccX-ALD accounts for ~35% of all cases of X-ALD. Another 35–40% of affected males are diagnosed with AMN as they present as young adults with stiffness, clumsiness, and slowly progressive paraparesis with sphincter disturbances. Approximately two-third of affected individuals develop adrenal insufficiency. At least 40–50% of AMN patients will demonstrate cerebral white matter lesions in T1 and T2 magnetic resonance (MR) images (cerebral AMN) and approximately 25% will follow a rapidly progressive neurodegenerative course similar to ccX-ALD. The rest of patients with AMN will continue to have the pure "uncomplicated" form without cerebral involvement.[98]

Other less common phenotypes include isolated adrenal insufficiency (Addison disease), adult-onset olivopontocerebellar degeneration syndrome and asymptomatic males. X-ALD carrier females are also at risk of developing mild neurologic deficits, which are present in about 50%, although symptomatic adrenal insufficiency is less likely to develop. While it is well established that more than one phenotype attributed to X-ALD can be seen in the same family, the exact genetic or environmental determinants of this phenotypic heterogeneity and lack of genotype–phenotype correlation are still unknown. However, in one study comparing patients with various forms of X-ALD (cc-ALD vs ac-ALD vs AMN), the c.776C> G variant of *TCN2* (transcobalamin 2) was identified as a risk factor for cerebral demyelination suggesting a possible role for methionine metabolism.[99] In addition, the *SOD2* (hypoactive) variant C47T (Ala16Val) may contribute to the development of cerebral demyelination in adolescent and adult X-ALD patients but not in those with childhood cerebral X-ALD.[100] Astrocytes and microglial cells from brain lesions of affected patients demonstrate increased expression of pro-inflammatory cytokines (IL-1, TNF-a) and intercellular adhesion molecules (ICAMs). Also, inducible nitric oxide synthase (iNOS) was demonstrated in the active edge of demyelinating plaques.[101]

Based on the cumulative evidence from the literature, Singh and Pujol proposed a three-hit model for the pathogenesis of X-ALD with oxidative stress being the initial requirement, which then triggers neuroinflammation (second hit) leading to cell death and demyelination via generalized peroxisomal dysfunction (third hit).[102,103] However, it should be noted that most lesions in human AMN (similar to an ALD KO mouse phenotype) and ALD, are noninflammatory with microglia being the dominant cell type. The myeloneuropathy of AMN is a central-peripheral distal (dying-back) axonopathy, perhaps caused by the perturbation of the membrane's microenvironment secondary to incorporation of VLCFA—gangliosides.[104] In addition to affecting the microglia, VLCFAs disrupt mitochondrial structure and function in *Abcd1*(-/-) oligodendrocytes and astrocytes albeit to a lesser extent.[105,106] It is still not clear mechanistically how the elevated levels of VLCFAs cause or contribute to the pathology seen in X-ALD since accumulation of VLCFA, per se, did not cause mitochondrial abnormalities (in skeletal muscle, brain, and isolated mitochondria, and skin fibroblasts) and mitochondrial abnormalities themselves do not cause the accumulation of VLCFA in X-ALD mice.[107] Nevertheless, there is evidence from different studies that there is secondary mitochondrial dysfunction using multiple approaches including transcriptomics, which revealed a common signature that is triggered by VLCFA increase and characterized by aberrations in oxidative phosphorylation, adipokine, and insulin signaling pathways.[108]

Oxidative stress is the hallmark not only of X-ALD, but also a number of other neurodegenerative diseases. Antioxidants were able to reverse the bioenergetic failure, together with the axonal degeneration and locomotor impairment displayed by *Abcd1* null mice, observations that may have therapeutic implications.[109–111]

11.3.3 CONTIGUOUS ABCD1/DXS1375E DELETION SYNDROME (CADDS)

Contiguous ABCD1/DXS1375E deletion syndrome (CADDS, MIM 300475) is a very rare X-linked contiguous gene microdeletion syndrome (Fig. 11.7) that spans three genes [centromere-*SLC2A8-BCAP31/DXS1375E-ABCD1*-telomere at Xq28]. Since the initial report by Corzo et al.[112] in 2002, a handful of additional patients have been described (recently reviewed by Calhoun and Raymond).[113–116] Each of the genes within the deleted segment can be mutated individually causing a clinically overlapping neurometabolic syndrome; however, the combined deletion of the three genes in this region is associated with a more severe phenotype. Deficiency of SLC6A8 causes cerebral creatine deficiency (MIM 300352), which is characterized by microcephaly, facial dysmorphism, neonatal hypotonia, developmental delay, severe speech delay, seizures, dystonia, and spasticity,[117] while the hallmarks of deficiency of the multifunction protein BCAP31 are deafness, dystonia, and hypomyelination with cerebral and cerebellar atrophy.[118] Hemizygous boys born with this microdeletion have severe neonatal hypotonia, growth and mental retardation, liver failure, and die early in life. They also have cerebral creatine deficiency and markedly elevated VLCFA levels. In some cases, the microdeletion can be maternally inherited, which is an extremely important issue for genetic counseling in these families.

11.3.4 ABCD2 DEFICIENCY

Although no human patients had been yet identified with ABCD2 deficiency, it is interesting to note the mouse phenotype that causes damage to the mitochondria, Golgi, and ER, and manifests clinically as late-onset cerebellar and sensory axonal ataxia, with loss of cerebellar Purkinje cells and dorsal root ganglia.[65]

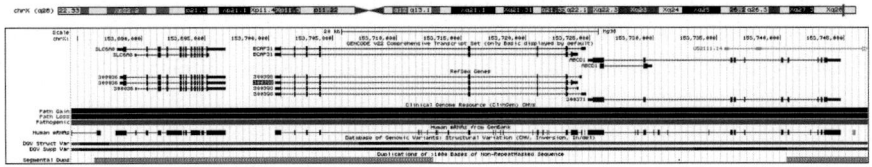

FIGURE 11.7

Schematic diagram showing the genomic region, which is deleted in patients with CADDS (Contiguous ABCD1/DXS1375E (BCAP31) deletion syndrome), and which maps to human chromosome Xq28 and includes *SLC6A8*, *BCAP31*, and *ABCD1* (cent-telo).

11.3.5 ABCD3 DEFICIENCY "A NOVEL BILE ACID BIOSYNTHESIS DISORDER"

In 2014, Ferdinandusse et al. reported the only patient with ABCD3 deficiency caused by a homozygous truncating mutation in *ABCD3*. A 4-year-old Turkish girl with normal growth and development presented with jaundice, hepatosplenomegaly, and anemia, which progressed to liver cirrhosis, portal hypertension, hepatopulmonary syndrome, and pancytopenia, secondary to hypersplenism. She died five days after undergoing liver transplantation. Laboratory studies showed elevated C27-bile acids (DHCA, THCA), C29-DCA (dicarboxylic acids), low C22:0, low but not deficient erythrocyte and fibroblast plasmalogens. Skin fibroblasts C26:0 VLCFA and pristanic acid oxidation was reduced while other peroxisomal β-oxidation enzyme activities were normal. Morphologically, there were reduced numbers of enlarged import-competent peroxisomes. Premortem liver biopsy showed cholestasis with portal–portal and portal–central fibrosis as well as pericellular fibrosis throughout the liver parenchyma.[67]

11.3.6 DISORDERS OF PEROXISOMAL FATTY ACID α-OXIDATION

11.3.6.1 Refsum disease

Refsum disease (MIM # 266500) was first described as a distinct clinical entity by Sigvald Refsum in 1946 with the hallmarks of the disorder being retinitis pigmentosa, cerebellar ataxia, polyneuropathy, and elevated cerebrospinal fluid protein level despite normal cell count. Skeletal malformations, such as shortening of the metacarpals and metatarsals, ichthyosis, sensorineural hearing loss, and anosmia are less common. In patients with Refsum disease, the clinical phenotype results from the accumulation of phytanic acid (C20:0 branched-chain fatty acid) in various body fluids and tissues as a result of recessive mutations in phytanoyl-CoA hydroxylase (*PHYH*), which is the first enzyme responsible for the peroxisomal α-oxidation (Fig. 11.3). Other biochemical markers of peroxisomal function including VLCFA levels are normal.[73,119]

In humans, phytanic acid is not synthesized de novo and rich dietary sources including meat, dairy products, fish, and ruminant fats are the exclusive source of this branched-chain fatty acid. As a result, restricting dietary intake of phytanic acid in patients with Refsum disease reduces and even normalizes their blood levels and is associated with improvement in disease-related symptoms such as the skin and electrocardiogram (ECG) abnormalities. Plasmapheresis is another therapeutic modality, which when combined with dietary measures results in more rapid and significant control of phytanic acid levels.[120]

11.3.7 DISORDERS OF PEROXISOMAL FATTY ACID β-OXIDATION

Four enzyme deficiencies are known to be responsible for peroxisomal fatty acid β-oxidation: 2-methylacyl-CoA racemase deficiency (AMACR, MIM 604489);

acyl-CoA oxidase deficiency (ACOX1, MIM 264470); DBP deficiency (HSD17B4, MIM 261515); and peroxisomal thiolase deficiency (sterol carrier protein 2, SCP2, MIM 184755).

11.3.7.1 2-Methylacyl-CoA racemase (AMACR) deficiency

AMACR deficiency was first reported by Freddendause et al. in two adults with late-onset axonal sensorimotor peripheral neuropathy, retinitis pigmentosa–like abnormalities, primary hypogonadism, and epilepsy.[121] Since then, this adult-onset, neurodegenerative phenotype has been expanded to include recurrent encephalopathy, demyelinating sensorimotor polyneuropathy, migraine, spasticity, and deep white matter abnormalities on brain magnetic resonance imaging (MRI). So far, only six cases had been reported in the literature and pristanic acid–restricted diet may be beneficial in some patients with this rare inborn error of metabolism.[122]

11.3.7.2 Acyl-CoA oxidase (ACOX1) deficiency

ACOX1 is the first enzyme in peroxisomal fatty acid β-oxidation. Unlike ACOX2 and ACOX3 (which are branched-chain and pristanoyl oxidases), ACOX1 is a straight chain peroxisomal oxidase. Autosomal recessive ACOX1 deficiency was first reported by Poll-The et al.[123] The clinical manifestations are similar to those of PBD. Owing to the clinical overlap with NALD, pseudo-neonatal adrenoleukodystrophy was initially used in ACOX1-deficient patients as a clinical diagnosis but has since been abandoned.

11.3.7.3 HSD17B4 (D-bifunctional protein) deficiency

While three biochemical phenotypes of autosomal recessive DBP deficiency had been identified (type I: combined hydratase and dehydrogenase deficiency; type II: isolated hydratase deficiency; type III: isolated dehydrogenase deficiency), the resulting clinical phenotypes (infantile-onset hypotonia, seizures, dysmorphic facial features, and death in early infancy) are clinically indistinguishable and show significant overlap with those of PBD.[124,125] In addition, autosomal recessive mutations in *HSD17B4* had been identified in some patients with Perrault syndrome, a molecularly heterogeneous neuro-endocrine disorder with variable expressivity. It is characterized by ovarian dysgenesis in females, sensorineural deafness in both males and females, and in some patients, neurological manifestations.[126] Cardinal endocrine features also include growth retardation, amenorrhea with low estradiol and elevated gonadotropin levels, and infertility. Additional neurological manifestations of Perrault syndrome include nystagmus, limited extraocular movements, cognitive impairment, ataxic gait, spastic diplegia, dysarthria, sensorimotor demyelinating or axonal peripheral neuropathy causing hypo/areflexia, and cerebellar atrophy (in some patients).

11.3.7.4 EHHADH (L-bifunctional protein) deficiency

Fanconi renotubular syndrome (FRTS) is a clinically and molecularly heterogeneous disorder that manifests as renal solute and water losses due to defective reabsorption in the proximal renal tubule. Biochemically, varying degrees of generalized amino aciduria, phosphaturia, glycosuria, and hypophosphatemic rickets or osteomalacia are detected. Clinical symptoms include polyuria, polydipsia, dehydration, and rickets. Mutations in FRTS1 (unknown gene), *SLC34A1* (FRTS2), *HNF4A* (FRTS4, with maturity-onset diabetes of the young), and most recently in *EHHADH* (FRTS3) cause the various clinical forms of FRTS. FRTS types 1, 3, and 4 are dominantly inherited while type 2 results from recessive mutations. The recently reported dominant negative mutation in *EHHADH* causes mistargeting of this peroxisomal enzyme to the mitochondria resulting in impaired oxidative phosphorylation and defects in the transport of fluids and a glucose analogue across the renal tubular epithelium, while *EHHADH* KO mice showed no abnormalities in their renal tubular cells.[127]

11.3.7.5 Peroxisomal thiolase deficiency

Two peroxisomal enzymes (AAC1 and SCP2) have thiolase activity and SCP2 is responsible for the breakdown of branched-chain fatty acids. Deficiency in the SCP2 only, but not AAC1, has been reported in two brothers.[128] The neurometabolic phenotype consists of early adulthood-onset dystonic head tremor and spasmodic torticollis, hypergonadotropic hypogonadism with azoospermia, hyposmia, and bilateral hyperintense signals involving the thalamus, pons, basal ganglia, and occipital region on MRI imaging. Plasma pristanic acid as well as urinary bile alcohol glucuronides are elevated.

11.3.8 DISORDERS OF ETHER PHOSPHOLIPID (PLASMALOGEN) BIOSYNTHESIS

Plasmalogens constitute 20% of total body phospholipid mass and are essential for normal prenatal development of fetal organs. They also appear to be important in adult life as they have been found to be deficient in various age-related diseases.[84] Classically, disorders of plasmalogen biosynthesis (Fig. 11.4) have been associated with the clinical syndrome RCDP, a neurometabolic multiple congenital anomalies syndrome characterized by prominent shortening of the proximal long bones of upper and lower extremities (rhizomelia), congenital contractures, short stature and even dwarfism, radiological skeletal abnormalities (metaphyseal cupping, abnormal ossification of long bones along with epiphyseal and extra-epiphyseal calcifications), ocular abnormalities (congenital cataract), and variable neurological deficits (spasticity and mental retardation).[129] Most RCDP patients have recessive mutations in the *PEX7* gene (RCDP1), which encodes the PTS2-receptor. PTS2 is essential for the correct targeting of a small group of proteins to the peroxisome. Both Alkyl-DHAP synthase (the second enzyme in the plasmalogen biosynthesis pathway) and phytanoyl-CoA hydroxylase are PTS2 proteins whose deficiency in RCDP1 patients explains the deficiency of plasmalogens and elevation of phytanic acid levels known to be present in these patients.[93] The enzymes, DHAPAT (dihydroxyacetone phosphate acyl-transferase) encoded by *GNPAT* (glycerone phosphate acyltransferase) and alkyl-DHAP synthase (ADHAPS) encoded by *AGPS* catalyze the first and second peroxisomal steps of plasmalogen synthesis, respectively. Deficiency of DHAPAT was first recognized in 1992 and it causes RCDP2[130] while deficiency of ADHAPS was identified in 1994 and it causes RCDP3.[131] More recently, two additional types of RCDP (4 and 5) caused by mutations in *FAR1* and *PEX5* (long isoform), respectively, have been described.

Buchert et al.[132] described three patients in two unrelated Syrian families with a novel and milder peroxisomal plasmalogen deficiency disorder characterized by severe intellectual disability, spasticity, epilepsy, congenital cataracts, microcephaly, and mild nonspecific facial dysmorphism, but without the characteristic rhizomelia or skeletal abnormalities that are typical of RCDP. Through exome sequencing and autozygosity mapping, two causative autosomal recessive mutations in *FAR1* (fatty acyl-CoA reductase 1) were identified. FAR1 and 2 reduce fatty acids to fatty alcohols used in the synthesis of plasmalogens.

In 2015, Barøy et al. described the newest form of RCDP (type 5), which they identified in four patients from two independent RCDP families of Pakistani origin. A homozygous recessive homozygous frame shift mutation in *PEX5L* (long isoform) segregated with the clinical phenotype. This novel mutation selectively caused loss of function of PEX5L, which specifically disrupts the import of PTS2-tagged proteins, thus causing RCDP instead of ZSD. Plasmalogen levels are also reduced. Clinically, affected individuals have congenital cataract, microcephaly, epilepsy, severe mental retardation, mild rhizomelia, short stature, demeyelinating motor and sensory peripheral neuropathy of upper and lower limbs, as well as radiographic features of RCDP.[133]

11.3.9 PRIMARY HYPEROXALURIA

In humans, three forms of primary hyperoxaluria exist, primary hyperoxaluria type 1 (PH1, MIM 259900), primary hyperoxaluria type 2 (PH2, MIM 260000) and primary hyperoxaluria type 3 (PH3, MIM 613616) with type 1 being more common while PH2 is less severe and less likely to cause renal failure. In patients with PH1, there is progressive renal deposition of calcium oxalate (CaOx) as urolithiasis and/or nephrocalcinosis that ultimately leads to renal failure.[134] On the other hand, systemic oxalosis results from progressive deposition of CaOx throughout the body in association with the progressive decline in renal function. PH1 results from inactivating recessive mutations in the liver-specific peroxisomal enzyme alanine:glyoxylate transferase (AGXT), which result in a biochemical profile characterized by hyperoxaluria and hyperglycolic aciduria. PH2 differs from PH1 in that there is combined hyperoxaluria with hyper-L-glyceric aciduria. A unique subset of patients with PH1 with high residual enzyme activity (within the heterozygous range) caused by *AGXT* mutations that results in mistargeting of AGXT to the mitochondria instead of the peroxisome matrix have been recognized. Normally, AGXT is targeted into the peroxisome via its PTS1 signal. However, through certain *AGXT* polymorphisms coupled with certain mutations, the mitochondrial sequence is enhanced causing mistargeting into the mitochondria. Other mutation classes affecting AGXT include intraperoxisomal aggregation, absence of catalytic activity, and combined absence of catalytic activity and immunoreactivity.[134] PH2 is caused by recessive mutations in glyoxylate reductase/hydroxypyruvate reductase (*GRHPR*), which is a cytosolic enzyme. In patients with PH3, homozygous or compound heterozygous mutations in *HOGA1* (4-hydroxy-2-oxoglutarate aldolase 1) have been identified. Liver transplantation or combined hepatorenal transplantation is considered the definitive treatment for patients with PH1. The combined hepatorenal transplantation approach is more advantageous as it replaces the biochemically defective organ as well as the pathophysiologically damaged and compromised kidney, which may ultimately lead to resolution of the effects of systemic oxalosis.[135,136]

11.3.10 ACATALASEMIA AND HYPOCATALASEMIA

Catalase is the main peroxisomal antioxidant that catalyzes the decomposition of hydrogen peroxide to oxygen and water. Acatalasemia or acatalasia is an inborn error of metabolism characterized by total or near total loss of catalase activity in erythrocytes, which appears to be the main regulator of both intracellular and extracellular hydrogen peroxide concentration. Catalase deficiency is also sometimes referred to as Takahara disease in recognition of the astute Japanese physician who recognized this diagnosis clinically when he observed in these patients the lack of bubble (oxygen) formation after rinsing an oral surgery site with hydrogen peroxide and the development of gum gangrene.[137]

The catalase gene (*CAT*) is closely linked to human WAGR (Wilms tumor, Aniridia, Genitourinary anomalies, and mental Retardation) locus on chromosome 11p13. A few patients with combined catalase deficiency and WAGR complex caused by heterozygous microdeletion involving this genomic region have been reported.[138]

Humans with hereditary acatalasemia/hypocatalasemia appear to have an increased risk of developing age-related diseases including diabetes, atherosclerosis, and cancer.[139] Their skin fibroblasts accumulate hydrogen peroxide and harbor signs of age-associated aberrant behaviors involving peroxisome protein import, growth and division, and ROS processing.[140] Similarly, acatalasemic mice have fewer pancreatic β-cells compared to normocatalasemic mice, along with accelerated severe atrophy and apoptosis resulting in faster development and higher frequency of diabetes mellitus. Such mice also have greater risk of developing different renal pathologies including renal and peritoneal fibrosis,[141,142] and adriamycin nephropathy.[143]

In most individuals with catalase deficiency, no mutation in the *CAT* gene has been identified suggesting genetic heterogeneity, epigenetic, or environmental causes as a possible explanation. Human (inherited or acquired) catalase deficiency may predispose to methemoglobinemia and hemolysis in patients receiving uric acid oxidase (rasburicase) therapy,[144] and most (85.1%) have one of the more common age-related chronic disorders such as senile graying of hair, diabetes mellitus, oral gangrene, schizophrenia, vitiligo, Parkinson's disease, arteriosclerosis, and hypertension.[145] However, catalase itself may be targeted by damaging oxidative stress leading to decreased enzyme activity and accumulation of hydrogen peroxide.[146]

11.3.11 MEVALONIC ACIDURIA

Isopentenyl pyrophosphate (IPP) and dimethylallyl pyrophosphate (DMAPP) are the building blocks for a diverse group of biomolecules (heme, cholesterol, vitamin K, CoQ10, steroids) whose synthesis starts with acetyl-CoA via the mevalonate kinase pathway (isoprenoid pathway or HMG-CoA reductase pathway).[147] The mevalonate kinase gene (*MVK*) encodes an ATP:mevalonate 5-phosphotransferase that is localized to the peroxisome. Mevalonic acid is synthesized from 3-hydroxy-3-methylglutaryl-CoA (HMG-CoA), a reaction catalyzed by HMG-CoA reductase, and is converted to mevalonate-5-phosphate by mevalonate kinase (ATP:mevalonate phosphotransferase).

Mutations in *MVK* have been found to be responsible for three clinically diverse human disorders: autosomal recessive hyper-IgD (immunoglobulin D) syndrome (MIM 260920), autosomal recessive mevalonic aciduria (MIM 610377), and autosomal dominant type 3 (Porokeratosis 3, MIM 175900). Patients with autosomal recessive mevalonic aciduria present with severe failure to thrive, recurrent febrile crises that decrease with age, developmental delay, anemia, hepatosplenomegaly, central cataracts, dysmorphic features, elevated serum IgD level, cerebral and cerebellar atrophy.[148] Patients with isolated autosomal recessive hyper-IgD syndrome present with recurrent and periodic febrile attacks, arthritis/arthralgia, and various vision abnormalities. The neurological deficits seen in patients with hyper-IgD syndrome are much less pronounced. Finally, porokeratosis is a clinically and molecularly heterogeneous genodermatosis characterized by annular, anhidrotic keratotic lesions located predominantly on sun-exposed areas and nail dystrophy in some patients.

11.3.12 DISORDERS OF PEROXISOMAL (AND MITOCHONDRIAL) PROLIFERATION/FISSION

MFF is a member of a protein complex (DNM1L and FIS1) that promotes mitochondrial and peroxisome fission. Using autozygosity mapping and exome sequencing in patients with mitochondrial encephalomyopathy, Shamseldin et al. identified a homozygous recessive truncating mutation in two affected Saudi Arabian brothers with consanguineous parents. Both mitochondria and peroxisomes had abnormal tubular morphology indicating failure of fission.[149]

11.3.13 PIPECOLIC ACIDEMIA

Human L-pipecolate oxidase (PIPOX, MIM 616713) is a peroxisomal enzyme that is responsible for the degradation of pipecolic acid, a product of L-lysine catabolism. PIPOX also degrades sarcosine but with a preference for L-pipecolic acid. Using various RNA expression techniques, PIPOX appears to be expressed in multiple tissues but translated in kidney and liver only and colocalizes with catalase in the peroxisomes in a punctate fashion.[150] Unlike secondary pipecolic acidemia due to PBD, isolated pipecolic acidemia is not linked directly to PIPOX deficiency.[151]

11.3.14 PEROXISOMAL MOSAICISM IN PEROXISOMAL DISORDERS

Peroxisomal mosaicism is a rare phenomenon that had been demonstrated in a few patients with PBD in whom clearly peroxisome deficient and competent cells coexisted, thus potentially causing diagnostic difficulties. Two types of peroxisomal mosaicism, type 1 and 2, have been recognized. Either one or both types may coexist in the same individual. In type 1, the biochemical profiles in body fluids and cultured fibroblasts are incongruent as fibroblasts demonstrate normal peroxisomal activity. The mechanism behind this phenomenon is not completely understood. In type 2, the mosaicism manifests in peroxisome morphology or ability to import matrix proteins in cultured or fixed tissue despite (seemingly) similar genotype.[152–154] In these patients with varying mosaicism, it would be potentially helpful to reassess their genotypes (mutation load) in DNA samples from various tissues using NGS (next generation sequencing), which may reveal true tissue-specific, postzygotic mosaicism, and explain this phenomenon.

11.4 LABORATORY DIAGNOSIS OF PEROXISOMAL DISORDERS

Various laboratory studies are available to help in confirming the diagnosis of peroxisomal disorders. The most commonly used studies with a reasonable turnaround time include measurement of plasma VLCFA (C22:0, C24:0, C26), phytanic and pristanic acids, plasma plasmalogens, pipecolic acid, and urinary bile acids. Table 11.2 provides the list of most common peroxisomal disorders and the expected associated laboratory abnormalities. Reference ranges for various (peroxisome-related) analytes taken from the literature are shown in Table 11.3.

11.4.1 VERY LONG CHAIN FATTY ACIDS

Elevated plasma and tissue VLCFA levels is the hallmark of almost all peroxisomal disorders especially X-ALD, which is the most common peroxisomal disorder including 85% of obligate heterozygous females for X-ALD. Elevated VLCFA levels can be detected at birth in affected male newborns and continue to be stably elevated throughout childhood and adulthood. They also correlate with the disease severity.[157] It is important to know that most circulating VLCFA and branched-chain fatty acids are mainly present in an esterified form and the free VLCFAs are bound to plasma proteins. VLCFAs are particularly stable especially when stored frozen. However, care is required to avoid sample contamination with waxes or grease as they interfere with the VLCFAs assay, which is quantified using gas chromatography-mass spectrometry (GC-MS) as well as electrospray ionization-tandem mass spectrometry (ESI-MS/MS).[155,156] In addition to plasma, measurement of VLCFA level can be performed in human skin fibroblasts where it is expected to be markedly elevated in patients with PBD but not in patients with RCDP. Elevated pipecolic acid level is another marker of peroxisome dysfunction. However, this occurs only in patients with generalized PBD. Thus the finding of elevated VLCFA and normal pipecolic acid level should point toward a peroxisome single enzyme deficiency.[158] If necessary, it is also possible to measure the phytanic acid (2S and 2R) diastereomers by GC/MS, which will confirm the diagnosis of AMACR (alpha-methylacyl-CoA racemase) deficiency as both isomers will be significantly elevated.[159]

Table 11.2 Laboratory Findings in Patients with Various Types of Peroxisomal Disorders

Phenotype			VLCFA	Phytanic Acid	Plasmalogens	Pipecolic Acid	Bile Acids
PBD/ZSD		ZS	↑↑↑	↑↑↑	↓↓↓	↑↑↑	↑↑↑
		NALD	↑↑	↑↑	↓↓	↑↑	↑↑
		IRD	↑	↑	↓	↑	↑
RCDP		RCDP-classical	Normal	↑↑↑	↓↓↓	↓↓	Normal
		RCDP-mild	Normal	↑↑↑	↓	↓	Normal
VLCFA transport		X-ALD	↑↑↑	Normal	Normal	Normal	Normal
Fatty Acid Oxidation (FAO)	α-FAO	ARD	Normal	↑↑↑	Normal	Normal	Normal
	β-FAO	AMACR deficiency*	Normal	Normal	Normal	Normal	↑↑
		ACOX1 deficiency	↑↑	Normal	Normal	Normal	Normal
		D-Bifunctional protein deficiency*	↑↑	Normal	Normal	Normal	↑
		Peroxisomal thiolase deficiency	↑	Normal	Normal	Normal	Normal

Abbreviations: ACOX1 deficiency, Acyl-CoA oxidase 1 deficiency; AMACR deficiency, Alpha-methylacyl-CoA racemase deficiency; ARD, Adult Refsum disease; IRD, Infantile Refsum disease; NALD, Neonatal adrenoleukodystrophy; PBD, Peroxisomal biogenesis disorder; RCDP, Rhizomelic chondrodysplasia punctata; X-ALD, X-linked adrenoleukodystrophy; ZS, Zellweger syndrome; ZSD, Zellweger syndrome spectrum disorder.
* Increased levels of bile acids intermediates.

Table 11.3 Reference Ranges for Biochemical Studies of Peroxisome Function

VLCFA	KFSHRC (µM)	Mayo♥ (µM)	KGI (Valianpour et al.) (Ref. 155)				Schutgens et al. 1993 (Ref. 156)			
			Normal	Males with X-ALD	X-ALD Female Carriers	Wanders RJ (n = 157 controls, µM)	Controls (109, mg/L)	ZS (n = 54, mg/mL)	X-ALD (n = 41, mg/mL)	RCDP (n = 20, mg/mL)
C22:0	40–119	≤96.3				40–119	25.3 (10.5–51.0)	6.3 (4.4–11.8)	20.8 (11.8–29.5)	18.3 (1.0–30.8)
C24:0	33–84	≤91.4				33–84	17.4 (8.5–35.7)	12.0 (7.7–22.4)	13.7 (7.0–21.1)	17.3 (1.0–27.3)
C26:0	0.45–1.32	≤1.30	0.67 ± 0.13	2.94 ± 0.87	1.54 ± 0.72	0.45–1.32	0.31 (0.11–0.62)	2.90 (1.66–4.45)	1.28 (0.82–1.71)	0.35 (0.02–0.83)
C24:0/C22:0 ratio	<1.2	≤1.39	0.86 ± 0.13	1.52 ± 0.21	1.18 ± 0.15	0.57–0.92	0.73 (0.48–0.89)	1.91 (1.55–2.40)	1.50 (1.18–1.74)	0.85 (0.68–1.03)
C26:0/C22:0 ratio	<0.028	≤0.023	0.01 ± 0.003	0.05 ± 0.02	0.02 ± 0.01	0.01–0.02	0.01 (0.00–0.02)	0.43 (0.25–0.63)	0.06 (0.04–0.09)	0.02 (0.01–0.04)
Pristanic acid	<12.01	0–4 months: ≤ 0.60 µM; ≥24 months: ≤ 2.98 µM	NA	NA	NA	NA	NR			
Phytanic acid	<2.98	0–4 months: ≤ 5.28 µM; ≥24 months: ≤ 9.88 µM	NA	NA	NA	NA	NR			
Pristanic/Phytanic acid ratio	NR	0–4 months: ≤ 0.35; ≥24 months: ≤ 0.39	NA	NA	NA	NA	NR			

KGI Kennedy-Krieger Institute, ♥ Mayo test catalogue (http://www.mayomedicallaboratories.com/test-catalog/, accessed on January 1, 2016), NR/NA not reported/not available.

11.4.2 MEASUREMENT OF PLASMALOGENS AND POLYUNSATURATED FATTY ACIDS

Plasmalogens are essential components of various membranes and structures of high fat content such as myelin and red blood cells (RBC). GC-based simultaneous measurement of dimethylacetals (DMA) and methylesters resulting from the transmethylation (hydrolysis) of plasmalogens and essential fatty acids ester bonds, respectively, is possible. Plasma, RBC, and cultured fibroblasts are used to determine total plasmalogens levels, which are expected to be markedly reduced in patients with PBD as well as most types of rhizomelic chondrodysplasia punctata. The plasmalogen values are not expressed in absolute numbers, rather as a percentage of the level of the corresponding fatty acid. For example, normal ranges ($n=25$ neonates and 15 children) for C16:0 DMA/C16:0 plasmalogens and C18:0 DMA/C18:0 plasmalogens are 6.6–9.4% and 13.5–21.5; 9.4–12.4 and 18.0–24.0%, respectively.[160–162] It should be remembered that normal plasmalogens levels may occur in mildly affected patients and that false-positive results (erroneously low plasmalogens levels) may occur due to incomplete sample transmethylation as well as RBC transfusion.

11.4.3 MEASUREMENT OF PEROXISOMAL ENZYMES ACTIVITY AND COMPLEMENTATION ANALYSIS

While analyte-based assays coupled with the clinical findings often confirm the diagnosis of a peroxisomal disorder, additional investigations including direct measurement of various peroxisomal enzymes usually in fibroblasts coupled with complementation studies and DNA mutation analysis together confirm the specific diagnosis. However, measurement of specific enzymes involved in α-, β-oxidation, or plasmalogen biosynthesis is available only in very few laboratories, is expensive and time- and labor-intensive process.[87,163,164] The advent and increasing implementation of NGS-based gene panels in various clinical molecular genetics laboratories is expected to shorten the time and lower the cost of such investigations. In Table 11.3, the reference ranges for the various peroxisomal biomarkers taken from the literature as well as our laboratory are listed.

Finally, magnetic resonance spectroscopy (MRS) may also be a useful diagnostic tool in patients with peroxisomal disorders. In eight patients with adrenoleukodystrophy (among a group of patients with demyelinating leukodystrophy), a distinctive profile of elevated Cho/NAA (>1.5) and Cho/Cr (>1.4) and reduced NAA/Cr (<1.1) was identified.[165]

11.4.4 NEWBORN SCREENING FOR X-LINKED ADRENOLEUKODYSTROPHY

The aim of newborn screening (NBS) is early identification of children born with clinically significant, treatable, and reversible medical disorders using reliable and cost-effective laboratory detection methods. Developing a simple, fast, cost-effective, and reliable NBS method for X-ALD using a disease-specific biomarker was necessary.[166] 1-Hexacosanoyl-2-lyso-sn-3-glycero-phosphorylcholine (C26:0-LysoPC) was identified as the disease-specific biomarker and efforts to quantify it using mass spectrometry began some years ago.[167–169] Initial reports demonstrated the utility of liquid chromatography-tandem mass spectrometry (LC-MS/MS) with multiple reaction monitoring (MRM) scanning as the method of choice for NBS. Further improvements to the technique were developed and it is now possible to reliably measure VLCFAs (C20, C22, C24, C26-LPCs) using a standard 3 mm dry blood spots (DBS) and a short analytical run of 1.5 minutes per sample by flow injection analysis-tandem mass spectrometry (FIA-MS/MS).[170]

Table 11.4 summarizes the results of the NBS efforts so far. Since C26:0-LysoPC is not specific for X-ALD, finding an elevated C26:0-LysoPC level may be the result of X-AMN, PBD, or peroxisomal single-enzyme deficiency. This is expected to complicate the process of follow-up of the results of NBS and therefore a post screening management protocol and guidelines is necessary to have. Early results from NBS for X-ALD suggest an incidence of 1/17,000 for X-ALD. ALD NBS is accomplished using a three-tier algorithm starting with MS/MS of C26:0, followed by measuring C26:0-LPC using HPLC–MS/MS (second tier). Third-tier testing involves full sequencing of the *ABCD1* gene.[171]

11.5 THERAPIES FOR PEROXISOMAL DISORDERS

The management of patients with complex disorders such as peroxisomal disorders requires the utilization of various therapeutic approaches including general supportive as well as more specific interventions based on the nature of the disorder being managed. General supportive therapies include physical and occupational therapy, ensuring adequate nutrition as well as routine medical care such as timely immunizations, gastrostomy tube feedings, antiepileptic therapy, and attending to intercurrent illnesses. Since patients with X-ALD and X-AMN are at risk of developing Addison disease causing potentially fatal adrenal insufficiency, steroid replacement therapy remains a very effective and essential treatment for these patients. Genetic counseling and providing prenatal and preimplantation genetic diagnosis to affected families are equally important. More specific therapeutic approaches may include dietary restriction of phytanic acid or its removal using plasmapheresis in patients with adult Refsum disease, dietary restriction, and enhanced omega oxidation of VLCFAs, supplementation with DHA, bile acids, plasmalogens in patients with impaired plasmalogen biosynthesis, induction of peroxisome proliferation using PPAR agonists, as well as induction of peroxin activity or bypassing defective peroxins.[172] The observation that orally administered labeled hexacosanoic acid accumulated in the brain of a terminally ill patient with childhood cerebral X-ALD suggested that restriction of oral intake of VLCFAs may result in clinical benefits. However, multiple clinical trials showed that dietary restriction of VLCFA in combination with oral supplementation with Lorenzo's oil (4:1 mixture of glyceryl trioleate (GTO) and glyceryl

Table 11.4 Studies of Newborn Screening for X-ALD

Study	Method	Population	Results	Reference Values	
Hubbard WC et al.[167]	LC-MSMS, MRM analysis of 26:0-lyso-PC with IS (d4-16:0-lyso-PAF)	1000 NBS samples	All were identified correctly except one false-positive case	C26:0 ng/blood spot Normal (n = 19) X-ALD & AMN (n = 25) PBD/ZSD (n = 9)	0.017 ± 0.008 0.170 ± 0.119 1.039 ± 0.661
Haynes CA and De Jesús[168]	Analyte-C26:0-LPC in DBS, 30-min-long run, simple extraction, isocratic (negative mode) HPLC-MS/MS	223 normal DBS, and 28 X-ALD		Normal range of C26:0-LPC: 0.09 ± 0.03 µmol/L whole blood; X-ALD: 1.13 ± 0.67 µmol/L	
Theda C et al.[169]	LC MS/MS, 2 minutes run time per sample, MRM transitions	4689 prospective newborns + 2 controls, 2 X-ALD males, 2 PBD per plate	No false positives	Newborn DBS: 0.36 ± 0.14 pmol/punch X-ALD DBS: 5.12 ± 0.91	
Turgeon CT et al.[170]	Measurement of C20, C22, C24, C26-LPCs using 3 mm DBS, methanol extraction, IS (d4-C26), FIA-MS/MS, SRM mode, 1.5-min run per sample	130 healthy newborn DBS, 20 adults, 16 X-ALD boys, 8 PBD, 12 X-ALD carriers	All were correctly identified. LC-MS/MS can be used a 2nd tier confirmatory test	NB controls X-ALD[a] NB-PBD Adult X-ALD Adult PBD	0.18 (0.12–0.23) 0.54 (0.47–0.67) 1.45 (1.33–1.58) 0.46 (0.28–0.77) 0.85 (0.27–1.07)

AMN adrenomyeloneuropathy; C26:0-LPC ; DBS dry blood spot; FIA-MS/MS flow injection analysis-tandem mass spectrometry; HPLC-MS/MS high pressure liquid chromatography-tandem mass spectrometry; MRM multiple reaction monitoring; NBS newborn screening; PBD peroxisome biogenesis disorder; SRM single reaction monitoring; X-ALD X-linked adrenoleukodystrophy; ZSD Zellweger spectrum disorder.

trierucate (GTE)) normalized plasma VLCFA levels, but did not result in clinical improvement, as it failed to halt the progression of the disease in various groups of patients with childhood cerebral ALD, AMN, and symptomatic heterozygous women. More recently, based on upto 15 years of follow up of asymptomatic boys with the X-ALD, the use of Lorenzo's oil appeared to be associated with reduced risk of developing MRI abnormalities.[173]

Since inflammation is known to be a prominent feature in childhood cerebral ALD, immunosuppressive therapy was also considered as another potentially helpful therapy. However, multiple antiinflammatory and immunosuppressive agents were found to be ineffective.[174] More recently, curative hematopoietic stem cell replacement therapy (HSCT) as well as experimental gene therapy have been performed in patients with cerebral X-ALD.[175] Depending on the severity of the disease process and degree of stem cell engraftment in the recipient's bone marrow and brain, and probably some other unknown factors, the efficacy of this therapeutic approach depends.[176–188] Clinical trials involving transplantation using matched unrelated donor bone marrow as well as umbilical cord blood and their outcomes are summarized in Table 11.5. More recently, autologous bone marrow transplantation after in vitro gene (therapy) correction using transduction with lentiviral vector was shown to be a promising and effective approach in a small number of boys with cerebral-X-ALD.[189,190]

Table 11.5 Clinical Trials and Outcomes of Hematopoietic Stem Cell Therapy (HSCT) and Umbilical Cord Blood Transplantation (UCBT) in Patients with Childhood Cerebral X-ALD

Study	Outcome	Reference
Bone marrow transplantation with hematopoietic stem cells (HSCT)		
1	6-year-old, unrelated donor, developed RPLS at 83 days, brain MRI: signal changes extending more peripherally into the subcortical and cortical regions of the occipital and temporal lobes, RPLS resolved with cessation of CSA.	176
2	126 boys (1982 to 1999; data analysis on 94): 56% survival at 5 and 8 years, 86% engraftment, visual and auditory processing deficits in many, baseline neurologic functional status predicted outcomes, disease progression was the main cause of death.	177
3	3 patients, nonmyeloablative (fludarabine) conditioning, smooth peri-BMT course, fast and stable engraftment. 3–5-year follow-up without neurological deterioration, variable VLCFA levels, MRI abnormalities improved in 1 patient.	178
4	1-year-old patient with early stage ALD, HLA-matched unrelated donor, fast and stable engraftment, plasma VLCFA decreased gradually and MRI changes improved, no neurological deterioration during 22 months follow-up.	179

(Continued)

Table 11.5 Clinical Trials and Outcomes of Hematopoietic Stem Cell Therapy (HSCT) and Umbilical Cord Blood Transplantation (UCBT) in Patients with Childhood Cerebral X-ALD   (Continued)

Study	Outcome	Reference
5	60 boys (2000–2009): median age at HSCT 8.7 years, different conditioning regimens and allograft sources, 78% ($n = 47$) alive at a median 3.7 years, 8% HSCT-related mortality at day 100, posttransplantation neurologic progression correlated with pre-HSCT neurologic status.	180
6	53 patients (1992–2008) with various inherited metabolic disorders, 22 received UCBT, 3 primary graft failures, 5-year overall was 78% for the cohort, and 73% for ALD patients, similar overall survival between unrelated marrow and unrelated cord blood donor groups.	181
Umbilical cord blood transplantation (UCBT)		
7	69 patients (1999–2004) with lysosomal storage and peroxisomal diseases including ($n = 8$) with X-ALD, 72% 1-year survival, 78% neutrophil engraftment by day 42 a median of 25 days, 36% had grade II– IV acute GVHD.	182
8	12 patients including 3 presymptomatic boys (1996–2005), chemotherapy-based myeloablative conditioning, 2 had acute GVHD (grade II–IV) and 2 had extensive chronic GVHD, 66.7% overall survival at 6 months, worse outcome in symptomatic patients.	183
9	6-year-old patient developed severe delayed alloimmune hemolytic anemia, immune-mediated neutropenia and thrombocytopenia, which responded to Campath-1H but not corticosteroids, cyclosporine, intravenous immune globulin, rituximab, and pentostatin.	184
10	2 patients developed EBV-related PTLD with a benign course.	185
11	1 patient with advanced CCALD, reduced-intensity conditioning, stable clinical and radiological course.	186
12	8-year-old boy, reduced-intensity conditioning, 11 months later developed immune-mediated axonopathy (sural nerve proven) due to cGVHD causing progressive walking difficulty and hand clumsiness.	187
13	2 patients received RIC, fast and stable engraftment without any serious complications.	188

Abbreviations: ALD, Adrenoleukodystrophy; BMT, Bone marrow transplantation; CCALD, Childhood cerebral adrenoleukodystrophy; CSA, Cyclosporine A; cGVHD, Chronic graft versus host disease; EBV, Epstein–Barr virus; GVHD, Graft versus host disease; HCST, Hematopoietic stem cell therapy; HLA, Human leukocyte antigen; PTLD, Posttransplant lymphoproliferative disorder; RIC, Reduced induced conditioning; RPLS, Reversible posterior leukoencephalopathy syndrome (headache, lethargy, acute visual loss, and focal seizures); UCBT, Umbilical cord blood transplantation; VLCFAs, Very long chain fatty acids; X-ALD, X-linked adrenoleukodystrophy.

Studies on animal models suggested potential novel therapies that need to be validated by human clinical studies and trials. For example, in the *Abcd1* mouse, oral treatment with pioglitazone, a PGC1α/PPARγ agonist restored mitochondrial bioenergetics and halted locomotor disability and axonal damage.[191] A similar observation was made about sirtuin 1 (SIRT1), which is one of the mitochondria's function master regulators,[192] the antioxidants (N-acetyl-cysteine, α-lipoic acid, and α-tocopherol,[193] valproic acid,[194] and the mTOR inhibitor, temsirolimus, which are able to restore the normal autophagic flux.[195] Restoration of normal or near-normal redox state by providing functioning targeted peroxisomal catalase enzyme replacement therapy might also be of clinical significance to patients with X-ALD.[25]

In addition to gene therapy using the lentiviral vector, which was performed in a couple of patients with ccX-ALD so far, other gene therapy approaches in the *Abcd1* mouse model seem to be promising.[196–198]

Finally, early studies using induced pleuripotent stem cells (iPSCs) derived from ccX-ALD patients' skin fibroblasts demonstrated the great potential this new approach may have toward better understanding of the disease pathogenesis and evaluating the effects of various pharmacological and biological therapeutics.[199–201]

REFERENCES

1. Lodhi IJ, Semenkovich CF. Peroxisomes: a nexus for lipid metabolism and cellular signaling. *Cell Metab* 2014;**19**(3):380–92.
2. Rhodin J. Correlation of ultrastructural organization and function in normal and experimentally changed peroxisomal convoluted tubule cells of the mouse kidney. *Dissertation, Aktiebolaget Godvil, Stockholm* 1954.
3. Vamecq J, Cherkaoui-Malki M, Andreoletti P, et al. The human peroxisome in health and disease: the story of an oddity becoming a vital organelle. *Biochimie* 2014;**98**:4–15.
4. De duve C. Functions of microbodies (peroxisomes). Abstr: Vth Meeting Am Soc Cell Biol. *J Cell Biol* 1965;**27**:25A.
5. Baudhuin P, Beaufay H, De Duve C. Combined biochemical and morphological study of particulate fractions from rat liver. Analysis of preparations enriched in lysosomes or in particles containing urate oxidase, D-amino acid oxidase, and catalase. *J Cell Biol* 1965;**26**(1):219–43.
6. De Duve C, Baudhuin P. Peroxisomes (microbodies and related particles). *Physiol Rev* 1966;**46**(2):323–57.
7. Goldfischer S, Moor CL, Johnson AB, et al. Peroxisomal and mitochondrial defects in cerebrohepatorenal syndrome. *Science* 1973;**182**:62–4.
8. Moser AE, Singh I, Brown FR, et al. The cerebrohepatorenal (Zellweger) syndrome. Increased levels and impaired degradation of very-long-chain fatty acids and their use in prenatal diagnosis. *N Engl J Med* 1984;**310**:1141–6.
9. Shimozawa N, Tsukamoto T, Suzuki Y, et al. A human gene responsible for Zellweger syndrome that affects peroxisome assembly. *Science* 1992;**255**:1132–4.
10. Rokka A, Antonenkov VD, Soininen R, et al. Pxmp2 is a channel-forming protein in Mammalian peroxisomal membrane. *PLoS One* 2009;**4**(4):e5090.
11. Visser WF, van Roermund CW, Waterham HR, et al. Identification of human PMP34 as a peroxisomal ATP transporter. *Biochem Biophys Res Commun* 2002;**299**(3):494–7.

12. Agrimi G, Russo A, Scarcia P, et al. The human gene SLC25A17 encodes a peroxisomal transporter of coenzyme A, FAD and NAD+ . *Biochem J* 2012;**443**(1):241–7.

13. Wanders RJ, Poll-The BT. Role of peroxisomes in human lipid metabolism and its importance for neurological development. *Neurosci Lett* 2015 pii: S0304-3940(15)00461-9.

14. Waterham HR, Ferdinandusse S, Wanders RJ. Human disorders of peroxisome metabolism and biogenesis. *Biochim Biophys Acta* 2015 pii: S0167-4889(15)00399-7.

15. Schlüter A, Fourcade S, Domènech-Estévez E, et al. PeroxisomeDB: a database for the peroxisomal proteome, functional genomics and disease. *Nucleic Acids Res* 2007;**35**(Database issue):D815–22.

16. Lazarow PB. Peroxisome biogenesis: advances and conundrums. *Curr Opin Cell Biol* 2003;**15**(4):489–97.

17. Dimitrov L, Lam SK, Schekman R. The role of the endoplasmic reticulum in peroxisome biogenesis. *Cold Spring Harb Perspect Biol* 2013;**5**(5):a013243.

18. Smith JJ, Aitchison JD. Peroxisomes take shape. *Nat Rev Mol Cell Biol* 2013;**14**:803–17.

19. Hettema EH, Erdmann R, van der Klei I, et al. Evolving models for peroxisome biogenesis. *Curr Opin Cell Biol* 2014;**29**:25–30.

20. Agrawal G, Subramani S. De novo peroxisome biogenesis: evolving concepts and conundrums. *Biochim Biophys Acta* 2015 pii: S0167-4889(15):00307-9.

21. van der Klei IJ, Veenhuis M. PTS1-independent sorting of peroxisomal matrix proteins by Pex5p. *Biochim Biophys Acta* 2006;**1763**(12):1794–800.

22. Ma C, Agrawal G, Subramani S. Peroxisome assembly: matrix and membrane protein biogenesis. *J Cell Biol* 2011;**193**(1):7–16.

23. Fransen M. Peroxisome dynamics: molecular players, mechanisms, and (dys)functions. *ISRN Cell Biol* 2012:24. Article ID 714192.

24. Young JM, Nelson JW, Cheng J, et al. Peroxisomal biogenesis in ischemic brain. *Antioxid Redox Signal* 2015;**22**(2):109–20.

25. Terlecky SR, Koepke JI. Drug delivery to peroxisomes: employing unique trafficking mechanisms to target protein therapeutics. *Adv Drug Deliv Rev* 2007;**59**(8):739–47.

26. Demarquoy J, Le Borgne F. Crosstalk between mitochondria and peroxisomes. *World J Biol Chem* 2015;**6**(4):301–9.

27. Honsho M, Yamashita SI, Fujiki Y. Peroxisome homeostasis: mechanisms of division and selective degradation of peroxisomes in mammals. *Biochim Biophys Acta* 2015 pii: S0167-4889(15)00344-4.

28. Schrader M, Bonekamp NA, Islinger M. Fission and proliferation of peroxisomes. *Biochim Biophys Acta* 2012;**1822**(9):1343–57.

29. Schrader M, Costello JL, Godinho LF, et al. Proliferation and fission of peroxisomes—An update. *Biochim Biophys Acta* 2015 pii: S0167-4889(15)00336-5.

30. Schrader M, Costello J, Godinho LF, et al. Peroxisome-mitochondria interplay and disease. *J Inherit Metab Dis* 2015;**38**(4):681–702.

31. Huber A, Koch J, Kragler F, et al. A subtle interplay between three Pex11 proteins shapes de novo formation and fission of peroxisomes. *Traffic* 2012;**13**(1):157–67.

32. Fagarasanu A, Fagarasanu M, Rachubinski RA. Maintaining peroxisome populations: a story of division and inheritance. *Annu Rev Cell Dev Biol* 2007;**23**:321–44.

33. Smith JJ, Aitchison JD. Regulation of peroxisome dynamics. *Curr Opin Cell Biol* 2009;**21**(1):119–26.

34. Knoblach B, Rachubinski RA. Sharing with your children: mechanisms of peroxisome inheritance. *Biochim Biophys Acta* 2015 pii: S0167-4889(15)00407-3.

35. Schrader M, Thiemann M, Fahimi HD. Peroxisomal motility and interaction with microtubules. *Microsc Res Tech* 2003;**61**:171–8.

36. Neuhaus A, Eggeling C, Erdmann R, et al. Why do peroxisomes associate with the cytoskeleton? *Biochim Biophys Acta* 2015 pii: S0167-4889(15)00406-1.

37. Ratushny AV, Saleem RA, Sitko K, et al. Asymmetric positive feedback loops reliably control biological responses. *Mol Syst Biol* 2012;**8**:577.

38. Varga T, Czimmerer Z, Nagy L. PPARs are a unique set of fatty acid regulated transcription factors controlling both lipid metabolism and inflammation. *Biochimica et Biophysica Acta* 2011;**1812**:1007–22.

39. Poulsen Ll, Siersbæk M, Mandrup S. PPARs: fatty acid sensors controlling metabolism. *Semin Cell Dev Biol* 2012;**23**(6):631–9.

40. Berger JP, Akiyama TE, Meinke PT. PPARs: therapeutic targets for metabolic disease. *Trends Pharmacol Sci* 2005;**26**(5):244–51.

41. Cheng L, Ding G, Qin Q, et al. Cardiomyocyte-restricted peroxisome proliferator-activated receptor-delta deletion perturbs myocardial fatty acid oxidation and leads to cardiomyopathy. *Nat Med* 2004;**10**(11):1245–50.

42. Kim HJ, Ham SA, Kim MY, et al. PPARδ coordinates angiotensin II-induced senescence in vascular smooth muscle cells through PTEN-mediated inhibition of superoxide generation. *J Biol Chem* 2011;**286**(52):44585–93.

43. Ticha I, Gnosa S, Lindblom A, et al. Variants of the PPARD gene and their clinicopathological significance in colorectal cancer. *PLoS One* 2013;**8**(12):e83952.

44. Latruffe N, Vamecq J, Cherkaoui Malki M. Genetic-dependency of peroxisomal cell functions - emerging aspects. *J Cell Mol Med* 2003;**7**(3):238–48.

45. Brubaker SW, Bonham KS, Zanoni I, et al. Innate immune pattern recognition: a cell biological perspective. *Annu Rev Immunol* 2015;**33**:257–90.

46. Dixit E, Boulant S, Zhang Y, et al. Peroxisomes are signaling platforms for antiviral innate immunity. *Cell* 2010;**141**:668–81.

47. Lazarow PB. Viruses exploiting peroxisomes. *Curr Opin Microbiol* 2011;**14**(4):458–69.

48. Mohan KV, Atreya CD. Novel organelle-targeting signals in viral proteins. *Bioinformatics* 2003;**19**(1):10–13.

49. Mohan KV, Som I, Atreya CD. Identification of a type 1 peroxisomal targeting signal in a viral protein and demonstration of its targeting to the organelle. *J Virol* 2002;**76**(5):2543–7.

50. Snyder F, Wood R. Alkyl and alk-1-enyl ethers of glycerol in lipids from normal and neoplastic human tissues. *Cancer Res* 1969;**29**:251–7.

51. Howard BV, Morris HP, Bailey JM. Ether-lipids, -glycerol phosphate dehydrogenase, and growth rate in tumors and cultured cells. *Cancer Res* 1972;**32**:1533–8.

52. Santos CR, Schulze A. Lipid metabolism in cancer. *FEBS J* 2012;**279**(15):2610–23.

53. Benjamin DI, Cozzo A, Ji X, et al. Ether lipid generating enzyme AGPS alters the balance of structural and signaling lipids to fuel cancer pathogenicity. *Proc Natl Acad Sci USA* 2013;**110**:14912–7.

54. Zhu Y, Liu XJ, Yang P, et al. Alkylglyceronephosphate synthase (AGPS) alters lipid signaling pathways and supports chemotherapy resistance of glioma and hepatic carcinoma cell lines. *Asian Pac J Cancer Prev* 2014;**15**(7):3219–26.

55. Louie SM, Roberts LS, Mulvihill MM, et al. Cancer cells incorporate and remodel exogenous palmitate into structural and oncogenic signaling lipids. *Biochim Biophys Acta* 2013;**1831**(10):1566–72.

56. Piano V, Benjamin DI, Valente S, et al. Discovery of inhibitors for the ether lipid-generating enzyme agps as anti-cancer agents. *ACS Chem Biol* 2015;**10**(11):2589–97.

57. Wu M, Ho SM. PMP24, a gene identified by MSRF, undergoes DNA hypermethylation-associated gene silencing during cancer progression in an LNCaP model. *Oncogene* 2004;**23**(1):250–9.

58. Zhang X, Wu M, Xiao H, et al. Methylation of a single intronic CpG mediates expression silencing of the PMP24 gene in prostate cancer. *Prostate* 2010;**70**(7):765–76.
59. van Roermund CW, Ijlst L, Wagemans T, et al. A role for the human peroxisomal half-transporter ABCD3 in the oxidation of dicarboxylic acids. *Biochim Biophys Acta* 2014;**1841**(4):563–8.
60. Kemp S, Theodoulou FL, Wanders RJ. Mammalian peroxisomal ABC transporters: from endogenous substrates to pathology and clinical significance. *Br J Pharmacol* 2011;**164**(7):1753–66.
61. Berger J, Albet S, Bentejac M, et al. The four murine peroxisomal ABC-transporter genes differ in constitutive, inducible and developmental expression. *Eur J Biochem* 1999;**265**(2):719–27.
62. Kobayashi T, Shinnoh N, Kondo A, et al. Adrenoleukodystrophy protein-deficient mice represent abnormality of very long chain fatty acid metabolism. *Biochem Bioph Res Co* 1997;**232**:631–6.
63. Lu JF, Lawler AM, Watkins PA, et al. A mouse model for X-linked adrenoleukodystrophy. *Proc Natl Acad Sci USA* 1997;**94**:9366–71.
64. Forss-Petter S, Werner H, Berger J, et al. Targeted inactivation of the X-linked adrenoleukodystrophy gene in mice. *J Neurosci Res* 1997;**50**:829–43.
65. Ferrer I, Kapfhammer JP, Hindelang C, et al. Inactivation of the peroxisomal ABCD2 transporter in the mouse leads to late-onset ataxia involving mitochondria, Golgi and endoplasmic reticulum damage. *Hum Mol Genet* 2005;**14**(23):3565–77.
66. Jimenez-Sanchez G, Hebron K, Thomas G, Valle D. Targeted disruption of the 70kDa peroxisomal membrane protein (PMP70) in mouse is associated with an increase in the related P70R protein, deficiency of hepatic glycogen and a dicarboxylic aciduria. *Pediatr Res* 1999;45:139A.
67. Ferdinandusse S, Jimenez-Sanchez G, Koster J, et al. A novel bile acid biosynthesis defect due to a deficiency of peroxisomal ABCD3. *Hum Mol Genet* 2015;**24**(2):361–70.
68. Min KT, Benzer S. Preventing neurodegeneration in the Drosophila mutant bubblegum. *Science* 1999;**284**(5422):1985–8.
69. Kirkby B, Roman N, Kobe B, et al. Functional and structural properties of mammalian acyl-coenzyme A thioesterases. *Prog Lipid Res* 2010;**49**(4):366–77.
70. Hunt MC, Siponen MI, Alexson SE. The emerging role of acyl-CoA thioesterases and acyltransferases in regulating peroxisomal lipid metabolism. *Biochim Biophys Acta* 2012;**1822**(9):1397–410.
71. Watkins PA, Ellis JM. Peroxisomal acyl-CoA synthetases. *Biochim Biophys Acta* 2012;**1822**(9):1411–20.
72. Jansen GA, Wanders RJ. Alpha-oxidation. *Biochim Biophys Acta* 2006;**1763**(12):1403–12.
73. Wanders RJ, Komen J, Ferdinandusse S. Phytanic acid metabolism in health and disease. *Biochim Biophys Acta* 2011;**1811**(9):498–507.
74. Wanders RJ. Peroxisomes, lipid metabolism, and peroxisomal disorders. *Mol Genet Metab* 2004;**83**(1–2):16–27.
75. Wanders RJ, Ferdinandusse S, Brites P, et al. Peroxisomes, lipid metabolism and lipotoxicity. *Biochim Biophys Acta* 2010;**1801**(3):272–80.
76. Dhaunsi GS, Al-Essa M, Ozand PT, et al. Carnitine prevents cyclic GMP-induced inhibition of peroxisomal enzyme activities. *Cell Biochem Funct* 2004;**22**(6):365–71.
77. Suzuki Y, Jiang LL, Souri M, et al. D-3-hydroxyacyl-CoA dehydratase/D-3-hydroxyacyl-CoA dehydrogenase bifunctional protein deficiency: a newly identified peroxisomal disorder. *Am J Hum Genet* 1997;**61**(5):1153–62.

78. Braiterman LT, Watkins PA, Moser AB, et al. Peroxisomal very long chain fatty acid beta-oxidation activity is determined by the level of adrenodeukodystrophy protein (ALDP) expression. *Mol Genet Metab* 1999;**66**(2):91–9.

79. Lines MA, Jobling R, Brady L, et al. Peroxisomal D-bifunctional protein deficiency: three adults diagnosed by whole-exome sequencing. *Neurology* 2014;**82**(11):963–8.

80. Jiang LL, Kurosawa T, Sato M, et al. Physiological role of D-3-hydroxyacyl-CoA dehydratase/D-3-hydroxyacyl-CoA dehydrogenase bifunctional protein. *J Biochem* 1997;**121**(3):506–13.

81. Suzuki Y, Shimozawa N, Yajima S, et al. Different intracellular localization of peroxisomal proteins in fibroblasts from patients with aberrant peroxisome assembly. *Cell Struct Funct* 1992;**17**(1):1–8.

82. Cheng JB, Russell DW. Mammalian wax biosynthesis. I. Identification of two fatty acyl-Coenzyme A reductases with different substrate specificities and tissue distributions. *J Biol Chem*;3;279(36):37789-37797.

83. Farooqui AA, Farooqui T, Horrocks LA. *Metabolism and Functions of Bioactive Ether Lipids in the Brain*. Springer; 2008:17–37.

84. Braverman NE, Moser AB. Functions of plasmalogen lipids in health and disease. *Biochim Biophys Acta* 2012;**1822**(9):1442–52.

85. Thai TP, Rodemer C, Jauch A, et al. Impaired membrane traffic in defective ether lipid biosynthesis. *Hum Mol Genet* 2001;**10**(2):127–36.

86. Razeto A, Mattiroli F, Carpanelli E, et al. The crucial step in ether phospholipid biosynthesis: structural basis of a noncanonical reaction associated with a peroxisomal disorder. *Structure* 2007;**15**(6):683–92.

87. Schrakamp G, Roosenboom CF, Schutgens RB, et al. Alkyl dihydroxyacetone phosphate synthase in human fibroblasts and its deficiency in Zellweger syndrome. *J Lipid Res* 1985;**26**(7):867–73.

88. Huyghe S, Mannaerts GP, Baes M, et al. Peroxisomal multifunctional protein-2: the enzyme, the patients and the knockout mouse model. *Biochim Biophys Acta* 2006;**1761**:973–94.

89. Bowen P, Lee CS, Zellweger H, et al. A familial syndrome of multiple congenital defects. *Bull Johns Hopkins Hosp* 1964;**114**:402–14.

90. Brown FR, McAdams AJ, Cummins JW, et al. Cerebro-hepato-renal (Zellweger) syndrome and neonatal adrenoleukodystrophy: similarities in phenotype and accumulation of very long chain fatty acids. *Johns Hopkins Med J* 1982;**151**:344–51.

91. Moser HW. Adrenoleukodystrophy: Phenotype, genetics, pathogenesis and therapy. *Brain* 1997;**120**:1485–508.

92. Heymans HSA, Schutgens RBH, Tan R, et al. Severe plasmalogen deficiency in tissues of infants without peroxisomes (Zellweger syndrome). *Nature* 1983;**306**:69–70.

93. Wanders RJ. Metabolic functions of peroxisomes in health and disease. *Biochimie* 2014;**98**:36–44.

94. Funato M, Shimozawa N, Nagase T, et al. Aberrant peroxisome morphology in peroxisomal beta- oxidation enzyme deficiencies. *Brain Dev* 2006;**28**(5):287–92.

95. Wiesinger C, Eichler FS, Berger J. The genetic landscape of X-linked adrenoleuko dystrophy:inheritance, mutations, modifier genes, and diagnosis. *Appl Clin Genet* 2015;**8**:109–21.

96. Horn MA, Retterstøl L, Abdelnoor M, et al. Adrenoleukodystrophy in Norway: high rate of de novo mutations and age-dependent penetrance. *Pediatr Neurol* 2013;**48**(3):212–9.

97. Eichler EE, Budarf ML, Rocchi M, et al. Interchromosomal duplications of the adrenoleukodystrophy locus: a phenomenon of pericentromeric plasticity. *Hum Mol Genet* 1997;**6**(7):991–1002.

98. Moser HW. Adrenoleukodystrophy: phenotype, genetics, pathogenesis and therapy. *Brain* 1997;**120**(Pt 8):1485–508.

99. Semmler A, Bao X, Cao G, et al. Genetic variants of methionine metabolism and X-ALD phenotype generation: results of a new study sample. *J Neurol* 2009;**256**(8):1277–80.

100. Brose RD, Avramopoulos D, Smith KD. SOD2 as a potential modifier of X-linked adrenoleukodystrophy clinical phenotypes. *J Neurol* 2012;**259**(7):1440–7.

101. Powers JM, Liu Y, Moser AB, et al. The inflammatory myelinopathy of adreno-leukodystrophy: cells, effector molecules, and pathogenetic implications. *J Neuropathol Exp Neurol* 1992;**51**:630–43.

102. Singh I, Pujol A. Pathomechanisms underlying X-adrenoleukodystrophy: a three-hit hypothesis. *Brain Pathol* 2010;**20**:838–44.

103. Fidaleo M. Peroxisomes and peroxisomal disorders: the main facts. *Exp Toxicol Pathol* 2010;**62**(6):615–25.

104. Powers JM, DeCiero DP, Ito M, et al. Adrenomyeloneuropathy: a neuropathologic review featuring its noninflammatory myelopathy. *J Neuropathol Exp Neurol* 2000;**59**(2):89–102.

105. Baarine M, Beeson C, Singh A, et al. ABCD1 deletion-induced mitochondrial dysfunction is corrected by SAHA: implication for adrenoleukodystrophy. *J Neurochem* 2015;**133**(3):380–96.

106. Kruska N, Schönfeld P, Pujol A. Astrocytes and mitochondria from adrenoleukodystrophy protein (ABCD1)-deficient mice reveal that the adrenoleukodystrophy-associated very long-chain fatty acids target several cellular energy-dependent functions. *Biochim Biophys Acta* 2015;**1852**(5):925–36.

107. Oezen I, Rossmanith W, Forss-Petter S, et al. Accumulation of very long-chain fatty acids does not affect mitochondrial function in adrenoleukodystrophy protein deficiency. *Hum Mol Genet* 2005;**14**(9):1127–37.

108. Schlüter A, Espinosa L, Fourcade S, et al. Functional genomic analysis unravels a metabolic-inflammatory interplay in adrenoleukodystrophy. *Hum Mol Genet* 2012;**21**(5):1062–77.

109. Galea E, Launay N, Portero-Otin M, et al. Oxidative stress underlying axonal degeneration in adrenoleukodystrophy: a paradigm for multifactorial neurodegenerative diseases? *Biochim Biophys Acta* 2012;**1822**(9):1475–88.

110. López-Erauskin J, Galino J, Bianchi P, et al. Oxidative stress modulates mitochondrial failure and cyclophilin D function in X-linked adrenoleukodystrophy. *Brain* 2012;**135**(Pt 12): 3584–98.

111. Fourcade S, López-Erauskin J, Ruiz M, et al. Mitochondrial dysfunction and oxidative damage cooperatively fuel axonal degeneration in X-linked adrenoleukodystrophy. *Biochimie* 2014;**98**:143–9.

112. Corzo D, Gibson W, Johnson K, et al. Contiguous deletion of the X-linked adrenoleukodystrophy gene (ABCD1) and DXS1357E: a novel neonatal phenotype similar to peroxisomal biogenesis disorders. *Am J Hum Genet* 2002;**70**(6):1520–31.

113. Calhoun AR, Raymond GV. Distal Xq28 microdeletions: clarification of the spectrum of contiguous gene deletions involving ABCD1, BCAP31, and SLC6A8 with a new case and review of the literature. *Am J Med Genet A* 2014;**164A**(10):2613–7.

114. Osaka H, Takagi A, Tsuyusaki Y, et al. Contiguous deletion of SLC6A8 and BAP31 in a patient with severe dystonia and sensorineural deafness. *Mol Genet Metab* 2012;**106**(1):43–7.
115. Iwasa M, Yamagata T, Mizuguchi M, et al. Contiguous ABCD1 DXS1357E deletion syndrome: report of an autopsy case. *Neuropathology* 2013;**33**(3):292–8.
116. van de Kamp JM, Betsalel OT, Mercimek-Mahmutoglu S, et al. Phenotype and genotype in 101 males with X-linked creatine transporter deficiency. *J Med Genet* 2013;**50**(7):463–72.
117. Anselm IA, Alkuraya FS, Salomons GS, et al. X-linked creatine transporter defect: a report on two unrelated boys with a severe clinical phenotype. *J Inherit Metab Dis* 2006;**29**(1):214–9.
118. Cacciagli P, Sutera-Sardo J, Borges-Correia A, et al. Mutations in BCAP31 cause a severe X-linked phenotype with deafness, dystonia, and central hypomyelination and disorganize the Golgi apparatus. *Am J Hum Genet* 2013;**93**(3):579–86.
119. Verhoeven NM, Jakobs C. Human metabolism of phytanic acid and pristanic acid. *Prog Lipid Res* 2001;**40**(6):453–66.
120. Baldwin EJ, Gibberd FB, Harley C, et al. The effectiveness of long-term dietary therapy in the treatment of adult Refsum disease. *J Neurol Neurosurg Psychiatry* 2010;**81**(9):954–7.
121. Ferdinandusse S, Denis S, Clayton PT, et al. Mutations in the gene encoding peroxisomal alpha-methylacyl-CoA racemase cause adult-onset sensory motor neuropathy. *Nat Genet* 2000;**24**(2):188–91.
122. Smith EH, Gavrilov DK, Oglesbee D, et al. An adult onset case of alpha-methyl-acyl-CoA racemase deficiency. *J Inherit Metab Dis* 2010;**33**(Suppl 3):S349–53.
123. Poll-The BT, Roels F, Ogier H, et al. A new peroxisomal disorder with enlarged peroxisomes and a specific deficiency of acyl-CoA oxidase (pseudo-neonatal adrenoleukodystrophy). *Am J Hum Genet* 1988;**42**:422–34.
124. Watkins PA, Chen WW, Harris CJ, et al. Peroxisomal bifunctional enzyme deficiency. *J Clin Invest* 1989;**83**(3):771–7.
125. Watkins PA, McGuinness MC, Raymond GV, et al. Distinction between peroxisomal bifunctional enzyme and acyl-CoA oxidase deficiencies. *Ann Neurol* 1995;**38**(3):472–7.
126. Pierce SB, Walsh T, Chisholm KM, et al. Mutations in the DBP-deficiency protein HSD17B4 cause ovarian dysgenesis, hearing loss, and ataxia of Perrault syndrome. *Am J Hum Genet* 2010;**87**(2):282–8.
127. Klootwijk ED, Reichold M, Helip-Wooley A, et al. Mistargeting of peroxisomal EHHADH and inherited renal Fanconi's syndrome. *N Engl J Med* 2014;**370**:129–38.
128. Ferdinandusse S, Kostopoulos P, Denis S, et al. Mutations in the gene encoding peroxisomal sterol carrier protein X (SCPx) cause leukencephalopathy with dystonia and motor neuropathy. *Am J Hum Genet* 2006;**78**(6):1046–52.
129. Poll-The BT, Gärtner J. Clinical diagnosis, biochemical findings and MRI spectrum of peroxisomal disorders. *Biochim Biophys Acta* 2012;**1822**(9):1421–9.
130. Wanders RJA, Schumacher H, Heikoop J, et al. Human dihydroxyacetonephosphate acyltransferase deficiency: a new peroxisomal disorder. *J Inherit Metab Dis* 1992;**15**:389–91.
131. Wanders RJA, Dekker C, Horvath VA, et al. Human alkyldihydroxyacetonephosphate synthase deficiency: a new peroxisomal disorder. *J Inherit Metab Dis* 1994;**17**:315–8.
132. Buchert R, Tawamie H, Smith C, et al. A peroxisomal disorder of severe intellectual disability, epilepsy, and cataracts due to fatty acyl-CoA reductase 1 deficiency. *Am J Hum Genet* 2014;**95**(5):602–10.

133. Barøy T, Koster J, Strømme P, et al. A novel type of rhizomelic chondrodysplasia punctata, RCDP5, is caused by loss of the PEX5 long isoform. *Hum Mol Genet* 2015;**24**(20):5845–54.

134. Danpure CJ. Primary hyperoxaluria type 1: AGT mistargeting highlights the fundamental differences between the peroxisomal and mitochondrial protein import pathways. *Biochim Biophys Acta* 2006;**1763**(12):1776–84.

135. Tasic V, Gucev Z. Nephrolithiasis and Nephrocalcinosis in children - metabolic and genetic factors. *Pediatr Endocrinol Rev* 2015;**13**(1):468–76.

136. Bacchetta J, Mekahli D, Rivet C, et al. Pediatric combined liver-kidney transplantation: a 2015 update. *Curr Opin Organ Transplant* 2015;**20**(5):543–9.

137. Takahara S. Progressive oral gangrene probably due to lack of catalase in the blood (acatalasaemia); report of nine cases. *Lancet* 1952;**2**(6745):1101–4.

138. Niikawa N, Fukushima Y, Taniguchi N, et al. Chromosome abnormalities involving 11p13 and low erythrocyte catalase activity. *Hum Genet* 1982;**60**:373–5.

139. Goth L, Eaton JW. Hereditary catalase deficiencies and increased risk of diabetes. *Lancet* 2000;**356**:1820–1.

140. Koepke JI, Wood CS, Terlecky LJ, et al. Progeric effects of catalase inactivation in human cells. *Toxicol Appl Pharmacol* 2008;**232**:99–108.

141. Kobayashi M, Sugiyama H, Wang DH, et al. Catalase deficiency renders remnant kidneys more susceptible to oxidant tissue injury and renal fibrosis in mice. *Kidney Int* 2005;**68**:1018–31.

142. Fukuoka N, Sugiyama H, Inoue T, et al. Increased susceptibility to oxidant-mediated tissue injury and peritoneal fibrosis in acatalasemic mice. *Am J Nephrol* 2008;**28**(4):661–8.

143. Takiue K, Sugiyama H, Inoue T, et al. Acatalasemic mice are mildly susceptible to adriamycin nephropathy and exhibit increased albuminuria and glomerulosclerosis. *BMC Nephrol* 2012;**13**:14.

144. Góth L, Bigler NW. Catalase deficiency may complicate urate oxidase (rasburicase) therapy. *Free Radic Res* 2007;**41**(9):953–5.

145. Góth L, Nagy T. Inherited catalase deficiency: is it benign or a factor in various age related disorders? *Mutat Res* 2013;**753**(2):147–54.

146. D'souza A, Kurien BT, Rodgers R, et al. Detection of catalase as a major protein target of the lipid peroxidation product 4-HNE and the lack of its genetic association as a risk factor in SLE. *BMC Med Genet* 2008;**9**:62.

147. Holstein SA, Hohl RJ. Isoprenoids: remarkable diversity of form and function. *Lipids* 2004;**39**(4):293–309.

148. Hoffmann G, Gibson KM, Brandt IK, et al. Mevalonic aciduria--an inborn error of cholesterol and nonsterol isoprene biosynthesis. *N Engl J Med* 1986;**314**(25):1610–4.

149. Shamseldin HE, Alshammari M, Al-Sheddi T, et al. Genomic analysis of mitochondrial diseases in a consanguineous population reveals novel candidate disease genes. *J Med Genet* 2012;**49**(4):234–41.

150. Dodt G, Kim DG, Reimann SA, et al. L-Pipecolic acid oxidase, a human enzyme essential for the degradation of L-pipecolic acid, is most similar to the monomeric sarcosine oxidases. *Biochem J* 2000;**345**(Pt 3):487–94.

151. Pasmant E, de Saint-Trivier A, Laurendeau I, et al. Characterization of a 7.6-Mb germline deletion encompassing the NF1 locus and about a hundred genes in an NF contiguous gene syndrome patient. *Eur J Hum Genet* 2008;**16**(12):1459–66.

152. Mandel H, Espeel M, Roels F, et al. A new type of peroxisomal disorder with variable expression in liver and fibroblasts. *J Pediatr* 1994;**125**(4):549–55.

153. Espeel M, Mandel H, Poggi F, et al. Peroxisome mosaicism in the livers of peroxisomal deficiency patients. *Hepatology* 1995;**22**(2):497–504.
154. Pineda M, Giros M, Roels F, et al. Diagnosis and follow-up of a case of peroxisomal disorder with peroxisomal mosaicism. *J Child Neurol* 1999;**14**(7):434–9.
155. Valianpour F, Selhorst JJ, van Lint LE, et al. Analysis of very long-chain fatty acids using electrospray ionization mass spectrometry. *Mol Genet Metab* 2003;**79**(3):189–96.
156. Schutgens RB, Bouman IW, Nijenhuis AA, et al. Profiles of very-long-chain fatty acids in plasma, fibroblasts, and blood cells in Zellweger syndrome, X-linked adrenoleukodystrophy, and rhizomelic chondrodysplasia punctata. *Clin Chem* 1993;**39**(8):1632–7.
157. Moser AB, Kreiter N, Bezman L, et al. Plasma very long chain fatty acids in 3,000 peroxisome disease patients and 29,000 controls. *Ann Neurol* 1999;**45**(1):100–10.
158. Peduto A, Baumgartner MR, Verhoeven NM, et al. Hyperpipecolic acidaemia: a diagnostic tool for peroxisomal disorders. *Mol Genet Metab* 2004;**82**(3):224–30.
159. Ferdinandusse S, Rusch H, van Lint AE, et al. Stereochemistry of the peroxisomal branched-chain fatty acid alpha- and beta-oxidation systems in patients suffering from different peroxisomal disorders. *J Lipid Res* 2002;**43**(3):438–44.
160. Labadaridis I, Moraitou M, Theodoraki M, et al. Plasmalogen levels in full-term neonates. *Acta Paediatr* 2009;**98**(4):640–2.
161. Takemoto Y, Suzuki Y, Horibe R, et al. Gas chromatography/mass spectrometry analysis of very long chain fatty acids, docosahexaenoic acid, phytanic acid and plasmalogen for the screening of peroxisomal disorders. *Brain Dev* 2003;**25**(7):481–7.
162. Moraitou M, Dimitriou E, Zafeiriou D, et al. Plasmalogen levels in Gaucher disease. *Blood Cells Mol Dis* 2008;**41**(2):196–9.
163. Schutgens RB, Romeyn GJ, Wanders RJ, et al. Deficiency of acyl-CoA: dihydroxyacetone phosphate acyltransferase in patients with Zellweger (cerebro-hepato-renal) syndrome. *Biochem Biophys Res Commun* 1984;**120**(1):179–84.
164. Wanders RJ, Kos M, Roest B, Meijer AJ, et al. Activity of peroxisomal enzymes and intracellular distribution of catalase in Zellweger syndrome. *Biochem Biophys Res Commun* 1984;**123**(3):1054–61.
165. Bizzi A, Castelli G, Bugiani M, et al. Classification of childhood white matter disorders using proton MR spectroscopic imaging. *Am J Neuroradiol* 2008;**29**(7):1270–5.
166. Raymond GV, Jones RO, Moser AB. Newborn screening for adrenoleukodystrophy: implications for therapy. *Mol Diagn Ther* 2007;**11**(6):381–4.
167. Hubbard WC, Moser AB, Liu AC, et al. Newborn screening for X-linked adrenoleukodystrophy (X-ALD): validation of a combined liquid chromatography-tandem mass spectrometric (LC-MS/MS) method. *Mol Genet Metab* 2009;**97**(3):212–20.
168. Haynes CA, De Jesús VR. Improved analysis of C26:0-lysophosphatidylcholine in dried-blood spots via negative ion mode HPLC-ESI-MS/MS for X-linked adrenoleukodystrophy newborn screening. *Clin Chim Acta* 2012;**413**(15-16):1217–21.
169. Theda C, Gibbons K, Defor TE, et al. Newborn screening for X-linked adrenoleukodystrophy: further evidence high throughput screening is feasible. *Mol Genet Metab* 2014;**111**(1):55–7.
170. Turgeon CT, Moser AB, Mørkrid L, et al. Streamlined determination of lysophosphatidylcholines in dried blood spots for newborn screening of X-linked adrenoleukodystrophy. *Mol Genet Metab* 2015;**114**(1):46–50.
171. Vogel BH, Bradley SE, Adams DJ, et al. Newborn screening for X-linked adrenoleukodystrophy in New York State: diagnostic protocol, surveillance protocol and treatment guidelines. *Mol Genet Metab* 2015;**114**(4):599–603.

172. Pai GS, Khan M, Barbosa E, et al. Lovastatin therapy for X-linked adrenoleukodystrophy: clinical and biochemical observations on 12 patients. *Mol Genet Metab* 2000;**69**(4):312–22.

173. Moser HW, Raymond GV, Lu SE, et al. Follow-up of 89 asymptomatic patients with adrenoleukodystrophy treated with Lorenzo's oil. *Arch Neurol* 2005;**62**(7):1073–80.

174. Naidu S, Bresnan MJ, Griffin D, et al. Childhood adrenoleukodystrophy. Failure of intensive immunosuppression to arrest neurologic progression. *Arch Neurol* 1988;**45**(8):846–8.

175. Berger J, Gärtner J. X-linked adrenoleukodystrophy: clinical, biochemical and pathogenetic aspects. *Biophysica Acta* 2006;**1763**:1721–32.

176. Chan AK, Bhargava R, Desai S, et al. Reversible posterior leukoencephalopathy syndrome in a child with cerebral X-linked adrenoleukodystrophy treated with cyclosporine after bone marrow transplantation. *J Inherit Metab Dis* 2003;**26**(6):527–36.

177. Peters C, Charnas LR, Tan Y, et al. Cerebral X-linked adrenoleukodystrophy: the international hematopoietic cell transplantation experience from 1982 to 1999. *Blood* 2004;**104**(3):881–8.

178. Resnick IB, Abdul Hai A, Shapira MY, et al. Treatment of X-linked childhood cerebral adrenoleukodystrophy by the use of an allogeneic stem cell transplantation with reduced intensity conditioning regimen. *Clin Transplant* 2005;**19**(6):840–7.

179. Okamura K, Watanabe T, Onishi T, et al. Successful allogeneic unrelated bone marrow transplantation using reduced-intensity conditioning for the treatment of X-linked adrenoleukodystrophy in a one-yr-old boy. *Pediatr Transplant* 2009;**13**(1):130–3.

180. Miller WP, Rothman SM, Nascene D, et al. Outcomes after allogeneic hematopoietic cell transplantation for childhood cerebral adrenoleukodystrophy: the largest single-institution cohort report. *Blood* 2011;**118**(7):1971–8.

181. Mitchell R, Nivison-Smith I, Anazodo A, et al. Outcomes of haematopoietic stem cell transplantation for inherited metabolic disorders: a report from the Australian and New Zealand Children's Haematology Oncology Group and the Australasian Bone Marrow Transplant Recipient Registry. *Pediatr Transplant* 2013;**17**(6):582–8.

182. Martin PL, Carter SL, Kernan NA, et al. Results of the cord blood transplantation study (COBLT): outcomes of unrelated donor umbilical cord blood transplantation in pediatric patients with lysosomal and peroxisomal storage diseases. *Biol Blood Marrow Transplant* 2006;**12**(2):184–94.

183. Beam D, Poe MD, Provenzale JM, et al. Outcomes of unrelated umbilical cord blood transplantation for X-linked adrenoleukodystrophy. *Biol Blood Marrow Transplant* 2007;**13**(6):665–74.

184. Chao MM, Levine JE, Ferrara JL, et al. Successful treatment of refractory immune hemolysis following unrelated cord blood transplant with Campath-1H. *Pediatr Blood Cancer* 2008;**50**(4):917–9.

185. Cheng FW, Lee V, To KF, et al. Post-transplant EBV-related lymphoproliferative disorder complicating umbilical cord blood transplantation in patients of adrenoleukodystrophy. *Pediatr Blood Cancer* 2009;**15;53**(7):1329–31.

186. Awaya T, Kato T, Niwa A, et al. Successful cord blood transplantation using a reduced-intensity conditioning regimen for advanced childhood-onset cerebral adrenoleukodystrophy. *Pediatr Transplant* 2011;**15**(6):E116–20.

187. Shibata M, Kato T, Awaya T, et al. Chronic immune-mediated axonal polyneuropathy following umbilical cord blood transplant for childhood-onset cerebral adrenoleukodystrophy. *Pediatr Transplant* 2012;**16**(8):E388–91.

188. Niizuma H, Uematsu M, Sakamoto O, et al. Successful cord blood transplantation with reduced-intensity conditioning for childhood cerebral X-linked adrenoleukodystrophy at advanced and early stages. *Pediatr Transplant* 2012;**16**(2):E63–70.
189. Cartier N, Hacein-Bey-Abina S, Bartholomae CC, et al. Hematopoietic stem cell gene therapy with a lentiviral vector in X-linked adrenoleukodystrophy. *Science* 2009;**326**(5954):818–23.
190. Cartier N, Hacein-Bey-Abina S, Bartholomae CC, et al. Lentiviral hematopoietic cell gene therapy for X-linked adrenoleukodystrophy. *Methods Enzymol* 2012;**507**:187–98.
191. Morató L, Galino J, Ruiz M, et al. Pioglitazone halts axonal degeneration in a mouse model of X-linked adrenoleukodystrophy. *Brain* 2013;**136**(Pt 8):2432–43.
192. Morató L, Ruiz M, Boada J, et al. Activation of sirtuin 1 as therapy for the peroxisomal disease adrenoleukodystrophy. *Cell Death Differ* 2015;**22**(11):1742–53.
193. López-Erauskin J, Fourcade S, Galino J, et al. Antioxidants halt axonal degeneration in a mouse model of X-adrenoleukodystrophy. *Ann Neurol* 2011;**70**(1):84–92.
194. Fourcade S, Ruiz M, Guilera C, et al. Valproic acid induces antioxidant effects in X-linked adrenoleukodystrophy. *Hum Mol Genet* 2010;**19**(10):2005–14.
195. Launay N, Aguado C, Fourcade S, et al. Autophagy induction halts axonal degeneration in a mouse model of X-adrenoleukodystrophy. *Acta Neuropathol* 2015;**129**(3):399–415.
196. Mastroeni R, Bensadoun JC, Charvin D, et al. Insulin-like growth factor-1 and neurotrophin-3 gene therapy prevents motor decline in an X-linked adrenoleukodystrophy mouse model.. *Ann Neurol* 2009;**66**(1):117–22.
197. Gong Y, Mu D, Prabhakar S, et al. Adenoassociated virus serotype 9-mediated gene therapy for x-linked adrenoleukodystrophy. *Mol Ther* 2015;**23**(5):824–34.
198. Biffi A, Bartolomae CC, Cesana D, et al. Lentiviral vector common integration sites in preclinical models and a clinical trial reflect a benign integration bias and not oncogenic selection. *Blood* 2011;**117**(20):5332–9.
199. Jang J, Kang HC, Kim HS, et al. Induced pluripotent stem cell models from X-linked adrenoleukodystrophy patients. *Ann Neurol* 2011;**70**(3):402–9.
200. Baarine M, Khan M, Singh A, Singh I. Functional characterization of ipsc-derived brain cells as a model for X-linked adrenoleukodystrophy. *PLoS One* 2015;**10**(11):e0143238.
201. Russo FB, Cugola FR, Fernandes IR, et al. Induced pluripotent stem cells for modeling neurological disorders. *World J Transplan* 2015;**5**(4):209–21.
202. Wood CS, Koepke JI, Teng H, et al. Hypocatalasemic fibroblasts accumulate hydrogen peroxide and display age-associated pathologies. *Traffic* 2006;**7**:97–107.
203. Takemoto K, Tanaka M, Iwata H, et al. Low catalase activity in blood is associated with the diabetes caused by alloxan. *Clin Chim Acta* 2009;**407**:43–6.

Disorders of purine and pyrimidine metabolism 12

L. Hubert[1,2] and V.R. Sutton[1,2,3]

[1]Baylor College of Medicine, Houston, TX, United States; [2]Baylor Genetics Laboratories, Houston, TX, United States; [3]Texas Children's Hospital, Houston, TX, United States

12.1 INTRODUCTION

Inborn errors of purine and pyrimidine metabolism are a group of disorders with a broad spectrum of clinical presentations characterized by abnormal concentrations of purines, pyrimidines, and their associated metabolites in body fluids.[1] The importance of purines and pyrimidines is highlighted by their roles in a diverse range of biological processes. These include serving as the basic structural components for DNA and RNA, regulation of cellular metabolism, energy conservation and transport, involvement in lipid and carbohydrate metabolism, and signal transduction and translation.[2,3] The production of purines and pyrimidines is the result of two pathways: *de novo* and salvage[4] (Figs 12.1 and 12.2). The *de novo* pathway is a multistep process that uses substrates such as CO_2, glycine, and glutamine to generate purines and pyrimidines, while the salvage pathway relies on the recycling of purine and pyrimidine catabolic products. Under normal conditions, the salvage pathway exerts feedback control over *de novo* synthesis.[2] The proper function of these individual processes and maintenance of intra-pathway communication is required for cellular homeostasis and prevention of disease.

The purine *de novo* pathway begins with phosphoribosylpyrophosphate (PRPP), synthesized by PRPP synthetase (PRS), leading to the production of the nucleotide inosine monophosphate (IMP). The pathway concludes with the conversion of IMP to adenosine and guanosine nucleotides. These mononucleotides are further processed into di- and tri-nucleotides, deoxyribonucleotides, and eventually incorporated into RNA and DNA. Alternatively, catabolism of purines results in production of uric acid by xanthine dehydrogenase. In the purine salvage pathway guanine, hypoxanthine and adenine are converted to mononucleotides by hypoxanthine-guanine phosphoribosyltransferase (HPRT) and adenine phosphoribosyltransferase (APRT), while deoxyguanosine and adenosine are functionally activated by enzyme-specific kinases. The pyrimidine *de novo* pathway is initiated by cytosolic carbamoylphosphate synthetase II in the production of carbamoylphosphate, and leading to the production of orotic

Biomarkers in Inborn Errors of Metabolism. DOI: http://dx.doi.org/10.1016/B978-0-12-802896-4.00009-2

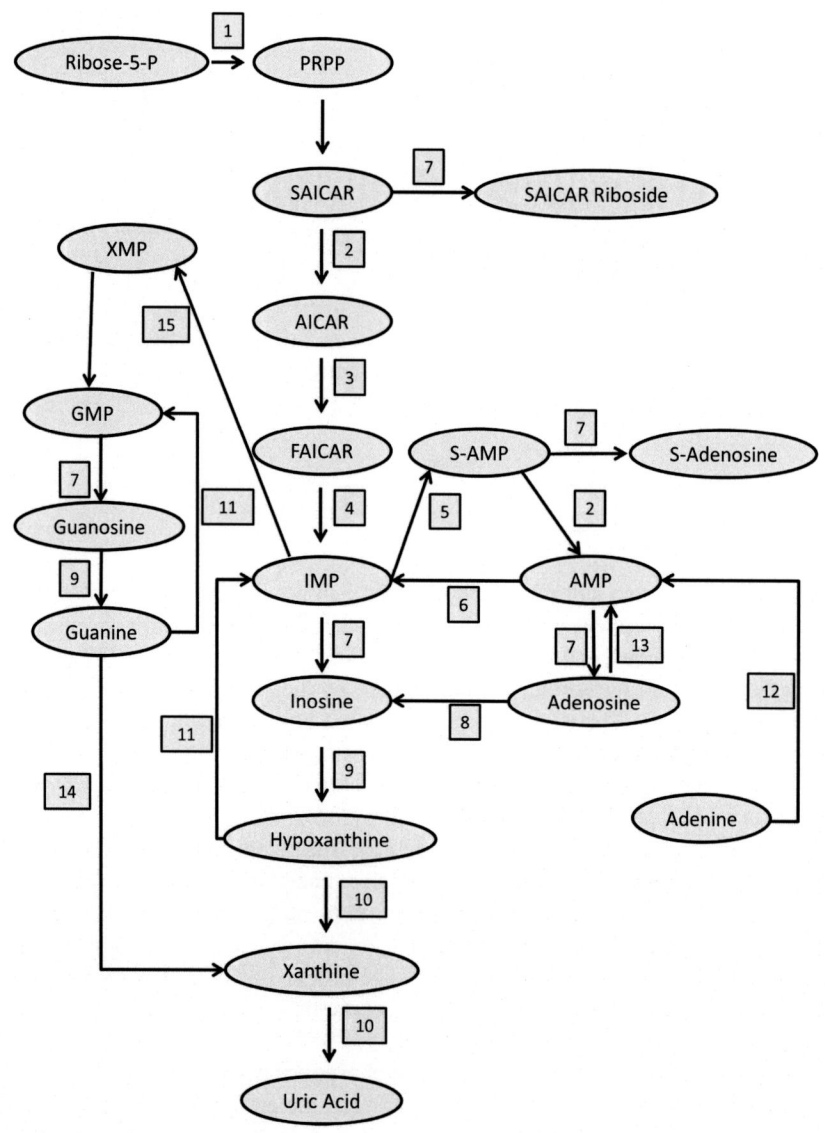

FIGURE 12.1

Purine metabolism pathway. PRPP: Phosphoribosylpyrophosphate; SAICAR: Succinylaminoimidazole carboxamide ribotide; AICAR: Aminoimidazole carboxamide ribotide; FAICAR: Formylaminoimidazole carboxamide ribotide; IMP: Inosine monophosphate; GMP: Guanosine monophosphate; AMP: Adenosine monophosphate; SAMP: Adenylosuccinate; S-Ado: Succinyladenosine; XMP: Xanthosine monophosphate. (1) PRPP synthetase; (2) adenylosuccinase (adenylosuccinate lyase); (3) AICAR transformylase; (4) IMP cyclohydrolase (3 and 4 form ATIC); (5) adenylosuccinate synthetase; (6) AMP deaminase; (7) 5′-nucleotidase(s); (8) adenosine deaminase; (9) purine nucleoside phosphorylase; (10) xanthine dehydrogenase; (11) hypoxanthine-guanine phosphoribosyltransferase; (12) adenine phosphoribosyltransferase; (13) adenosine kinase; (14) guanase; (15) IMP dehydrogenase.

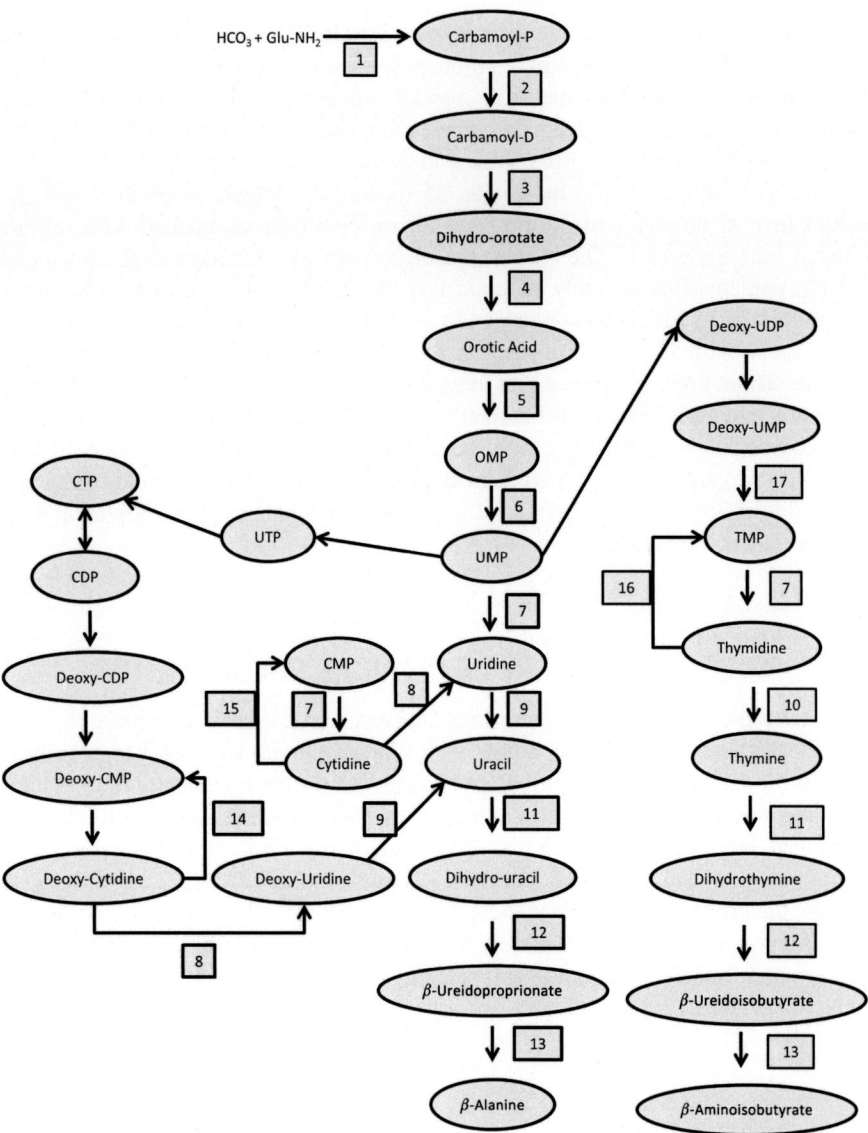

FIGURE 12.2

Pyrimidine metabolism pathway. Glu-NH2: Glutamine; Carbamoyl-P: Carbamoyl-phosphate; Carbamoyl-Asp: Carbamoyl-aspartate; OMP: Orotidine monophosphate; PRPP: Phosphoribosyl-pyrophosphate; UMP: Uridine monophosphate; CMP: Cytidine monophosphate; CTP: Cytidine triphosphate; TMP: Thymidine monophosphate; pyrimidine synthesis: (1) carbamoylphosphate synthetase II; (2) ATCase; (3) dihydroorotase (1, 2, and 3 comprise CAD); (4) dihydroorotate dehydrogenase; (5) orotate phosphoribosyl-transferase; (6) OMP decarboxylase (5 and 6 comprise UMP synthase); (7) pyrimidine-5′-nucleotidase; (8) cytidine deaminase; (9) uridine phosphorylase; (10) thymidine phosphorylase; (11) dihydropyrimidine dehydrogenase; (12) dihydropyrimidinase; (13) ureidopropionase; (14) deoxy-cytidine kinase; (15) uridine/cytidine kinase; (16) thymidine kinase; (17) thymidylate synthetase.

acid (OA) by dihydroorotate dehydrogenase (DHODH). Using orotic acid, uridine 5′-monophosphate (UMP) synthase produces the centralized nucleotide UMP, which serves as a branch point for metabolic breakdown and the salvage pathway. During catabolism, uracil and thymine are processed into β-alanine and β-aminoisobutyrate, which serve as precursors for the citric acid cycle.[5]

Enzymatically, there are more than 35 recognized defects associated with the metabolism of purines and pyrimidines but only half are associated with serious clinical consequences.[1,6] The current prevalence of these disorders is unknown and the last epidemiological study reported less than 1000 patients in a population of 435 million in 18 European countries.[7] In another study, 28 patients with purine disorders and 1 with a pyrimidine disorder were diagnosed over a three-year period in Poland.[8] These findings suggest that these disorders occur at a higher frequency than originally thought, although still remain individually rare. The number of new inborn errors of metabolism, including purine and pyrimidine disorders, increases each year and given the gamut of associated clinical presentations, clinicians should have a low threshold for interrogating purine and pyrimidine metabolism in an individual with various phenotypes (Table 12.1).

12.2 BRIEF DESCRIPTION OF CLINICAL PRESENTATION

Originally, these disorders were presumed to be pediatric diseases but more recently have been shown to present in adults with milder symptoms. Their broad clinical presentation is fueled by the global involvement of purine- and pyrimidine-associated metabolites in essential cellular processes. As a result the related perturbations may lead to functional aberrations observed in immunological, hematological, neurological, musculoskeletal, and renal systems (Tables 12.1 and 12.2).[7] Because of this, the clinical indicators of these disorders are often broad-based, increasing the difficulty of diagnosis. To address this problem, analytical techniques including tandem mass spectrometry and genome analysis with association studies are being explored (Tables 12.3 and 12.4).

12.3 DISORDERS OF PURINE AND PYRIMIDINE METABOLISM

12.3.1 DISORDERS OF DE NOVO PURINE BIOSYNTHESIS

12.3.1.1 Phosphoribosylpyrophosphate synthetase 1 (PRS-1) deficiency

Abnormalities in PRS-1 enzyme activity or expression levels can result in several distinct disorders. In disorders of PRS-1 deficiency, disease severity is directly correlated to loss of enzymatic activity. The least severe PRS-1 deficiency is X-linked

Table 12.1 Clinical Features of Purine Disorders

Disease/Feature	Seizures	ID	Ataxia	SNHL	Gout/Stones	Lens Dislocation	SCID
Molybdenum cofactor disease	X	X				X	
Adenylosuccinase deficiency	X	X					
Lesch–Nyhan disease		X			X		
PRPS (superactivity-infantile form and deficiency Arts syndrome)	−/+	X	X	X	X		
APRT deficiency					X		
Xanthine oxidase deficiency					X		
ADA deficiency							X
PNP deficiency							X

Table 12.2 Clinical Features of Pyrimidine Disorders

Disorder/Feature	Megaloblastic Anemia	Immune Deficiency	ID	Seizures	GI Problems	Macrocephaly/Dysmorphic
UMP synthetase deficiency	X	X	X	X		
Dihydropyrimidine dehydrogenase deficiency[a]			X	X		X
Dihydropyrimidinase deficiency			X	X	X	
Ureidopropionase deficiency[a]			X	X		
Thymidine phosphorylase deficiency			X		X	

[a]Denotes conditions where the severity can be very broad.

Table 12.3 Analyte Abnormalities in Purine Disorders

Disease	Metabolites Present[a]
Molybdenum cofactor disease	Xanthine, hypoxanthine
Adenylosuccinase deficiency	Succinyladenosine
Lesch–Nyhan disease	Xanthine, hypoxanthine
PRPS deficiency	Low hypoxanthine
APRT	Adenine
Xanthinuria	Xanthine
Elevated Uric Acid	**Low Uric Acid**
Lesch–Nyhan disease	Molybdenum cofactor disease
PRPS superactivity	PRPS deficiency

[a]Table refers to elevated levels unless otherwise stated.

Table 12.4 Analyte Abnormalities in Pyrimidine Disorders

Disorder	Analyte Abnormalities
UMP synthetase deficiency	Orotic acid and orotidine
Dihydropyrimidine dehydrogenase deficiency	Uracil and thymine
Dihydropyrimidinase deficiency	Uracil, thymine, dihydrouracil, and dihydrothymine
β-Ureidopropionase deficiency	Dihydrouracil, dihydrothymine, urediopropionic, and uredioisobutyric
Thymidine phosphorylase deficiency	Thymidine and deoxyuridine

nonsyndromic sensorineural deafness (DFN2), followed by Charcot–Marie–Tooth disease X-5 (CMTX5) with the most severe being Arts syndrome where the phenotype includes intellectual disability, seizures, ataxia, peripheral neuropathy, optic atrophy, sensorineural hearing loss, and susceptibility to pulmonary infections.[9–11] In addition, pathogenic variants in the open reading frame of *PRPS1* result in superactivity of PRS-1. The dysregulation of purine metabolism results in a phenotype similar to that of enzyme deficiency, including intellectual disability and hearing loss. Currently, laboratory diagnostic methods are designed to quantify urine hypoxanthine, plasma uric acid, and erythrocyte guanosine-5′-triphosphate (GTP) and nicotinamide adenine dinucleotide (NAD) levels.

12.3.1.2 *Adenylosuccinate lyase (ADSL) deficiency*

Adenylosuccinate lyase (ADSL) is responsible for the conversion of succinylaminoimidazolecarboxamide (SAICA)-ribotide to AICA-ribotide and convert succinyl-AMP (adenosine monophosphate) to AMP.[12] Deficiency of ADSL can result in three different subtypes characterized by age on onset and disease severity.[13–15] The neonatal form presents with early-onset seizures, developmental delay, and microcephaly, whereas later onset forms may just have intellectual disability or autism. Diagnosis can be achieved by measurement of urine or cerebrospinal fluid (CSF) succinyladenosine or related compounds.

12.3.1.3 Inosine monophosphate dehydrogenase 1 (IMPDH1) deficiency

Inosine monophosphate dehydrogenase (IMPDH) oxidizes IMP to xanthosine-monophosphate. Defects in IMPDH1 are associated with Leber congenital amaurosis-11 and retinitis pigmentosa 10.[16] Measurement of IMP and guanosine monophosphate (GMP) in urine or other body fluids are used for diagnosis.

12.4 DISORDERS OF PURINE CATABOLISM

12.4.1 MYELOADENYLATE DEAMINASE (MADA) DEFICIENCY

A variant in the *AMPD1* gene that encodes myeloadenylate deaminase (MADA) (p.Gln12*) is found in about 12% of Caucasians. The majority of individuals who are homozygous for this allele are asymptomatic and this appears to be the result of alternate splicing of the gene. MADA converts the deamination of AMP to IMP and ammonia in skeletal muscle and plays an important role in purine nucleotide interconversions. The clinical phenotype of MADA includes exercise-induced muscle pain and rhabdomyolysis.[17] The diagnosis may be suspected because of a lack of rise in venous ammonia on the forearm ischemia test; definitive diagnosis required either DNA analysis or muscle biopsy for histochemical analysis of MADA.

12.4.2 ADENOSINE DEAMINASE 1 (ADA1) DEFICIENCY

ADA1 catalyzes deamination of nucleosides adenosine and deoxyadenosine to inosine and deoxyinosine, respectively. Deficiency of ADA1 results in early-onset severe combined immunodeficiency (SCID) and late-onset combined immune-deficiency clinical immune deterioration.[18] Increased activity of ADA1 is seen as a secondary phenomenon in Diamond–Blackfan anemia.[19] A diagnosis is made by finding increased levels of adenosine and deoxyadenosine in urine or through enzyme analysis.

12.4.3 ADENOSINE DEAMINASE 2 (ADA2) DEFICIENCY

Adenosine deaminase 2 (ADA2) is an isoform of ADA1 with lower substrate affinity.[20] ADA2 has been shown in model organisms to be a growth factor for the development and differentiation of both endothelial cells and leukocytes. ADA2 deficiency is characterized by a combination of vasculopathy and immune dysfunction. Signs and symptoms include intermittent fevers, early-onset lacunar strokes, livedoid rash (a mottled, reticulated rash in a vascular pattern), hepatosplenomegaly, hypogammaglobulinemia, and low immunoglobulin M (IgM) levels due to B-cell dysfunction and death.[21] Diagnosis may be achieved by DNA analysis.

12.4.4 PURINE NUCLEOSIDE PHOSPHORYLASE (PNP DEFICIENCY)

Purine nucleoside phosphorylase (PNP) is responsible for transforming inosine and guanosine and their deoxy counterparts to their respective bases, hypoxanthine and guanine. This results in overproduction of purine nucleosides. PNP deficiency is characterized by decreased T-cell function that results in immunodeficiency and intellectual disability is seen in about two-thirds of individuals.[22,23] Diagnostic biomarkers include elevations in inosine and guanosine in urine or other body fluids. Enzyme analysis may also be done. Newborn screening for SCID utilizing quantitative analysis of T-cell Receptor Excision Circles (TRECs) in newborn screening blood spots identifies individuals with PNP deficiency.

12.4.5 PURINE 5'-NUCLEOTIDASE DEFICIENCY

Purine nucleotidase converts IMP, AMP, and GMP to their corresponding nucleosides. Purine 5'-nucleotidase deficiency has a wide-ranging clinical presentation including behavioral problems, developmental delay/intellectual disability, seizures, ataxia, aggressive behavior, and recurrent infections of the sinuses and middle ear.[24] Purine nucleoside levels are normal but urinary urate concentration is low. DNA analysis is required for confirmation of the diagnosis.

12.4.6 XANTHINE OXIDASE/DEHYDROGENASE (XOD) DEFICIENCY

Xanthine oxidase/dehydrogenase (XOD) converts xanthine to urate. Primary deficiency of XOD is also known as type I xanthinuria. In XOD deficiency, xanthine precipitates in urine as crystals and forms renal stones. Symptoms in infancy include irritability and hematuria; older individuals have symptoms related to renal stones, including pain, hematuria, and urinary tract infections, and ultimately chronic renal failure may occur. Diagnosis is made by finding high levels of xanthine and hypoxanthine in urine.

12.4.7 MOLYBDENUM COFACTOR (MoCo) DEFICIENCY

Molybdenum cofactor (MoCo) deficiency, also known as type III xanthinuria, is characterized by deficiency of xanthine sulfite and aldehyde oxidases.[25,26] Molybdenum cofactor synthase (MOCS1), molybdopterin synthase (MOCS2), and gephyrin protein (GPHN) are involved in the processing of the cofactor molybdenum and have been implicated in MoCo deficiency. Infants with MoCo deficiency present with complex neonatal seizures, microcephaly, developmental brain abnormalities, and severe hypotonia. There is often a rapid decline that results in neonatal death. Those that survive have lens dislocation.[27] Analysis of urine reveals significant elevations in xanthine, hypoxanthine, and S-sulfocysteine. Total plasma homocysteine is typically low.

12.5 DISORDERS OF THE PURINE SALVAGE PATHWAY

12.5.1 HYPOXANTHINE-GUANINE PHOSPHORIBOSYL TRANSFERASE (HPRT) DEFICIENCY

HPRT converts hypoxanthine to IMP and guanine to GMP. Defects of HPRT are responsible for Lesch–Nyhan syndrome and HPRT-related gout.[28–30] Lesch–Nyhan syndrome is characterized by hyperuricemia, psychomotor delay, dystonia, progressive neurologic decline, self-mutilation, increase aggressiveness, and megaloblastic anemia. Full-scale IQ is generally in the 60–70 range, which is higher than one might expect given the seizures and self-mutilation. Milder forms of HPRT deficiency present with adult-onset gout, dystonia, spasticity, dysarthria, and spinocerebellar ataxia; they may also have mild cognitive problems. Diagnostic biomarkers include more commonly urine but also plasma levels of uric acid, hypoxanthine, and xanthine.

12.5.2 ADENINE PHOSPHORIBOSYL TRANSFERASE (APRT) DEFICIENCY

APRT converts adenine to AMP. APRT deficiency results in dihydroxyadeninuria type I and II. Clinical presentations of these disorders include nephrolithiasis, crystalluria, and renal failure due to the crystallization and precipitation of 2,8-dihydroxyadenine.[31] Diagnostic biomarkers include urinary adenine.

12.5.3 ADENOSINE KINASE (ADK) DEFICIENCY

Adenosine kinase (ADK) phosphorylates adenosine to AMP. Clinical presentations of ADK deficiency include global developmental delay that gradually gets progressively worse, early-onset seizures, mild dysmorphic features, and hypermethioninemia.[32] Diagnostic biomarkers include plasma and CSF methionine, S-adenosyl methionine (SAMe) and S-adenosyl homocysteine (SAH), and urine adenosine.

12.5.4 S-ADENOSYL HOMOCYSTEINE HYDROLASE (SAHH) DEFICIENCY

S-adenosyl homocysteine hydrolase (SAHH) deficiency is due to abnormal methionine metabolism and presents with growth failure, mental and motor retardation that is slowly progressive, facial dysmorphism with abnormal hair and teeth, and cardiomyopathy.[32] Diagnostic biomarkers include methionine, SAH, and SAMe.

12.5.5 ADENYLATE KINASE 1 (AMPK1) DEFICIENCY

Adenylate kinase (AMPK) controls the interconversion of adenine nucleotides.[33] AMPK deficiency presents with nonspherocytic hemolytic anemia with possible intellectual delay or psychomotor impairment.

12.5.6 ADENYLATE KINASE 2 (AK2) DEFICIENCY

Adenylate kinase (AK2) catalyzes the conversion of adenosine triphosphate (ATP) to adenosine diphosphate (ADP).[34] Most cells express both AK1 and AK2 with the exception of cells in the reticuloendothelial system and inner ear, which only express AK2. Individuals with AK2 deficiency have hypoplasia of thymic and other lymphoid tissue that results in absence of both lymphoid tissue and granulocytes in peripheral blood resulting in SCID. Sensorineural hearing loss is also seen.

12.5.7 DEOXYGUANOSINE KINASE (DGUOK) DEFICIENCY

Deoxyguanosine kinase (DGUOK) converts deoxyguanosine to deoxy-GMP and provides precursors for mitochondrial DNA biosynthesis.[35–37] The mitochondrial DNA depletion in DGUOK deficiency typically results in early-onset progressive liver failure, developmental delay, hypoglycemia, and increased lactate in body fluids. Increased hepatic iron levels have been reported and may lead to a misdiagnosis of neonatal hemochromatosis.

12.6 DISORDERS OF URIC ACID TRANSPORT

12.6.1 UROMODULIN (UMOD); RENIN (REN); HEPATOCYTE NUCLEAR FACTOR-1-BETA (HNF1B) DEFICIENCIES

Uromodulin (UMOD), renin (REN), and hepatocyte nuclear factor-1-beta (HNF1B) are all involved in urate transport.[38–41] Haploinsufficiency of any of these proteins is associated with juvenile onset hyperuricemia, gout, and progressive renal failure. The diagnostic biomarker for these defects is elevated serum uric acid.

12.7 DISORDERS OF DE NOVO OF PYRIMIDINE BIOSYNTHESIS

12.7.1 DIHYDROOROTATE DEHYDROGENASE (DHODH) DEFICIENCY

DHODH converts dihydroorotate (DHO) to OA. DHODH deficiency causes Miller syndrome, a condition with severe micrognathia, cleft lip, eyelid colobomas, supernumerary nipples, and ulnar ray developmental defects.[42] Diagnostic biomarkers include urine orotic acid and plasma dihydroorotate.

12.7.2 URIDINE MONOPHOSPHATE SYNTHASE (UMPS) DEFICIENCY

Hereditary orotic aciduria is caused by the deficiency of uridine monophosphate synthase (UMPS). UMPS is a bifunctional enzyme consisting of orotate phosphoribosyltransferase and orotidine-5-monophosphate decarboxylase. UMPS catalyzes conversion of orotate to uridine monophosphate. The initial presenting findings are macrocytic anemia that is refractory to folic acid and vitamin B12 treatment. If not diagnosed and properly treated, growth, and developmental delays ensue.[43] Diagnostic biomarkers include urine orotic acid and orotidine.

12.8 DISORDERS OF PYRIMIDINE CATABOLISM

12.8.1 THYMIDINE PHOSPHORYLASE (TP) DEFICIENCY

Deficiency of thymidine phosphorylase causes *mi*tochondrial *n*eurogastro*i*ntestinal *e*ncephalopathy (MNGIE) disease. Thymidine phosphorylase (TP) catalyzes the breakdown of pyrimidine nucleosides deoxythymidine and deoxyuridine to thymine and uracil. Clinical presentations include ptosis, progressive external ophthalmoplegia (PEO), gastrointestinal dysmotility, cachexia, diffuse leukoencephalopathy, peripheral neuropathy, and mitochondrial dysfunction. The age of onset is in the teenage to early adulthood years. Muscle biopsy may reveal ragged red fibers, decreased cytochrome c oxidase activity, and other histochemical and enzymatic evidence of respiratory chain dysfunction.[44] Diagnostic biomarkers include increased urinary and plasma thymidine (Tables 12.2 and 12.4).

12.8.2 DIHYDROPYRIMIDINE DEHYDROGENASE (DPD) DEFICIENCY

Dihydropyrimidine dehydrogenase (DPD) converts uracil and thymine to dihydrouracil and dihydrothymine. DPD deficiency presents with seizures with delayed motor development and intellectual disability.[45] Diagnostic biomarkers include plasma and urinary thymine and uracil.

12.8.3 DIHYDROPYRIMIDINASE HYDROLASE (DPH) DEFICIENCY

Dihydropyrimidinase hydrolase (DPH) converts dihydrouracil and dihydrothymine to β-ureidopropionate and β-ureidoisobutyrate. DPH deficiency presents with seizures and developmental delay/intellectual disability; some also have growth retardation and microcephaly.[46] Diagnostic biomarkers include thymine, uracil, dihydrouracil, and dihydrothymine.

12.8.4 β-UREIDOPROPIONASE (βUP) DEFICIENCY

β-ureidopropionase (βUP) converts β-ureidopropionate and β-ureidoisobutyrate to β-alanine and β-aminoisobutyric acid, respectively. βUP deficiency presents with developmental brain abnormalities, including white matter disease, seizures, intellectual disability, developmental defects of the eyes (microphthalmia, hypoplasia of the optic nerves and retinal degeneration), and genitourinary malformations.[47] Diagnostic biomarkers include elevated plasma and urine, uracil, and thymine.

12.8.5 URIDINE MONOPHOSPHATE HYDROLASE 1 (UMPH1) DEFICIENCY

Uridine monophosphate hydrolase 1 (UMPH1) catalyzes the dephosphorylation of UMP and cytidine monophosphate (CMP) to their corresponding nucleosides. UMPH1 deficiency presents with mild-to-moderate hemolytic anemia with reticulocytosis; peripheral smear reveals basophilic stippling due to the accumulation of high concentrations of pyrimidine nucleotides within the erythrocyte.[48] Diagnostic biomarkers include erythrocytic pyrimidine nucleotides.

12.9 DISORDERS OF THE PYRIMIDINE SALVAGE PATHWAY

12.9.1 THYMIDINE KINASE 2 (TK2) DEFICIENCY

Thymidine kinase 2 (TK2) is responsible for the phosphorylation of deoxythymidine. TK2 deficiency is characterized by impaired mtDNA replication and thus, represents a mitochondrial DNA depletion syndrome.[49,50] Clinical presentations in include early-onset muscle weakness associated with depletion of mtDNA in skeletal muscle.

12.10 BIOMARKERS FOR DETECTION OF PURINE AND PYRIMIDINE METABOLISM

The decision to investigate for inborn errors of purine and pyrimidine metabolism is often difficult to make, even for the most attentive clinician. This diagnostic dilemma exist because of the lack of awareness, varied clinical presentations of associated disorders, and unavailability of proper analytical resources.[51] Currently, the majority of diagnoses are accomplished by analyzing urinary excretion profiles. When urine is not available, blood and CSF may be used for testing but are not as reliable due to lower concentrations of diagnostic compounds.[52] In addition, tissue-specific enzymatic-based assays offer another investigative opinion.

12.11 URINE AND PLASMA URIC ACID

Measurement of the concentration of uric acid, the end-product of purine metabolism, in urine or plasma is the primary indicator for many disorders. Significantly elevated or reduced uric acid concentration may indicate several disorders of purine metabolism including HPRT, XOD, PNP deficiencies, PRS-1 superactivity, familial juvenile hyperuricemia nephropathy (FJHN), and hereditary renal hypouricemia.[4] Accurate diagnosis is dependent on the establishment of control ranges for both adults and children with considerations for diet and sample handling. It should also be noted that children have a higher uric acid clearance and therefore, may have normal uric acid levels despite purine overproduction.[7] Renal dysfunction may lead to false negatives when analytical testing is correlated to creatinine concentrations. Once a correct diagnosis is achieved, confirmation by enzymatic or DNA testing may be employed to confirm a specific diagnosis. However, uric acid concentration is not exclusively correlated with purine disorders, therefore elevations should always be followed up while normal uric acid levels do not rule out a possible purine disorder.[2]

12.12 URINE PURINE AND PYRIMIDINE PROFILES

Nucleotides cannot be directly measured since they do not ordinarily exist outside of the cell. To test for perturbations of purine and pyrimidine metabolism, associated nucleosides and bases are targeted. This is possible because intracellular nucleotides are broken down into nucleosides and then excreted in urine. Owing to this phenomena, analysis of urinary excretion profiles can be used for the diagnosis of most of these disorders and is preferred over plasma and CSF.[53] A classic example of this is adenylosuccinate lyase deficiency, which is diagnosed by the detection of the elevated nucleosides succinyladenosine and SAICA-riboside in urine, a result of the accumulation of nucleotides, succinyl-AMP and SAICA-ribotide, in the cell. To accurately assess purine and pyrimidine levels, a variety of techniques are used including high-performance liquid chromatography (HPLC) with diode array UV detection, thin-layer chromatography (TLC), proton nuclear magnetic resonance (H-NMR), gas chromatography–mass spectrometry (GC/MS) and liquid chromatography–tandem mass spectrometry (LC/MS/MS).

12.13 BRIEF DESCRIPTION OF TREATMENT

Fundamentally, therapeutic efforts for inborn errors of purine and pyrimidine metabolism should be focused on preventing the accumulation of toxic compounds or replacing those that are deficient. Theoretically, this can be accomplished through pharmaceutical manipulation of biosynthesis or recycling, or through gene therapy.[4,54] Unfortunately, because purine and pyrimidine metabolism is involved in such diverse physiological roles, this has been proven difficult. Of the more than 30 known associated defects, only a small number of them have treatments with bone marrow transplantation or enzyme replacement for ADA and PNP deficiency, allopurinol for adenine phosphoribosyl transferase deficiency and uridine for orotic aciduria.[4] Because of limited therapeutic options, clinical symptoms are often targeted. For patients with ADA or PNP deficiency, bone marrow transplantation is effective.[55,56] This reduces levels of toxic nucleosides and nucleotides by providing B- and T-cells with supplemental enzymatic function. Another treatment option for these patients has been enzyme replacement therapy with bovine ADA complexed with polyethylene glycol. Attempts at gene therapy for ADA-deficient patients has had limited success in the past but a new treatment, Strimvelis, shows great promise.[57] Patients with a deficiency of XDH (xanthinuria type I), APRT, FJHN, HPRT or partial HPRT (HPRT with neurological dysfunction (HRND), HPRT-related hyperuricemia (HRH)), or patients with a superactivity of *PRPS1* should be treated by inhibiting xanthine oxidase with allopurinol, which decreases the production of uric acid leading to accumulation of more soluble compounds, xanthine and hypoxanthine. Further treatment measures may include dietary restrictions and treatment with bicarbonate or citrate for the alkalinization of the urine.[4] It should be noted that the neurological and behavioral features of HPRT deficiency are not affected by allopurinol and must be addressed separately. Specifically, patients may require muscle relaxants, removal of teeth, and/or physical restraints to prevent self-injurious behavior.[3] AMP deaminase-deficient patients are reported to benefit from ribose treatment to improve loss of muscular strength and endurance.[58] Treatment of UMP synthase deficiency with uridine by-passes the enzyme defect but should be monitored to obtain minimal orotic acid production.[4] As previously mentioned, therapeutic options are limited and ongoing research and development is needed to address this group of disorders.

12.14 CONFOUNDING CONDITIONS

The most commonly identified confounding conditions are disorders of the urea cycle that result in elevated urinary orotic acid levels. The differentiating factor for the pyrimidine disorders is the lack of hyperammonemia and the very high levels of orotic acid in the urine. Diets high in purines (liver, game meats, some nuts) can result in subsequent increases in purines and their derivatives, including uric acid. Medications and vitamins that can lead to increases in urinary purine excretion include allopurinol and niacin. Uric acid may also be elevated in glycogen storage disease Ia/Ib, fructose-1-6 bisphosphatase deficiency, fatty acid oxidation disorders, and other conditions with lactic acidemia. Circulating purines and pyrimidines (uric acid, hypoxanthine, uridine) have been reported in individuals suffering from multiple sclerosis.[59] Low levels of uric acid may be seen in renal Fanconi syndrome, while elevated levels of purines and pyrimidines may be identified in renal failure. High levels of uric acid can be seen in patients on thiazide diuretics, aspirin, cytotoxic agents, and cyclosporine.[60]

12.15 CONCLUSIONS

Inborn errors of purine and pyrimidine metabolism are a diverse group of disorders that may present with a wide range of phenotypes but neurologic abnormalities, hematologic abnormalities, and nephrolithiasis/gout are recurring features of these disorders. Owing to their broad spectrum of clinical presentations, rarity, and lack of a general biomarker of disease, they can often be diagnostically challenging. These characteristics have led to their largely unknown prevalence in the general population. This in itself is problematic as early recognition is critical for treatment that may be lifesaving or have the potential to increase the quality of life for affected individuals with many of these disorders. For certain disorders, metabolites such as uric acid that is widely available in clinical diagnostic labs, may provide a clue to pursue diagnostic evaluation for purine disorders; however, many of the disorders have no such "common biomarker" and measurement of specific purine and pyrimidine analytes in biological fluids is necessary for diagnosis. It is important for the clinician and laboratorian to be aware of the phenotypes of these diverse disorders and perform diagnostic testing for individuals whose clinical phenotype is consistent with perturbed purine and/or pyrimidine metabolism.

REFERENCES

1. Kelley RE, Andersson HC. Disorders of purines and pyrimidines. *Handb Clin Neurol* 2014;**120**:827–38.
2. Cameron JS, Moro F, Simmonds HA. Gout, uric acid and purine metabolism in paediatric nephrology. *Pediatr Nephrol* 1993;**7**(1):105–18.
3. van Gennip AH, van Kuilenburg AB. Defects of pyrimidine degradation: clinical, molecular and diagnostic aspects. *Adv Exp Med Biol* 2000;**486**:233–41.
4. Jurecka A. Inborn errors of purine and pyrimidyne metabolism. *Postepy Biochem* 2011;**57**(2):172–82.
5. Berg MTJ, Stryer L. Biosynthesis of nucleotides. *Biochemistry* 2002:602–26.
6. Bakker JA, Bierau J. Purine and pyrimidine metabolism: still more to learn. *Ned Tijdschr Klin Chem Labgeneesk* 2012;**37**:3–6.
7. Simmonds HA, Duley JA, Fairbanks LD, McBride MB. When to investigate for purine and pyrimidine disorders. Introduction and review of clinical and laboratory indications. *J Inherit Metab Dis* 1997;**20**(2):214–26.
8. Jurecka A, Zikanova M, Tylki-Szymanska A, et al. Clinical, biochemical and molecular findings in seven Polish patients with adenylosuccinate lyase deficiency. *Mol Genet Metab* 2008;**94**(4):435–42.
9. de Brouwer AP, Williams KL, Duley JA, et al. Arts syndrome is caused by loss-of-function mutations in PRPS1. *Am J Hum Genet* 2007;**81**(3):507–18.
10. Maruyama K, Ogaya S, Kurahashi N, et al. Arts syndrome with a novel missense mutation in the PRPS1 gene: a case report. *Brain Dev* 2016;**38**(10):954–8.
11. Synofzik M, Muller vom Hagen J, Haack TB, et al. X-linked Charcot-Marie-Tooth disease, Arts syndrome, and prelingual non-syndromic deafness form a disease continuum: evidence from a family with a novel PRPS1 mutation. *Orphanet J Rare Diseases* 2014;**9**:24.
12. Fernandes J. *Inborn metabolic diseases: diagnosis and treatment*. Heidelberg: Springer; 2006.
13. Mouchegh K, Zikanova M, Hoffmann GF, et al. Lethal fetal and early neonatal presentation of adenylosuccinate lyase deficiency: observation of 6 patients in 4 families. *J Pediatr* 2007;**150**(1):57–61.e2.
14. Spiegel EK, Colman RF, Patterson D. Adenylosuccinate lyase deficiency. *Mol Genet Metab* 2006;**89**(1–2):19–31.
15. Lundy CT, Jungbluth H, Pohl KR, et al. Adenylosuccinate lyase deficiency in the United Kingdom pediatric population: first three cases. *Pediatr Neurol* 2010;**43**(5):351–4.
16. Bowne SJ, Sullivan LS, Mortimer SE, et al. Spectrum and frequency of mutations in IMPDH1 associated with autosomal dominant retinitis pigmentosa and leber congenital amaurosis. *Invest Ophthalmol Vis Sci* 2006;**47**(1):34–42.
17. Morisaki T, Gross M, Morisaki H, Pongratz D, Zollner N, Holmes EW. Molecular basis of AMP deaminase deficiency in skeletal muscle. *Proc Natl Acad Sci USA* 1992;**89**(14):6457–61.
18. Arredondo-Vega FX, Santisteban I, Daniels S, Toutain S, Hershfield MS. Adenosine deaminase deficiency: genotype-phenotype correlations based on expressed activity of 29 mutant alleles. *Am J Hum Genet* 1998;**63**(4):1049–59.
19. Cowan MJ, Brady RO, Widder KJ. Elevated erythrocyte adenosine deaminase activity in patients with acquired immunodeficiency syndrome. *Proc Natl Acad Sci USA* 1986;**83**(4):1089–91.

20. Zhou Q, Yang D, Ombrello AK, et al. Early-onset stroke and vasculopathy associated with mutations in ADA2. *N Engl J Med* 2014;**370**(10):911–20.

21. Woollard KJ, Geissmann F. Monocytes in atherosclerosis: subsets and functions. *Nat Rev Cardiol* 2010;**7**(2):77–86.

22. Camici M, Micheli V, Ipata PL, Tozzi MG. Pediatric neurological syndromes and inborn errors of purine metabolism. *Neurochem Int* 2010;**56**(3):367–78.

23. Giblett ER, Ammann AJ, Wara DW, Sandman R, Diamond LK. Nucleoside-phosphorylase deficiency in a child with severely defective T-cell immunity and normal B-cell immunity. *Lancet* 1975;**1**(7914):1010–3.

24. Page T, Yu A, Fontanesi J, Nyhan WL. Developmental disorder associated with increased cellular nucleotidase activity. *Proc Natl Acad Sci USA* 1997;**94**(21):11601–6.

25. Raivio KO, Saksela M, Lapatto R. Xanthine oxidoreductase: role in human pathophysiology and in hereditary xanthinuria. 2001.

26. Ichida K, Matsumura T, Sakuma R, Hosoya T, Nishino T. Mutation of human molybdenum cofactor sulfurase gene is responsible for classical xanthinuria type II. *Biochem Biophys Res Commun* 2001;**282**(5):1194–200.

27. Reiss J, Hahnewald R. Molybdenum cofactor deficiency: mutations in GPHN, MOCS1, and MOCS2. *Hum Mutat* 2011;**32**(1):10–18.

28. Kelley WN, Rosenbloom FM, Henderson JF, Seegmiller JE. A specific enzyme defect in gout associated with overproduction of uric acid. *Proc Natl Acad Sci USA* 1967;**57**(6):1735–9.

29. Yamada Y. Deficiencies of hypoxanthine guanine phosphoribosyltransferase (HPRT). *Nihon Rinsho* 2008;**66**(4):687–93.

30. Nguyen KV, Naviaux RK, Paik KK, Nyhan WL. Novel mutations in the human HPRT gene. *Nucleosides Nucleotides Nucleic Acids* 2011;**30**(6):440–5.

31. Bollee G, Dollinger C, Boutaud L, et al. Phenotype and genotype characterization of adenine phosphoribosyltransferase deficiency. *J Am Soc Nephrol* 2010;**21**(4):679–88.

32. Bjursell MK, Blom HJ, Cayuela JA, et al. Adenosine kinase deficiency disrupts the methionine cycle and causes hypermethioninemia, encephalopathy, and abnormal liver function. *Am J Hum Genet* 2011;**89**(4):507–15.

33. Toren A, Brok-Simoni F, Ben-Bassat I, et al. Congenital haemolytic anaemia associated with adenylate kinase deficiency. *Br J Haematol* 1994;**87**(2):376–80.

34. Noma T. Dynamics of nucleotide metabolism as a supporter of life phenomena. *J Med Invest* 2005;**52**(3–4):127–36.

35. Spinazzola A, Invernizzi F, Carrara F, et al. Clinical and molecular features of mitochondrial DNA depletion syndromes. *J Inher Metab Dis* 2009;**32**(2):143–58.

36. Dimmock DP, Zhang Q, Dionisi-Vici C, et al. Clinical and molecular features of mitochondrial DNA depletion due to mutations in deoxyguanosine kinase. *Hum Mutat* 2008;**29**(2):330–1.

37. Al-Hussaini A, Faqeih E, El-Hattab AW, et al. Clinical and molecular characteristics of mitochondrial DNA depletion syndrome associated with neonatal cholestasis and liver failure. *J Pediatr* 2014;**164**(3):553–559.e1-2.

38. Bollee G, Dahan K, Flamant M, et al. Phenotype and outcome in hereditary tubulointerstitial nephritis secondary to UMOD mutations. *Clin J Am Soc Nephrol* 2011;**6**(10): 2429–38.

39. Zivna M, Hulkova H, Matignon M, et al. Dominant renin gene mutations associated with early-onset hyperuricemia, anemia, and chronic kidney failure. *Am J Hum Genet* 2009;**85**(2):204–13.

40. Piret SE, Danoy P, Dahan K, et al. Genome-wide study of familial juvenile hyperuricaemic (gouty) nephropathy (FJHN) indicates a new locus, FJHN3, linked to chromosome 2p22.1-p21. *Hum Genet* 2011;**129**(1):51–8.

41. Horikawa Y, Iwasaki N, Hara M, et al. Mutation in hepatocyte nuclear factor-1 beta gene (TCF2) associated with MODY. *Nat Genet* 1997;**17**(4):384–5.

42. Ng SB, Buckingham KJ, Lee C, et al. Exome sequencing identifies the cause of a mendelian disorder. *Nat Genet* 2010;**42**(1):30–5.

43. Bailey CJ. Orotic aciduria and uridine monophosphate synthase: a reappraisal. *J Inherit Metab Dis* 2009;**32**(Suppl. 1):S227–33.

44. Fairbanks LD, Marinaki AM, Carrey EA, Hammans SR, Duley JA. Deoxyuridine accumulation in urine in thymidine phosphorylase deficiency (MNGIE). *J Inherit Metab Dis* 2002;**25**(7):603–4.

45. Van Kuilenburg AB, Vreken P, Abeling NG, et al. Genotype and phenotype in patients with dihydropyrimidine dehydrogenase deficiency. *Hum Genet* 1999;**104**(1):1–9.

46. van Kuilenburg AB, Dobritzsch D, Meijer J, et al. Dihydropyrimidinase deficiency: phenotype, genotype and structural consequences in 17 patients. *Biochim Biophys Acta* 2010;**1802**(7–8):639–48.

47. van Kuilenburg AB, Dobritzsch D, Meijer J, et al. ss-ureidopropionase deficiency: phenotype, genotype and protein structural consequences in 16 patients. *Biochim Biophys Acta* 2012;**1822**(7):1096–108.

48. Rees DC, Duley J, Simmonds HA, et al. Interaction of hemoglobin E and pyrimidine 5′ nucleotidase deficiency. *Blood* 1996;**88**(7):2761–7.

49. Oskoui M, Davidzon G, Pascual J, et al. Clinical spectrum of mitochondrial DNA depletion due to mutations in the thymidine kinase 2 gene. *Arch Neurol* 2006;**63**(8):1122–6.

50. Mancuso M, Salviati L, Sacconi S, et al. Mitochondrial DNA depletion: mutations in thymidine kinase gene with myopathy and SMA. *Neurology* 2002;**59**(8):1197–202.

51. Valik D, Jones JD. Hereditary disorders of purine and pyrimidine metabolism: identification of their biochemical phenotypes in the clinical laboratory. *Mayo Clin Proc* 1997;**72**(8):719–25.

52. Duran M, Dorland L, Wadman SK, Berger R. Group tests for selective screening of inborn errors of metabolism. *Eur J Pediatr* 1994;**153**(7 Suppl. 1):S27–32.

53. Strange RC. *Techniques in diagnostic human biochemical genetics: a laboratory manual.* Amsterdam: Elsevier B.V.; 1992;280–1.

54. Torres-Torronteras J, Gomez A, Eixarch H, et al. Hematopoietic gene therapy restores thymidine phosphorylase activity in a cell culture and a murine model of MNGIE. *Gene Ther* 2011;**18**(8):795–806.

55. Carpenter PA, Ziegler JB, Vowels MR. Late diagnosis and correction of purine nucleoside phosphorylase deficiency with allogeneic bone marrow transplantation. *Bone Marrow Transplant* 1996;**17**(1):121–4.

56. Cicalese MP, Ferrua F, Castagnaro L, et al. Update on the safety and efficacy of retroviral gene therapy for immunodeficiency due to adenosine deaminase deficiency. *Blood* 2016.

57. Tartibi HM, Hershfield MS, Bahna SL. A 24-year enzyme replacement therapy in an adenosine-deaminase-deficient patient. *Pediatrics* 2016;**137**(1).

58. Wagner DR, Gresser U, Zollner N. Effects of oral ribose on muscle metabolism during bicycle ergometer in AMPD-deficient patients. *Ann Nutr Metab* 1991;**35**(5):297–302.

59. Tavazzi B, Batocchi AP, Amorini AM, et al. Serum metabolic profile in multiple sclerosis patients. *Mult Scler Int* 2011;**2011**:167156.

60. Scott JT. Drug-induced gout. *Bailliere's Clin Rheumatol* 1991;**5**(1):39–60.

Biomarkers for the study of catecholamine and serotonin genetic diseases

13

A. Ormazabal, M. Molero-Luis, A. Garcia-Cazorla and R. Artuch

Hospital Sant Joan de Déu, Barcelona, Spain

13.1 BRIEF DESCRIPTION OF THE DISORDER AND PATHWAY

The neurotransmitter family is varied and includes inhibitory amino acids (gamma-aminobutyric acid (GABA) and glycine), excitatory amino acids (aspartate and glutamate), acetylcholine, monoamines (adrenaline, noradrenaline, dopamine, and serotonin), and purines (adenosine and adenosine mono-, di-, and triphosphate), among others. Several genetic diseases affecting metabolism and function of these neurotransmitters have been reported in the last decades. In this chapter, we will focus on the laboratory biomarkers of the serotonin and catecholamine genetic defects, including those affecting its metabolism (biosynthesis and catabolism of monoamines and of its obligatory cofactor tetrahydrobiopterin (BH_4)) and transport of dopamine.

Serotonin and catecholamines are involved in motor, perceptual, cognitive, and emotional brain functions, as well as in some other functions such as vascular tone, temperature, endocrine system, or swallowing regulation.[1] The pathways involved in their synthesis are shown in Fig. 13.1. The amino acids tyrosine and tryptophan are the precursors of dopamine and serotonin, respectively. After a common rate-limiting enzymatic step catalyzed by two hydroxylases dependent on BH_4, L-dopa, and 5-hydroxytryptophan are synthesized. Then, after a common decarboxylation step catalyzed by L-aromatic amino acid decarboxylase (whose cofactor is pyridoxal-phosphate), the active neurotransmitters dopamine and serotonin are formed. Finally, several catabolic steps lead to the generation of the main end-stable metabolites homovanillic (HVA) and 5-hydroxyindoleacetic (5-HIAA) acids, which are the most useful biomarkers for diagnosis. Other active compounds are also synthesized from serotonin and dopamine, such as melatonin or catecholamines (Fig. 13.1). Ten disorders of monoamine metabolism and two in monoamine transport will be discussed.[1] Of the 10 genetic conditions related to monoamine metabolism, 2 specifically affect

BIOCHEMICAL PATHWAYS OF NEUROTRANSMITTERS AND PTERINS

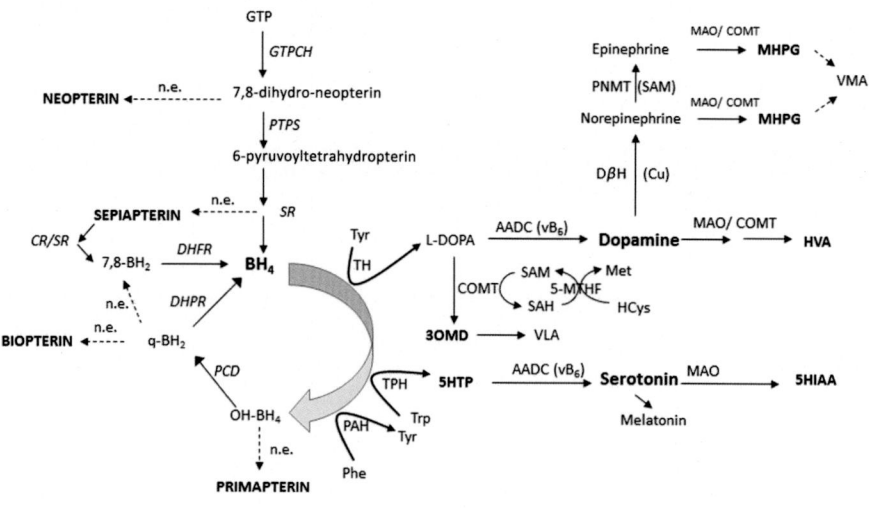

FIGURE 13.1

Metabolic pathways for the synthesis and catabolism of monoamines and pterins. The key metabolites for neurotransmitters and pterins are marked in bold and capital letters. Enzymes appear in italics.

biosynthesis of catecholamines: Tyrosine hydroxylase deficiency (TH: MIM *191290) impairs synthesis of dihydroxyphenylalanine (L-dopa)-causing dopamine deficiency and a neurological disease with prominent extrapyramidal signs;[2] and dopamine-β-hydroxylase deficiency (DBH: MIM *609312), which impairs catecholamine biosynthesis (epinephrine and norepinephrine), with its clinical hallmark of severe orthostatic hypotension with sympathetic failure.[3] Two other disorders of monoamine metabolism involve both catecholamine and serotonin metabolism: Aromatic L-amino acid decarboxylase deficiency (AADC: MIM *107930) is located upstream of the neurotransmitter amines and causes a combined deficiency of dopamine and serotonin that leads to a complex clinical picture that may include muscle hypotonia, oculogyric crises, movement disorders, and autonomic features (excessive sweating and temperature instability),[4] and the X-linked monoamine oxidase-A deficiency (MAO-A: MIM *309850), located downstream from dopamine and serotonin, which is the only defect in monoamine catabolism, that causes isolated severe behavioral disturbances.[5]

BH₄ is synthesized from guanosine-5′-triphosphate (GTP) in a three-step reaction involving GTP cyclohydrolase I (GTPCH-I), 6-pyruvoyltetrahydropterin synthase, and sepiapterin reductase (SR). The BH₄ salvage pathway is also important, and includes pterin 4-alpha carbinolamine dehydratase and dihydropteridine reductase (DHPR) enzymes (Fig. 13.1). There are six defects in BH₄ cofactor biosynthesis, the essential coenzyme for both serotonin and catecholamine generation in the rate-limiting enzymatic step of tyrosine and tryptophan hydroxylation (Fig. 13.1): the dominant form of GTPCH-I deficiency (MIM *600225)[6] and the recessively inherited SR deficiency (MIM *182125)[7] that cause mainly movement disorders, with different degrees of serotonin-related clinical disturbances. BH_4 is also required in the liver for the conversion of phenylalanine to tyrosine in a reaction catalyzed by phenylalanine hydroxylase, and, for this reason, several defects affecting BH_4 metabolism lead to hyperphenylalaninemia (PKU (phenylketonuria)) because of BH_4 deficiency. These include recessively inherited GTPCH-I, 6-pyruvoyltetrahydropterin synthase (PTPS), pterin 4-alpha carbinolamine dehydratase (PCD), and DHPR deficiencies.[1] These defects also present alterations in biogenic amines in the central nervous system, but they can be detected in neonatal screening programs by means of phenylalanine quantification in Guthrie cards.

In the last years, two genetic conditions affecting synaptic transporter functions have been reported, opening a new avenue in the research of monoamine deficiencies: the dopamine transporter 1 (DAT1: MIM *126455) deficiency[8] and the vesicular monoamine transporter type 2 (VMAT2: MIM *193001) defect,[9] both causing early Parkinsonism-dystonia. DAT1 removes dopamine from the synaptic cleft, thereby terminating its action on post- and presynaptic receptors. VMAT2 translocates dopamine and serotonin into synaptic vesicles and is essential for the correct functions of biogenic amines.

13.2 BRIEF DESCRIPTION OF TREATMENT

Different treatment approaches have been trialed for the above-mentioned genetic diseases. Since the pathophysiology of the disorders differs, treatment strategies must be necessarily different. In general, some of the diseases may respond well to therapy, and the clinical outcome may be, in some cases, excellent. Unfortunately, for most of the monoamine diseases, treatment is not fully effective and new therapeutic approaches must be investigated.[10]

TH deficiency can be treated with L-dopa in combination with an L-dopa decarboxylase inhibitor, with the rationale to restore brain dopamine values. The response is variable, ranging from complete remission to mild improvement of signs and symptoms.[11] Therapy should be started with low doses to prevent dyskinesia, which may be successfully treated with amantadine.[12] Treatment of AADC deficiency is aimed at stimulating residual AADC activity, stimulating postsynaptic receptors, or preventing degradation of the limited neurotransmitters that are produced.[13] Various strategies have been used, including cofactor supplementation (pyridoxal-phosphate), MAO inhibitors, high-dose L-dopa as "substrate therapy," serotoninergic agents, or combinations of these and anticholinergic drugs. Treatment may be beneficial, but the effects are limited, and long-term prognosis is poor. In fact, only some patients with relatively mild forms clearly improved on a combined therapy with pyridoxal-phosphate, dopamine agonists, and monoamine oxidase B inhibitors.[14] Gene therapy is being tested with promising results.[1] Concerning DBH deficiency, therapy with

L-dihydroxyphenylserine (L-Dops) is available. This compound can be directly converted by AADC into noradrenaline, thereby bypassing the defective enzyme. The prognosis on therapy is satisfactory to good.[15] For MAO-A deficiency, no effective treatment is known at present. In the case of transportopathies, the experience is very limited because they are recently discovered and extremely rare diseases. For DAT1 deficiency, the clinical picture shows progressive Parkinsonism-dystonia that is medically refractory.[8] In VMAT2, treatment with L-dopa was associated with worsening, whereas dopamine agonists may improve the symptoms.[9]

The best examples of a good clinical response to treatment are those of BH$_4$ disturbances, especially the dominant form of GTPCH-I deficiency. Patients have been treated successfully with a combination of low doses of L-dopa and a dopa decarboxylase inhibitor. In general, there is normally a complete or near-complete response of motor problems soon after the start of the therapy. In cases of action dystonia and adult-onset cases, L-dopa does not always show complete effects.[1] For SR, therapeutic approaches involve dopamine and serotonin precursor supplementation, and most patients respond well to L-dopa and 5-hydroxytryptophan combination.[16] For the BH$_4$ defects causing PKU (recessively inherited GTPCH-I, PTPS, PCD, and DHPR deficiencies) current treatments include the combination of L-dopa and 5-hydroxytryptophan (to ameliorate neurotransmitter deficiencies) plus BH$_4$ (except for DHPR deficiency) and, if required, dietary phenylalanine restriction to decrease blood phenylalanine values up to a safe range.

13.3 BIOMARKERS FOR DIAGNOSIS

13.3.1 PERIPHERAL MARKERS

In general, biomarkers in peripheral biological fluids (blood and urine) are not suitable for diagnosis of most monoamine disorders. However, under some circumstances, they may provide useful information. Here we review the most widely used biomarkers, highlighting their limitations. The most important biomarkers and their concentration in different biological fluids according to the disease are stated in Table 13.1.

13.3.1.1 Catecholamines in plasma and urine

Catecholamines (dopamine, norepinephrine (noradrenaline), and epinephrine (adrenaline)) act as neurotransmitters and hormones at central and peripheral levels. The involvement of these neurotransmitters in multiple regulatory systems and metabolic processes supports their important use as biomarkers.[17]

In DBH deficiency, a near-complete absence of norepinephrine and epinephrine together with high dopamine concentration (and its metabolites) in plasma and urine are characteristic. However, no experience or positive results have been confirmed for the other genetic conditions affecting monoamine metabolism. In fact, normal or even hyperdopaminuria has been reported for TH- and AADC-deficient patients.[11]

Table 13.1 Biogenic Amines and Pterin Patterns Observed in Cerebrospinal Fluid and Biomarkers in Urine or Blood in the Inherited Disorders Affecting Catecholamine and Serotonin Metabolism

Disorder	Cerebrospinal Fluid								Blood/Urine
	HVA	5HIAA	HVA/5HIAA ratio	3OMD	BH4	BP	NP	SP	
TH	↓/↓↓	N	↓↓	N	N	N	N	N	↑ VLA urine
AADC	↓↓	↓↓	N	↑	N	N	N	N	↓↓ E, NE, ↑ Dopamine Urine/plasma
DBH*	↑	N	↑	N	N	N	N	N	
MAO	↓↓	↓↓	N	N	N	N	N	N	
DAT1	↑	N	↑↑	N	N	N	N	N	
VMAT2	N	N	N	N	N	N	N	N	
GTPCH (Recessive)	↓↓	↓↓	N	N	↓↓	↓↓	↓↓	N	↑ Blood Phe; ↓ urine BP, NP
GTPCH (Dominant)	↓	↓/N	N	N	↓	↓	↓	N	Phe loading test
PTPS	↓↓	↓↓	N	N	↓↓	↓↓	↑↑	N	↑ Blood Phe; ↓ urine BP, ↑ NP
SR	↓↓	↓↓	N	N	↓↓	↑	N	↑↑	Phe loading test; ↑ urine SP
PCD	↓/N	↓/N	N	N	N	N	N	N	↑ Blood Phe; ↑ urine primapterin
DHPR	↓	↓	N	N	↓/N	↑	N	N	↑ Blood Phe; ↓ DHPR activity

GTPCH: GTP cyclohydrolase; PTPS: 6-Pyruvoyltetrahydropterin synthase; SR: Sepiapterin reductase; PCD: Pterin 4-alpha carbinolamine dehydratase; DHPR: Dihydropteridine reductase; TH: Tyrosine hydroxylase; AADC: Aromatic L-amino acid decarboxylase; DBH: Dopamine beta hydroxylase; MAO: Monoamine oxidase; DAT: Dopamine transporter; BH₄: Tetrahydrobiopterin; BP: Biopterin; NP: Total neopterin; SP: Sepiapterin; Phe: Phenylalanine; HVA: Homovanillic acid; 5HIAA: 5-Hydroxyindoleacetic acid; 3OMD: 3-O-methyldopa; N: Normal; ↓: Decreased; ↓↓: Very decreased; ↑: Elevated; ↑↑: Very elevated; *: Predicted.

Catecholamines exist in biological samples at extremely low concentrations, demanding specific and very sensitive analytical methods. Moreover, they are chemically unstable, prone to spontaneous oxidation, and decompose easily at high pH levels (pH of urine should be less than 4.0). Solid-phase extraction is the sample preparation methodology most widely used for the extraction and preconcentration of catecholamines. Among the earliest techniques are the radioenzymatic and immunological assays, which have been replaced by more sensitive and selective chromatographic methods such as high-performance liquid chromatography (HPLC) with electrochemical detection, capillary electrophoresis with fluorescence, electrochemical, ultraviolet (UV), or mass spectrometry (MS) detection.[17]

13.3.1.2 Monoamines and organic acids in urine

In general, analysis of monoamines in urine is not suitable for diagnosis of these genetic disorders because 5-HIAA or HVA may be highly variable depending on external factors. In fact, this potential utility has not yet been reported.

An abnormal profile of organic acids could be detected in some patients with AADC and in vitamin B_6 deficiencies. Urinary vanillactic acid (VLA) elevation has been described, but also increased vanilpyruvic acid, N-acetyl-vanilalanine, and N-acetyl-tyrosine have been reported in some patients.[14,18,19] Urine organic acid analysis may be performed using gas chromatography/MS or by liquid chromatography/tandem mass spectrometry (LC/Ms-MS). Both methods are robust, and supported by much experience in different laboratories.[20]

13.3.1.3 Pterins

The analysis of pterins in urine is done in all patients with elevated blood phenylalanine levels detected by newborn screening programs to delineate the differential diagnosis of PKU. This includes the analysis of neopterin, biopterin, and primapterin in urine[10,21] (Table 13.1). Recently, a new method for the quantification of sepiapterine in urine has been described. This new approach allows the diagnosis of SR deficiency in a peripheral sample, avoiding the lumbar puncture.[22] For pterin analysis, the urine sample should be protected from light to prevent degradation, and some authors suggest oxidizing before storing the sample. Samples should be immediately stored at −80°C until analysis.

Pterins are determined mainly by chromatographic techniques (HPLC with fluorescence or electrochemical detection).[23] This approach is single step, cost-effective, and allows the differentiation of the different genetic conditions related to BH_4 deficiency (together with few additional tests). Further, more sophisticated methods have been described, such as capillary electrophoresis using fluorescence detection, an online UV-photoirradiation HPLC system, using a diode array and fast scanning fluorescence detectors and ultra-PLC with fluorescence detection.[23–26]

13.3.1.4 Phenylalanine loading test

Several reports have demonstrated the usefulness of the phenylalanine loading test in the diagnosis of autosomal dominant GTPCH-I and SR deficiencies.[10,27]

This test is based on stressing hepatic phenylalanine hydroxylase with a phenylalanine load, which is not converted into tyrosine at a normal rate because of the partial BH_4 deficiency in the liver, resulting in an increased phenylalanine/tyrosine ratio. The phenylalanine loading test consists of administering 100 mg/kg phenylalanine and subsequently measuring the phenylalanine/tyrosine ratio in plasma or blood spot samples at different time intervals (baselines 1, 2, 4, and 6h after loading). In patients with mutations in either *GCH1* or *SR* genes, this phenylalanine challenge results in an increased phenylalanine/tyrosine ratio in the blood at 1–6h after phenylalanine administration. This test is particularly useful when lumbar puncture and cerebrospinal fluid (CSF) analyses are not possible. However, false-negative and false-positive results have been reported and do not allow differentiation between GTPCH-I and SR deficiencies. Phenylalanine and tyrosine concentrations may be analyzed by ion pair HPLC with UV detection or liquid chromatography tandem mass chromatography (LC-MS/MS) procedures.[10,27]

13.3.2 CENTRAL NERVOUS SYSTEM MARKERS

CSF is the most suitable biological sample for the diagnosis of most of the monoamines disorders. In Table 13.1, the analyses of biogenic amines and pterins in CSF and the diagnostic value for the different genetic conditions are stated. A typical chromatogram of a control subject and several patients with defects in TH, AADC, MAO-A, and BH_4 (SR and GTPCH-I) deficiencies is presented in Fig. 13.2.

13.3.2.1 Catecholamines in CSF

Dopamine and serotonin can be analyzed indirectly by measuring their main stable end-metabolites, HVA and 5-HIAA, respectively. Their concentrations in CSF provide insight into the turnover of dopamine and serotonin in those brain areas where they are synthesized. Therefore, HVA and 5-HIAA can be used as indirect markers of the functioning of dopamine and serotonin pathways in the brain. The analyses of 3-ortomethyldopa and methoxyhyroxyphenylglycol (as dopamine and norepinephrine metabolites) and 5-hydroxytryptophan, as a serotonin precursor metabolite (Fig. 13.1), allow not only the identification but also the differentiation of the biogenic amine disorders in one analysis. Defects in monoamine biosynthesis show decreased CSF HVA and 5-HIAA (TH, AADC, and BH_4 deficiencies), and in AADC deficiency together with grossly elevated precursors (3-orthomethydopa and 5-hydroxytryptophan). DBH and MAO-A defects usually display high HVA values (Fig. 13.1). DAT1 deficiency also displays increased CSF HVA values because of an accelerated degradation of dopamine in the synaptic cleft, whereas VMAT2 defect does not show a clearly impaired biogenic amine profile.

Protocolized lumbar puncture collection is required for reliable analysis of biogenic amines. Since there is a rostrocaudal gradient (the concentration of some metabolites is higher in the last fractions of the CSF when compared with the first collected cerebrospinal fluid), it is important to compare the patient's values to reference values established using the same CSF fraction. Since red blood cell lysis

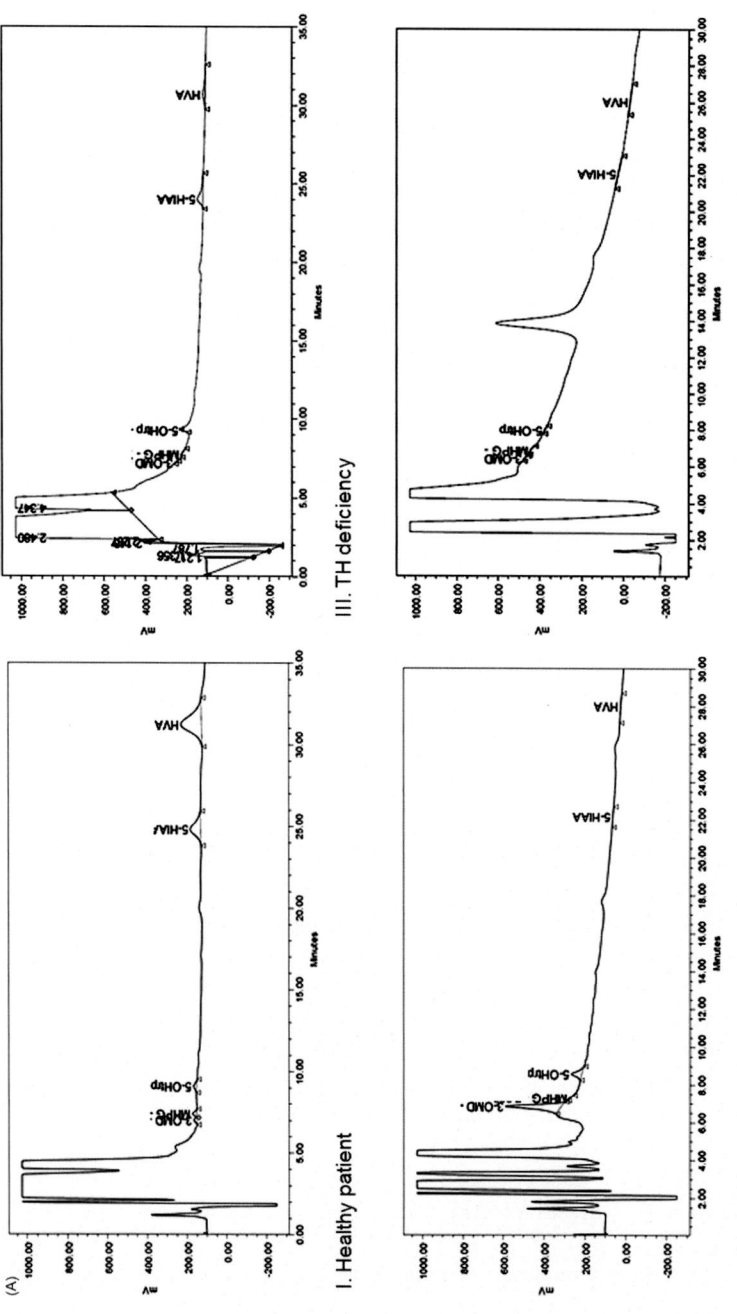

FIGURE 13.2

Chromatograms of neurotransmitters and pterins in cerebrospinal fluid. (A) Cerebrospinal fluid neurotransmitter chromatograms. Chromatogram I shows a normal neurotransmitter profile in CSF. The other chromatograms show pathological profiles. Chromatogram II shows an AADC pattern with very low homovanillic (HVA) and 5-hydroxyindoleacetic (5-HIAA) acids with high 3-O-methyldopa (3OMD) values. Chromatogram III represents a TH deficiency profile with low HVA and 3OMD with normal 5-OH-trp and 5-HIAA values. In chromatogram IV, a MAO-A deficiency pattern, with very low values of HVA and 5-HIAA without accumulation of dopamine and serotonin precursors is presented. Genetic studies of *DDC*, *TH*, and *MAO* genes confirmed the biochemical findings. (B) Cerebrospinal fluid pterin chromatograms. The chromatograms show CSF pterin profiles in different situations. Chromatogram I depicts a normal profile from a healthy control. In chromatogram II, a patient with dominant GTPCH deficiency is presented, showing of neopterin and biopterin concentrations. Through another specific HPLC method it is possible to analyze sepiapterin. Chromatogram III shows a normal CSF profile (no detectable sepiapterin), and chromatogram IV depicts a CSF profile from a patient with SR deficiency SP accumulation). Genetic studies of *GTPCH* and *SPR* genes confirmed the biochemical findings.

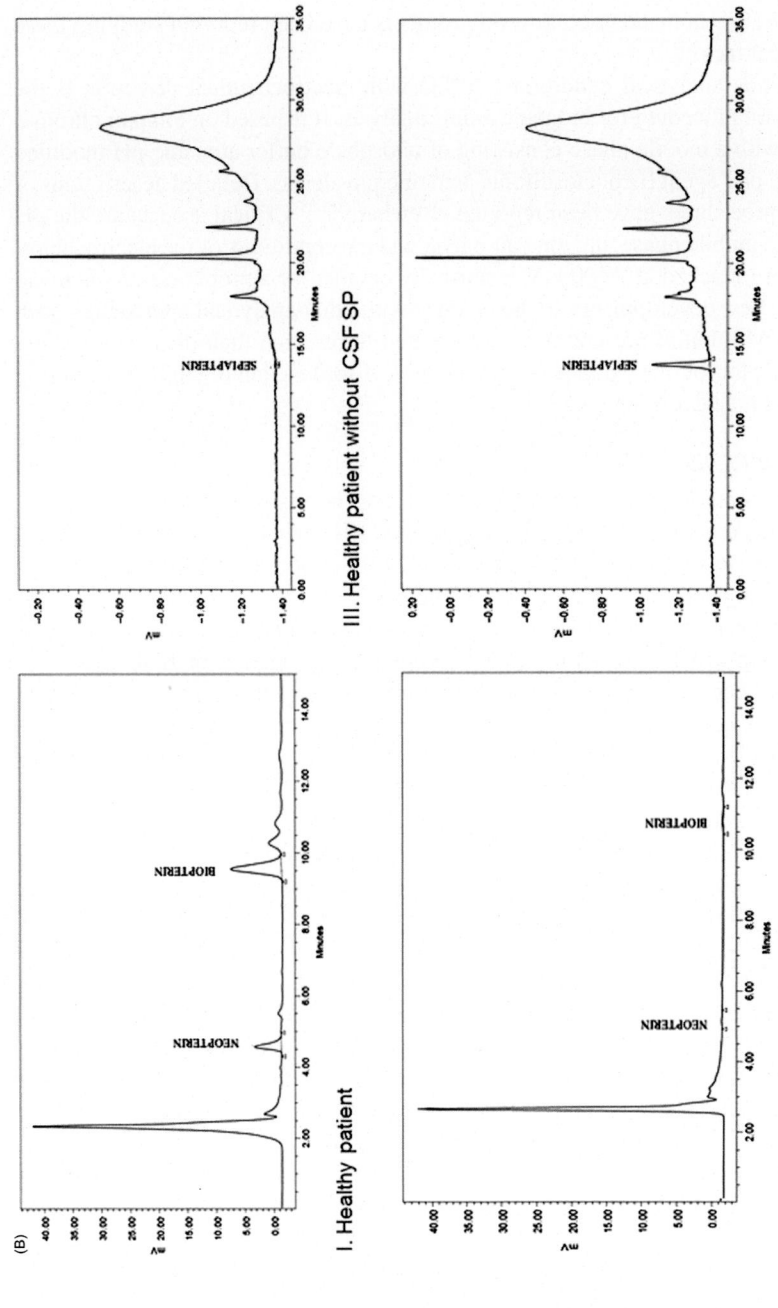

FIGURE 13.2

(Continued)

causes oxidation of amine metabolites, blood-contaminated samples must be centrifuged immediately, and the clear CSF supernatant transferred to a new tube. Sample storage at –80°C is mandatory. Several protocols have been reported studying these preanalytical factors.[26,28]

As regards analytical conditions, HPLC with electrochemical detection is the gold standard procedure for biogenic amine analysis. It is based on ion pair chromatography, with a mobile phase consisting of phosphate buffer at acidic pH modified with an ion pair agent (heptanosulfonic acid or equivalents). Detailed descriptions of analytical procedures have been reported elsewhere.[26,28] Critical aspects are the pH value of the mobile phase, the ion pair agent, and the conditions of the electrochemical detector (attached at +400 mV is normally enough for a proper electrochemical detection). New developments are being done with other analytical approaches, such as LC/MS-MS, but at present are more devoted to research than diagnosis and are not available for routine diagnosis of monoamine disorders, but it will be a promising approach in the near future.

13.3.2.2 Pterins

Neopterin, biopterin, sepiapterin, BH_2, and BH_4 may be analyzed in CSF, and they are useful biomarkers for the differential diagnosis of BH_4 metabolism genetic disorders with normal blood phenylalanine values (SR and the dominant form of GTPCH-I defects are shown in Fig. 13.1). GTPCH-I deficiency shows mildly decreased neopterin and biopterin values, whereas sepiapterin reductase deficiency shows increased CSF biopterin concentrations because of increased degradation of BH_4. The other BH_4 defects can be detected through newborn screening programs for PKU, and the specific diagnosis is reached by the analysis in urine of neopterin, biopterin, and primapterin (Table 13.1). As we will explain in the last part of this chapter, neopterin is also a powerful tool for identification of inflammatory and immune conditions in the central nervous system.[29]

Preanalytical conditions are worthy of consideration. For the measurement of neopterin, biopterin, and sepiapterin, the most common practice is the CSF sample oxidation with manganese dioxide or iodine, and sample protection from light.[23] To measure BH_2 and BH_4, CSF sample storage with the stabilizing agent (dithioerythritol or diethylenetriaminpentaacteic acid) is required. CSF neopterin and biopterin can be analyzed using reverse-phase HPLC with fluorescence detector.[26] The procedure is single and consists of a mobile phase with phosphate buffer and methanol. Fluorescence detection occurs at 350 nm (excitation) and 450 nm (emission) (Fig. 13.2). For sepiapterin analysis, the analytical conditions are similar but a sample concentration is required.[30] For BH_4 and BH_2 quantification, HPLC with electrochemical detector is the gold standard procedure.[23] However, for a first-line diagnosis of all of the genetic conditions related to BH_4 disturbances, HPLC with fluorescence detection is a single step, reliable procedure. Typical chromatograms from controls and from patients with different pterin disorders are presented in Fig. 13.2.

13.3.3 OTHER BIOMARKERS IN CSF

As complementary exams to improve the diagnosis efficacy, vitamins and other biomarkers may be analyzed. In fact, an expanding number of biomarkers are being identified in CSF as potential diagnostic targets, allowing the diagnosis of other conditions. For example, and directly related to biogenic amine metabolism, CSF pyridoxal-phosphate may be quantified by reverse-phase HPLC with fluorescence detection, as previously reported.[31] Pyridoxal-phosphate is the active form of vitamin B_6 and is the essential cofactor of AADC, a key enzyme to synthesize dopamine and serotonin. Those defects that cause low pyridoxal-phosphate levels or pyridoxal-phosphate sequestration (pyridoxamine 5-prime-phosphate oxidase, PNPO *MIM 603287 and antiquitin defects *MIM 107323, respectively) cause a secondary AADC deficiency (low HVA and 5-HIAA values with an elevation of the precursors 3-orthomethyldopa and 5-hydroxytryptophan) associated with different degrees of CSF pyridoxal-phosphate deficiency. CSF amino acid concentrations (threonine and glycine) may be increased in these conditions. Urine VLA excretion may be increased as well.[32]

Further, 5-methyltetrahydrofolate (5-MTHF) may be measured by HPLC with fluorescence detection,[33] and it serves for the diagnosis of cerebral folate deficiency. Since 5-MTHF is the cofactor of catechol-orthomethyltransferase enzyme (Fig. 13.1), secondary cerebral folate deficiencies after L-dopa treatment are frequently observed as a result of increased folate consumption.

A large list of other biomarkers may be interesting for differential diagnosis, and may include glucose (for diagnosis of glucose transporter type 1 (GLUT-1) deficiency), lactate (energy metabolism problems), amino acids (hyperglycinemia and serine deficiency), GABA, or thiamine (diagnosis of basal ganglia disorder responsive to biotin), among others.

13.3.4 ENZYME ACTIVITY ANALYSES

Enzyme activity measurements can help to diagnose monoamine deficiencies, although only the genetic analysis will provide the definitive diagnosis. The only enzymatic test routinely done in specialized clinical laboratories is DHPR activity measurement in blood spots for differential diagnosis of PKU.[34] Regarding the monoamine defects detailed in this chapter, several enzyme activities may be analyzed to support the genetic diagnosis. However, in some cases, decreased enzyme activities have been demonstrated with no mutations in the candidate genes.

AADC activity: Analysis of AADC activity may be measured in plasma samples.[35] This technique consists of measuring the production of dopamine by HPLC with electrochemical detection after the incubation of the sample with the dopamine precursor L-dopa in the presence of pyridoxal-phosphate.[36] Since AADC is also responsible for serotonin synthesis, 5-hydroxytryptophan as precursor and subsequent serotonin determination can also be used for analyzing the AADC activity.

However, AADC activity is much higher using L-dopa as a substrate, and the latter is therefore preferable.[37]

GTPCH-I activity: Measurement of GTPCH-I activity is rather difficult because this enzyme is not present in blood cells or fibroblasts. Therefore, it is necessary to induce the expression of this enzyme with recombinant human interferon-gamma and tumoral necrosis factor-α.[38] The assay monitors the conversion of guanosine triphosphate to neopterin triphosphate, which is detected as neopterin (Fig. 13.1), using HPLC with fluorescence detection. Particularly, the measurement of GTPCH-I activity is useful in patients with dominant inheritance of the disease to support the diagnosis. It has been demonstrated that patients harboring one mutation at the *GCH1* gene causing the typical symptoms of the disease have less enzyme activity than those asymptomatic carriers.[39] This fact is due to a classic dominant negative effect of some mutations that lead to a destabilizing effect in the protein.[40]

SR activity: The assay monitors the conversion of sepiapterin to BH_4, which is then measured as the oxidized product, biopterin, using HPLC with fluorescence detection.[41] SR activity may be assayed in skin fibroblasts, chorionic villi, and various blood fractions including stimulated mononuclear blood cells.

DBH activity: The activity of this enzyme, which is involved in dopamine conversion to noradrenaline, can be analyzed in plasma samples. However, its measurement is not routinely used because the biochemical hallmarks of the diseases (low levels of norepinephrine and epinephrine in plasma, and 5–10-fold elevated plasma levels of dopamine) are very sensitive for diagnosis.[42] In addition, there is a common polymorphism in the *DBH* gene (1021 C> T) that causes an undetectable plasma DBH activity with normal values of norepinephrine, epinephrine, and dopamine. The normal quantity of norepinephrine is difficult to explain, but one hypothesis is that only a residual DBH activity is needed to ensure normal catecholamine formation.[42]

DHPR activity: For the differential diagnosis of PKU, DHPR activity is regularly measured because some patients can present with normal urine pterins. The study of DHPR activity is done in dried blood spots on filter paper, and it uses the BH_4-dependent reduction of ferricytochrome c in the presence of reduced nicotinamide adenine dinucleotide.[34]

The other enzymes or proteins causing genetic monoamine deficiencies (MAO-A, TH DAT1, and VMAT2) cannot be measured routinely in clinical laboratories, mainly because no expression of these proteins is available human biological samples (e.g., TH activity is expressed in the central nervous system and adrenal glands but not in easily available biological samples).

13.3.5 GENETIC DIAGNOSIS

Mutational analysis should be done to confirm the diagnosis of monoamine neurotransmitter defects. As occurs with other monogenic diseases, the confirmation of mutations permits patients to start with specific therapies or to have genetic counseling for affected families.

Although most of the genes have been studied using a single gene testing approach (Sanger sequencing), next-generation sequencing (NGS) (targeted gene panel diagnosis) is increasingly used in clinical laboratories, allowing a quicker diagnosis. Through whole exome and genome sequencing, new genes causing impaired monoamine status are being discovered.[43] The enormous complexity of synaptic transmission, where hundreds of proteins with different functions are involved, strongly suggests that massive sequencing of large series of patients with undiagnosed neurological diseases will lead to the discovery of new genes involved in human diseases. In this section, we report the main features of the different genes implicated in monoamine disorders.

13.3.5.1 Tyrosine hydroxylase (TH)

The *TH* gene is located on chromosome 11p15.5 and it contains 14 exons. There are four splicing variants (TH1 to TH4).[44] Several mutations are reported, including missense mutations in codifying regions, splicing, and intronic mutations (see database on www.biopku.org). Approximately 100 mutations have been reported, most of them slightly deleterious mutations, suggesting that a total loss of TH activity is incompatible with life.[11] However, some severe mutations leading to protein truncation have been reported.[11] A founder effect has been demonstrated, and some mutations are more common in Greek (c.707 C> T)[45] and Dutch populations (c.698 G> A).[11] Promoter mutations seem to be more usual in TH-deficiency type A (the mild phenotype of the disease). Patients harboring promoter mutations usually demonstrate a good response to L-dopa treatment.[11,46] Genotype–phenotype correlations are scarce, although in the largest series of patients studied, the division into two phenotypes is proposed,[11] even if the actual trend is to consider the TH-deficiency phenotype as a continuum.[1]

13.3.5.2 L-aromatic amino acid decarboxylase (DDC)

The *DDC* gene is located on chromosome 7p12.3–p12.1 and it codifies for 15 exons that encode an amino acid sequence of 480 amino acid residues.[47] There are two AADC forms differing in their *5′* untranslated regions (5′-UTRs). To date, there is no reported genotype–phenotype correlation.[14] With the exception of the Chinese population, in which there is a common founder mutation (IVS6 + 4A> T), most patients harbor private mutations expanded through the entire *DDC* gene. Brun et al. reported a large cohort of AADC-deficient patients, showing that the most frequent mutations are IVS6+ 4A> T (allele frequency of 45%), followed by p.S250F (allele frequency of 6%), p.G102S (allele frequency of 8%), and p.R462P (allele frequency 6%).[14] These patients are registered in the *Jointly Administered Knowledge Environment (*JAKE) database (www.biopku.org).

Kinetic analyses have been done for the p.G102S mutation, showing a 60-fold decreased AADC enzyme affinity for L-dopa.[48]

13.3.5.3 Dopamine beta hydroxylase (DBH)

The *DBH* gene is composed of 12 exons and is localized on chromosome 9q34.[49] There are two cDNA variants of the DBH gene (type A and B), which encode the same sequence of 603 amino acids. Few mutations have been published, including missense variants, one single-base pair deletion, and splice-site mutations.[47] Since there are few patients with DBH deficiency, there are no studies about the genotype–phenotype correlation.

13.3.5.4 Monoamino oxidase (MAO-A)

MAO protein can exist in two different forms, MAO-A and MAO-B, sharing 70% identity at the amino acid level and exhibiting an equal organization of their 15 exons. Their position on chromosome X (p11.23–11.4 region) is very close to the Norrie disease gene (*NDP*), and some reports about patients with microdeletions at this position present loss of the *NDP* gene leading to a syndrome characterized by congenital blindness, hearing loss, and mental disability (Norrie disease, OMIM *310600).[50] Deletions in the three genes (*MAO-A, MAO-B,* and *NDP*),[51] or deletions affecting *MAO-B* and *NDP* genes,[52] or deletions in *MAO-A* and *MAO-B*[50] have been described, but there are no described patients with isolated MAO-B defects. Therefore, it is thought that MAO-A is the most important enzyme for the biogenic amine catabolism, and the one responsible for the behavioral disturbances in these syndromes.

13.3.5.5 Dopamine transporter type I (SLC16A3)

The *SLC16A3* gene codifies human DAT1; it is located on chromosome 5p15.3 and it contains 15 exons. To date, a variety of mutations have been published, including missense mutations, nonsense mutations, splice-site variants, and deletions,[53] all showing a typical CSF profile of DAT1 deficiency (remarkably increased values of the HVA/5-HIAA ratio, Table 13.1). Since there are few reported patients, there are no reported genotype–phenotype correlations.

13.3.5.6 Vesicular monoamine transporter 2 (SLC18A2)

VAMT2 is encoded by the *SLC18A2* gene and is localized in 10q25.3. Rilstone and colleagues reported a Saudi family with about eight members with symptoms and signs related to deficiencies in dopamine, serotonin, norepinephrine, and epinephrine. Interestingly, patients displayed no remarkable alterations in CSF monoamine profile, but all of them presented with mutations in the *SLC18A2* gene.[9]

13.3.5.7 GTP cyclohydrolase I (GCH1)

GTPCH-I enzyme is the first involved in the synthesis of BH4. It is encoded by the *GCH1* gene, which is localized in 14q22.1-q22.2 and contains six exons.[54] Mutations in this gene can be inherited in either an autosomal recessive or dominant form, causing dopa-responsive dystonia or Segawa disease, the most common among the monoamine diseases. In the autosomal dominant form, a mutation in one allele together with the wild-type allele coexists. In contrast to other BH4 deficiencies, the dominant form, together with SR deficiency, is not detected by newborn screening programs.[55] More than 140 mutations have been described in this gene, including missense mutations, nonsense mutations, frameshift mutations, intronic splice site in the promoter region, and one nonsense-to-sense mutation (www.biopku.org[55]). Studies about the association between genotype and phenotype are unclear, and it seems that the autosomal dominant GCH-1 form shows low penetrance and a female predominance.[55]

13.3.5.8 6-Pyruvoyltetrahydropterin synthase (PTS)

The PTPS enzyme participates in the second step of the synthesis of BH4. It is codified by the *PTS* gene, which has 6 exons and is localized in 11q22.3-q23.3. There are approximately 50 mutations distributed across all six exons and the first three introns. Although substitutions are the most common mutations, insertions, deletions, and splice-site mutations are also stated.[55] The majority of described mutations cause severe (or central) PTPS deficiency form; the mild form is less frequent. There are specific mutations more common in the severe form such as R25G, and other ones are more frequently associated with the mild form (R16C and L26F).[55] However, the limited available data show no correlation between genotype and phenotype. PTPS deficiency is the most prevalent (in the order of 56%, 21) and most heterogeneous form of BH4 metabolism defects.[56]

13.3.5.9 Sepiapterin reductase (SPR)

The *SPR* gene is localized to 2p13 and encompasses three exons. There are fewer than 10 published mutations stated on the www.biopku.org database. This disease is the most recently described defect in BH_4 metabolism.[38] Diagnosis is made through neurotransmitter metabolite studies in CSF because plasma phenylalanine levels are within normal reference ranges (unlike autosomal dominant GTPCH-I deficiency). For this reason, it is believed that this is probably an underdiagnosed condition. The IVS2-2A4G variant, at the splice site consensus sequence in intron 2, has been shown to result from a founder effect in a Maltase population.[57]

13.3.5.10 Pterin-4αα-carbinolamine dehydratase (PCBD1)

PCD (or DCoH) protein is encoded by the *PCBD1* gene, which is located on chromosome 10q22 and contains four exons.[58] Studies have shown that the *PCBD* gene has an identical human paralog with the same numbers of exons[59] called *DCoH2*. The few known mutations (less than 10) are all present in exon 4, and all patients with these mutations display increased urinary excretion of primapterin and transient hyperphenylalaninemia. It is hypothesized that the mild symptoms of patients with PCD defect are due to a compensatory effect of the DCoH2 isozyme.[60]

13.3.5.11 Dihydropteridine reductase (QDPR)

DHPR deficiency is caused by mutations in the *QDPR* gene, which contains seven exons and is located on chromosome 4p15.3. The reported mutations are distributed over all exons and two introns, including missense mutations, nonsense mutations, frameshift mutations, splice-site mutations, and insertions. Most of the patients present the severe DHPR deficiency form, whereas the few patients presenting with the mild form have only affected serotonin metabolism.[55]

13.4 BIOMARKERS FOLLOWED FOR TREATMENT EFFICACY

Few experiences are currently reported regarding this issue.[1] The number of known patients for each condition is very small, and there are no international clinical trials to study the clinical utility of potential available biomarkers for treatment monitoring. Since the clinical response after therapy may be extremely variable, the analysis of biochemical markers for treatment monitoring seems important. Here we have classified the available biomarkers as peripheral (analyzed in urine or blood samples) and central (requires lumbar puncture and CSF collection for the analysis).

Concerning *peripheral markers*, several possibilities exist and should be trialed for treatment monitoring, since they avoid repeated lumbar punctures. In general, for dopamine deficiency, plasma prolactin analysis should be considered during patient follow-up. The rationale is that dopamine is the natural inhibitor of prolactin excretion, and thus, in cases of dopamine deficiency, plasma prolactin values are high. Several reports have dealt with this aspect in different genetic dopamine deficiencies.[61,62] An important limitation of plasma prolactin monitoring is that a single prolactin evaluation can be misleading because of the dependency of prolactin fluctuations on the L-dopa administration schedule.[61] Short prolactin profiling has been demonstrated as suitable for monitoring these patients, even in patients treated with dopamine agonists.[61] Another important consideration is that prolactin is highly variable among different individuals according to age, sex, and other factors. Accurate reference values for a pediatric population have been recently established, opening the possibility to use prolactin for both diagnostic and treatment monitoring purposes.[63] Regarding methodologies for prolactin quantification, they are available in most clinical chemistry laboratories, and rely on automated immunochemical procedures. Monitoring of other peripheral markers such as urinary HVA or dopamine or other biogenic amines in blood is not an alternative because their concentration may be strongly variable and uninformative (e.g., paradoxical normal or even high urinary dopamine excretion have been reported in TH- and AADC-deficient patients).[11]

For serotonin deficiency treatment monitoring, urinary 5-HIAA or blood serotonin levels are not useful tools. An interesting alternative may be the analysis of melatonin or some of its metabolites (6-sulfatoxymelatonin) in blood, urine, or saliva. The rationale for this is that melatonin is synthesized from serotonin exclusively in the pineal gland, thus being a good biomarker for the estimation of serotonin concentrations in the brain. Although there is not enough experience in melatonin analysis in blood or urine for treatment monitoring in primary genetic neurotransmitter deficiencies, its utility for PKU treatment monitoring has been reported.[64] Difficulties in data interpretation may be important. It is especially important during sample collection to consider that melatonin levels fluctuate (the melatonin peak occurs during the night). First morning urine samples are suitable for 6-sulfatoxymelatonin analysis as an estimation of brain serotonin status.[64] Thus, it may be a promising alternative for serotonin deficiency treatment monitoring. The most commonly used method for melatonin analysis in body fluids is commercially available enzyme-linked immunosorbent assay (ELISA) kits.[64]

As regards *central nervous system biomarkers*, classically, the most common practicum for treatment monitoring of neurotransmitter disorders has been CSF collection to measure serial biogenic amines over the treatment follow-up period. It is difficult to determine when CSF should be collected. A lumbar puncture to monitor biogenic amine concentrations (mainly HVA and 5-HIAA) may be recommended for the patient with a poor clinical outcome after treatment. In patients with TH and pterin-related disorders, treatment with either L-dopa or 5-hydroxytryptophan usually restores CSF HVA, and 5-HIAA values.[1,11] Thus, if normal values are not reached, incremental increases in L-dopa dosage may be advisable. For AADC, MAO, DAT1, and VMAT deficiencies, this strategy is probably not as useful as it is in the other diseases because, in most cases, HVA and 5-HIAA will remain essentially unchanged irrespective of the clinical response. CSF pterin analysis will not be useful for treatment monitoring because BH_4 is not used as treatment in these conditions, and no modifications of pterin values in CSF are expected after the current treatments are employed. Other biomarker studies may be useful, such as CSF pyridoxal-phosphate, because it is used as coadjuvant therapy in AADC deficiency, or CSF 5-MTHF, because cerebral folate deficiency may appear as a secondary event after L-dopa therapy.[1,16] These vitamins will be discussed in another chapter in this book.

13.5 BIOMARKERS FOLLOWED FOR DISEASE PROGRESSION

Available information regarding this topic is very scarce. To the best of our knowledge, there is no consensus or large series of patients reported in a complete study regarding disease progression. The only work dealing with this matter was done for TH deficiency.[11] The conclusion of the authors after studying the largest series of TH-deficient patients was that the HVA/5HIAA ratio in CSF may be used to predict L-dopa responsiveness and neurological outcome.[11] Patients displaying mild phenotypes present the highest HVA values when compared with patients with the most severe form of TH deficiency. Therefore, the only predictors for these diseases would be the CSF concentrations of HVA and 5-HIAA as markers of dopamine and serotonin status, considering that the lower the biogenic amine concentrations in CSF are, the more severe the dopamine and serotonin deficiency will be. However, this approach should be carefully considered, and new biomarkers for investigating disease progression should be investigated.

13.6 CONFOUNDING CONDITIONS AFFECTING BIOMARKER EXPRESSION

In this part of the chapter, we will focus on changes in the best-established biomarkers analyzed in CSF, including biogenic amines and pterins (neopterin). Importantly, many patients without specific diagnoses but who present with motor disturbances or dystonic symptoms have low HVA values in CSF, suggesting that dopaminergic depletion should be investigated.[65]

13.6.1 BIOGENIC AMINES IN ENVIRONMENTAL AND GENETIC CONDITIONS

Both HVA and 5-HIAA are the most informative biogenic amines regarding the identification of dopamine and serotonin deficiency, respectively. However, they represent end-stable metabolites of neurotransmitters of which concentrations may be influenced by several genetic and environmental conditions. As waste metabolites, once HVA and 5-HIAA have been synthesized by the action of several enzymes (Fig. 13.1), they are removed from the central nervous system to the blood (and finally excreted in the urine) mainly through the organic anionic transporter 3 (OAT3) located in the choroid plexus. The choroid plexus forms the blood–CSF barrier and protects the brain from circulating metabolites, drugs, and toxins. It is involved in both transport from essential molecules from blood to CSF (folate, ascorbic acid)[66] and removing some waste metabolites from CSF to blood, such as HVA and 5-HIAA. Dysfunction in this tissue has been described to increase biogenic amine concentrations in CSF, as reported for Kearns–Sayre syndrome, a mitochondrial disorder in which one of the target organs is choroid plexus.[67]

Some environmental (nongenetic diseases) may impair biogenic amine concentrations as well. For example, in perinatal asphyxia, altered HVA concentrations have been described. A marked increase of HVA levels during the first days of life was observed, followed by an important decline of this metabolite in CSF,[68] probably explained by the damage of dopaminergic neurons. Traumatic lesions, infections, or neurodegenerative processes can also cause destruction of dopaminergic and serotoninergic areas in the brain (e.g., substantia nigra and rafe nucleus), leading to decreased concentrations of HVA and 5-HIAA.[28,69] In this sense, radiological alterations such as cortical atrophy or white matter disturbances are associated with low 5-HIAA or HVA values, respectively.[69–71] Some other studies have reported that patients with low HVA values in CSF may be associated with having epilepsy or epileptic encephalopathies.[72,73] However, those findings are still controversial because other studies have demonstrated normal HVA values in patients with epilepsy.[71,74]

As regards to genetic diseases, a wide variety of disorders have been associated with biogenic amine deficiencies, and in most cases, the pathophysiological mechanisms are not well understood.[71] There is a large list of genetic disorders that can present with reductions in HVA and 5-HIAA values in CSF, such as pontocerebellar hypoplasia type 2,[72] leukodystrophies,[69] mitochondrial disorders,[70,75] Rett syndrome,[76] vanishing white matter disease, Miller–Fisher syndrome, Steinert disease, or Angelman syndrome,[68,71] among others. However, not all patients diagnosed with these diseases show consistent HVA or 5-HIAA alterations, meaning that these biomarkers might be a nonspecific finding in these disorders.[71] Moreover, not all patients with these disorders have symptoms of dopamine and serotonin deficiency. Recently, decreased levels of biogenic amines have been described in two patients with voltage-gated sodium channelopathies with no basal ganglia lesions. These alterations have been postulated to be due to decreased neurotransmitter release from vesicles dependent on Ca^{2+} influx,[43] opening a new avenue in the elucidation of the pathophysiological basis of some monoamine defects of unknown etiology.

13.6.2 INBORN ERRORS OF METABOLISM MIMICKING MONOAMINES DISTURBANCES

Several reports reinforce the presence of secondary alterations in biogenic amines in the CSF of neurological patients affecting between 6–20% of the studied patients.[70–72,77] Some patients with neurometabolic diseases (and also the above-mentioned secondary alterations) might show low HVA and 5-HIAA in CSF, even in concentrations lower than primary defects, meaning that an overlap can exist in the biogenic amine values of primary and secondary defects. Therefore, in general terms, it is important to have the clinical, radiological, and, obviously, genetic information to make a final diagnosis.[71]

Several inborn errors of metabolism can display alterations in CSF biogenic amine values. Vitamin B_6 metabolism disturbances cause a secondary decreased activity of AADC (PNPO (*MIM 603287) and antiquitin (*MIM 107323) defects). Deficiency of PNPO enzyme presents with very low CSF pyridoxal-phosphate values, causing an alteration in PLP-dependent enzymes such as AADC, threonine dehydratase, or glycine cleavage system. The blockage in the AADC reaction causes a deficiency in the synthesis of dopamine and serotonin in the central nervous system and, therefore, low values of HVA and 5-HIAA in CSF. The difference between AADC and PNPO deficiencies is that, in the latter, very low CSF PLP values can be observed, along with other biochemical alterations such as an elevation of CSF and plasma threonine and glycine values. Clinically, patients with PNPO deficiency respond dramatically to PLP suppression of seizures.[78] Antiquitin (or aminoadipic semialdehyde dehydrogenase) deficiency (*ALDH7A1* gene) is a recessive disease that causes a chemical inactivation of pyridoxal-phosphate.[79] Although it can present biochemically with low biogenic amines in CSF, there are biomarkers that are more specific, such as α-amino adipic semialdehyde (AASA) or pipecolic acid. AASA is a product of lysine catabolism and is in chemical equilibrium with piperidine-6-caborxylate. The metabolite forms an adduct with pyridoxal-phosphate, which becomes inactive in B6-dependent reactions, such as AADC.

Folate transport and metabolism defects can also affect the synthesis of biogenic amines. Further, 5-MTHF is essential for the synthesis of S-adenosyl-methionine, which represents the preferred methyl group donor in many reactions (Fig. 13.1). L-dopa and dopamine depend on 5-MTHF availability to follow its normal catabolism (Fig. 13.1). Thus, decreased values of central nervous system folate can affect dopamine metabolism, presenting with low HVA values in CSF.[80] Genetic conditions causing cerebral folate deficiency are methylenetetrahydrofolate reductase (*MIM 607093) and dyhydrofolate reductase (*MIM 126060) deficiencies, and folate receptor 1 (*MIM 136430) and proton-coupled folate transporter defects (*MIM 611672).[81–84]

Mitochondrial energy metabolism diseases (oxidative phosphorylation defects) are commonly associated with alterations in biogenic amine values.[75] Neurotransmission is an energetically demanding process;[85] therefore, some energy metabolism defects can affect the biosynthesis and transport of monoamines and consequently lead to decreased concentrations of neurotransmitters. Some authors have reported that

L-dopa treatment in patients with early-onset mitochondrial defects causes little or no clinical improvement.[75] However, adult patients with Parkinsonism because of mitochondrial defects can respond to low L-dopa doses.[86] On the contrary, there are mitochondrial defects that can present with high biogenic amine values,[71] Kearns–Sayre syndrome being the clear example, with high values of HVA and 5-HIAA in CSF. Disturbances in exporting HVA and 5-HIAA out from CSF by energetically dependent transporter OAT3 may explain the accumulation of these metabolites in this fluid.[67]

There is evidence that Lesch–Nyhan disease (MIM*30800) is associated with a presynaptic dopaminergic deficit.[87] Postmortem human brain tissue shows a 60–90% decrease in basal ganglia dopamine levels, whereas other neurotransmitter systems are preserved.[88] These results are corroborated in other studies that report HVA alterations in CSF in patients with Lesch–Nyhan disease.[89] Literature regarding L-dopa treatment in Lesch–Nyhan disease is heterogeneous, whereas early initiation of treatment can contribute to a better short-term outcome,[89] there is no evidence that supports long-term L-dopa treatment in patients with this disorder.

Other inborn errors of metabolism are reported, even anecdotally, with alterations in end-metabolites of dopamine (HVA) and serotonin (5-HIAA). Since not all patients diagnosed with these diseases show consistently decreased values of CSF HVA and 5-HIAA, these biomarkers might be a nonspecific finding in these disorders.[71] Among the diseases that can be associated with impaired CSF biogenic amine values are nonketotic hyperglycinemia, oligosaccharidosis, Niemann–Pick type C, occipital horn syndrome, serine deficiency, thiamine transporter type 2, and carbamoyl phosphate synthetase deficiency.[71]

In any case, the therapy with L-dopa, 5-hydroxytryptophan, or both, should be considered in those patients with consistent low 5-HIAA and HVA values in CSF, particularly in patients during the first decade of life, when maturation and the formation of the correct neuronal net are actively occurring.

13.6.3 CEREBROSPINAL FLUID NEOPTERIN IN IMMUNE AND INFLAMMATORY PROCESSES

Neopterin is produced by lymphocytes, macrophages, dendritic cells, and probably neurons after stimulation by interferon-γ. Therefore, high neopterin concentration in plasma or CSF is widely considered as a sensitive but nonspecific biomarker of immune-mediated and inflammatory disorders. Elevated CSF neopterin has been described in active inflammation, demyelination, metabolic stress, neuronal injury, viral and bacterial infections, certain malignancies, allograft rejection, and autoimmune and neurodegenerative diseases.[29,90] Recent studies on cultured cells have demonstrated a potential cytoprotective role of neopterin in the central nervous system against damage or inflammation.[91] The high diagnostic sensitivity of CSF neopterin analysis for immune and inflammatory conditions is strongly advisable in the routine determination of this metabolite in CSF samples because it may discriminate a genetic–metabolic condition from an immune-mediated process. It must be taken into account that frequently the neurological phenotypes in both groups of disorders may overlap. Further, inflammatory response in some genetic conditions can be detected after neopterin analysis,[29] opening the possibility to modulate it by means of antiinflammatory therapies. A cut-off value of 61 nmol/L of CSF neopterin has been proposed to detect immune and inflammatory-mediated reactions. Further investigations in this area are necessary because neopterin may display a wide range of concentrations in immune-mediated disorders (ranging from 61 to more than 2,000 nmol/L), depending on the disease. Thus, the predictive value of neopterin regarding diagnosis (viral or bacterial infections, autoimmune processes) or even prognosis should be investigated.

13.7 OTHER BIOMARKERS: LESS ESTABLISHED, FUTURE

Biochemical markers: Identification of novel biomarkers for diagnosis and treatment responses through metabolomics and proteomics techniques will expand our knowledge in the following years and, in combination with the rapidly expanding data arising from NGS approaches, may provide novel insights into the functional consequences of the genetic variants detected. These high-throughput technologies are becoming available in some specialized laboratories (LC/MS-MS for untargeted metabolomics) and can analyze thousands of molecules with microliter volumes of body fluids.[92] Bioinformatic analyses are essential tools to annotate correctly all of the compounds detected.[93] Thus, the metabolomic approach has the potential to lead to the identification not only of novel biomarkers not yet discovered because of the lack of methodology, but also of already known biomarkers not previously associated with the neurotransmitter deficiencies. CSF proteomic analysis is also being revealed as a very useful tool to better understand the complex pathophysiology of the synapses in genetic monoamine deficiencies.[94]

Genetic markers: The list of genetic diseases with alterations in biogenic amines is growing. It may be possible that in near future, through NGS, such as targeted exome or whole exome/genome sequencing, either new inborn errors of metabolism related to neurotransmitter pathways or new phenotypes associated with monoamine diseases will be defined. These techniques are becoming more economical and accessible, and will undoubtedly expand the clinical phenotypes that are associated with mutation of specific genes and thus will improve the diagnosis of monoamine neurotransmitter disorders.[1] Whole exome sequencing has identified syndromic intellectual disability as a new phenotype of AADC deficiency that is associated with Marfanoid features and facial dysmorphism.[95] The immense amount of data generated after NGS may make the effect of the different variants predictable in treatment response in the prognosis of the disease.

Imaging techniques: Although this approach is beyond the scope of the chapter, it is important to note that this field is rapidly progressing, and both *in vivo* and *in vitro* neuroimaging techniques, such as magnetic resonance spectroscopy for patient study, or nuclear magnetic resonance imaging for biological sample analysis, are tools with immense potential. An interesting book about the current applications of nuclear magnetic resonance imaging in the investigation of metabolic diseases in different biological fluid has been published.[96]

In conclusion, biomarkers for the study of the different neurometabolic conditions reviewed in this chapter may provide important information for diagnosis, treatment monitoring, and, to a lesser extent, for the prognosis and clinical outcomes of patients with these diseases. The rapid identification of monoamine disturbances by means of biochemical analysis opens the possibility of early therapeutic efforts that may dramatically improve the clinical outcome in some patients. However, treatment is, in general, not satisfactory, and further developments on this issue are guaranteed. The main limitation we have at present for the biochemical analysis is that CSF probably does not fully reflect the extreme complexity of the biochemical processes occurring in the synapses. With the availability of high-throughput technologies, such as NGS, metabolomic, and proteomic approaches, in all likelihood, our knowledge about these complex diseases will improve in the next few years. Further, discovery of new diseases and genes affecting neurotransmission is expected.

13.8 ABBREVIATIONS

AADC	Aromatic L-amino acid decarboxylase
7,8-BH2	7,8-Dihydrobiopterin
BH$_4$	Tetrahydrobiopterin
COMT	Catechol O-methyltransferase
CR	Carbonyl reductase
DHFR	Dihydrofolate reductase
DHPR	Dihydropteridine reductase
DBH	Dopamine beta hydroxylase
GTP	Guanosine triphosphate
GTPCH	GTP cyclohydrolase I
5HIAA	5-Hydroxyindoleacetic acid
5HTP	5-Hydroxytryptophan
5-MTHF	5-Methyltetrahydrofolate
HCys	Homocysteine
HVA	Homovanillic acid
L-dopa	3,4-Dihydroxyphenylalanine
MAO	Monoamine oxidase
Met	Methionine
MHPG	3-Methoxy-4-hydroxyphenylglycol
n.e.	Nonenzymatic
3OMD	3-O-methyldopa
OH-BH4	Hydroxy-tetrahydrobiopterin
PCD	Pterin-4a-carbinolamine dehydratase
PNMT	Phenylethanolamine N-methyltransferase
PTPS	6-Pyruvoly-tetrahydropterin synthase
q-BH2	Quinoide-dihydrobiopterin

SAH	S-adenosylhomocysteine
SAM	S-adenosyl-methionine
SR	Seapiapterin reductase
TPH	Tryprophan-5-hydroxylase
TH	Tyrosine 3-hydroxylase
VLA	Vanillactic acid
VMA	Vanillmandelic acid
vB_6	Vitamin B_6

REFERENCES

1. Ng J, Papandreou A, Heales SJ, Kurian MA. Monoamine neurotransmitter disorders--clinical advances and future perspectives. *Nat Rev Neurol* 2015;**11**(10):567–84.
2. Lüdecke B, Knappskog PM, Clayton PT, et al. Recessively inherited L-dopa-responsive parkinsonism in infancy caused by a point mutation (L205P) in the tyrosine hydroxylase gene. *Hum Mol Genet* 1996;**5**:1023–8.
3. Man in 't Veld AJ, Boomsma F, Moleman P, Schalekamp MA. Congenital dopamine-beta-hydroxylase deficiency. A novel orthostatic syndrome. *Lancet* 1987;**1**:183–8.
4. Hyland K, Surtees RAH, Rodeck C, Clayton PT. Aromatic L-amino acid decarboxylase deficiency: clinical features, diagnosis, and treatment of a new inborn error of neurotransmitter amine synthesis. *Neurology* 1988;**42**:1980–8.
5. Brunner HG, Nelen MR, Breakefield XO, et al. Abnormal behaviour associated with a point mutation in the structural gene for monoamine oxidase A. *Science* 1993;**262**:578–80.
6. Ichinose H, Ohye T, Takahashi E, et al. Hereditary progressive dystonia with marked diurnal fluctuation caused by mutations in the GTP cyclohydrolase I gene. *Nat Genet* 1994;**8**:236–42.
7. Friedman J, Roze E, Abdenau JE, et al. Sepiapterin reductase deficiency: a treatable mimic of cerebral palsy. *Ann Neurol* 2012;**71**:520–30.
8. Kurian MA, Zhen J, Cheng SY, et al. Homozygous loss-of-function mutations in the gene encoding the dopamine transporter are associated with infantile parkinsonism-dystonia. *J Clin Invest* 2009;**119**(6):1595–603.
9. Rilstone JJ, Alkhater RA, Minassian BA. Brain dopamine-serotonin vesicular transport disease and its treatment. *N Engl J Med* 2013;**368**(6):543–50.
10. Wijemanne S, Jankovic J. Dopa-responsive dystonia—clinical and genetic heterogeneity. *Nat Rev Neurol* 2015;**11**:414–24.
11. Willemsen MA, Verbeek MM, Kamsteeg EJ, et al. Tyrosine hydroxylase deficiency: a treatable disorder of brain catecholamine biosynthesis. *Brain* 2010;**133**(Pt 6):1810–22.
12. Pons R, Syrengelas D, Youroukos S, Orfanou I, et al. Levodopa-induced dyskinesias in tyrosine hydroxylase deficiency. *Mov Disord.* 2013;**28**:1058–63.
13. Manegold C, Hoffmann GF, Degen I, et al. Aromatic L-amino acid decarboxylase deficiency: clinical features, drug therapy and follow-up. *J Inherit Metab Dis* 2009;**32**(3):371–80.
14. Brun L, Ngu LH, Keng WT, et al. Clinical and biochemical features of aromatic L-amino acid decarboxylase deficiency. *Neurology* 2010;**75**(1):64–71. 6.
15. Robertson D, Garland EM. Dopamine beta-hydroxylase deficiency. In: Pagon RA, Bird TC, Dolan CR, Stephens K, editors. *GeneReviews [Internet]*. Seattle (WA): University of Washington, Seattle; 2005.

16. Marecos C, Ng J, Kurian M. What is new in neurotransmitter disorders? *J Inherit Metab Dis* 2014;**37**:619–26.
17. Bicker J, Fortuna A, Alves G, Falcão A. Liquid chromatographic methods for the quantification of catecholamines and their metabolites in several biological samples--a review. *Anal Chim Acta* 2013;**768**:12–34.
18. Abdenur JE, Abeling N, Specola N, Jorge L, Schenone AB, van Cruchten AC, et al. Aromatic l-aminoacid decarboxylase deficiency: unusual neonatal presentation and additional findings in organic acid analysis. *Mol Genet Metab* 2006;**87**(1):48–53.
19. Arnoux JB, Damaj L, Napuri S, Serre V, Hubert L, Cadoudal M, et al. Aromatic L-amino acid decarboxylase deficiency is a cause of long-fasting hypoglycemia. *J Clin Endocrinol Metab* 2013;**98**(11):4279–84.
20. Heales S. Biogenic amines. In: Blau N, Duran M, Gibson KM, editors. *Laboratory guide to the methods in biochemical genetics*. Berlin-Heidleberg: Springer-Verlag; 2008. p. 703–16.
21. Opladen T, Hoffmann GF, Blau N. An international survey of patients with tetrahydrobiopterin deficiencies presenting with hyperphenylalaninaemia. *J Inherit Metab Dis* 2012;**35**(6):963–73.
22. Carducci C, Santagata S, Friedman J, Pasquini E, Carducci C, Tolve M, et al. Urine sepiapterin excretion as a new diagnostic marker for sepiapterin reductase deficiency. *Mol Genet Metab* 2015;**115**(4):157–60.
23. Blau N, Thöny B. Pterins and related enzymes. In: Blau N, Duran M, Gibson KM, editors. *Laboratory guide to the methods in biochemical genetics*. Berlin-Heidleberg: Springer-Verlag; 2008. p. 703–16.
24. Tomšíková H, Solich P, Nováková L. Sample preparation and UHPLC-FD analysis of pteridines in human urine. *J Pharm Biomed Anal* 2014;**95**:265–72.
25. Cañada-Cañada F, Espinosa-Mansilla A, Muñoz de la Peña A, Mancha de Llanos A. Determination of marker pteridins and biopterin reduced forms, tetrahydrobiopterin and dihydrobiopterin, in human urine, using a post-column photoinduced fluorescence liquid chromatographic derivatization method. *Anal Chim Acta* 2009;**648**(1):113–22.
26. Ormazabal A, García-Cazorla A, Fernández Y, Fernández-Alvarez E, Campistol J, Artuch R. HPLC with electrochemical and fluorescence detection procedures for the diagnosis of inborn errors of biogenic amines and pterins. *J Neurosci Methods* 2005;**142**(1):153–148. PubMed PMID: 15652629.
27. López-Laso E, Ormazabal A, Camino R, Gascón FJ, Ochoa JJ, Mateos ME, et al. Oral phenylalanine loading test for the diagnosis of dominant guanosine triphosphate cyclohydrolase 1 deficiency. *Clin Biochem* 2006;**39**(9):893–7.
28. Hyland K, Surtees RA, Heales SJ, Bowron A, Howells DW, Smith I. Cerebrospinalfluid concentrations of pterins and metabolites of serotonin and dopamine in a pediatric reference population. *Pediatr. Res.* 1993;**34**(1):10–14.
29. Molero-Luis M, Fernández-Ureña S, Jordán I, Serrano M, Ormazábal A, Garcia-Cazorla À, et al. Neopterin Working Group. Cerebrospinal fluid neopterin analysis in neuropediatric patients: establishment of a new cut off-value for the identification of inflammatory-immune mediated processes. *PLoS One* 2013;**8**(12):e83237. http://dx.doi.org/10.1371/journal.pone.0083237. 24367586.
30. Zorzi G, Redweik U, Trippe H, Penzien JM, Thöny B, Blau N. Detection of sepiapterin in CSF of patients with sepiapterin reductase deficiency. *Mol Genet Metab* 2002;**75**(2):174–7. PubMed PMID: 11855937.

31. Ormazabal A, Oppenheim M, Serrano M, García-Cazorla A, Campistol J, Ribes A, et al. Pyridoxal 5'-phosphate values in cerebrospinal fluid: reference values and diagnosis of PNPO deficiency in paediatric patients. *Mol Genet Metab* 2008;**94**(2):173–7.

32. Plecko B, Stöckler S. Vitamin B6 dependent seizures. *Can J Neurol Sci* 2009;**36**(Suppl 2): S73–7. Review. PubMed PMID: 19760909.

33. Ormazábal A, Perez-Dueñas B, Sierra C, Urreitzi R, Montoya J, Serrano M, et al. Folate analysis for the differential diagnosis of profound cerebrospinal fluid folate deficiency. *Clin Biochem* 2011;**44**(8–9):719–21.

34. Narisawa K, Arai N, Hayakawa H, Tada K. Diagnosis of dihydropteridine reductase deficiency by erythrocyte enzyme assay. *Pediatrics* 1981;**68**(4):591–2.

35. Boomsma F, van der Hoorn FA, Schalekamp MA. Determination of aromatic-L-amino acid decarboxylase in human plasma. *Clin Chim Acta* 1986;**2**:173–83.

36. Hyland K, Clayton PT. Aromatic L-amino acid decarboxylase deWciency: diagnostic methodology. *Clin Chem* 1992;**12**:2405–10.

37. Verbeek MM, Geurtz PB, Willemsen MA, Wevers RA. Aromatic L-amino acid decarboxylase enzyme activity in deficient patients and heterozygotes. *Mol Genet Metab* 2007;**90**(4):363–9.

38. Bonafé L, Thöny B, Leimbacher W, Kierat L, Blau N. Diagnosis of dopa-responsive dystonia and other tetrahydrobiopterin disorders by the study of biopterin metabolism in fibroblasts. *Clin Chem* 2001;**47**(3):477–85. PubMed PMID: 11238300.

39. Segawa M. Autosomal dominant GTP cyclohydrolase I (AD GCH 1) deficiency (Segawa disease, dystonia 5; DYT 5). *Chang Gung Med J* 2009;**32**(1):1–11. Review. PubMed PMID: 19292934.

40. Suzuki T, Ohye T, Inagaki H, Nagatsu T, Ichinose H. Characterization of wild-type and mutants of recombinant human GTP cyclohydrolase I: relationship to etiology of dopa-responsive dystonia. *J Neurochem* 1999;**73**:2510–6.

41. Ferre J, Naylor EW. Sepiapterin reductase in human amniotic and skin fibroblasts, chorionic villi, and various blood fractions. *Clin Chim Acta* 1988;**174**:271–82.

42. Timmers HJ, Deinum J, Wevers RA, Lenders JW. Congenital dopamine-beta-hydroxylase deficiency in humans. *Ann N Y Acad Sci* 2004;**1018**:520–3. Review. PubMed PMID: 15240410.

43. Horvath GA, Demos M, Shyr C, Matthews A, Zhang L, Race S, et al. Secondary neurotransmitter deficiencies in epilepsy caused by voltage-gated sodium channelopathies: A potential treatment target? *Mol Genet Metab* 2015; S1096-7192(15):30078-0.

44. Kaneda N, Kobayashi K, Ichinose H, Kishi F, Nakazawa A, Kurosawa Y, et al. Isolation of a novel cDNA clone for human tyrosine hydroxylase: alternative RNA splicing produces four kinds of mRNA from a single gene. *Biochem Biophys Res Commun* 1987;**146**: 971–5.

45. Pons R, Serrano M, Ormazabal A, et al. Tyrosine hydroxylase deficiency in three Greek patients with a common ancestral mutation. *Mov Disord* 2010;**25**:1086–90.

46. Ribasés M, Serrano M, Fernández-Alvarez E, Pahisa S, Ormazabal A, García-Cazorla A, et al. A homozygous tyrosine hydroxylase gene promoter mutation in a patient with dopa-responsive encephalopathy: clinical, biochemical and genetic analysis. *Mol Genet Metab* 2007;**92**(3):274–7. Epub 2007 Aug 14. PubMed PMID: 17698383.

47. Haavik J, Blau N, Thöny B. Mutations in human monoamine-related neurotransmitter pathway genes. *Hum Mutat* 2008;**29**(7):891–902. http://dx.doi.org/10.1002/humu.20700. Review. PubMed PMID: 18444257.

48. Chang YT, Sharma R, Marsh JL, McPherson JD, Bedell JA, Knust A, et al. Levodopa-responsive aromatic L-amino acid decarboxylase deficiency. *Ann Neurol* 2004;**55**(3):435–8. PubMed PMID: 14991824.

49. Craig SP, Buckle VJ, Lamouroux A, Mallet J, Craig IW. Localization of the human dopamine beta hydroxylase (DBH) gene to chromosome 9q34. *Cytogenet Cell Genet* 1988;**48**(1):48–50. PubMed PMID: 3180847.

50. Whibley A, Urquhart J, Dore J, Willatt L, Parkin G, Gaunt L, et al. Deletion of MAOA and MAOB in a male patient causes severe developmental delay, intermittent hypotonia and stereotypical hand movements. *Eur J Hum Genet.* 2010;**18**(10):1095–9. http://dx.doi.org/10.1038/ejhg.2010.41. 20485326.

51. Lenders JW, Eisenhofer G, Abeling NG, Berger W, Murphy DL, Konings CH, et al. Specific genetic deficiencies of the A and B isoenzymes of monoamine oxidase are characterized by distinct neurochemical and clinical phenotypes. *J Clin Invest* 1996;**97**(4):1010–9. PubMed PMID: 8613523; PubMed Central PMCID: PMC507147.

52. Rodriguez-Revenga L, Madrigal I, Alkhalidi LS, Armengol L, González E, Badenas C, et al. *Am J Med Genet A* 2007;**143A**(9):916–20.

53. Kurian MA, Li Y, Zhen J, Meyer E, Hai N, Christen HJ, et al. Clinical and molecular characterisation of hereditary dopamine transporter deficiency syndrome: an observational cohort and experimental study. *Lancet Neurol* 2011;**10**(1):54–62. http://dx.doi.org/10.1016/S1474-4422(10)70269-6. Epub 2010 Nov 25. PubMed PMID: 21112253; PubMed Central PMCID: PMC3002401.

54. Ichinose H, Ohye T, Takahashi E, Seki N, Hori T, Segawa M, et al. Hereditary progressive dystonia with marked diurnal fluctuation caused by mutations in the GTP cyclohydrolase I gene. *Nat Genet* 1997;**8**:236–42.

55. Thöny B, Blau N. Mutations in the BH4-metabolizing genes GTP cyclohydrolase I, 6-pyruvoyl-tetrahydropterin synthase, sepiapterin reductase, carbinolamine-4a-dehydratase, and dihydropteridine reductase. *Hum Mutat.* 2006;**27**(9):870–8. PubMed PMID: 16917893.

56. Burlina A, Balu N. Tehtrahydrobiopterin disorders presenting with hyperphenylalanemia. In: Hoffmann GF, Blau N, editors. *Congenital neurotransmitters disorders. Nova Science Publishers, Inc*; 2014 p. 39–50.

57. Farrugia R, Felice AE 2004. BH4 deficiency in a small island population. Human Genome Meeting, Berlin, Germany (Abstract).

58. Thöny B, Heizmann CW, Mattei MG. Chromosomal location of two human genes encoding tetrahydrobiopterinmetabolizing enzymes: 6-pyruvoyl-tetrahydropterin synthase maps to 11q22.3–q23.3, and pterin-4a-carbinolamine dehydratase maps to 10q22. *Genomics* 1994;**19**:365–8.

59. Rose RB, Pullen KE, Bayle JH, Crabtree GR, Alber T. Biochemical and structural basis for partially redundant enzymatic and transcriptional functions of DCoH and DCoH2. *Biochemistry* 2004;**43**:7345–55.

60. Hevel JM, Stewart JA, Gross KL, Ayling JE. Can the DCoHalpha isozyme compensate in patients with 4a-hydroxy-tetrahydrobiopterin dehydratase/DCoH deficiency? *Mol Genet Metab* 2006;**88**(1):38–46.16423549.

61. Porta F, Ponzone A, Spada M. Short prolactin profile for monitoring treatment in BH4 deficiency. *Eur J Paediatr Neurol* 2015;**19**(3):360–3. http://dx.doi.org/10.1016/j.ejpn.2015.01.010. 25707872.

62. Concolino D, Muzzi G, Rapsomaniki M, Moricca MT, Pascale MG, Strisciuglio P. Serum prolactin as a tool for the follow-up of treated DHPR-deficient patients. *J Inherit Metab Dis* 2008;**31**(Suppl 2):S193–7.

63. Aitkenhead H, Heales SJ. Establishment of paediatric age-related reference intervals for serum prolactin to aid in the diagnosis of neurometabolic conditions affecting dopamine metabolism. *Ann Clin Biochem* 2013;**50**(Pt 2):156–8.

64. Yano S, Moseley K, Azen C. Large neutral amino acid supplementation increases melatonin synthesis in phenylketonuria: a new biomarker. *Pediatr* 2013;**162**(5):999–1003. 23164313.

65. Kurian MA. What is the role of dopamine in childhood neurological disorders? *Dev Med Child Neurol* 2013;**55**(6):493–4.23496203.

66. Spector R, Keep RF, Robert Snodgrass S, Smith QR, Johanson CE. A balanced view of choroid plexus structure and function: Focus on adult humans. *Exp Neurol* 2015;**267**:78–86. 25747036.

67. Tondo M, Málaga I, O'Callaghan M, Serrano M, Emperador S, Ormazabal A, et al. Biochemical parameters to assess choroid plexus dysfunction in Kearns-Sayre Syndrome patients. *Mitochondrion* 2011;**11**(6):867–70. 21745599.

68. Serrano M, Ormazábal A, Pérez-Dueñas B, Artuch R, Coroleu W, Krauel X, et al. Perinatal asphyxia may cause reduction in CSF dopamine metabolite concentrations. *Neurology* 2007;**69**(3):311–3.

69. De Grandis E, Serrano M, Pérez-Dueñas B, Ormazábal A, Montero R, Veneselli E, et al. Cerebrospinal fluid alterations of the serotonin product, 5-hydroxyindolacetic acid, in neurological disorders. *J Inherit Metab Dis* 2010;**33**(6):803–9. 20852934.

70. García-Cazorla A, Serrano M, Pérez-Dueñas B, González V, Ormazábal A, Pineda M, et al. Secondary abnormalities of neurotransmitters in infants with neurological disorders. *Dev Med Child Neurol* 2007;**49**(10):740–4. 17880642.

71. Molero-Luis M, Serrano M, Ormazábal A, Pérez-Dueñas B, García-Cazorla A, Pons R, et al. Neurotransmitter Working Group. Homovanillic acid in cerebrospinalfluid of 1388 children with neurological disorders. *Dev Med Child Neurol* 2013;**55**(6): 559–66. 23480488.

72. Van Der Heyden JC, Rotteveel JJ, Wevers RA. Decreased homovanillic acid concentrations in cerebrospinal fluid in children without a known defect in dopamine metabolism. *Eur J Paediatr Neurol* 2003;**7**(1):31–7. 12615172.

73. Giroud M, Dumas R, Dauvergne M, D'Athis P, Rochette L, Beley A, et al. 5-Hydroxyindoleacetic acid and homovanillic acid in cerebrospinal fluid of children with febrile convulsions. *Epilepsia* 1990;**31**(2):178–81.

74. Devinsky O, Emoto S, Goldstein DS, Stull R, Porter RJ, Theodore WH, et al. Cerebrospinal fluid and serum levels of dopa, catechols, and monoamine metabolites in patients with epilepsy. *Epilepsia* 1992;**33**(2):263–70.

75. Garcia-Cazorla A, Duarte S, Serrano M, Nascimento A, Ormazabal A, Carrilho I, et al. Mitochondrial diseases mimicking neurotransmitter defects. *Mitochondrion* 2008;**8**(3):273–8.

76. Temudo T, Rios M, Prior C, Carrilho I, Santos M, Maciel P, et al. Evaluation of CSF neurotransmitters and folate in 25 patients with Rett disorder and effects of treatment. *Brain Dev* 2009;**31**(1):46–51.

77. Mercimek-Mahmutoglu S, Sidky S, Hyland K, Patel J, Donner EJ, Logan W, et al. Prevalence of inherited neurotransmitter disorders in patients with movement disorders and epilepsy: a retrospective cohort study. *Orphanet J Rare Dis* 2015;**10**:12.

78. Clayton PT. B6-responsive disorders: a model of vitamin dependency. *J Inherit Metab Dis* 2006;**29**(2–3):317–26. Review 16763894.

79. Burlina A, Balu N. Tehtrahydrobiopterin disorders presenting with hyperphenylalane-mia. In: Hoffmann GF, Blau N, editors. *Congential Neurotransmitters disorders*. Nova Science Publishers, Inc; 2014. p. 39–50.

80. Cario H, Smith DE, Blom H, Blau N, Bode H, Holzmann K, et al. Dihydrofolate reductase deficiency due to a homozygous DHFR mutation causes megaloblastic anemia and cerebral folate deficiency leading to severe neurologic disease. *Am J Hum Genet* 2011;**88**(2):226–31.

81. Watkins D, Rosenblatt DS. Update and new concepts in vitamin responsive disorders of folate transport and metabolism. *J. Inherit Metab Dis* 2012;**35**(4):665–70.

82. Banka S, Blom HJ, Walter J, et al. Identification and characterization of an inborn error of metabolism caused by dihydrofolate reductase deficiency. *Am J.J Hum Genet* 2011;**88**(2):216–25.

83. Steinfeld R, Grapp M, Kraetzner R, et al. Folate receptor alpha defect causes cerebral folate transport deficiency: a treatable neurodegenerative disorder associated with disturbed myelin metabolism. *Am J Hum Genet* 2009;**85**(3):354–63.

84. Qiu A, Jansen M, Sakaris A, et al. Identification of an intestinal folate transporter and the molecular basis for hereditary folate malabsorption. *Cell* 2006;**127**(5):917–28.

85. Ly CV, Verstreken P. Mitochondria at the synapse. *Neuroscientist* 2006;**12**(4):291–9. Review 16840705.

86. Bandettini di Poggio M, Nesti C, Bruno C, Meschini MC, Schenone A, Santorelli FM. Dopamine-agonist responsive Parkinsonism in a patient with the SANDO syndrome caused by POLG mutation. *BMC Med Genet* 2013;**14**:105.

87. Visser JE, Schretlen DJ, Bloem BR, Jinnah HA. Levodopa is not a useful treatment for Lesch-Nyhan disease. *Mov Disord* 2011;**26**(4):746–9.

88. Shirley TL, Lewers JC, Egami K, Majumdar A, Kelly M, Ceballos-Picot I, et al. A human neuronal tissue culture model for Lesch-Nyhan disease. *J Neurochem* 2007;**101**(3):841–53. 17448149.

89. Serrano M, Pérez-Dueñas B, Ormazábal A, Artuch R, Campistol J, Torres RJ, et al. Levodopa therapy in a Lesch-Nyhan disease patient: pathological, biochemical, neuroimaging, and therapeutic remarks. *Mov Disord* 2008;**23**(9):1297–300.

90. Dale RC, Brilot F. Biomarkers of inflammatory and auto-immune central nervous system disorders. *Curr Opin Pediatr* 2010;**22**(6):718–25.

91. Ghisoni K, Martins Rde P, Barbeito L, Latini A. Neopterin as a potential cytoprotective brain molecule. *J Psychiatr Res* 2015;**71**:134–9.

92. Rao JU, Engelke UF, Sweep FC, Pacak K, Kusters B, Goudswaard AG, et al. Genotype-specific differences in the tumor metabolite profile of pheochromocytoma and paraganglioma using untargeted and targeted metabolomics. *J Clin Endocrinol Metab* 2015;**100**(2):E214–22.

93. Engel J, Blanchet L, Bloemen B, van den Heuvel LP, Engelke UH, Wevers RA, et al. Regularized MANOVA (rMANOVA) in intargeted metabolomics. *Anal Chim Acta* 2015;**899**:1–12.

94. Ortez C, Duarte ST, Ormazábal A, Serrano M, Pérez A, Pons R, et al. Cerebrospinal fluid synaptic proteins as useful biomarkers in tyrosine hydroxylase deficiency. *Mol Genet Metab* 2015;**114**(1):34–40.

95. Graziano C, Wischmeijer A, Pippucci T, Fusco C, Diquigiovanni C, Nõukas M, et al. Syndromic intellectual disability: a new phenotype caused by an aromatic amino acid decarboxylase gene (DDC) variant. *Gene* 2015;**559**(2):144–8.
96. Wevers R, Engelke U, Moolenaar S. Proton NMR spectroscopy of body fluids. In: Blau N, Duran M, Blascovics ME, Gibson M, editors. *Physician's Guide to the Laboratory Diagnosis of Metabolic Diseases*. Springer Berlin Heidelberg; 2003. p. 77–85.

Cerebral creatine deficiency syndromes

14

Q. Sun

Baylor College of Medicine, Houston, TX, United States

14.1 INTRODUCTION

Creatine is critical for temporal and spatial regulation of the intracellular adenosine triphosphate (ATP) energy pool.[1–3] In humans, half of creatine comes from diet and half from endogenous biosynthesis. Creatine, which is synthesized principally in the liver and pancreas, is distributed through the bloodstream, and actively transported into muscle and brain where it participates in the high-energy phosphate buffering system. Creatine is known to be an energy source for muscle and brain functions. Some creatine is converted to creatine phosphate by accepting a high-energy bond from ATP under the action of creatine kinase (CK). This reaction is reversible. The high energy of creatine phosphate can exchange with adenosine diphosphate (ADP) to generate ATP. In this way, the creatine phosphate cycle links ATP consumption with ATP generation in various cellular locations. Three cytosolic CK isoforms, brain BB-CK, muscle type MM-CK, and the MB-CK heterodimer, replenish ATP, maintaining a stable ATP/ADP ratio in cytoplasm. On the other hand, two mitochondrial CK isoforms recharge creatine with high energy. The creatine/creatine phosphate cycle regenerates and buffers ATP. This ensures sustainable energy reserve whenever a spiked ATP is required. In cerebral creatine deficiency syndromes, creatine supply is reduced and the creatine/creatine phosphate cycle is impaired.

14.2 BRIEF DESCRIPTION OF CLINICAL PRESENTATION

Individuals with cerebral creatine deficiency syndromes manifest a diverse spectrum of neurological phenotypes. The most common features include seizures, intellectual disability (ID), autism, and speech delay. While there is a significant amount of phenotypic overlap, the disorders are distinct in their presentation, pathogenesis, and treatment, and therefore will be discussed individually.

14.3 CEREBRAL CREATINE DEFICIENCY SYNDROMES

Cerebral creatine deficiency syndromes include defects in both creatine synthesis and creatine membrane transporters.[4-9] A short two-step pathway of *de novo* creatine biosynthesis involves two enzymes: arginine:glycine amidinotransferase (AGAT) and guanidinoacetate methyltransferase (GAMT). In addition, an X-linked creatine transporter (XCrT) is critical to maintain the physiological levels in cytosol (see Fig. 14.1). Creatine and creatine phosphate are nonenzymatically converted to creatinine, which is excreted in urine. Approximately 1.5% of body creatine is turned into creatinine daily.

14.3.1 ARGININE:GLYCINE AMIDINOTRANSFERASE DEFICIENCY (OMIM 612718)

Arginine:glycine amidinotransferase (AGAT) is the first enzyme in creatine biosynthesis. It converts arginine and glycine to guanidinoacetate (GAA) and ornithine. AGAT deficiency is an autosomal recessive disorder caused by mutations in the gene *GATM*, which is located on chromosome 15q15. This is the rate-limiting step. AGAT is subject to feedback inhibition by creatine and ornithine. The reaction is predominantly located in the mitochondria intermembrane space in the kidney.[10]

Fewer than 20 AGAT-deficient patients have been reported. Clinically, AGAT deficiency is characterized with delayed psychomotor development, mild-to-moderate ID, and speech delay. Other presentations include myopathy/proximal muscle

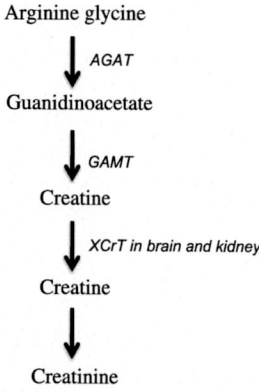

FIGURE 14.1

Creatine metabolic pathways. Pathway of creatine biosynthesis and transport. *AGAT,* Arginine:glycine amidinotransferase; *GAMT,* guanidinoacetate methyltransferase; *XCrT,* X-linked creatine transporter.

weakness, and autistic behavior. Myopathy is unique to AGAT among cerebral creatine deficiency syndromes. In addition, only a few AGAT patients were reported as having occasional seizures. This is greatly different from GAMT and XCrT deficiencies in which movement disorders and seizures are more common.[11–16]

Recently, a mouse AGAT knockout model has been created to study creatine depletion effects in skeletal muscle. In AGAT$^{-/-}$ mice, myoatrophy was exhibited. Levels of ATP and activities of proton-pumping respiratory chain enzymes (Complex III and IV) were reduced while overall mitochondrial contents and ATPase (Complex V) were increased. All muscle abnormalities were reversed within 24 hours by creatine supplementation.[17] On the other hand, it was found that brain creatine concentration took up to 20 days to restore to predepletion levels. GAA depletion is proposed to lead to unique myopathy in AGAT patients since GAA is suggested as an alternative substrate for creatine phosphate kinase. Depletion of this high-energy reservoir in muscle was suggested as the consequence of missing GAA in AGAT deficiency.[18]

14.3.2 GUANIDINOACETATE METHYLTRANSFERASE DEFICIENCY (OMIM 612736)

Guanidinoacetate methyltransferase (GAMT) is the second enzyme in the creatine synthesis pathway. It transfers a methyl group to GAA, producing creatine and S-adenosyl homocysteine (SAH). The reaction occurs mainly in the liver. Interestingly, this enzyme reaction consumes 40% of the cellular methyl donor S-adenosylmethionine (SAM). GAMT deficiency is inherited in an autosomal recessive fashion. The gene *GAMT* is located on chromosome 19p13.

The estimated incidence of GAMT deficiency was 1:250,000, with a carrier frequency of 1 in 250, according to a pilot study using newborn screening dry blood spots performed in the Netherlands. In other studies, carrier frequency of this disorder was determined to be between 1 in 812 to 1 in 1475 in British Columbia, Canada, by variants reported in the Exome Variant Server database or targeted mutation screening.[19–21] The higher carrier frequency obtained in the first study is possibly due to a high consanguinity rate in a mixed ethnic background of the Dutch population in comparison to the general population.

GAMT deficiency was the first inborn error in creatine biosynthesis discovered.[22] Predominant clinical symptoms of GAMT deficiency are central nervous system (CNS)-related development delay, especially in movement and speech development, ataxia, and seizures. Muscle hypotonia is also frequent in GAMT patients. Although presentations are heterogeneous, the onset is usually in early childhood.[23–29] Accumulation of GAA in this disorder is toxic for the brain.[30] GAA has been found to interact with GABA$_A$ (γ-aminobutyric acid type A) receptors in murine brain studies. This provides a possible mechanism explaining the neurological phenotypes in GAMT deficiency.[31]

14.3.3 X-LINKED CREATINE TRANSPORTER DEFICIENCY (MIM 300352)

The X-linked membrane creatine transporter (XCrT) is encoded by *SLC6A8*, located at Xq28. The transporter is ubiquitously expressed and responsible for the uptake of creatine into the cell cytoplasm in brain and muscle. The transporter is also critical for renal reabsorption of creatine.[32,33] The deficiency is estimated to have a prevalence of 0.3–0.5% in males.[34]

Clinical features are mainly ID, severe motor and language delay, cognitive retardation, seizures, ataxia, hypotonia, and autistic behaviors in males. Dysmorphic findings, such as short stature, microcephaly, and mid-face hypoplasia have been described.[6,29,35–37] Mutations in *SLC6A8* were also found to be prevalent in causing male ID, second only to Fragile X syndrome.[38] As in other X-linked disorders, up to 50% of female carriers may be symptomatic. Note that carrier women may have normal urine creatine/creatinine ratios. Thus, it is recommended that molecular testing should be performed if female carrier diagnosis is suspected.[34]

Creatine has been implicated to function as an antagonist on $GABA_A$ and NMDA (N-methyl-D-aspartate) receptors.[39] Permeation of creatine through the blood–brain barrier in mature brain was limited. In consequence, the brain needs to synthesize its own creatine. It has been perplexing why the levels of endogenously synthesized creatine by AGAT and GAMT is not sufficient for the brain energy requirement in patient with a creatine transporter deficiency. It has been demonstrated that the entire creatine synthesis pathway is available in only 12% of CNS cells. In approximately 43% of cells, only AGAT or GAMT enzymatic activity, but not both, is present. The remaining CNS cells contain neither AGAT nor GAMT. It has been suggested that an intercellular transportation of GAA and creatine is required. *SLC6A8* may play this essential role in CNS cells.[32,40,41]

14.4 SECONDARY CONDITIONS THAT CAN CAUSE CREATINE OR GAA ABNORMALITIES

14.4.1 ORNITHINE METABOLISM DISORDERS: ORNITHINE δ-AMINOTRANSFERASE DEFICIENCY AND HYPERORNITHINEMIA-HYPERAMMONEMIA-HOMOCITRULLINURIA

Ornithine δ-aminotransferase (OAT) deficiency is also known as gyrate atrophy (GA) of the choroid and retina (OMIM 258870). This autosomal recessive condition presents with progressive chorioretinal degeneration, myopia, night blindness, and eventually complete blindness in the fourth or fifth decade. OAT maintains a stable ornithine level in mitochondria. In OAT deficiency, hyperornithinemia inhibits AGAT, causing creatine deficiency. A study of seven OAT-deficient patients, aged from 11 to 27 years, revealed a profound plasma and urinary creatine, and GAA deficiency in all seven patients.[42] The marked deficiency of creatine was confirmed with cerebral proton magnetic resonance spectroscopy (MRS). Interestingly two patients in this small cohort had normal intelligence.

Hyperornithinemia-hyperammonemia-homocitrullinuria (HHH, OMIM 238970) is an autosomal recessive disease caused by deficiencies in mitochondrial ornithine transporter SLC25A15. Cytosolic ornithine produced by arginase in urea cycle has to be transported inside mitochondria to replenish a new cycle of ammonia elimination. It combines with carbamoyl phosphate to form citrulline at the step catalyzed by ornithine transcarbamylase (OTC). In HHH, lack of local ornithine inside mitochondria results in deficiency of OTC substrate and block of the urea cycle, thus causing hyperammonemia. Accumulated carbamoyl phosphate combines with lysine to form homocitrulline. In addition, elevations of cytosolic ornithine inhibit AGAT as in OAT deficiency above. Absence of brain creatine in addition to ammonia toxicity could contribute to the IDs and other neurological presentations in HHH.[43,44]

14.4.2 UREA CYCLE DISORDERS

Ornithine and arginine are involved in both the urea cycle and creatine biosynthesis. Arginine is not only the guanidino group donor for creatine synthesis, but is also the substrate for protein building and nitric oxide formation. When their concentrations are disturbed, due to one of urea cycle disorders, a secondary creatine deficiency could be the consequence. Ornithine may be elevated and arginine decreased in OTC deficiency (OMIM 311250) and argininosuccinate synthetase (ASS) deficiency (OMIM 207900). Creatine deficiencies have been reported in OTC- or ASS-deficient patients.[43,45] On the contrary, plasma arginine is elevated in arginase deficiency (OMIM 207800). Arginine supplementation is also a common treatment for urea cycle disorders. Elevated arginine levels can lead to secondary GAA accumulation.[46]

14.4.3 HOMOCYSTEINE METHYLATION CYCLE

Interestingly, changes in guanidinoacetate and/or creatine excretion are also reported in disorders in which one-carbon methyl group metabolism is disturbed. Examples include S-adenosyl homocysteine hydrolase (SAHH) deficiency and cobalamin deficiency.[47,48] Since 40% of the methyl donor SAM is consumed in the second step of creatine synthesis, it is understandable that restriction of the methyl donor can lead to secondary creatine deficiency. In SAHH deficiency, cerebrospinal fluid (CSF) GAA was observed to be increased and creatine was diminished. On the other hand, in cobalamin-deficient (CblC) patients, plasma GAA, methylmalonic acid, SAM, and SAH were all increased while creatine was in the low-reference range. Patients' cerebral creatine levels are also normal.

14.5 BIOMARKERS FOR DIFFERENTIAL DIAGNOSIS OF CEREBRAL CREATINE DEFICIENCY SYNDROMES

Since the presentations of cerebral creatine deficiency syndromes typically include commonly found neurological symptoms such as IDs and seizures, it is difficult to reach a definitive diagnosis clinically. The biomarker assays in the laboratory are usually the first-tier clinical testing (see Table 14.1 and Fig. 14.2). Brain creatine level, as identified by MRS or nuclear magnetic resonance (NMR), is also utilized in the process. Finally DNA analyses of mutations in the targeted gene confirm the diagnosis.

Table 14.1 Guanidinoacetate (GAA) and Creatine (CRT) Changes in Cerebral Creatine Deficiency Syndromes

Disorders	Plasma (µM)		Urine (mmoles/mole Creatinine)	
	GAA	CRT	GAA	CRT
AGAT deficiency	Low	Low	Low	Normal/Low
GAMT deficiency	High	Low	Normal/High	Normal/Low
CRT transporter defect	Normal	Normal/low	Normal	High

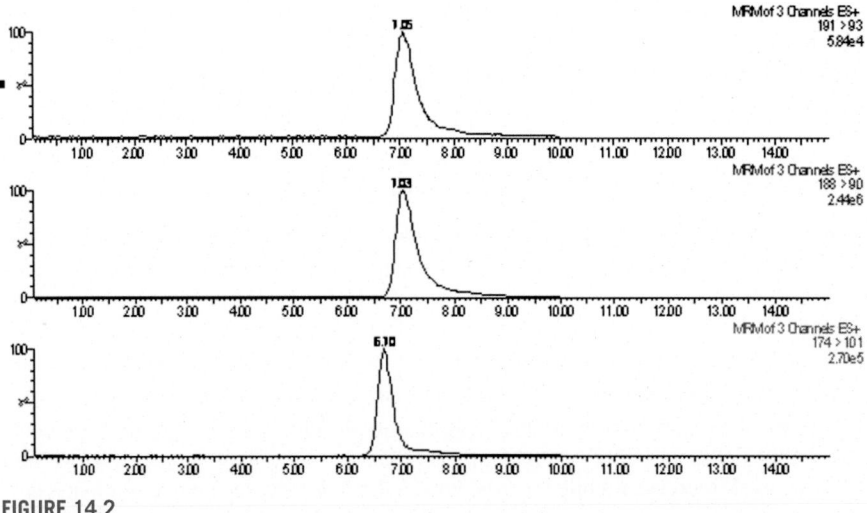

FIGURE 14.2

Chromatogram of LC-MS/MS analyses of a sample. The individual traces of MRM transitions are as follows: top panel, D3-Creatine (*m/z* 191 > 93); middle, Creatine (*m/z* 188 > 90) at about 7.0 minutes, and bottom, GAA (*m/z* 174 > 101) at 6.7 minutes.

14.5.1 GUANIDINOACETATE

Plasma or serum guanidinoacetate (GAA) measurement is essentially utilized to differentiate between the two creatine *de novo* synthesis disorders, AGAT and GAMT deficiencies. In AGAT deficiency, GAA is usually absent in plasma and low in urine. In GAMT deficiency, GAA is typically several times higher than the high concentration of the normal range. However, in rare GAMT cases modest GAA elevations were shown. Follow-up of plasma GAA concentrations and DNA confirmation are necessary.

Secondary GAA increases are demonstrated in argininemia, SAHH deficiency, and cobalamin disorders. Arginine supplementation is also known to contribute to mild GAA increases.

Mild GAA decreases in urine are frequently observed, and thus urinary GAA concentration is not a specific biomarker for AGAT and GAMT deficiencies. As most urinary assays, GAA values are normalized to creatinine concentrations of specimens. Extremely diluted or concentrated urines can cause biased GAA concentrations. Plasma or serum GAA level, to follow-up on initial urinary GAA abnormalities, is needed to confirm the AGAT or GAMT deficiency diagnosis.

Several groups have reported on newborn screening methods using residual dried blood spot cards. GAMT deficiency patients were identified with elevated GAA in newborn blood spots.[21,49,50] Prenatal diagnosis is possible by measuring guanidinoacetate in amniotic fluid.[51] It was reported that early diagnoses of this creatine deficiency can lead to early treatment and prevention of IDs and seizures.

14.5.2 CREATINE

MRS of the brain of AGAT, GAMT, and XCrT-deficient patients reveals CNS creatine depletion.[28,52,53] With AGAT deficiency, biochemical testing reveals extremely low creatine and creatinine in urine. For patients with GAMT deficiency, creatine is low to within normal limits in infancy. Creatine is present in foods such as meat and fish, so when affected infants start eating solid food, their creatine levels are typically in the normal range. However, the level declines if the proband is on strict vegetarian diet.

An elevated urinary creatine/creatinine ratio is the most helpful biomarker in diagnosing XCrT deficiency. Van de Kamp et al. investigated 101 male patients with transporter deficiency. Urine creatine/creatinine ratio, brain MRS, molecular studies, and creatine fibroblast uptake assays were all reliable in diagnosing the disorder. CSF creatine levels were normal or increased.[37] Mild mutations with residual activities showed lower creatine/creatinine ratios in the urine. For women carriers, this urine test is not recommended due to skewed X-inactivation.

14.6 BIOMARKERS FOLLOWED FOR TREATMENT EFFICACY AND DISEASE PROGRESSION

High creatine concentrations in urine and plasma are the consequences of creatine supplementation in creatine-deficient patients. In GAMT deficiency patients, GAA levels have been shown to be reduced when treated by arginine restriction and ornithine administration, but are not corrected to the normal range.[23] Mild GAA increases are observed in patients with argininemia or under arginine supplementation. Brain creatine levels are increased in AGAT- and GAMT-deficient patients after creatine therapy.

14.7 BRIEF DESCRIPTION OF TREATMENT

Creatine monohydrate supplementation is the major treatment for all the three disorders. High-dose creatine has been shown to decrease seizure activity and to improve movement symptoms. In addition, brain creatine levels have been restored as shown by MRS in AGAT-deficient patients. Myopathy was significantly improved.[16] For GAMT deficiency, ornithine supplementation and arginine restriction were employed to reduce GAA, which has been suggested to be neurotoxic.[23] Improvements in both behavior and language development in treated patients has been demonstrated. Notably, early diagnosis and treatment in both AGAT and GAMT patients, some presymptomatically, has been reported to result in normal or almost normal cognitive and behavior development. This encouraging outcome argues for adding treatable GAMT deficiency to the newborn screening list.

Creatine transporter patients received supplementation of creatine (creatine monohydrate or cyclocreatine), and/or in combination with L-arginine and glycine. Dunbar et al. reported that only a small percentage of patients responded to the therapy.[54] Patients receiving these treatments early in life (<9 years) are more likely to demonstrate positive responses with elevated cerebral creatine levels or improved clinical symptoms.

14.8 CONCLUSIONS

Cerebral creatine deficiency syndromes result in defective brain and muscle creatine supplies, leading to insufficient cellular ATP storage. Plasma and urinary measurements of creatine and guanidinoacetate are used in the diagnosis of creatine disorders and differentiating them from secondary conditions implicated in creatine metabolism. Early treatment of GAMT deficiency has prevented ID and seizures in patients. Including this disease in the newborn screening could result in better prognosis.

REFERENCES

1. Monge C, Beraud N, Kuznetsov AV, et al. Regulation of respiration in brain mitochondria and synaptosomes: restrictions of ADP diffusion in situ, roles of tubulin, and mitochondrial creatine kinase. *Mol Cell Biochem* 2008;**318**(1–2):147–65.
2. Saks V, Kaambre T, Guzun R, et al. The creatine kinase phosphotransfer network: thermodynamic and kinetic considerations, the impact of the mitochondrial outer membrane and modelling approaches. *Subcell Biochem* 2007;**46**:27–65.

3. Saks V, Kuznetsov A, Andrienko T, et al. Heterogeneity of ADP diffusion and regulation of respiration in cardiac cells. *Biophys J* 2003;**84**(5):3436–56.
4. Ganesan V, Johnson A, Connelly A, Eckhardt S, Surtees RA. Guanidinoacetate methyltransferase deficiency: new clinical features. *Pediatr Neurol* 1997;**17**(2):155–7.
5. Item CB, Stockler-Ipsiroglu S, Stromberger C, et al. Arginine:glycine amidinotransferase deficiency: the third inborn error of creatine metabolism in humans. *Am J Hum Genet* 2001;**69**(5):1127–33.
6. Salomons GS, van Dooren SJ, Verhoeven NM, et al. X-linked creatine-transporter gene (SLC6A8) defect: a new creatine-deficiency syndrome. *Am J Hum Genet* 2001;**68**(6):1497–500.
7. van der Knaap MS, Verhoeven NM, Maaswinkel-Mooij P, et al. Mental retardation and behavioral problems as presenting signs of a creatine synthesis defect. *Ann Neurol* 2000;**47**(4):540–3.
8. Stockler S, Hanefeld F, Frahm J. Creatine replacement therapy in guanidinoacetate methyltransferase deficiency, a novel inborn error of metabolism. *Lancet* 1996;**348**(9030):789–90.
9. Stockler S, Marescau B, De Deyn PP, Trijbels JM, Hanefeld F. Guanidino compounds in guanidinoacetate methyltransferase deficiency, a new inborn error of creatine synthesis. *Metabolism* 1997;**46**(10):1189–93.
10. Tormanen CD. Comparison of the properties of purified mitochondrial and cytosolic rat kidney transamidinase. *Int J Biochem* 1990;**22**(11):1243–50.
11. Bianchi MC, Tosetti M, Fornai F, et al. Reversible brain creatine deficiency in two sisters with normal blood creatine level. *Ann Neurol* 2000;**47**(4):511–3.
12. Battini R, Alessandri MG, Leuzzi V, et al. Arginine:glycine amidinotransferase (AGAT) deficiency in a newborn: early treatment can prevent phenotypic expression of the disease. *J Pediatr* 2006;**148**(6):828–30.
13. Edvardson S, Korman SH, Livne A, et al. L-arginine:glycine amidinotransferase (AGAT) deficiency: clinical presentation and response to treatment in two patients with a novel mutation. *Mol Genet Metab* 2010;**101**(2–3):228–32.
14. Ndika JD, Johnston K, Barkovich JA, et al. Developmental progress and creatine restoration upon long-term creatine supplementation of a patient with arginine:glycine amidinotransferase deficiency. *Mol Genet Metab* 2012;**106**(1):48–54.
15. Nouioua S, Cheillan D, Zaouidi S, et al. Creatine deficiency syndrome. A treatable myopathy due to arginine-glycine amidinotransferase (AGAT) deficiency. *Neuromuscul Disord* 2013;**23**(8):670–4.
16. Stockler-Ipsiroglu S, Apatean D, Battini R, et al. Arginine:glycine amidinotransferase (AGAT) deficiency: clinical features and long term outcomes in 16 patients diagnosed worldwide. *Mol Genet Metab* 2015.
17. Nabuurs CI, Choe CU, Veltien A, et al. Disturbed energy metabolism and muscular dystrophy caused by pure creatine deficiency are reversible by creatine intake. *J Physiol* 2013;**591**(Pt 2):571–92.
18. Fitch CD, Chevli R. Inhibition of creatine and phosphocreatine accumulation in skeletal muscle and heart. *Metabolism* 1980;**29**(7):686–90.
19. Mercimek-Mahmutoglu S, Pop A, Kanhai W, et al. A pilot study to estimate incidence of guanidinoacetate methyltransferase deficiency in newborns by direct sequencing of the GAMT gene. *Gene* 2016;**575**(1):127–31.
20. Desroches CL, Patel J, Wang P, et al. Carrier frequency of guanidinoacetate methyltransferase deficiency in the general population by functional characterization of missense variants in the GAMT gene. *Mol Genet Genomics* 2015;**290**(6):2163–71.

21. Mercimek-Mahmutoglu S, Sinclair G, van Dooren SJ, et al. Guanidinoacetate methyl-transferase deficiency: first steps to newborn screening for a treatable neurometabolic disease. *Mol Genet Metab* 2012;**107**(3):433–7.

22. Stockler-Ipsiroglu S. Creatine deficiency syndromes: a new perspective on metabolic dis-orders and a diagnostic challenge. *J Pediatr* 1997;**131**(4):510–1.

23. Stockler-Ipsiroglu S, van Karnebeek C, Longo N, et al. Guanidinoacetate methyltrans-ferase (GAMT) deficiency: outcomes in 48 individuals and recommendations for diagno-sis, treatment and monitoring. *Mol Genet Metab* 2014;**111**(1):16–25.

24. Mercimek-Mahmutoglu S, Ndika J, Kanhai W, et al. Thirteen new patients with guanidi-noacetate methyltransferase deficiency and functional characterization of nineteen novel missense variants in the GAMT gene. *Hum Mutat* 2014;**35**(4):462–9.

25. Gordon N. Guanidinoacetate methyltransferase deficiency (GAMT). *Brain Dev* 2010;**32**(2):79–81.

26. Dhar SU, Scaglia F, Li FY, et al. Expanded clinical and molecular spectrum of guanidi-noacetate methyltransferase (GAMT) deficiency. *Mol Genet Metab* 2009;**96**(1):38–43.

27. Caldeira Araujo H, Smit W, Verhoeven NM, et al. Guanidinoacetate methyltransferase deficiency identified in adults and a child with mental retardation. *Am J Med Genet A* 2005;**133A**(2):122–7.

28. Schulze A, Hess T, Wevers R, et al. Creatine deficiency syndrome caused by guanidinoac-etate methyltransferase deficiency: diagnostic tools for a new inborn error of metabolism. *J Pediatr* 1997;**131**(4):626–31.

29. Comeaux MS, Wang J, Wang G, et al. Biochemical, molecular, and clinical diag-noses of patients with cerebral creatine deficiency syndromes. *Mol Genet Metab* 2013;**109**(3):260–8.

30. Schulze A, Ebinger F, Rating D, Mayatepek E. Improving treatment of guanidinoacetate methyltransferase deficiency: reduction of guanidinoacetic acid in body fluids by argi-nine restriction and ornithine supplementation. *Mol Genet Metab* 2001;**74**(4):413–9.

31. Neu A, Neuhoff H, Trube G, et al. Activation of GABA(A) receptors by guanidinoac-etate: a novel pathophysiological mechanism. *Neurobiol Dis* 2002;**11**(2):298–307.

32. Braissant O, Henry H. AGAT, GAMT and SLC6A8 distribution in the central nerv-ous system, in relation to creatine deficiency syndromes: a review. *J Inherit Metab Dis* 2008;**31**(2):230–9.

33. Guimbal C, Kilimann MW. A Na(+)-dependent creatine transporter in rabbit brain, muscle, heart, and kidney. cDNA cloning and functional expression. *J Biol Chem* 1993;**268**(12):8418–21.

34. van de Kamp JM, Mancini GM, Pouwels PJ, et al. Clinical features and X-inactivation in females heterozygous for creatine transporter defect. *Clin Genet* 2011;**79**(3):264–72.

35. Bizzi A, Bugiani M, Salomons GS, et al. X-linked creatine deficiency syndrome: a novel mutation in creatine transporter gene SLC6A8. *Ann Neurol* 2002;**52**(2):227–31.

36. Kleefstra T, Rosenberg EH, Salomons GS, et al. Progressive intestinal, neurological and psychiatric problems in two adult males with cerebral creatine deficiency caused by an SLC6A8 mutation. *Clin Genet* 2005;**68**(4):379–81.

37. van de Kamp JM, Betsalel OT, Mercimek-Mahmutoglu S, et al. Phenotype and gen-otype in 101 males with X-linked creatine transporter deficiency. *J Med Genet* 2013;**50**(7):463–72.

38. Clark AJ, Rosenberg EH, Almeida LS, et al. X-linked creatine transporter (SLC6A8) mutations in about 1% of males with mental retardation of unknown etiology. *Hum Genet* 2006;**119**(6):604–10.

39. Royes LF, Fighera MR, Furian AF, et al. Neuromodulatory effect of creatine on extracellular action potentials in rat hippocampus: role of NMDA receptors. *Neurochem Int* 2008;**53**(1-2):33–7.

40. Braissant O. Creatine and guanidinoacetate transport at blood-brain and blood-cerebrospinal fluid barriers. *J Inherit Metab Dis* 2012;**35**(4):655–64.

41. Braissant O, Cagnon L, Monnet-Tschudi F, et al. Ammonium alters creatine transport and synthesis in a 3D culture of developing brain cells, resulting in secondary cerebral creatine deficiency. *Eur J Neurosci* 2008;**27**(7):1673–85.

42. Valayannopoulos V, Boddaert N, Mention K, et al. Secondary creatine deficiency in ornithine delta-aminotransferase deficiency. *Mol Genet Metab* 2009;**97**(2):109–13.

43. Boenzi S, Pastore A, Martinelli D, et al. Creatine metabolism in urea cycle defects. *J Inherit Metab Dis* 2012;**35**(4):647–53.

44. Dionisi Vici C, Bachmann C, Gambarara M, Colombo JP, Sabetta G. Hyperornithinemia-hyperammonemia-homocitrullinuria syndrome: low creatine excretion and effect of citrulline, arginine, or ornithine supplement. *Pediatr Res* 1987;**22**(3):364–7.

45. Arias A, Garcia-Villoria J, Ribes A. Guanidinoacetate and creatine/creatinine levels in controls and patients with urea cycle defects. *Mol Genet Metab* 2004;**82**(3):220–3.

46. Brosnan JT, Brosnan ME. Creatine metabolism and the urea cycle. *Mol Genet Metab* 2010;**100**(Suppl 1):S49–52.

47. Buist NR, Glenn B, Vugrek O, et al. S-adenosylhomocysteine hydrolase deficiency in a 26-year-old man. *J Inherit Metab Dis* 2006;**29**(4):538–45.

48. Bodamer OA, Sahoo T, Beaudet AL, et al. Creatine metabolism in combined methylmalonic aciduria and homocystinuria. *Ann Neurol* 2005;**57**(4):557–60.

49. Pasquali M, Schwarz E, Jensen M, et al. Feasibility of newborn screening for guanidinoacetate methyltransferase (GAMT) deficiency. *J Inherit Metab Dis* 2014;**37**(2):231–6.

50. El-Gharbawy AH, Goldstein JL, Millington DS, et al. Elevation of guanidinoacetate in newborn dried blood spots and impact of early treatment in GAMT deficiency. *Mol Genet Metab* 2013;**109**(2):215–7.

51. Cheillan D, Salomons GS, Acquaviva C, et al. Prenatal diagnosis of guanidinoacetate methyltransferase deficiency: increased guanidinoacetate concentrations in amniotic fluid. *Clin Chem* 2006;**52**(4):775–7.

52. Carducci C, Birarelli M, Leuzzi V, et al. Guanidinoacetate and creatine plus creatinine assessment in physiologic fluids: an effective diagnostic tool for the biochemical diagnosis of arginine:glycine amidinotransferase and guanidinoacetate methyltransferase deficiencies. *Clin Chem* 2002;**48**(10):1772–8.

53. Mencarelli MA, Tassini M, Pollazzon M, et al. Creatine transporter defect diagnosed by proton NMR spectroscopy in males with intellectual disability. *Am J Med Genet A* 2011;**155A**(10):2446–52.

54. Dunbar M, Jaggumantri S, Sargent M, Stockler-Ipsiroglu S, van Karnebeek CD. Treatment of X-linked creatine transporter (SLC6A8) deficiency: systematic review of the literature and three new cases. *Mol Genet Metab* 2014;**112**(4):259–74.

Congenital disorders of glycosylation

15

R. Ganetzky, F.J. Reynoso and M. He

University of Pennsylvania, Philadelphia, PA, United States

15.1 INTRODUCTION

Congenital disorders of glycosylation (CDGs), is a relatively recently discovered category of inherited metabolic disease. The number of identified CDGs has been expanding exponentially. These diseases result from mutations affecting the addition of sugars to proteins and/or lipids. There are at least 10 pathways involved in protein glycosylation, each involving multiple enzymes, resulting in over a hundred known CDGs. Each disorder is distinct in phenotypic features and biochemical abnormalities.

The majority of CDG patients have a genetic defect that affects N-linked protein glycosylation.[1] In this process, glycans are added to the amide group of asparagine (Asn) residues. Glycans are developed by the addition of individual nucleotide-bound sugar moieties to dolichol on the cytosolic side of the endoplasmic reticulum (ER).[1,2] All N-linked glycans begin with a chain of two N-acetylglucosamine moieties, nine mannose moieties distributed in three branches, and three glucose moieties.[2] This structure is finalized on the luminal side of the ER and transferred to the target Asn[3] on nascent proteins. Following this transfer, the glycan is remodeled by the removal of some sugar moieties, especially glucose.[2] The modified protein is then transferred to the Golgi apparatus and further remodeled by the addition of additional sugar moieties and other secondary modifications.[1,2] Disorders can occur in dolichol synthesis, dolichol processing, transport between the cytoplasmic and luminal side of the ER, in addition to sugar moieties (type I disorders) or in transport to the Golgi apparatus, formation of the Golgi apparatus, or secondary remodeling (type II disorders[1]). For N-linked glycoproteins, which represent approximately more than 10% of all proteins, glycosylation is critical for proper protein folding, inter- and intracellular trafficking, interaction with other proteins and functioning.[1]

O-glycosylation occurs at the hydroxyl group of serine or threonine and sugars are added directly to form single sugar or complexed carbohydrate modification. This is most medically recognized in the O-mannosylation of dystroglycan, which is important for normal muscular scaffolding formation and the O-xylosylation of glycosaminoglycans for proteoglycans, which are important in connective tissue.[4] O-glycosylation chains are more variable than N-glycosylation chains and several distinct enzymatic processes are involved for the different O-linked glycoproteins, in contrast to the consensus initial glycan in N-glycosylation.[5] A number of O-linked protein glycosylation processes occur exclusively in the Golgi apparatus.

CDGs also occur in the lipid-based glycosylation pathways; the disorders in the glycosylphosphatidylinositol (GPI) anchor biosynthesis pathway are a major group of glycosylation disorders affecting glycolipid biosynthesis. This is an important posttranslational modification that occurs ubiquitously in all eukaryotes. The GPI anchor is a complex structure comprising a phosphoethanolamine linker, a glycan core, and a phospholipid tail.[6,7] The formation of this very complex structure begins with the synthesis of precursor molecules in the ER membrane. Then the assembly of the GPI anchor occurs in sequential steps in the endoplasmic reticulum with subsequent remodeling in the Golgi apparatus after it is attached to the C-terminus of proteins.[6] GPI anchoring provides proteins with a diverse set of functions including signal transduction, cell adhesion, and antigen presentation.

Finally, genetic defects affecting the availability of nucleotide sugars or dolichol-linked sugars as a result of abnormal biosynthesis or transport of these activated monosaccharides; affecting cellular trafficking, secretory pathways, or defects in general, Golgi apparatus functioning can affect multiple glycosylation pathways.[1]

15.2 BRIEF DESCRIPTION OF CLINICAL PRESENTATION

Because of the diversity of glycosylation pathways and targeted proteins, there is a wide diversity of anticipated presentation of congenital disorders of glycosylation. Because of the targeting of multiple proteins in most cases, multiorgan system involvement is common. Similarly, because of the high biosynthetic demand of the central nervous system, neurologic involvement is present in almost all CDGs.[8,9]

Common features in the N-linked CDGs include developmental delay,[9] failure to thrive,[9,10] microcephaly,[8] coagulopathy,[8,10] hyperinsulinemic hypoglycemia,[11] congenital brain malformations (most commonly cerebellar atrophy[12]), abnormal fat distribution,[13] inverted nipples,[13] and immune dysfunction. Some clinical features in CDG patients could present at birth and stay static or improve with time, while some (such as cerebellar dysplasia) are progressive and may not be apparent during infancy.

A substantial category of O-linked CDGs are those where glycosylation of dystroglycan is affected, resulting in a range of symptoms from congenital muscular dystrophy to muscle-eye-brain disorder that includes brain and eye involvement to Walker–Warburg syndrome, which additionally can feature severe brain malformations such as lissencephaly, hydrocephaly, or encephalocele.[14,15]

GPI anchoring biogenesis defects can present as multiple congenital anomaly syndromes with severe neurologic impairment and early death. To date, 12 genes in this pathway have been associated with human disease (*PIGA, PIGM, PIGN, PIGV, PIGL, PIGO, PIGT, PGAP2, PIGW, PGAP1, PGAP3, ST2GAL5*). This is a rapidly growing group of disorders with many of them being characterized within the last 5 years. Prior to that the only GPI anchor biogenesis defect that was known was due to somatic mutations in *PIGA*, which results in paroxysmal nocturnal hemoglobinuria (PNH).[1,16]

It is important to note that the full clinical spectrum of CDGs is not known, because there still exist multiple genes that have not yet been associated with human disease and very few patients have been reported in the majority of the CDG subtypes; moreover, no single diagnostic test is sensitive for all CDGs and many known CDGs subtypes are likely underdiagnosed, based on the projected frequencies of disease from known allele frequencies.[1,17] Therefore, CDG should be considered in all patients with unexplained multisystem or neurologic presentations.

15.3 SELECTED DISORDERS OF GLYCOSYLATION

The CDGs can be grouped into N-glycosylation disorders, multiple glycosylation disorders, O-linked glycosylation disorders, and glycolipid biosynthesis disorders. The official nomenclature of CDGs is to refer to the disorders by the defective enzyme/gene; however, the original nomenclature in which disorders were labeled type I or type II followed by a letter still persists in clinical use and is included here parenthetically. Selected disease-causing genes and N-glycosylation pathways are shown in Fig. 15.1.

15.3.1 PMM2-CDG (CDG-Ia)

PMM2-CDG is the most common form of CDG.[18] The role of PMM2 is to convert mannose-6-phosphate to mannose-1-phosphate, the form necessary for producing guanosine diphosphate (GDP)-mannose for mannosylation of glycans. Nine mannose moieties must be added to the original sugar chain for all N-glycosylation species. Inability to add mannose to the glycan chain results in hypoglycosylation. Major features of disease include neurologic involvement, including cerebellar hypotrophy, hypotonia, strabismus, epilepsy, failure to thrive, feeding difficulties and developmental delay.[18,19] Relatively specific occasional features include hyperinsulinemic hypoglycemia, coagulopathy and ascites resulting from abnormal lymphatic drainage and hypoalbuminemia.[18,20–22] Physical exam can be notable for abnormal fat distribution with suprapubic or buttock fat pads and nipple inversion.[13,21] A severe infantile onset form is often fatal within the first 2 years of life, whereas later-onset forms may result in nonprogressive intellectual disability and normal life expectancy.[23] These clinical features are frequently seen in many other type I disorders of N-glycosylation, including ALG3-CDG, ALG6-CDG, ALG9-CDG, ALG11-CDG, ALG12-CDG, GRFT1-CDG.[12,13,24–29]

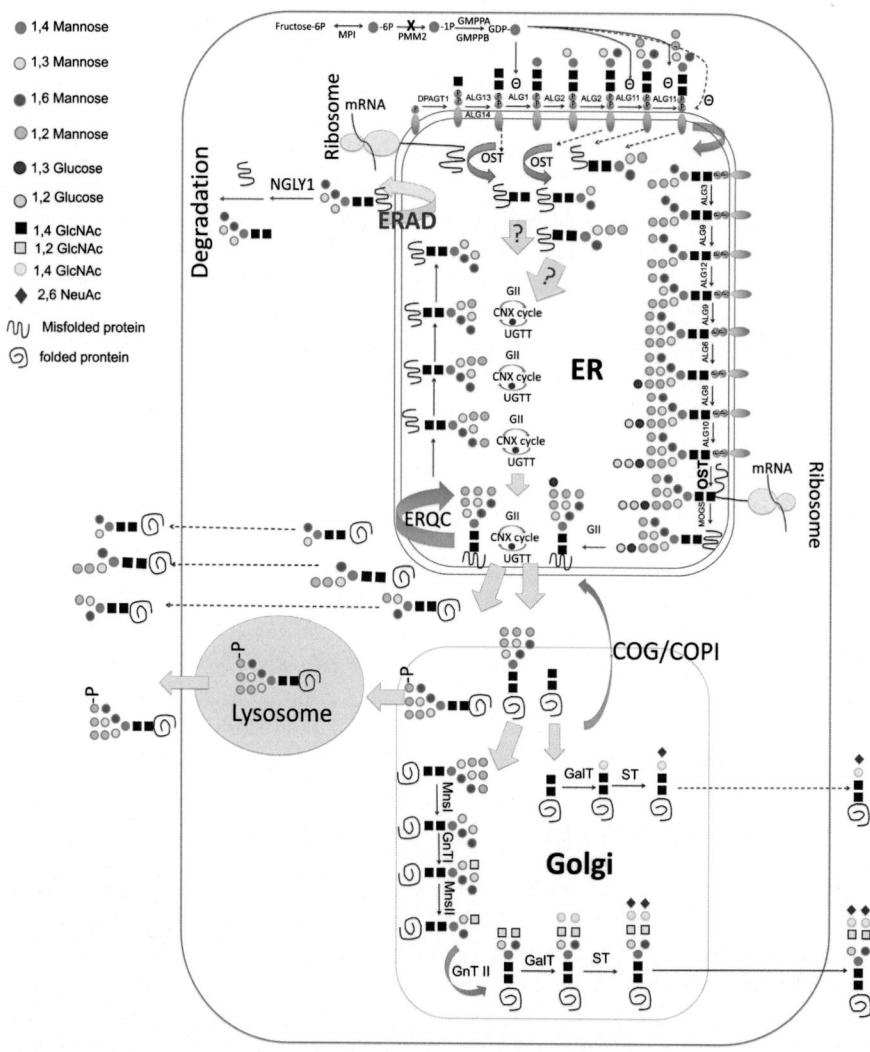

FIGURE 15.1

N-glycosylation pathway and biomarkers for diagnosing PMM2-CDG.

15.3.2 MPI-CDG (CDG-Ib)

MPI-CDG is distinct from most other CDGs in two striking ways: first, MPI-CDG has no or minimal neurologic features.[30] The initial phenotype is most notably protein-losing enteropathy, which can include chronic diarrhea and failure to thrive.[30] Hepatic fibrosis, coagulopathy, and hypoglycemia are also frequent findings.[31] Secondly, MPI-CDG is mostly treatable, using supplemental mannose.[30] This circumvents the role of MPI, which is providing mannose by conversion from fructose.[30] The much rarer CDG-ALG8 has been reported in one patient to be a phenocopy of MPI-CDG with protein-losing enteropathy and hepatomegaly;[32] however, most ALG8-CDG patients additionally have facial dysmorphology and severe neurologic symptoms.[33]

15.3.3 ALG1-CDG (CDG-Ik)

ALG1-CDG is one of the most common CDGs in Western Europe after CDG-PMM2.[34] Most reported patients have isolated neurologic abnormalities, including developmental delay, acquired microcephaly, and seizures.[34] Severe, infantile onset has been reported to be associated with optical atrophy and facial dysmorphia. About 10% of ALG1-CDG patients present with inverted nipples, which is a much less frequent finding comparing to PMM2-CDG; however, milder cases may have no "red flags," emphasizing the importance of screening for CDGs in patients with isolated neurodevelopmental abnormalities.[34] It is important to be aware that there are 14 pseudo-genes of ALG1 in the human genome, which presents a technical challenge for next-generation sequencing-based technology.[35] Therefore, unfortunately this frequent subtype of type I CDG is often not included in clinical molecular genetic panels for CDG offered by several commercial laboratories. Specialized expertise and experience are also essential in the interpretation of rare variants in this gene by whole exome sequencing.

15.3.4 CDGs PRESENTING AS CONGENITAL MYASTHENIA (ALG2-CDG, ALG14-CDG, DPAGT1-CDG, GFPT1-CDG)

The acetylcholine receptor at the neuromuscular junction requires N-linked glycosylation for proper assembly, localization, and sensitization.[36–39] Therefore, many of the type I N-linked CDGs have been reported to present as a myasthenic syndrome with a broad range of severity within each disorder from the Pena-Shokier-like phenotype, with fetal akinesia and arthogryposis, to more mild adult-onset myasthenia.[40–42] It appears that these groups of CDGs are mainly involved in the early assembling of high mannose glycan before the assembling of Man6GlcNAc2. The severe infantile forms of these disorders have additional findings reported, with cataracts, iris colobomas, and hypomyelination reported in ALG2-CDG,[43] and cataracts and arthrogryposis reported in DPAGT1-CDG.[44]

15.3.5 ALG3-CDG (CDG-Id), ALG9-CDG (CDG-Il), AND ALG12-CDG (CDG-Ig)

ALG3, ALG9, and ALG12 are involved in the assembling of Man6-Man9GlcNAc2 in ER lumen. Skeletal dysplasia with shortening of limbs is a frequent clinical feature reported in both ALG9 and ALG12-CDG.[26,28] Hypogammaglobulinemia and immunodeficiency are relatively common in ALG9 and ALG12-CDG.[28] Hepatosplenomegaly and cystic renal disease are interesting clinical features reported in ALG9-CDG.[26] ALG9-CDG may be relatively common in Canada and the United Kingdom compared to other countries due to a founder mutation Y286C.[45] These CDG subtypes could be diagnosed by N-glycan analysis. Very few ALG3-CDG cases have been reported; colobomas and arthrogryposis are unusual features reported in ALG3-CDG.[46]

15.3.6 DISORDERS OF GLYCOSYLATION IN ER ALG6-CDG (CDG-Ic), ALG8-CDG (CDG-Ih)

The final steps of glycosylation before the glycan is transferred from dolichol to the nascent polypeptide are the addition of three glucose moieties. These glucose moieties are often trimmed off by ER glucosidases during protein-folding quality control. Their presence on mature glycoproteins is not well recognized, but these moieties are important in several glycoproteins in the nervous system and selected other glycoproteins, including coagulation proteins, immunoglobulins, and lipoproteins. ALG6, and the less common ALG8-CDG, present primarily with neurologic features such as intellectual disability, ataxia and seizures, coagulopathy, and hypogammaglobulinemia.[25,32,33] ALG6 also features hypocholesterolemia.[25] Since these glucose moieties are removed from majority of the mature glycans on glycoproteins, glycosylation analysis of blood is often unrevealing[47] of glycan structural abnormality.

15.3.7 MOGS-CDG (CDG-IIb)

MOGS encodes glucosidase I, which is responsible for trimming glucose moieties off of N-linked glycoproteins. Two families have been reported with MOGS-CDG.[48,49] Consensus features include developmental delay, dysmorphic facial features, hypotonia, and hypoplastic genitalia.[48,49] Like ALG6- and ALG8-CDG, MOGS-CDG is difficult to diagnosis using transferrin analysis alone; however, an abnormal Glc3Man1 tetrasaccharide is abundant on urine glycans[49] and glucosylated N-glycan could also be detected in plasma N-glycan profile in this disease.

15.3.8 DISORDERS OF THE OLIGOSACCHARYLTRANSFERASE (OST) AND TRANSLOCON-ASSOCIATED PROTEIN (TRAP) COMPLEXES (DDOST-CDG, MAGT1-CDG (IAP-CDG), STT3A-CDG, STT3B-CDG, TUSC3-CDG, SSR4-CDG)

The oligosaccharyltransferase (OST) complex transfers the oligosaccharide from dolichol to the nascent polypeptide. Disorders have been described in the catalytic subunits, STT3A and STT3B, several noncatalytic subunits (such as TUSC3 or MAGT1), and components of the translocon-associated protein (TRAP) complex, such as SSR4,[50] resulting in global hypoglycosylation.[51–53] These disorders have nonspecific symptoms, primarily intellectual disability. Other common features include hypotonia, strabismus, and seizures,[51] and abnormal fat distribution. It is important to note that MAGT1-CDG, and SSR4-CDG are X-linked and should be considered in families with apparent nonsyndromic X-linked intellectual disability.[53] Hypoglycosylation may be subtle or nondetectable on transferrin analysis and N-glycans from these patients often have normal structure;[51] a flow cytometry method using overexpression of glycosylated green fluorescent protein in fibroblasts may be a more reliable functional assay to detect these disorders.

15.3.9 DISORDERS OF THE CONSERVED OLIGOMERIC GOLGI (COG) COMPLEX AND GOLGI MEMBRANE PROTEINS (COG1-CDG, COG4-CDG, COG5-CDG, COG6-CDG, COG7-CDG, COG8-CDG, TMEM165-CDG, ATP6V0A2-CDG)

These rare type II CDGs occur due to abnormal retrograde protein trafficking between Golgi apparatus and ER, therefore disrupt multiple glycosylation pathways that are associated with Golgi apparati. A variety of symptoms have been reported, including microcephaly, global developmental delay, facial dysmorphia, cerebral or cerebellar atrophy, hypotonia, muscular dystrophy, feeding abnormalities,[54] and wrinkled skin. The clinical spectrum of conserved oligomeric Golgi (COG) deficiency varies from mild nonsyndromic intellectual disability to early-onset multiple system disorder in almost all known COG subtypes. Bone dysplasia and periodic fever are interesting features in TMEM165-CDG, a defect in a Golgi apparatus membrane protein.[55] ATP6V0A2-CDG is also known as cutis laxa type IIA, a disorder with wrinkled skin as its key feature.[56] ATP6V0A2 is a subunit of V-type H+ ATPase complex that is known to regulate intracellular pH gradient.[56] ATP6V0A2-CDG is the first CDG described in H+ ATPase complexes.

15.3.10 DISORDERS OF O-MANNOSYLATION (POMT1-CDG, POMT2-CDG, POMGNT1-CDG, FKRP-CDG, FKTN-CDG, LARGE-CDG)

The disorders of O-glycosylation are more protean than the disorders of N-glycosylation; however, a majority of the disorders that affect O-mannosylation present with congenital muscular dystrophy due to abnormal mannosylation of alpha-dystroglycan.[57] These range in severity from Walker–Warburg syndrome (congenital muscular dystrophy with structural brain abnormalities), muscle-eye-brain disease, limb girdle muscular dystrophy, with or without intellectual impairment to apparently isolated dilated cardiomyopathy prior to clinical recognition of muscular dystrophy.[14,58,59] It is important to note that O-mannosylation is initiated in ER and matured in the Golgi apparatus. Disorders that affect the biosynthesis of mannose-linked dolichol or general Golgi apparatus functions could manifest features of muscular dystrophy, cardiomyopathy, or structural brain abnormalities that are typically seen in O-mannosylation CDG as described above.

15.3.11 DISORDERS OF O-XYLOSYLATION OF PROTEOGLYCANS (EXT1-CDG, EXT2-CDG, CHST14-CDG, CHSY1-CDG, B3GAT3-CDG, CHST3-CDG, B4GALT7-CDG, SLC35D1-CDG)

Glycosaminoglycans are an important component of skin and bone connective tissue that require O-glycosyation using an O-xylosylation linker.[4,60] Therefore, disorders of O-xylosylation present as skeletal and connective tissue abnormalities, many of which were well-described clinical genetic entities prior to understanding of the underlying glycosylation abnormalities. These include hereditary multiple exostoses (EXT1-, EXT2-CDG), musculocontractural, and progeroid-type Ehlers–Danlos syndrome (CHST14-CDG, B4GALT7-CDG).[60]

15.3.12 NGLY1-CDG AND GMPPA-CDG

NGLY1-CDG is a congenital disorder of deglycosylation. A defect in cytosolic N-glycanase cleaves N-linked glycan chains from misfolded glycoproteins that exit from ER. This step is important for the degradation of misfolded and incorrectly glycosylated glycoproteins.[61] Patients with NGLY1-CDG have storage of misfolded glycoproteins in their liver, which appears as cytoplasmic storage or vacuolization on liver biopsy.[61] Clinical manifestations include global developmental delay, micropcephaly, a-/hypolacrima, hyporeflexia, seizures, hypotonia, and liver dysfunction.[61] Interestingly, patients with GMPPA-CDG, a defect that appears to upregulate GDP-mannose synthesis, also present with alacrima, achalasia, microcephaly, developmental delay, ataxia, and hypotonia.[62] Both NGLY1-CDG and GMPPA-CDG are not deficiencies in glycan synthesis, rather, it is possible that regulation of intracellular glycoprotein levels is disrupted in these disorders.

15.4 OTHER INBORN DEFECTS ASSOCIATED WITH ABNORMAL GLYCOSYLATION

15.4.1 GALACTOSEMIA

Secondary glycosylation defects occur in galactosemia (deficiency of the galactose-1-phosphate uridyltransferase enzyme) due to inhibition of galactosyltransferases by high galactose levels. Transferrin analysis shows undersialyation, with elevated mono-/diglycosylation and a-/diglycosylation ratios and N-glycan analysis shows a diversity of species, with increased high mannose species and hypogalactosylation.[63,64] The glycosylation profile normalizes with appropriate dietary restriction.[64] However, this has never been studied in galactokinase deficiency or galactose epimerase deficiency.

15.4.2 FRUCTOSEMIA

Secondary glycosylation defects occur in fructosemia (or hereditary fructose intolerance, caused by the deficiency of aldolase B) due to inhibition of phosphomannose isomerase by elevated fructose-1-phosphate levels.[65] This results in a glycosylation pattern that mimics MPI-CDG; these two conditions have phenotypic overlap with hepatic involvement and coagulopathy and clinical recognition of fructose aversion may lag diagnosis, so it is important to consider the possibility of fructosemia in the differential diagnosis for MPI-CDG.[65] This glycosylation pattern normalizes with appropriate dietary fructose restriction.[65]

15.5 CONFOUNDING CONDITIONS THAT CAN CAUSE ABNORMAL GLYCOSYLATION PATTERNS

Alcohol consumption: Hypoglycosylation of transferrin occurs in patients with moderate alcohol consumption in a dose-dependent manner related to the average daily intake of alcohol, beginning roughly around 40 grams of alcohol consumer per day.[66] The exact reason for this phenomenon is unknown, but alcohol seems to inhibit sialyl transferase and promote sialidase activity.[67] In adult patients, there are reported cases of difficulty distinguishing alcohol-related-hypoglycosylation pattern from CDG.[68]

Transferrin variation: Polymorphisms in the gene encoding transferrin results in changes in how transferrin runs on electrophoretic gels, which can interfere with the diagnosis of CDG in a few possible ways: transferrin isoform D can be mistaken as hyposialyted transferrin; transferrin isoform B when hyposialyted can be mistaken for normally sialyted transferrin, alternately, heterozygosity for two rare transferrin isoforms can result in multiple bands that are difficult to interpret.[69,70] Iron saturation of transferrin can also cause differences in isoelectric focusing and result in false-positive banding patterns.[70] This particularly interferes with electrophoresis-based assays for carbohydrate-deficient transferrin; more recent accurate-mass mass spectrometry analytic methods are more able to differentiate hyposialylation from rare transferrin isoforms.

Chronic disease: A number of chronic diseases, including, in particular, end-stage liver disease have been reported to cause false-positive elevations of hyposialyted or hypoglycosylated transferrin[71]; however, this seems to be more commonly seen with immunoassays and is not consistently reproducible using modern high-performance *liquid chromatography* (HPLC) and/or capillary electrophoresis methods.[71–73]

Pregnancy: Hyposialyation or hypersialylation of transferrin has been observed in pregnancy, as well as in patients on estrogen replacement therapy.[74]

15.6 BIOMARKERS FOR DIAGNOSIS OF CONGENITAL DISORDERS OF GLYCOSYLATION

Several methods have been developed to analyze glycosylation patterns. No single method is completely sensitive to all CDGs. Multiple algorithms have been devised to address this clinical challenge.[75,76] It is also important to note that in several CDGs, particularly SLC35A2-CDG, the abnormal glycosylation pattern may decrease in abundance over time, reducing the sensitivity of analysis,[77] while in other type II CDG subtypes, such as TMEM165-CDG, the abnormal pattern of protein glycosylation may also change over time, switching from hyposialylation early in life to hypogalactosylation later in life.[78]

15.6.1 CARBOHYDRATE-DEFICIENT TRANSFERRIN

Normal transferrin glycosylation has two glycosylation sites, each with an asparagine-linked biantennary complex.[79] In type I CDGs, where there is impairment of forming and transferring N-glycans to glycoproteins, there is an increase of α- or mono-glycosylated transferrin with decrease of di-glycosylated transferrin due to one or both glycosylation sites being underglycosylated. In contrast, in type II CDGs, where the impairment is glycoprotein processing, there are glycans at each glycosylation site, but with abnormal structures, so there is increased tri-sialo and other truncated glycan species.[79] Transferrin sialylation can be measured by isoelectric focusing, HPLC, or mass spectrometry.[71,79,80] Other methods, such as immunoassays, have fallen out of favor due to false-positive results.[71,73] It has been recently recognized that abnormal glycan structures are also identified in majority of patients with type I CDGs and some of which could be observed by transferrin analysis by acute-mass mass spectrometry.[81] Although transferrin analysis is the most common biomarker used to diagnose CDG, it is important to note that it does not have sufficient sensitivity to detect several CDG subtypes, including all disorders of O-glycosylation (see Table 15.1).[79]

15.6.2 APOLIPOPROTEIN CIII ANALYSIS

Apolipoprotein CIII normally undergoes O-glycosylation, with a mucin core 1 glycan profile, so is informative to O-linked CDGs that affect those processes.[82] Similarly to transferrin glycosylation, apolipoprotein CIII glycosylation can be measured either by isoelectric focusing or by mass spectrometry.[82,83] It is important to note that since there are not common enzymes to all O-glycosylation, this testing is limited to detect defects in enzymes involved in O-linked glycosylation of apolipoprotein CIII.[83]

15.6.3 N-GLYCAN ANALYSIS

N-Glycan analysis can be performed by enzymatically cleaving N-linked glycans from total glycoproteins. The glycan species can then be purified and analyzed using Matrix-Assisted Laser Desorption/Ionization-Time of Flight Mass Spectroscopy (MALDI-TOF MS).[77] Detection of abnormal glycan species or levels can indicate a CDG.[77] Since this process analyzes glycans released from all glycoproteins, it can detect the abnormalities of N-glycan types that are not present on transferrin molecules such as glycosylated species, high mannose N-glycans, and hybrid N-glycan species.[77] It is underrecognized that many subtypes of type I CDG have abnormal levels of high mannose species, which could be detected by N-glycan analysis but not transferrin analysis. In addition, by analyzing the glycan species directly, the resolution and sensitivity of N-glycan analysis is much higher than analyzing monosaccharide changes on a glycoprotein, commonly transferrin. N-glycan analysis can be helpful in differentiating among different subtypes of CDGs with the same transferrin profile, including distinguishing between ALG1-CDG, PMM2-CDG[81] or MPI-CDG (Fig. 15.1), ALG3-CDG, ALG9-CDG, and ALG12-CDG, as well as detecting

Table 15.1 Examples of Biomarkers in Type I, Type II, and Mixed Type I and II CDG Subtypes

Disorders	Plasma or Serum CDT	Plasma or Serum N-Glycan	Plasma or Serum O-Glycan	Other Testing
PMM2-CDG	Abnormal	Abnormal	Normal	Enzyme in fibroblast
MPI-CDG	Abnormal	Abnormal	Normal	Enzyme in fibroblast
ALG1-CDG	Abnormal	Abnormal	Normal	
ALG12-CDG	Abnormal	Abnormal	Normal	
MAN1B1-CDG	Abnormal	Abnormal	Normal	
DPAGT1-CDG	Abnormal	Normal	Normal	
ALG3-CDG	Abnormal	Abnormal	Normal	
ALG9-CDG	Abnormal	Abnormal	Normal	
ALG8-CDG	Abnormal/ Normal	Normal	Normal	
MOGS-CDG	Normal/ Abnormal	Abnormal	Normal	Abnormal urine free glycans
DDOST-CDG and other OST complex subunit	Abnormal/ Normal	Normal	Normal	Reduced ICAM-1 cell surface expression in fibroblast by FACS
ATP6V0A2-CDG	Abnormal/ normal	Abnormal	Abnormal	
Disorders of COG	Abnormal/ normal	Abnormal	Abnormal	
Disorders of O-mannosylation	Normal	Normal	Normal	Glycosylated dystroglycan staining by immuno-histochemistry
Disorders of O-xylosylation	Normal	Normal	Normal	
GNE-CDG	Normal	Normal	Abnormal	
PGM3-CDG	Normal	Abnormal/ normal	Abnormal	
PGM1-CDG	Abnormal	Abnormal	Abnormal	
NGLY1-CDG	Normal	Normal	Normal	ddVenus assay in fibroblast

glycosylated species in MOGS-CDG. In contrast, because it does not analyze the glycoproteins directly, it is unable to detect disorders that affect the transfer of structurally normal glycans to glycoproteins, such as defects in OST or TRAP complexes or DPAGT1-CDG (CDG-Ij).

15.6.4 O-GLYCAN ANALYSIS

O-glycan analysis is performed analogously to N-glycan analysis[77] using beta elimination to chemically cleave O-linked glycans from total glycoproteins in plasma or serum. In particular, there are a few key O-glycan species that can be analyzed in plasma or serum: mucin core 1 and mucin core 2. Both of these can be mono- or disialylated; hypoglycosylation of O-glycan or truncation of O-glycan is often indicative of CDG.[77] This is typically abnormal in combined glycosylation disorders and can be beneficial in further differentiating CDGs with a type II transferrin pattern and/or abnormal N-glycan analysis.[77,84] O-glycan analysis is generally more informative than apolipoprotein C testing, as apolipoprotein C does not have core 2 glycans.[77] It is also more sensitive for screening of defects in nucleotide-sugar synthesis as Km of glycotransferases in O-glycosylation is often higher than that of N-glycosylation. Because of the diversity in O-glycosylation, O-glycan analysis does not detect all the disorders of O-glycosylation and importantly plasma-based O-glycan analysis does not detect the disorders of O-mannosylation,[84] as O-mannosylation are almost exclusively found on glycoproteins in muscle or brain.

It is important to note that O-linked protein glycosylation in circulation are also highly dynamic and regulated by many factors. O-glycosylation abnormalities found in plasma or serum need to be confirmed in another tissue, such as fibroblast or by another test, such as molecular genetic testing.

15.6.5 IMMUNOHISTOCHEMISTRY

Immunohistochemistry can be performed on muscle biopsy specimens with an antibody specific for glycosylated alpha-dystroglycan to detect disorders of O-mannosylation,[85] and antibodies targeting glycosaminoglycans could be used to detect defects in O-linked proteoglycans by immunohistochemistry or immunofluorescence staining of related tissues.

15.6.6 URINE GLYCANS

Some CDGs have increased free glycans due to the accumulation of abnormal intermediates from glycoprotein synthesis. In these disorders, excess free glycans can be found in the urine.[77] Urine identification of glycan species using MALDI-TOF MS can be performed.[86] This technique is particularly diagnostically useful for MOGS-CDG.[49]

15.6.7 FLUORESCENCE-ACTIVATED CELL SORTING (FACS)

Fluorescence-activated cell sorting (FACS) can be a useful method to study GPI anchor expression, which can be affected in the GPI anchoring biogenesis defects as well as defects affecting the synthesis of the GPI anchor precursors. The most studied GPI-anchored proteins include CD55, CD16b, CD59, and FLAER

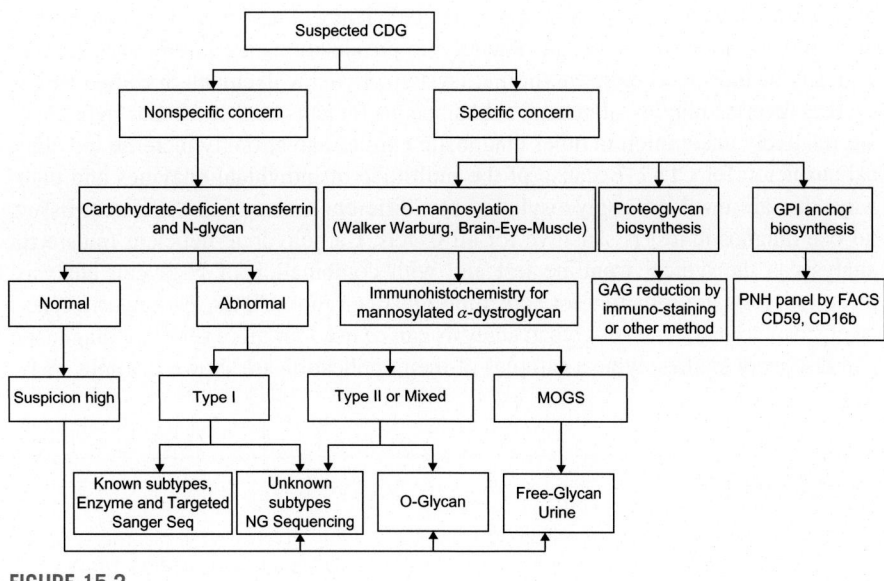

FIGURE 15.2

Diagnostic flow chart for CDG testing.

(fluorescein-labeled proaerolysin) that binds to the GPI anchor. It is important to keep in mind that expression of these proteins can vary among different cell types.[16,87] In peripheral blood, there is often only a fraction of cells that show reduction of surface GPI anchor protein staining in GPI anchor biosynthesis disorder.

15.7 ANTICIPATED CHANGES IN DIAGNOSIS AND MANAGEMENT OF CDG

The congenital disorders of glycosylation are a diverse, protean, and rapidly expanding category of disorders. As our diagnostic capabilities expand, next-generation sequencing allows for the discovery of genetic cause of disease in an unbiased manner and we continue to expand our understanding of glycosylation pathways the number of CDGs will continue to grow. A suggested diagnostic flow chart is shown in Fig. 15.2.

15.8 CONCLUSIONS

The CDGs encompass a broad and diverse group of disorders. The best characterized CDGs are defects in N-glycosylation; other described diseases affect O-glycosylation, GPI anchors, or multiple glycosylation process such as remodeling of glyco-conjugates in the Golgi apparatus, deficiency of activated monosaccharide, or deglycosylation in cytoplasm. Phenotypic presentations are highly variable, but typically include neurologic and/or multisystem organ involvement. Specific features such as inverted nipples, abnormal subcutaneous fat pads, and cerebellar hypoplasia are relatively uncommon in other diagnostic entities and strongly increase the clinical suspicion for CDG. Because of the multitude of individual enzymes and pathways that are involved in glycosylation at a different time and in a different tissue, no one diagnostic test is sensitive for all CDGs. Carbohydrate-deficient transferrin analysis is the typical frontline test and with combination of N-glycan analysis, these two tests are sensitive for screening most common CDGs, particularly type I N-glycosylation defects; O-glycan analysis can be used for more sensitive diagnostic and discovery studies, typical samples of their application are shown in Table 15.1.

REFERENCES

1. Freeze HH, Chong JX, Bamshad MJ, Ng BG. Solving glycosylation disorders: fundamental approaches reveal complicated pathways. *Am J Hum Genet* 2014;**94**:161–75.
2. Stanley P, Schachter H, Taniguchi N. N-Glycans. In: Varki A, Cummings RD, Esko JD, editors. *Essentials of Glycobiology* 2nd edn. Cold Spring Harbor Laboratory Press; 2009.
3. Hanover JA, Lennarz WJ. N-Linked glycoprotein assembly. Evidence that oligosaccharide attachment occurs within the lumen of the endoplasmic reticulum. *J Biol Chem* 1980;**255**:3600–4.
4. Bourdon MA, Krusius T, Campbell S, Schwartz NB, Ruoslahti E. Identification and synthesis of a recognition signal for the attachment of glycosaminoglycans to proteins. *Proc Natl Acad Sci U S A* 1987;**84**:3194–8.
5. Freeze HH, Haltiwanger RS. Other Classes of ER/Golgi-derived Glycans. In: Varki A, Cummings RD, Esko JD, editors. *Essentials of Glycobiology* 2nd edn. Cold Spring Harbor: Cold Spring Harbor Laboratory Press; 2009.
6. Fujita M, Kinoshita T. GPI-anchor remodeling: potential functions of GPI-anchors in intracellular trafficking and membrane dynamics. *Biochim Biophys Acta* 2012;**1821**:1050–8.
7. Paulick MG, Bertozzi CR. The glycosylphosphatidylinositol anchor: a complex membrane-anchoring structure for proteins. *Biochemistry* 2008;**47**:6991–7000.
8. Funke S, Gardeitchik T, Kouwenberg D, et al. Perinatal and early infantile symptoms in congenital disorders of glycosylation. *Am J Med Genet A* 2013;**161A**:578–84.
9. Freeze HH, Eklund EA, Ng BG, Patterson MC. Neurology of inherited glycosylation disorders. *Lancet Neurol* 2012;**11**:453–66.
10. Freeze HH. Congenital disorders of glycosylation and the pediatric liver. *Semin Liver Dis* 2001;**21**:501–15.
11. Kapoor RR, James C, Hussain K. Hyperinsulinism in developmental syndromes. *Endocr Dev* 2009;**14**:95–113.
12. Barone R, Fiumara A, Jaeken J. Congenital disorders of glycosylation with emphasis on cerebellar involvement. *Semin Neurol* 2014;**34**:357–66.
13. Rymen D, Jaeken J. Skin manifestations in CDG. *J Inherit Metab Dis* 2014;**37**:699–708.
14. Meilleur KG, Zukosky K, Medne L, et al. Clinical, pathologic, and mutational spectrum of dystroglycanopathy caused by LARGE mutations. *J Neuropathol Exp Neurol* 2014;**73**:425–41.

15. Michele DE, Barresi R, Kanagawa M, et al. Post-translational disruption of dystroglycan-ligand interactions in congenital muscular dystrophies. *Nature* 2002;**418**:417–22.

16. Ng BG, Freeze HH. Human genetic disorders involving glycosylphosphatidylinositol (GPI) anchors and glycosphingolipids (GSL). *J Inherit Metab Dis* 2015;**38**:171–8.

17. Schollen E, Kjaergaard S, Legius E, Schwartz M, Matthijs G. Lack of Hardy-Weinberg equilibrium for the most prevalent PMM2 mutation in CDG-Ia (congenital disorders of glycosylation type Ia). *Eur J Hum Genet* 2000;**8**:367–71.

18. Jaeken J. Congenital disorders of glycosylation. *Handb Clin Neurol* 2013;**113**:1737–43.

19. Monin M-L, Mignot C, De Lonlay P, et al. 29 French adult patients with PMM2-congenital disorder of glycosylation: outcome of the classical pediatric phenotype and depiction of a late-onset phenotype. *Orphanet J Rare Dis* 2014;**9**:207.

20. Arnoux JB, Boddaert N, Valayannopoulos V, et al. Risk assessment of acute vascular events in congenital disorder of glycosylation type Ia. *Mol Genet Metab* 2008;**93**:444–9.

21. Wolthuis DFGJ, van Asbeck EV, Kozicz T, Morava E. Abnormal fat distribution in PMM2-CDG. *Mol Genet Metab* 2013;**110**:411–3.

22. Truin G, Guillard M, Lefeber DJ, et al. Pericardial and abdominal fluid accumulation in congenital disorder of glycosylation type Ia. *Mol Genet Metab* 2008;**94**(4):481.

23. Sparks SE, Krasnewich DM. PMM2-CDG (CDG-Ia) *GeneReviews*. Seattle: University of Washington; 2015.

24. Riess S, Reddihough DS, Howell KB, et al. ALG3-CDG (CDG-Id): clinical, biochemical and molecular findings in two siblings. *Mol Genet Metab*; 110: 170–175.

25. Dercksen M, Crutchley AC, Honey EM, et al. ALG6-CDG in South Africa: Genotype-Phenotype Description of Five Novel Patients. *JIMD Rep* 2013;**8**:17–23.

26. AlSubhi S, AlHashem A, AlAzami A, et al. Further Delineation of the ALG9-CDG Phenotype. *JIMD Rep* 2015 published online Oct 10. http://dx.doi.org/10.1007/8904_2015_504.

27. Thiel C, Rind N, Popovici D, et al. Improved diagnostics lead to identification of three new patients with congenital disorder of glycosylation-Ip. *Hum Mutat* 2012;**33**:485–7.

28. Chantret I, Dupré T, Delenda C, et al. Congenital disorders of glycosylation type Ig is defined by a deficiency in dolichyl-P-mannose: Man7GlcNAc2-PP-dolichyl mannosyltransferase. *J Biol Chem* 2002;**277**:25815–22.

29. Vleugels W, Haeuptle MA, Ng BG, et al. RFT1 deficiency in three novel CDG patients. *Hum Mutat* 2009;**30**:1428–34.

30. Niehues R, Hasilik M, Alton G, et al. Carbohydrate-deficient glycoprotein syndrome type Ib. *Phosphomannose isomerase deficiency and mannose therapy. J Clin Invest* 1998;**101**:1414–20.

31. Vuillaumier-Barrot S, Le Bizec C, de Lonlay P, et al. Protein losing enteropathy-hepatic fibrosis syndrome in Saguenay-Lac St-Jean, Quebec is a congenital disorder of glycosylation type Ib. *J Med Genet* 2002;**39**:849–51.

32. Chantret I, Dancourt J, Dupré T, et al. A deficiency in dolichyl-P-glucose:Glc1Man9GlcNAc2-PP-dolichyl alpha3-glucosyltransferase defines a new subtype of congenital disorders of glycosylation. *J Biol Chem* 2003;**278**:9962–71.

33. Höck M, Wegleiter K, Ralser E, et al. ALG8-CDG: novel patients and review of the literature. *Orphanet J Rare Dis* 2015;**10**:73.

34. Dupré T, Vuillaumier-Barrot S, Chantret I, et al. Guanosine diphosphate-mannose:GlcNAc2-PP-dolichol mannosyltransferase deficiency (congenital disorders of glycosylation type Ik): five new patients and seven novel mutations. *J Med Genet* 2010;**47**:729–35.

35. Rohlfing A-K, Rust S, Reunert J, et al. ALG1-CDG: a new case with early fatal outcome. *Gene* 2014;**534**:345–51.

36. Ramanathan VK, Hall ZW. Altered glycosylation sites of the delta subunit of the acetylcholine receptor (AChR) reduce alpha delta association and receptor assembly. *J Biol Chem* 1999;**274**:20513–20.

37. Nishizaki T. N-glycosylation sites on the nicotinic ACh receptor subunits regulate receptor channel desensitization and conductance. *Brain Res Mol Brain Res* 2003;**114**:172–6.

38. Romero-Fernandez W, Borroto-Escuela DO, Perez Alea M, Garcia-Mesa Y, Garriga P. Altered trafficking and unfolded protein response induction as a result of M3 muscarinic receptor impaired N-glycosylation. *Glycobiology* 2011;**21**:1663–72.

39. Rodríguez Cruz PM, Palace J, Beeson D. Inherited disorders of the neuromuscular junction: an update. *J Neurol* 2014;**261**:2234–43.

40. Belaya K, Finlayson S, Cossins J, et al. Identification of DPAGT1 as a new gene in which mutations cause a congenital myasthenic syndrome. *Ann N Y Acad Sci* 2012;**1275**:29–35.

41. Zoltowska K, Webster R, Finlayson S, et al. Mutations in GFPT1 that underlie limb-girdle congenital myasthenic syndrome result in reduced cell-surface expression of muscle AChR. *Hum Mol Genet* 2013;**22**:2905–13.

42. Cossins J, Belaya K, Hicks D, et al. Congenital myasthenic syndromes due to mutations in ALG2 and ALG14. *Brain* 2013;**136**:944–56.

43. Thiel C, Schwarz M, Peng J, et al. A new type of congenital disorders of glycosylation (CDG-Ii) provides new insights into the early steps of dolichol-linked oligosaccharide biosynthesis. *J Biol Chem* 2003;**278**:22498–505.

44. Ganetzky R, Izumi K, Edmondson A, et al. Fetal akinesia deformation sequence due to a congenital disorder of glycosylation. *Am J Med Genet A* 2015;**167A**:2411–7.

45. Vleugels W, Keldermans L, Jaeken J, et al. Quality control of glycoproteins bearing truncated glycans in an ALG9-defective (CDG-IL) patient. *Glycobiology* 2009;**19**:910–7.

46. Körner C, Knauer R, Stephani U, Marquardt T, Lehle L, von Figura K. Carbohydrate deficient glycoprotein syndrome type IV: deficiency of dolichyl-P-Man:Man(5)GlcNAc(2)-PP-dolichyl mannosyltransferase. *EMBO J* 1999;**18**:6816–22.

47. Westphal V, Xiao M, Kwok P-Y, Freeze HH. Identification of a frequent variant in ALG6, the cause of Congenital Disorder of Glycosylation-Ic. *Hum Mutat* 2003;**22**:420–1.

48. Sadat MA, Moir S, Chun T-W, et al. Glycosylation, hypogammaglobulinemia, and resistance to viral infections. *N Engl J Med* 2014;**370**:1615–25.

49. De Praeter CM, Gerwig GJ, Bause E, et al. A novel disorder caused by defective biosynthesis of N-linked oligosaccharides due to glucosidase I deficiency. *Am J Hum Genet* 2000;**66**:1744–56.

50. Losfeld ME, Ng BG, Kircher M, et al. A new congenital disorder of glycosylation caused by a mutation in SSR4, the signal sequence receptor 4 protein of the TRAP complex. *Hum Mol Genet* 2014;**23**:1602–5.

51. Shrimal S, Ng BG, Losfeld M-E, Gilmore R, Freeze HH. Mutations in STT3A and STT3B cause two congenital disorders of glycosylation. *Hum Mol Genet* 2013(22):4638–45.

52. Jones MA, Ng BG, Bhide S, et al. DDOST mutations identified by whole-exome sequencing are implicated in congenital disorders of glycosylation. *Am J Hum Genet* 2012;**90**:363–8.

53. Molinari F, Foulquier F, Tarpey PS, et al. Oligosaccharyltransferase-subunit mutations in nonsyndromic mental retardation. *Am J Hum Genet* 2008;**82**:1150–7.

54. Foulquier F. COG defects, birth and rise! *Biochim Biophys Acta* 2009;**1792**:896–902.

55. Zeevaert R, de Zegher F, Sturiale L, et al. Bone Dysplasia as a Key Feature in Three Patients with a Novel Congenital Disorder of Glycosylation (CDG) Type II Due to a Deep Intronic Splice Mutation in TMEM165. *JIMD Rep* 2013;**8**:145–52.

56. Fischer B, Dimopoulou A, Egerer J, et al. Further characterization of ATP6V0A2-related autosomal recessive cutis laxa. *Hum Genet* 2012;**131**:1761–73.

57. Wells L. The o-mannosylation pathway: glycosyltransferases and proteins implicated in congenital muscular dystrophy. *J Biol Chem* 2013;**288**:6930–5.

58. Yamamoto T, Hiroi A, Kato Y, Shibata N, Osawa M, Kobayashi M. Possible Diverse Roles of Fukutin: More Than Basement Membrane? In: Hegde M, Ankala A, editors. *Muscular Dystrophy*. InTech; 2012. http://dx.doi.org/10.5772/1242.

59. Murakami T, Hayashi YK, Noguchi S, et al. Fukutin gene mutations cause dilated cardiomyopathy with minimal muscle weakness. *Ann Neurol* 2006;**60**:597–602.

60. Asteggiano CG, Delgado MA, Millón MBB, de Kremer RD. Heparan sulfate proteoglycans and congenital disorder of O-linked glycosylation. In: Manuel Mora-Montes H, editor. *Biochemical and molecular bases of multiple osteochondromatosis*. Glycans: Biochemistry, Characterization and Applications; 2012. p. 103–20.

61. Enns GM, Shashi V, Bainbridge M, et al. Mutations in NGLY1 cause an inherited disorder of the endoplasmic reticulum-associated degradation pathway. *Genet Med* 2014;**16**:751–8.

62. Koehler K, Malik M, Mahmood S, et al. Mutations in GMPPA cause a glycosylation disorder characterized by intellectual disability and autonomic dysfunction. *Am J Hum Genet* 2013;**93**:727–34.

63. Charlwood J, Clayton P, Keir G, Mian N, Winchester B. Defective galactosylation of serum transferrin in galactosemia. *Glycobiology* 1998;**8**:351–7.

64. Sturiale L, Barone R, Fiumara A, et al. Hypoglycosylation with increased fucosylation and branching of serum transferrin N-glycans in untreated galactosemia. *Glycobiology* 2005;**15**:1268–76.

65. Moraitou M, Dimitriou E, Mavridou I, et al. Transferrin isoelectric focusing and plasma lysosomal enzyme activities in the diagnosis and follow-up of hereditary fructose intolerance. *Clin Chim Acta* 2012;**413**:1714–5.

66. Schellenberg F, Schwan R, Mennetrey L, Loiseaux M-N, Pagès JC, Reynaud M. Dose-effect relation between daily ethanol intake in the range 0-70 grams and %CDT value: validation of a cut-off value. *Alcohol Alcohol* 2005;**40**:531–4.

67. Sillanaukee P, Strid N, Allen JP, Litten RZ. Possible reasons why heavy drinking increases carbohydrate-deficient transferrin. *Alcohol Clin Exp Res* 2001;**25**:34–40.

68. Helander A, Jaeken J, Matthijs G, Eggertsen G. Asymptomatic phosphomannose isomerase deficiency (MPI-CDG) initially mistaken for excessive alcohol consumption. *Clin Chim Acta* 2014;**431**:15–18.

69. Albahri Z, Marklová E, Vanícek H, Minxová L, Dédek P, Skálová S. Genetic variants of transferrin in the diagnosis of protein hypoglycosylation. *J Inherit Metab Dis* 2005;**28**:1184–8.

70. Marklová E, Albahri Z. Transferrin D protein variants in the diagnosis of congenital disorders of glycosylation (CDG). *J Clin Lab Anal* 2009;**23**:77–81.

71. Bergström JP, Helander A. HPLC evaluation of clinical and pharmacological factors reported to cause false-positive carbohydrate-deficient transferrin (CDT) levels. *Clin Chim Acta* 2008;**389**:164–6.

72. Arndt T, Meier U, Nauck M, Gressner AM. Primary biliary cirrhosis is not a clinical condition for increased carbohydrate-deficient transferrin: experience with four independent CDT analysis methods. *Clin Chim Acta* 2006;**372**:184–7.

73. Arndt T, Gressner A, Herwig J, Meier U, Sewell AC. Argininosuccinate lyase deficiency (ASL) and carbohydrate-deficient transferrin (CDT): experience with four independent CDT analysis methods--misleading results given by the %CDT TIA assay. *Clin Chim Acta* 2006;**373**:117–20.

74. Sillanaukee P, Alho H, Strd N, Jousilahti P, Vartiainen E, Olsson U. Effect of hormone balance on carbohydrate-deficient transferrin and gamma-glutamyltransferase in female social drinkers. *Alcohol Clin Exp Res* 2000;**24**:1505–9.

75. He M, Matern D, Raymond K, Wolfe L. The Congenital Disorders of Glycosylation. In: Garg U, Smith L, Heese BA, editors. *Laboratory Diagnosis of Inherited Metabolic Disease*. AACC Press; 2012. p. 167–86.

76. Supraha Goreta S, Dabelic S, Dumic J. Insights into complexity of congenital disorders of glycosylation. *Biochem Medica* 2012:156–70.

77. Xia B, Zhang W, Li X, et al. Serum N-glycan and O-glycan analysis by mass spectrometry for diagnosis of congenital disorders of glycosylation. *Anal Biochem* 2013;**442**:178–85.

78. Althoff SS, Grüneberg M, Reunert J, et al. TMEM165 Deficiency: Postnatal Changes in Glycosylation. *JIMD Rep* 2015 published online Aug 4. http://dx.doi.org/10.1007/8904_2015_455.

79. Van Scherpenzeel M, Willems E, Lefeber DJ. Clinical diagnostics and therapy monitoring in the congenital disorders of glycosylation. *Glycoconj J* 2016 published online Jan 7. http://dx.doi.org/10.1007/s10719-015-9639-x.

80. Wada Y. Mass spectrometry for congenital disorders of glycosylation, CDG. *J Chromatogr B Analyt Technol Biomed Life Sci* 2006;**838**:3–8.

81. Zhang W, James PM, Ng BG, et al. A Novel N-Tetrasaccharide in Patients with Congenital Disorders of Glycosylation, Including Asparagine-Linked Glycosylation Protein 1, Phosphomannomutase 2, and Mannose Phosphate Isomerase Deficiencies. *Clin Chem* 2016;**62**:208–17.

82. Wopereis S, Grünewald S, Morava E, et al. Apolipoprotein C-III isofocusing in the diagnosis of genetic defects in O-glycan biosynthesis. *Clin Chem* 2003;**49**:1839–45.

83. Wada Y, Kadoya M, Okamoto N. Mass spectrometry of apolipoprotein C-III, a simple analytical method for mucin-type O-glycosylation and its application to an autosomal recessive cutis laxa type-2 (ARCL2) patient. *Glycobiology* 2012;**22**:1140–4.

84. Faid V, Chirat F, Seta N, Foulquier F, Morelle W. A rapid mass spectrometric strategy for the characterization of N- and O-glycan chains in the diagnosis of defects in glycan biosynthesis. *Proteomics* 2007;**7**:1800–13.

85. Sparks S, Quijano-Roy S, Harper A, et al. Congenital Muscular Dystrophy Overview. In: Pagon RA, Adam MP, Ardinger HH, editors. *GeneReviews*. University of Washington, Seattle; 2012.

86. Vakhrushev SY, Snel MF, Langridge J, Peter-Katalinić J. MALDI-QTOFMS/MS identification of glycoforms from the urine of a CDG patient. *Carbohydr Res* 2008;**343**:2172–83.

87. Yang H-S, Yang M, Li X, Tugulea S, Dong H. Diagnosis of paroxysmal nocturnal hemoglobinuria in peripheral blood and bone marrow with six-color flow cytometry. *Biomark Med* 2013;**7**:99–111.

Disorders of vitamins and cofactors

16

L.D. Smith[1] and U. Garg[2,3]

[1]*University of North Carolina School of Medicine, Chapel Hill, NC, United States;*
[2]*University of Missouri School of Medicine, Kansas City, MO, United States;*
[3]*Children's Mercy Hospitals and Clinics, Kansas City, MO, United States*

Vitamins are organic compounds that are required for a number of biochemical functions, mainly as cofactors for proper functioning of many enzymes. They are required in small quantities to maintain health and development, and the majority of them are not synthesized by humans and must be obtained exogenously. They must be transported to appropriate intracellular compartments. A number of inborn errors of metabolism that result from defects in intracellular recycling or storage have been described. With the likely implementation of metabolomics techniques to identify and follow biomarkers of diseases other than inborn errors of metabolism, it is important to recognize that overlap can occur between disorders of simple deficiency or excess and disorders that affect biochemical processes as inborn errors.[1] In this chapter, several vitamin responsive disorders, excluding BH4, folate (discussed in Chapter 12), and the fat-soluble vitamins D, A, K, and E are discussed.

16.1 THIAMINE (VITAMIN B1)

Thiamine is present in many foods, of which the major source is unrefined cereal grains, liver, heart, and kidney. Thiamine pyrophosphate (TPP) is the biologically active cofactor that is important in the generation of cellular energy. Inherited defects of thiamine metabolism have only recently been identified, despite recognition of dietary thiamine deficiency as the underlying etiology of beriberi since the early 1900s.[2] Defects in cellular uptake, thiamine activation, and attachment of the active cofactor to target enzymes are now recognized.[3] Clinical presentation of affected individuals does not exactly recapitulate nutritionally related beriberi. Beriberi, which is rare in developed countries, can either be "wet" or "dry." The former presents with cardiac and circulatory system involvement (tachycardia, vasodilatation with high output cardiac failure, dyspnea on exertion, paroxysmal nocturnal dyspnea, peripheral edema) with mortality associated with the weakening of capillary walls leading to systemic edema aggravated by high output heart failure. Dry beriberi results from impairment of and damage to peripheral nerves that result in muscle wasting and partial paralysis (ataxia, numbness of hands/feet, loss of deep tendon reflexes, mental confusion, dysarthria, pain, nystagmus, and vomiting). Beriberi can progress to fulminate Wernicke–Korsakoff syndrome (encephalopathy and psychosis).

Thiamine is absorbed in the small intestine by either of two closely related, widely distributed transporters that facilitate high-affinity transport across cell membranes[4,5]: THTR1 (*SLC19A2)* and THTR2 (*SLC19A3*). THTR2 allows for transport of thiamine into the cell, while THTR1 appears to be responsible for release of free thiamine into the circulation.[3] There is an additional transport mechanism, RFC1 (reduced folate carrier 1), that transports TPP and TMP (thiamine monophosphate) into the circulation.[6]

TPP is the intracellularly active form of thiamine and is necessary for the function of many different enzymes. Free thiamine is converted to TPP by the action of thiamine pyrophosphokinase in the cytoplasm. While immediately available to cytoplasmic enzymes, it is also required as a cofactor in the mitochondrial compartment, hence, an inner mitochondrial membrane TTP transporter also exists. TPP is further used within the peroxisome and must be bound to hydroxyacyl-CoA (coenzyme A) lyase apoprotein to facilitate this transport.[3]

In addition to thiamine-responsive pyruvate dehydrogenase deficiency and thiamine-responsive maple syrup urine disease, which represent disorders of attachment of active cofactor to the enzyme and will not be discussed in detail here, the majority of inherited defects disrupt either thiamine transport or activation.

Thiamine absorption, transport, and metabolism are shown in Fig. 16.1.

16.1.1 THTR1 DEFICIENCY

Defects in THTR1 cause thiamine-responsive megaloblastic anemia, which typically presents in infancy or childhood with megaloblastic anemia, diabetes mellitus, and sensorineural hearing loss.[7–9] While these constitute the core symptoms, other clinical findings may include thrombocytopenia, ringed sideroblasts, short stature, cardiac arrhythmias, structural heart defects, cardiomyopathy, ophthalmologic manifestations (optic atrophy, retinal abnormalities), and stroke-like episodes. In addition, lactic acid levels in both blood and cerebrospinal fluid (CSF) can be elevated, demonstrating the important role that α-ketoacid dehydrogenase complexes, which require TPP as a cofactor, play in energy metabolism.

16.1.1.1 Diagnostic tests

Blood thiamine levels are generally within reference range. Diagnosis requires suspicion, with confirmation by DNA-sequencing analysis.

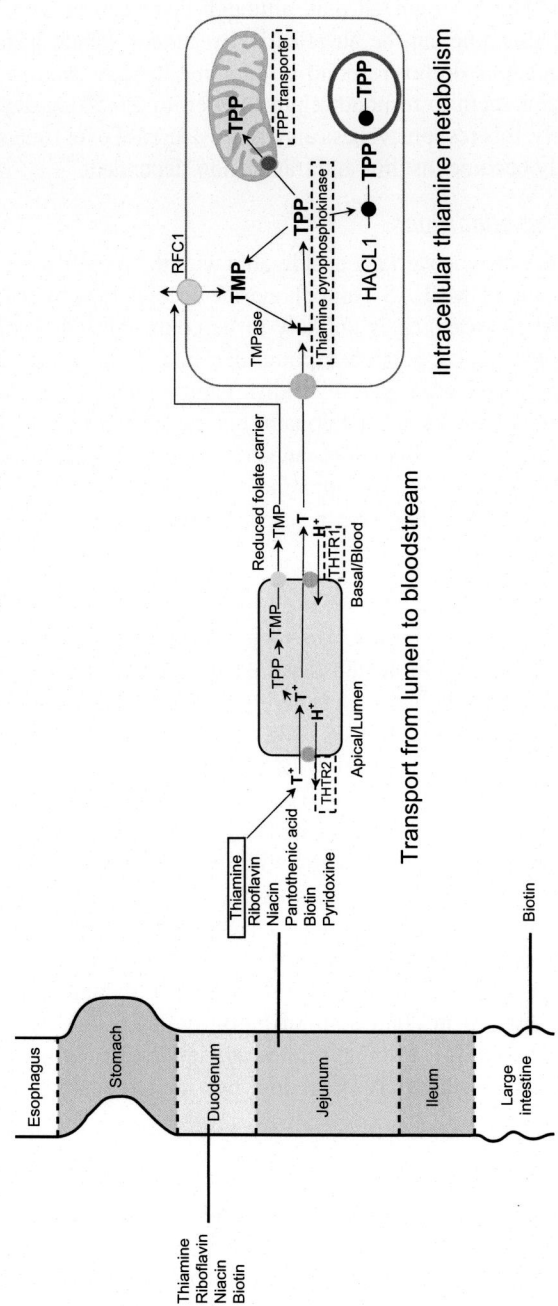

FIGURE 16.1

Sites of intestinal absorption of factors. Pathway of thiamine transport, including known defects in the thiamine pathway (dashed boxes).

16.1.1.2 Treatment

Once diagnosed, it has been recognized that, although there can be variability in response, provision of thiamine can be an effective treatment. While hearing loss and neurologic complications do not respond to thiamine therapy, anemia, cardiac arrhythmias, and diabetes seem to respond relatively well to 25–50 mg/day of thiamine.[3,9,10] Unfortunately, this responsiveness appears to decrease over time such that adult patients ultimately become insulin- and transfusion-dependent.[9]

16.1.1.3 Confounding conditions

Symptoms of THTR1 deficiency overlap considerably with the presentation of mitochondrial disorders, such as MELAS (mitochondrial encephalopathy with lactic acidosis and stroke-like episodes). It is unlikely to be confused with beriberi that typically results from poor intake, poor absorption (diarrhea, diuretic use), impaired use (liver disease), or excessive use (hyperthyroidism) and presents with either nervous system involvement (Wernicke encephalopathy) or cardiovascular involvement. Differentiation from mitochondrial disorders cannot be made on biochemical laboratory results alone, although response to supplementation with thiamine in THTR1 deficiency, if identified early, may lead one to suspect the diagnosis.

16.1.2 THTR2 DEFICIENCY

Defective function of THTR2 has been reported as either a subacute encephalopathy with symmetrical basal ganglia lesions in the caudate nucleus and putamen, or an early-onset, fatal encephalopathy with cerebral atrophy and symmetric thalamic, basal ganglia, and brain stem lesions. While there is some variability in the clinical and biochemical presentations of what is now called thiamine metabolism dysfunction syndrome 2 (OMIM 607483), encephalopathy, and basal ganglia lesions appear to be universal.[11–15] Patients with this autosomal recessive condition often experience episodic encephalopathy with febrile illnesses with seizures, external ophthalmoplegia, dysphagia, and confusion. Coma and death may occur. Presentation may also mimic a mitochondrial encephalopathy. In the originally described patients, a rapid response to biotin was seen and patients did well, if identified and treated early.[14] The response to biotin can be explained by control of *SLC19A3* gene expression: in conditions of biotin deficiency, *SLC19A3* gene expression is down-regulated. It is felt that limited availability of biotin aggravates the condition, the effects of which are overcome by supplementation with both biotin and thiamine.[16–18]

16.1.2.1 Diagnostic tests

Biochemical testing may reveal lactic acidemia with elevated CSF lactic acid levels and diminished pyruvate dehydrogenase and α-ketoglutarate dehydrogenase activity on muscle biopsy samples.[19,20] Magnetic resonance imaging (MRI) findings typically include changes in the basal ganglia as noted above. Biochemical testing cannot be used to confirm the diagnosis, which can be suspected if a response is seen to the provision of biotin and thiamine. Genetic testing with the demonstration of pathogenic variants in *SLC19A3* is necessary to confirm the diagnosis.[19,20]

16.1.2.2 Treatment

No clear genotype–phenotype relationship exists to direct treatment although some patients respond to thiamine or biotin alone. Provision of biotin (2–10 mg/day) and thiamine (100–400 mg/day) has been commonly used.[3,11,15]

16.1.2.3 Confounding conditions

Unlike THTR1 deficiency, THTR2 deficiency may present very similarly to dry beriberi resulting from poor intake, poor absorption (diarrhea, diuretic use), impaired use (liver disease), or excessive use (hyperthyroidism), and presents with either nervous system involvement (Wernicke encephalopathy) or cardiovascular involvement. Even age of presentation may not be particularly helpful as adolescent and adult onset of the disorder has been documented.[12,13,21] There is also overlap with the presentation of mitochondrial disorders, such as Leigh syndrome.[19–21] Differentiation from mitochondrial disorders cannot be made on biochemical laboratory results alone, although response to supplementation with thiamine in THTR1 deficiency, if identified early, may lead one to suspect the diagnosis.

16.1.3 THIAMINE PYROPHOSPHOKINASE DEFICIENCY

This rare autosomal recessive condition, caused by mutations in the *TPK1* gene, presents with childhood onset of episodic ataxia, dystonia, and psychomotor retardation after normal development although a Leigh-like syndrome has also been reported.[22,23] TPP is a required cofactor for many enzymes, although deficiency affects pyruvate dehydrogenase and α-ketoglutarate dehydrogenase most appreciably.[3]

16.1.3.1 Diagnostic tests

Diagnostic tests are most informative during symptomatic episodes with elevated blood and CSF lactic acid levels and increased α-ketoglutarate on urine organic acid profile. TPP levels in blood and muscle are consistently low. Demonstration of low blood TPP concentrations is highly suggestive of the diagnosis although confirmation by DNA sequencing of the *TPK1* gene should be considered.

16.1.3.2 Treatment

Treatment with 100–200 mg/day thiamine and a high-fat diet has been reported to be effective in reducing symptoms.[22,23]

16.1.3.3 Confounding conditions

As with THTR2 deficiency, TPP deficiency can present similarly to either dry beriberi or mitochondrial disorders. Demonstration of low blood TPP levels is highly suggestive of TPP deficiency.

16.1.4 MITOCHONDRIAL TPP TRANSPORTER DEFICIENCY

Originally described in its most severe form as Amish lethal microcephaly,[24–26] it has become apparent that less severe forms of mitochondrial TPP transporter deficiency exist.[27] Amish lethal microcephaly is an autosomal recessive condition that presents with extreme microcephaly, micrognathia, contractures, a nearly absent cranial vault, and absence of anterior and posterior fontanels. Hepatomegaly may also be present. In addition to the contractures and limb hypertonia, there is truncal hypotonia and limited psychomotor development. Brain MRI demonstrates no gyral development, partial agenesis of the corpus callosum, and cerebellar and pons hypoplasia. Spiegel et al.[27] reported on four siblings with illness-associated episodes of flaccid paralysis and encephalopathy, followed by residual weakness and a progressive polyneuropathy without cognitive impairment (bilateral striatal necrosis with chronic progressive polyneuropathy). Brain MRI revealed basal ganglia involvement of the caudate nucleus and putamen, sparing the globus pallidus.

16.1.4.1 Diagnostic tests

In patients with the more severe form of the disorder, urine organic acid profiles demonstrate variably increased excretion of α-ketoglutarate and lactate. Lactic acidosis is present during episodes of intercurrent illness, particularly viral infection. Laboratory findings are not as pronounced in the less severe forms of the disorder. Elevated CSF lactic acid concentrations have been observed during acute episodes without increased urinary α-ketoglutarate. No laboratory test, other than the identification of pathogenic variants in the *SLC25A19* gene, is diagnostic.

16.1.4.2 Treatment

There is no evidence that supplementation with high-dose thiamine is effective in treating this disorder although it has been tried in those patients identified with bilateral striatal necrosis and chronic progressive polyneuropathy in the hopes of preventing acute episodes and slowing progression.[27]

16.1.4.3 Confounding conditions

As with other thiamine deficiency disorders, TPP deficiency has overlap with disorders of mitochondrial dysfunction. Syndromic and nonsyndromic genetic and environmental causes of microcephaly must also be considered. The finding of intermittent lactic acidosis with intercurrent illness may help to direct diagnosis. Thiamine-responsive pyruvate dehydrogenase deficiency may present similarly to the milder form of the disorder with both ataxia and lactic acidemia.

16.2 RIBOFLAVIN (VITAMIN B2)

Historically, riboflavin, or lactochrome as it was called, was first isolated from whey in 1879. Riboflavin functions as a cofactor in a number of enzymatic reactions. The flavins, riboflavin 5′-phosphate mononucleotide (FMN) and riboflavin 5′-adenosine diphosphate (FAD) are necessary for the proper functioning of flavin coenzyme systems that are involved in the regulation of cellular metabolism as well as carbohydrate, amino acid, and fatty acid metabolism. Riboflavin is not stored and hence, a constant dietary supply is needed. Riboflavin is needed for conversion of folic acid and pyridoxine to their active forms, is required for proper folding of proteins in the endoplasmic reticulum, is important in immune function, is necessary for acyl-CoA dehydrogenation reactions (fatty acid oxidation, branched-chain amino acid catabolism), and is needed for the production of glutathione.[28–32] Deficiency results in fatigue, night blindness, cataracts, migraine headaches, peripheral neuropathy, anemia, growth retardation, developmental anomalies such as cleft lip/palate and congenital heart defects, and dermatologic symptoms (cheilosis, glossitis, scaly skin rashes confined to scrotum and vulva, and chapped/fissured lips).

While deficiency is rare and is usually of dietary origin, and is thus seen in situations of multiple nutrient deficiencies, riboflavin transporter defects are known to cause Brown–Vialetto–Van Laere syndrome (BVVLS) and Fasio–Londe (FL) syndrome.[33–37] First described in 1894, these very rare neurodegenerative disorders have variable age of onset (from infancy to adulthood) and present with sensorineural hearing loss, bulbar palsy, and respiratory compromise. Presentation of these disorders, now felt to represent one condition, differs only in that hearing loss is not part of FL syndrome.

Interestingly, milk and eggs are the best dietary source for free riboflavin as other foodstuffs tend to contain FAD and FMN. FAD and FMN must be hydrolyzed to free riboflavin by nonspecific phosphatases in order for absorption to occur. Absorption is achieved via active transport, primarily in the small intestine, using specific riboflavin transporters. Both free riboflavin and FMN may enter the plasma: free riboflavin is bound to albumin and immunoglobulins. After cellular uptake, almost all of the riboflavin is bound to enzymes. Unbound flavins are rapidly hydrolyzed and free riboflavin diffuses out of the cell and is excreted.[38]

Three human transporters have been identified: hRFVT-1, hRFVT-2, and hRFVT-3, which are encoded by the *SLC52A1*, *SLC52A2*, and *SLC52A3* genes, respectively.[39] While similar in structure and function, they have different tissue expression and transport capacities. The predominant transporter for the brain is hRFVT-3, although it is now known that mutations in any of the transporters can cause BVVLS.[34,40] Inheritance of BVVLS is autosomal recessive in nature. Biochemically, BVVLS and FL syndromes mimic multiple acyl-CoA dehydrogenase deficiency (MADD).[28,41] Fig. 16.2 shows the transport and metabolism of riboflavin.

16.2.1 DIAGNOSTIC TESTS

Since FAD generated from riboflavin is an electron acceptor for acyl-CoA dehydrogenation reactions in branched-chain amino acid catabolism and mitochondrial fatty acid oxidation, laboratory testing results often mimic those seen in mild MADD.[28,34,41] Thus, urine organic acid profiles may demonstrate mild elevations in ethylmalonic acid, adipic acid, 2-hydroxyglutaric acid and suberic acid. Hexonylglycine and isovalerylglycine may also be elevated. Acylcarnitine profiles may also appear similarly to milder forms of MADD with elevations of C4, C5, C6,

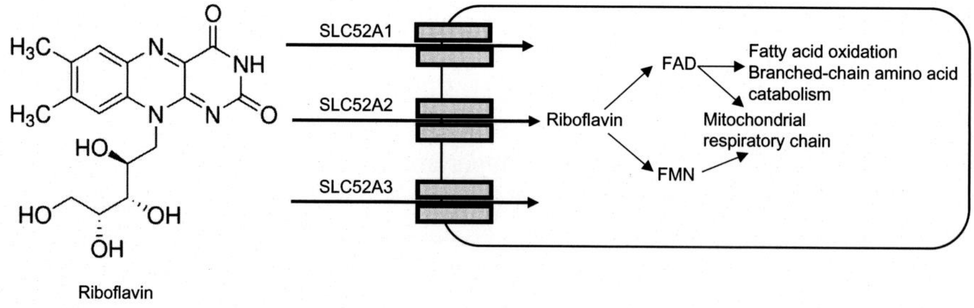

FIGURE 16.2

Riboflavin uptake defect. There are three riboflavin transporters; human disease has been associated with mutations in SLC52A2 and SLC52A3. Biochemical findings of riboflavin deficiency reflect deficiencies of FAD and FMN, although abnormalities are not always present in Brown–Vialetto–Van Laere syndrome and Fazio–Londe disease caused by diminished transport of riboflavin in the central nervous system.

C8, C10, C12, and C14. However, these elevations may not be seen.[34,42] Plasma flavin levels (riboflavin, FMN, and FAD) are also low in untreated patients. Reduced red blood cell glutathione reductase activity points toward riboflavin deficiency. Deficiency may results in false positive elevations of urinary catecholamines (dopamine, norepinephrine, epinephrine) and urine urobilinogen.

16.2.2 TREATMENT

Supplementation with riboflavin (10 mg/kg/day up to 450 mg/day) results in improvement in muscle strength, motor function, hearing, vision, and respiration. In some, recovery is swift, while in others it may be more gradual.[35,43] If there is little-to-no response to riboflavin supplementation, then symptoms are unlikely to result from mutations in the riboflavin transporter genes.

16.2.3 CONFOUNDING CONDITIONS

Primary riboflavin deficiency results from inadequate dietary intake. Secondary riboflavin deficiency can be seen with chronic diarrhea, conditions with malabsorption (inflammatory bowel disease, gluten intolerance), chronic liver disease, hemo- and peritoneal dialysis, long-term use of barbiturates, and chronic alcoholism.[44,45] While dietary deficiency more typically presents with a peripheral neuropathy rather than central nervous system (CNS) involvement, there is at least one reported pediatric case of a reversible neurodegenerative disease in a child with moderate riboflavin deficiency.[46] In addition, similar clinical and biochemical findings may be seen in ethylmalonic encephalopathy (ethylmalonic aciduria) and mild MADD. Both are autosomal recessive conditions. The former results from mutations in the *ETHE1* gene and the latter from mutations in *ETFDH*, *ETFA*, or *ETFB* genes. Finally, maternal riboflavin deficiency and riboflavin transporter haploinsufficiency have both been associated with transient neonatal-onset glutaric aciduria type II.[47,48]

16.3 NIACIN (VITAMIN B3)

The functional forms of niacin include nicotinic acid, nicotinamide, and any derivative that can be converted to nicotinamide adenine dinucleotide (NAD) or nicotinamide adenine dinucleotide phosphate (NADP). Hence, niacin is essential for all cells to function in that both NAD and NADP are involved in myriad biochemical reactions ranging from glycolysis to sterol biosynthesis. Niacin deficiency results in pellegra (diarrhea, dermatitis, dementia, and death), a disease that is most often associated with nutritionally marginal corn-based diets,[49] because of the low concentration of both free niacin and tryptophan in maize. *In vivo*, tryptophan is converted to niacin and hence, its deficiency can also lead to development of pellegra. Pyridoxine is a cofactor necessary for the synthesis of niacin from tryptophan so pyridoxine deficiency can also result in niacin deficiency.

While there are no specifically identified inherited disorders of niacin biosynthesis, niacin deficiency can result from defects in *SLC6A19*, a neutral amino acid transporter present in the intestine and the kidney, which is responsible for Hartnup disease.[50–52] In this disorder, the sodium-dependent transporter fails to absorb or reabsorb neutral amino acids, including tryptophan, resulting in an aminoaciduria and loss of amino acids in feces.[53] The neutral amino acid transporter, B^0AT1, requires either collectrin (TMEM27) in the kidney or angiotensin-converting enzyme 2 (ACE2) in the intestinal tract for stabilization of tertiary structure and cell surface expression.[54,55] Fig. 16.3 shows the absorption and metabolism of niacin.

16.3.1 DIAGNOSTIC TESTS

If clinically suspected, diagnosis of Hartnup disease can be made by comparison of urine and plasma amino acid profiles. Urine should have an excess of neutral amino acids (Gln, Val, Phe, Leu, Asn, Ile, Thr, Ala, Ser, His, Tyr, Trp), citrulline and indican with low-to-normal plasma concentrations. Urinary proline, hydroxyproline, and arginine should not be elevated, differentiating Hartnup disease from other forms of aminoaciduria. While tryptophan loading results in an increase in urinary indole excretion, genetic testing is available for this autosomal recessive disorder. Niacin plasma levels can also be measured by chromatographic techniques.

16.3.2 TREATMENT

Treatment involves provision of a high-protein diet and niacin supplementation.

16.3.3 CONFOUNDING CONDITIONS

Conditions that result in poor absorption of tryptophan and/or niacin can present with pellegra-like symptoms. Thus, inflammatory bowel disease, alcoholism, and prolonged treatment with isoniazid can also present similarly. In children, inflammatory bowel disease with poor absorption would be the most likely confounding diagnosis, although identification of a neutral aminoaciduria would suggest Hartnup disease.

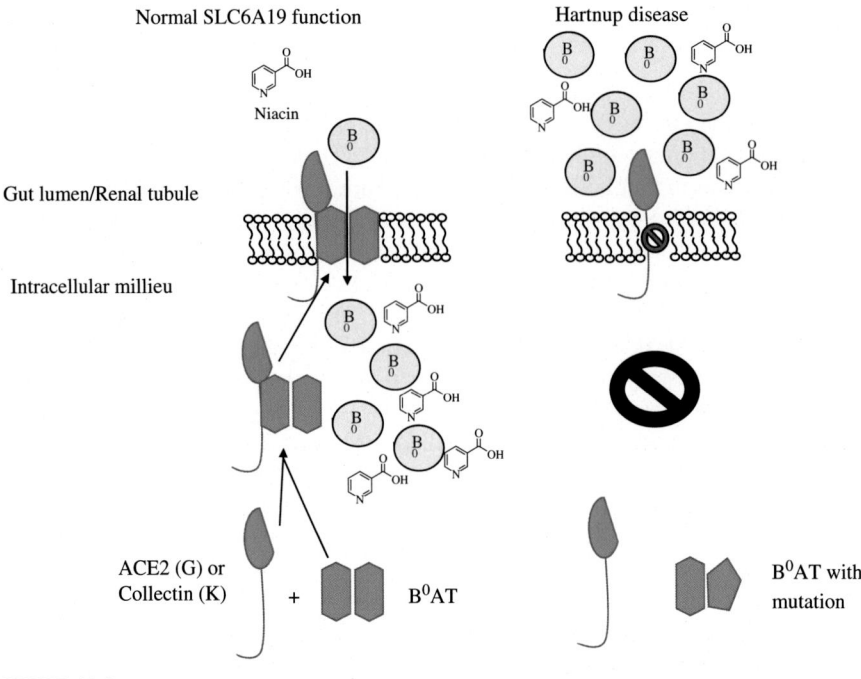

Normal SLC6A19 function

Hartnup disease

Niacin

Gut lumen/Renal tubule

Intracellular millieu

ACE2 (G) or Collectin (K)

B^0AT

B^0AT with mutation

FIGURE 16.3

Niacin absorption and metabolism. B^0 = neutral amino acid. B^0AT = neutral amino acid transporter.

16.4 PANTOTHENIC ACID (VITAMIN B5)

There is a paucity of published literature on human disorders associated with the essential vitamin pantothenic acid. Pantothenic acid is found in many foods and dietary deficiency is very rare and usually accompanies other nutritional deficiencies.[56] Signs and symptoms of isolated pantothenate deficiency have been experimentally induced, resulting in mood changes, postural hypotension, tachycardia with exertion, anorexia, and numbness and tingling of the hands and feet.[57–59]

Physiologically, pantothenate is absolutely required for the generation of CoA that functions as an acyl-group carrier. A phosphorylated derivative, phosphopantetheine is also integral to function of acyl carrier protein in the fatty acid synthase complex. Dietary CoA is hydrolyzed to dephospho-CoA, phosphopantetheine, and pantetheine in the intestinal lumen. Subsequent hydrolysis to pantothenic acid is necessary for cellular uptake by active transport. Cellular uptake of pantothenate, biotin, and lipoic acid are all mediated by the sodium-dependent multivitamin transporter (SMVT) encoded by the *SLC5A6* gene. SMVT is required for transport of both biotin and pantothenate across cell membranes, including the blood–brain barrier where it is preferentially expressed at the luminal membrane of brain capillary endothelial cells, resulting in a 50-fold increase in concentration of these vitamins in the CSF as compared to plasma.[60,61] A conditional knockout mouse model has been developed which, when in the homozygous state, results in impaired biotin and pantothenate uptake by the gut.[62] Homozygous knockout mice have a multitude of phenotypic findings related to lack of biotin and pantothenic acid uptake including postnatal growth retardation, abnormal appendicular skeletal morphology, lethargy, hunched posture, and abnormal intestinal mucosal morphology.[62] It may be that mutations in this transporter may be incompatible with life, as none have been identified in humans. Once in the blood stream, cellular uptake is also mediated by SMVT, although several other possible biotin transporters have been postulated.[60] Biotin and pantothenate are structurally similar and it has been shown that drugs or supplements with similar structures (a carboxyl group bound to a carbon chain without a polar functional group between the carboxyl group and a ring structure or a long carbon chain without a ring structure) can interfere with uptake.[60] For example, salicylic acid competes with and prevents pantothenate uptake by this transporter. Reye syndrome has been linked to CNS pantothenate deficiency,[63,64] suggesting that the neurometabolic deficiency in the condition may be a vitamin deficiency. Other nonsteroidal antiinflammatory medications also exert an inhibitory effect on the transporter.[60] Thus, this finding may inform the use and dosage of such medications to avoid side effects.

After transport into the cytosol, pantothenate is converted to CoA by pantothenate kinase, regulation of which is maintained by feedback inhibition of activity by CoA and acyl-CoA. CoA and acyl-CoA play important physiologic roles as noted above. To complete the process, CoA is then hydrolyzed to pantothenate, which is then eliminated by urinary excretion.

While deficiency results in pathologic symptoms, no toxicity has been associated with excessive intake.

In humans, there are four functional pantothenate kinases, encoded by three different genes (*PANK1*, *PANK2*, and *PANK3*). Compound heterozygous or homozygous mutations in one of these, *PANK2*, result in pantothenate kinase-associated neurodegeneration (PKAN).[65] This enzyme transits first to the cell nucleus and then to the mitochondrial intermembranous space, where it is postulated to act as a CoA sensor in order to monitor intercompartmental energy balance and CoA synthesis, which occurs in both cytosolic and mitochondrial compartments.[66,67] Features of this autosomal recessive condition include childhood onset of dystonia, spasticity, and a pigmentary retinopathy, with rapid progression. *PANK2* mutations can also lead to adult-onset parkinsonism and dystonia.[68,69] Biochemical testing does not provide a diagnosis, although it is possible to measure blood pantothenic acid levels.[70] The underlying pathologic process resulting in PKAN has not yet been elucidated, but diagnosis depends on suspicion as well as demonstration of distinctive findings on brain MRI: a classic finding on T2-weighted sequences of the basal ganglia demonstrates hypointensity of the globus pallidus with an anteromedial region of hyperintensity, although this finding is not completely pathognomonic as it can be seen as a result of carbon monoxide poisoning and other neuroferritinopathies.[66,69] There is a concomitant accumulation of iron in the globus pallidus as well. Interestingly, even though it would be predicted that CoA deficiency might be the underlying biochemical basis for this disease, there is no specific scientific evidence.[66] A second inborn error of CoA synthesis, CoA synthetase deficiency (CoPAN), caused by mutations in the *CoASY* gene, has been described with a similar phenotypic presentation.[71]

16.4.1 DIAGNOSTIC TESTS

There are currently no recommended diagnostic biochemical tests for identification of pantothenic acid deficiency, given the rarity of the condition. History, physical examination, and brain MRI scans with particular attention to T2-weighted scans suggest the diagnosis. Sequencing of *PANK2* and/or *CoASY* confirms the diagnosis.

16.4.2 TREATMENT

Treatment of PKAN and CoPAN is supportive and symptomatic.

16.4.3 CONFOUNDING CONDITIONS

Pantothenic acid deficiency is quite rare and is usually associated with multivitamin, multinutrient deficiency. The constitutional symptoms of deficiency are not specific, including headache, insomnia, fatigue, intestinal upset, and peripheral neuropathy. Thus, unless there is a high suspicion for an isolated deficiency, other diagnoses should be considered. It is likely, with more general availability of whole exome and whole genome sequencing modalities, that more disorders of pantothenic acid metabolism may be discovered. The MRI findings seen in PKAN and CoPAN are similar to those seen with other causes of neurodegeneration with brain iron accumulation, thus these disorders should also be considered in any differential diagnosis. For further discussion, the reader is directed to the excellent review by Hogarth.[69]

16.5 PYRIDOXINE (VITAMIN B6)

The active form of pyridoxine is pyridoxal 5′-phosphate (PLP), which is an essential vitamin obtained from the diet.[72] It cannot be synthesized *de novo* but can, similarly to biotin, be recycled in a pathway that includes adenosine triphosphate (ATP)-dependent pyridoxal kinase, flavin mononucleotide-dependent pyridoxine oxidase, and several phosphatases.[73,74] The intestine and the portal circulation are critical to B6 metabolism.[75] Hence, the conditions that affect intestinal integrity will affect B6 uptake and metabolism. PLP is not transported directly into the CNS, rather it is converted to pyridoxal by a membrane associated tissue nonspecific alkaline phosphatase (TNSALP), transported across the blood–brain barrier, enters the neuron and is rephosphorylated intracellularly. PLP is required for the activity of more than 160 enzymes that are involved in the gamut of intermediary metabolic pathways. Inherited disorders of PLP-enzyme defects are not specific to PLP. In many of those identified, PLP has been assigned a chaperone or cofactor role. Other disorders result from accumulation of metabolites and subsequent formation of complexes with PLP, affecting its bioavailability and chemical activity.[76,77] As such, these will not be discussed in detail in this chapter, but are presented in Table 16.1. Pyridox(am)ine 5′-phosphate oxidase and TNSALP deficiency will be discussed in more detail as they directly affect conversion of the B6 vitamers (pyridoxine, pyridoxamine, pyridoxal) to intracellular PLP.[78–81] Various forms of vitamin B6, and their metabolism are shown in Fig. 16.4.

Table 16.1 Vitamin B6 (Pyridoxine)-Related Disorders, Symptoms, and Biochemical Findings

Disease	Symptoms	Enzyme	Gene	Inheritance	Biochemical Findings
Aromatic L-amino acid decarboxylase deficiency OMIM 608643	Psychomotor delay, dystonia, choreoathetosis, oculogyric crisis, temperature instability with onset in early infancy, and diurnal fluctuation of symptoms	Dopa decarboxylase	DDC	AR	↓ CSF HVA, 5-HIAA ↓ Plasma catecholamines ↓ Whole blood serotonin ↑ CSF, plasma and urinary L-dopa, %HTP, 3-OMD, 3-methoxytyrosine Paradoxical ↑ urinary dopamine and dopamine metabolites ↓DDC activity
Cystothionuria OMIM 219500	Majority with normal cognition Liver fibrosis	Hepatic γ-cystathionase	CTH	AR	↑ Urinary cystathionine ↓ CTH activity
Homocystinuria OMIM 236200	Nl-tall stature Ectopia lentis/myopia/glaucoma High arched palate Pectus excavatum/carinatum Kyphoscoliosis Arachnodactyly Psychiatric disorders Thromboembolism	Cystathionine-β-synthase	CBS	AR	↑ Urinary homocysteine and methionine ↓ CBS activity
Ornithine aminotransferase deficiency OMIM 258870	Progressive chorioretinal degeneration with night blindness & myopia Progressive loss of peripheral vision Proximal muscle weakness	Ornithine aminotransferase	OAT	AR	↑ Plasma ornithine Nl plasma ammonia levels ↑ Urinary ornithine, lysine, arginine ↓ Plasma lysine, glutamic acid, glutamine ↓ OAT activity
Primary hyperoxaluria type I OMIM 259900	Optic atrophy, retinopathy, choroidal neovascularization (Peripheral vascular insufficiency Arterial spasm Arterial occlusion Intermittent claudication) Calcium oxalate urolithiasis, nephrocalcinosis Hematuria Renal failure	Alanine-glyoxylate Aminotransferase	AGXT	AR	Metabolic acidosis ↑ Urinary oxalate, glycolic acid ↑ Plasma oxalate Tissue deposition of calcium oxalate ↓ AGT activity
X-linked sideroblastic anemia OMIM 300751	Variable age of onset, often in childhood Hypochromic, microcytic anemia Sideroblastic anemia Macrocytic anemia in manifesting females Variable age of onset	δ-Aminolevulinate synthase 2	ALAS2	X-linked recessive	↓ Hemoglobin Perinuclear mitochondrial iron deposition in erythrocyte precursors Systemic iron overload
Pyridoxine-dependent epilepsy OMIM 266100	Neonatal/infantile onset epileptic encephalopathy	α-Aminoadipic semialdehyde dehydrogenase (Antiquitin)	ALDH7A1	AR	↑ Serum & CSF pipecolic acid ↑ Serum, CSF and urinary α-Aminoadipic semialdehyde

(Continued)

Table 16.1 Vitamin B6 (Pyridoxine)-Related Disorders, Symptoms, and Biochemical Findings (Continued)

Disease	Symptoms	Enzyme	Gene	Inheritance	Biochemical Findings
PLP-responsive epileptic encephalopathy OMIM 610090	Progressive microcephaly Neonatal epileptic encephalopathy (NEE) Burst suppression on EEG Seizures Myoclonus Truncal hypotonia	Pyridoxamine 5′-phosphate oxidase	PNPO	AR	Metabolic acidosis ↑ Blood lactate Hypoglycemia Nl-↑ to plasma glycine, threonine ↓ Plasma arginine ↑ Urine vanillactic acid (VLA) ↓ CSF homovanillic acid (HVA) 5-Hydroxyindoleacetic acid (5-HIAA) ↑ CSF 3-methoxytyrosine (3-MT) ↑ CSF glycine, threonine, taurine, histidine ↓ CSF arginine ↓ CSF pyridoxal, pyridoxal 5-prime-phosphate (PLP)
Hypophosphatasia OMIM 241500 OMIM 146300	Infantile form: Short limb dwarfism Blue sclera Poorly formed teeth Rachitic rosary/rib fractures Small thoracic cage Nephrocalcinosis Lack of boney ossification Seizures Adult onset form: Poor dentition, premature tooth loss Rickets, fractures May be asymptomatic	Tissue nonspecific alkaline phosphatase	ALPL	AR AR/AD	↑ Plasma calcium ↑ Urinary calcium ↑ Urinary phosphoethanolamine ↑ Plasma and urinary inorganic pyrophosphate ↓ Tissue and serum AP activity ↑ Urinary phosphoethanolamine ↓ Serum AP activity
Familial hyperphosphatasia with mental retardation OMIM 239300	Dysmorphic facial features Cleft palate Plagiocephaly Hypoplastic digits Hypotonia Seizures Cognitive impairment	Phosphatidyl-inositol glycan, class V	PIGV	AR	↑ Alkaline phosphatase ↑ Plasma phosphate
Hyperprolinemia type 2 OMIM 239510	Recurrent seizures Cognitive impairment	δ-1-Pyrroline-5-carboxylate dehydrogenase	P5CDH	AR	↑ Plasma proline, δ-1-pyrroline-5-carboxylate ↑ Urinary δ-1-pyrroline-5-carboxylate, δ-1-pyrroline-3-hydroxy--5-carboxylate Aminoaciduria ↑ Urinary proline, hydroxy-proline, glycine ↓ δ-1-Pyrroline-5-carboxylate dehydrogenase in fibroblasts/leukocytes

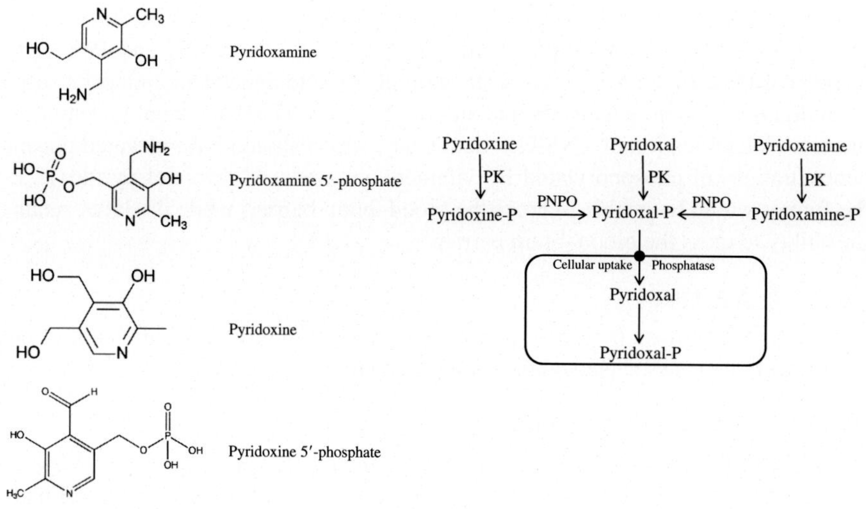

FIGURE 16.4

Various forms of vitamin B6 and their metabolism.

16.5.1 PYRIDOX(AM)INE 5′-PHOSPHATE OXIDASE (PNPO) DEFICIENCY

Deficiency of PNPO is a recessive condition caused by mutations in the *PNPO* gene. Deficiency of this enzyme results in a severe neonatal epileptic encephalopathy due to the inability of affected individuals to synthesize PLP from dietary pyridoxine or to recycle pyridoxamine phosphate, which leads to reduction in PLP-dependent reactions in the CNS. By and large, the most prominent clinical features are treatment-resistant fetal to neonatal-onset seizures in a burst-suppression pattern, including treatment with antiepileptics and pyridoxine. Low levels of PLP directly affect activity of the glycine cleavage system, threonine dehydratase, aromatic amino acid decarboxylase, and histidine decarboxylase.

16.5.1.1 Diagnostic tests

While not particularly sensitive or specific for the disorder, several biochemical tests can direct further investigation, such as consideration of confirmatory *PNPO* gene sequencing. Identification of vanillyl-lactate in the urine as well as decreased levels of CSF homovanillic acid, 5-hydroxyindoleacetic acid accompanied by elevated CSF glycine, threonine, histidine, 3-methoxytyrosine, taurine, and low-plasma arginine are suggestive of low intracellular levels of PLP. More recently, liquid chromatography tandem mass chromatography (LC-MS/MS) methods for measurement of all plasma B6 vitamers has been demonstrated as a potential method to identify PNPO deficiency, even in the face of treatment with B6.[82] Accumulation of pyridoxamine(PM), pyridoxamine 5′-phosphate(PMP), pyridoxine(PN), and pyridoxine 5′-phosphate(PMP) were observed with a reduced pyridoxal 5′-phosphate(PLP) to pyridoxal(PL) ratio in comparison to controls. Significantly, PLP, PL, PA, PN, MMP, and PM levels could be differentiated from individuals with pyridoxine-dependent epilepsy caused by antiquitin deficiency. This method, although not tested *per se*, should be applicable to the identification of TNSALP deficiency, which should have elevated plasma concentrations of phosphorylated B6 vitamers with reduced levels of pyridoxal, as the former would be unable to cross the blood–brain barrier, while the latter retains the ability to cross the blood–brain barrier.[82]

16.5.1.2 Treatment

Provision of high-dose pyridoxal phosphate results in improved seizure control but has little effect on associated cognitive impairment.

16.5.1.3 Confounding conditions

As LC-MS/MS protocols become available for the identification of plasma B6 vitamer levels, biochemical identification may become more refined. While clinical symptoms associated with pyridoxine-dependent epilepsy (PDE) may be similar, biochemical findings are substantially different in PDE in that levels of serum and CSF pipecolic acid and serum, CSF, and urinary α-aminoadipic semialdehyde are increased. The condition that could most easily be confused with PNPO deficiency is aromatic L-amino acid decarboxylase (AADC) deficiency and would be confused with the more severe form, although dysmorphic features are not commonly seen. CSF HVA and 5-hydroxyindoleacetic acid (5-HIAA) are decreased and urinary vanillyl-lactic acid is increased. However, the two can be distinguished by elevations of L-dopa, 5-hydroxytryptophan (5-HTP), and 3-ortho-methyldopa in AADC deficiency, while CSF amino acid profiles are abnormal in PNPO deficiency. With a burst-suppression electroencephalogram (EEG) pattern and elevated CSF and plasma glycine concentrations, the diagnosis of a glycine encephalopathy could also be considered; however, in this condition, there is an isolated elevation of CSF, plasma, and urinary glycine levels, and the other biochemical abnormalities seen in PNPO deficiency are not observed. While TNSALP deficiency also affects B6 metabolism, it would not likely be confused with PNPO deficiency, since the major clinical findings tend to be skeletal in nature.

16.5.2 TISSUE NONSPECIFIC ALKALINE PHOSPHATASE (TNSALP) DEFICIENCY

Deficiency of TNSALP was first described by Rathburn in 1948.[83] Clinical presentation is variable and can be differentiated into seven different forms based on age at which skeletal involvement is identified,[84] ranging from the severe perinatal form with skeletal deformities and pathognomonic radiographic findings with early death to a very mild form with isolated dental malformations (odontohypophosphatasia). For the purposes of this section, discussion will be limited to the infantile onset form, which can be confused with pyridoxine-responsive seizures. TNSALP primarily plays a role in bone growth and mineralization[85] by hydrolyzing inorganic phosphate, which can inhibit bone mineralization. One of many dephosphorylating enzymes, TNSALP is encoded by the *TNSALP* gene,[86] is ubiquitous,[87] and also plays a role in regulation of neurotransmission in the cerebral cortex.[88] It is essential for the conversion of pyridoxal 5′ phosphate, which is unable to cross the blood–brain barrier, to pyridoxal, which is then reconverted to PLP. In addition to other functions, PLP regulates γ-aminobutyric acid (GABA) synthesis.[89] When the inhibitory effect of GABA is diminished, excitatory neurotransmitters result in seizure activity.[90] The more severe forms of the disorder tend to be autosomal recessive in inheritance. Along with skeletal abnormalities (rickets, fractures, poorly mineralized cranium, micromelia), recurrent lung infections, respiratory compromise, and seizures can be present. A report by Belachew et al.[91] reinforces the fact that skeletal anomalies and other phenotypic features may not be overt, at least initially.

16.5.2.1 Diagnostic tests

If the diagnosis is suspected, in addition to clinical findings, serum alkaline phosphatase activity will be low or absent. Urinary phosphoethanolamine and serum inorganic pyrophosphate (PPi) and pyridoxal-5′-phosphate are elevated. Hypercalcemia and hypercalciuria, along with nephrocalcinosis may also be present.

16.5.2.2 Treatment

Historically, treatment was relatively ineffective and limited to calcitonin and chlorothiazide for hypercalcemia/hypercalciuria, although seizures respond to the provision of pyridoxine.[90,91] Enzyme replacement therapy with asofotase alpha (Strensiq) is currently under review for the treatment of infantile and juvenile-onset hypophosphatasia,[92,93] the use of which obviates the need for pyridoxine treatment.

16.5.2.3 Confounding conditions

While skeletal anomalies would likely suggest the diagnosis, given the variability in the phenotype, other conditions that may mimic TNSALP deficiency include those that reduce serum alkaline phosphatase activity, including zinc deficiency, hypothyroidism, hypoparathyroidism, folic acid deficiency, pyridoxine deficiency, and malnutrition. While celiac disease may result in low alkaline phosphatase activity, this condition tends to have a later onset and does not result in the associated radiographic skeletal anomalies. If serum calcium levels are low, then hypoparathyroidism should be suspected, rather than TNSALP.

16.6 BIOTIN (VITAMIN B7)

Unlike several of the trace elements and vitamins that are required for the function of hundreds of enzymes, the water soluble vitamin biotin is required for the function of only five enzymes, all carboxylases. These carboxylases catalyze biocarbonate fixation in organic acids and, as such, are necessary for fatty acid, amino acid, and glucose metabolism. It is also now known that biotin plays a role in the regulation of transcription by covalently binding to histone proteins as well as playing a role in genome stability.[94,95]

The role of biotin in metabolism was elucidated in microorganism and rat models initially since nutritional biotin deficiency is rare.[49] Rats and chicks fed raw egg white developed a condition called "egg white injury" with severe dermatitis, a kangaroo-like posture with spastic gait, alopecia, and death in four to six weeks[96]; however, biotin was not identified as the missing factor until the 1940s, at which time it was also determined that the cause of the disorder was tight binding of biotin by the egg white protein avidin.[97–101]

The enzymes for which biotin is a cofactor are acetyl-CoA carboxylase-α, acetyl-CoA carboxylase-β, propionyl-CoA carboxylase, 3-methylcrotonyl-CoA carboxylase (3-MCC), and pyruvate carboxylase. Acetyl-CoA carboxylase-α is the only carboxylase found in the cytoplasm where it is critical for the generation of malonyl-CoA, which is required for the biosynthesis of fatty acids. The other four carboxylases are localized to the mitochondrial matrix. Acetyl-CoA carboxylase-β plays a role in the regulation of fatty acid oxidation. Propionyl-CoA carboxylase is necessary for leucine, valine, odd-chain fatty acid, and cholesterol catabolism. 3-MCC plays a role in leucine catabolism. Pyruvate carboxylase is necessary for gluconeogenesis as well as participating in tricarboxylic acid anapleurisis, glucose-induced insulin release, and lipogenesis. Consequently, biotin plays a particularly important role in maintaining cardiac muscle and brain function.[95,102]

Dietary biotin exists in both protein-bound and free forms. Biotin-containing protein is digested in the gastrointestinal tract, with release of biocytin and biotin-containing peptides. Biotinidase is secreted by the pancreas with subsequent release of free biotin from the biocytin and peptides, although some biotinidase may be derived from intestinal flora. Free biotin is then transported across intestinal cell membranes via the SMVT, which is also responsible for the transport of pantothenic acid.[103,104] This transporter is also present in liver and peripheral tissues. There appears to be a role for monocarboxylate transporter 1 for biotin uptake by lymphatic cells. In the blood stream, biotin is bound to biotinidase for transport to other tissues. After transport across the cell membrane, again using the SMVT transporter, specific lysine residues in dependent carboxylases and histones are biotinylated by the enzyme holocarboxylase synthase. Biotin can be stored in the liver by binding to mitochondrial acetyl-CoA carboxylase-β. The majority of biotin is found in the cytoplasm and mitochondria although between 0.7% and 1% of intracellular biotin can be found in the nucleus.[95,102] The SCL19A3 transporter (folate transporter, member 3) is necessary for transport of biotin and thiamine across the blood–brain barrier.[105] Holocarboxylases are degraded to biocytin and small peptides from which free biotin is recycled and released by biotinidase (Fig. 16.5).

Clinical findings of biotin deficiency include a periorbital dermatitis, conjunctivitis, alopecia (including eyebrows), ataxia, hypotonia, seizures and skin infections. Developmental delay may also be identified.[106–108] Biochemically, deficiency leads to an anion gap metabolic acidosis with ketosis and lactic acidosis.

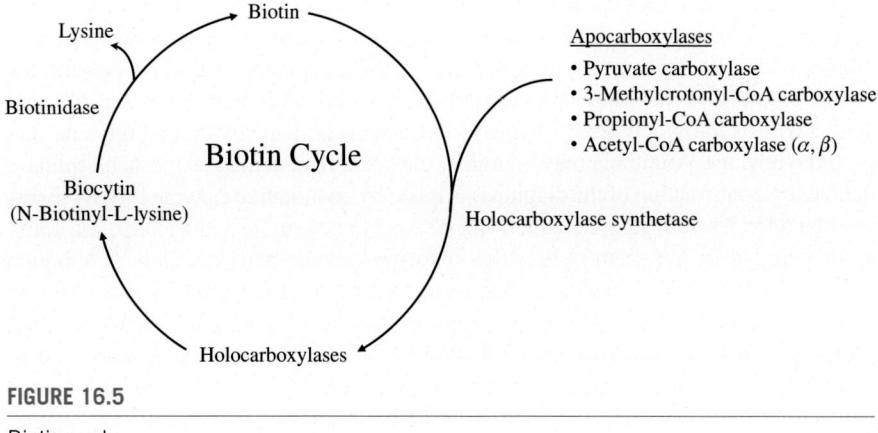

FIGURE 16.5

Biotin cycle.

16.6.1 BIOTINIDASE DEFICIENCY

Biotinidase is required to recycle biotin from degraded carboxylases as well as to release free biotin from biocytin. Both profound and partial biotinidase deficiency can occur, depending on the type of mutation present in the *BTD* gene, as well as the amount of residual biotinidase activity that is present. Individuals with profound deficiency have less than 10% of normal biotinidase activity and tend to present earlier than those with partial deficiency (those with 10–30% of normal activity).[106,107] Those with profound deficiency present with the classic clinical findings of biotin deficiency, within the first 1 week to 2 years of life and, unless identified early and treated, may have irreversible sensorineural hearing loss and vision loss with optic atrophy.[109,110] Those with partial deficiency tend to present later or during periods of physical stress, such a underlying illness, often with skin findings and no neurologic symptoms.[111,112] There can also be variability in presentation as there have been cases of asymptomatic adults with severe deficiency as well as delayed-onset profound deficiency.[113,114] The combined incidence of partial and profound biotinidase deficiency has been estimated to be 1 in 60,000 births with 1 in 123 individuals worldwide predicted to be carriers of this recessively inherited disorder.[95] At the present time, the effect of biotinidase deficiency on histone biotinylation is less clear: it is likely that holocarboxylase may be more important for this function. Abnormal histone biotinylation has been associated with decreased lifespan and heat resistance in *Drosophila melanogaster*[115,116]; however, no similar phenotype has been observed in humans.

16.6.1.1 Diagnostic tests

Newborn screening for biotinidase deficiency is on the recommended core panel of disorders.[117] Semiquantitative assessment of biotinidase activity is performed on dried blood spots as a colorimetric assay.[118–120] This disorder can be missed on tandem mass spectrometry since up to 20% of affected individuals will not have a demonstrable organic aciduria, even when symptomatic.[121,122] When organic aciduria is present, the profile is similar to that seen with holocarboxylase deficiency with elevations of lactic acid, 3-hydroxypropionic acid, 3-hydroxyisovaleric acid, 3-methylcrotonylglycine, and propionylglycine. Ammonia may be mildly elevated. If screening suggests biotinidase deficiency, confirmation of the diagnosis is made by quantitative enzyme activity measured on a fresh serum sample, which can be used to determine residual enzyme activity.[123] There does not seem to be strict genotype–phenotype correlation,[124] although it is clear that insertion/deletion mutations that result in frameshifts or premature stop codons are common.[125,126] Missense mutations in conserved amino acids that result in profound deficiency have also been identified.[127] Partial biotindase deficiency is usually observed in individuals with compound heterozygosity for a D444H mutation and another mutation, although compound heterozygosity for the D444H and A171T mutations results in profound deficiency.[106]

16.6.1.2 Treatment

Since biotinidase deficiency results in the inadequate recycling of biotin and release of free biotin from biocytin and biotin-containing peptides, it can easily be treated with exogenous free biotin, usually between 5 and 20 mg daily for life.

16.6.1.3 Confounding conditions

Expanded newborn screening for biotinidase deficiency should allow for differentiation from other causes of biotin deficiency. However, biotin deficiency can result from holocarboxylase synthase deficiency and SMVT defects. In addition, Mardach *et al.* have postulated that there may be other biotin transporters as they have reported on a child with biotin dependency that does not appear to be related to defective SMVT.[128] As previously mentioned, urine organic acid profiles can be completely normal in many individuals with biotinidase deficiency, which is an unlikely scenario in the case of holocarboxylase synthetase (HCS) deficiency. Acylcarnitine profiles, likewise, will be abnormal in HCS deficiency with elevations of C5-OH (3-hydroxyisovalerylcarnitine), C5:1 (tiglylcarnitine), and C3 (propionylcarnitine). Deficient transport of biotin secondary to SMVT dysfunction has also been reported to result in clinical and biochemical findings similar to those seen with HCS deficiency, although findings do not become apparent until intercurrent illness.[128] Other causes of biotin deficiency include prolonged treatment with anticonvulsants such as phenytoin, primidone, carbamazipine, phenobarbital, and valproic acid, as well as ingestion of high doses of lipoic acid, long-term use of antibiotics, excessive alcohol consumption, and habitual or regular consumption of raw egg whites.[102]

16.6.2 HOLOCARBOXYLASE SYNTHETASE DEFICIENCY

The enzyme HCS is absolutely required for the incorporation of biotin into the apocarboxylases pyruvate carboxylase, propionyl-CoA carboxylase, 3-methylcrotonyl-CoA carboxylase, and acetyl-CoA carboxylase. This rare autosomal recessive disorder results from mutations in the *HCLS* gene, occurring much less frequently than biotinidase deficiency. The majority of causative mutations have been localized to the putative biotin-binding region resulting in reduced biotin-binding affinity,[129,130] while others have been localized to the N-terminus, leading to reduced maximal velocity of enzyme activity with subsequently reduced levels of the active forms of the four biotin-dependent carboxylases.[131]

As with the majority of inborn errors of metabolism, holocarboxylase deficiency also has variability in age of onset, although most will present within the first days of life. Presenting symptoms are nonspecific: tachypnea with Kussmaul breathing, severe metabolic acidosis, ketosis, and hyperammonemia.[132] Those with less severe forms may present later with recurrent metabolic acidosis, precipitated by intercurrent illness, increased protein intake, or catabolic stress.[133] Skin findings include hair loss and an erythematous scaly rash in the intertriginous areas resembling seborrhea.

16.6.2.1 Diagnostic tests

While multiple carboxylase deficiency may be on the differential of elevated C5-OH (3-hydroxyisovaleryl) acylcarnitine on newborn screening, this is certainly not diagnostic and is most commonly seen with isolated 3-methylcrotonyl-CoA carboxylase deficiency. Other conditions with elevated C5-OH include 3-hydroxy-3-methylglutaryl (HMG)-CoA lyase deficiency (which also has elevated C6-DC), 3-methylglutaconyl-CoA hydratase deficiency and, rarely, biotinidase deficiency. Confirmation of a suspected diagnosis requires acylcarnitine profile, urine organic acid profile, and until the recent ubiquitous use of DNA sequence analysis, enzyme assay of carboxylase activities in lymphocytes that is not correctable by preincubation with biotin.[134] Biotin concentrations and biotinidase activity levels are within reference ranges. Urine may have an unpleasant cat urine odor. Urinary and plasma levels of lactic, pyruvic, 3-hydroxypropionic, 3-hydroxyisovaleric, and methylcitric acids, along with propionyl-, tiglyl-, and 3-methylcrotonylglycines are elevated. Plasma acylcarnitine profile demonstrates elevated C5-OH (3-hydroxyisovalerylcarnitine), C5:1 (tiglylcarnitine), and C3 (propionylcarnitine) levels. These findings reflect absent activities of 3-methylcrotonyl-CoA carboxylase, pyruvate carboxylase, propionyl-CoA carboxylase, and acetyl-CoA carboxylase. Mutational analysis of the *HLCS* gene can confirm the diagnosis.[135]

16.6.2.2 Treatment

Most cases of holocarboxylase deficiency are responsive to pharmacologic doses of biotin ranging from 10 to 20 mg/day, although some require treatment with significantly higher doses (40–200 mg/day).[136–138] Protein restriction is not usually necessary except in very severe cases with decreased responses to provision of biotin. Interestingly, biochemical abnormalities do not resolve with treatment and abnormal metabolites continue to be excreted in an inverse correlation to the carboxylase activity in lymphocytes.[136,139] Prognosis is generally good if identified and treated. Biotin supplementation is lifelong. Hearing and vision loss, as are seen in biotinidase deficiency, are not sequelae of this disorder.

16.6.2.3 Confounding conditions

As noted earlier, an elevated C5-OH on expanded newborn screening can be seen with holocarboxylase deficiency; however, this moiety can also be a finding in 3-MCC deficiency, HMG-CoA lyase deficiency, biotinidase deficiency, 3-oxothiolase deficiency, and 2-methyl-3-hydroxybutyryl-CoA dehydrogenase deficiency. As isolated conditions, these can generally be differentiated from holocarboxylase deficiency by specific urine organic acid and acylcarnitine profile analyses or examination of biotinidase activity levels (Table 16.2). Acquired biotin deficiency may also present with similar clinical and biochemical features but has the findings of normal biotinidase activity, decreased lymphocyte carboxylase activities that normalize after a single dose of oral biotin or, if performed *in vitro*, after preincubation with biotin, and low plasma and urine biotin levels.[134]

16.6.3 BIOTIN-RESPONSIVE BASAL GANGLIA DISEASE

This disorder is discussed in more depth in the section on thiamine, as it is caused by autosomal recessive mutations in the thiamine transporter encoded by *SLC19A3*,[140] the expression of which is regulated by biotin.[18]

16.6.4 BIOTIN TRANSPORTER DEFECT

While the SMVT transporter has been identified as the primary free biotin transporter in the gut endothelium, there is a single report of a patient with biotin dependency with neither defective SMVT, biotinidase, or holocarboxylase function nor nutritional biotin deficiency.[128] This patient presented with an acute-onset encephalopathy at 18 months of age. In addition, the urine organic acid profile was consistent with biotin-dependent carboxylase deficiency. All testing, including fibroblast and lymphocyte carboxylase activities and *SVMT* gene sequencing, was uninformative except that biotin uptake in primary blood lymphocytes was reduced by about 90 percent. Results from parental cells was suggestive of an autosomal recessive condition. To date, no definitive transporter has been identified.

16.7 COBALAMIN (VITAMIN B12)

Vitamin B12, also called cobalamin, is a cobalt containing vitamin that is synthesized only by microorganisms. In the human diet, animal products are the only source of vitamin B12. It was noted that B12 deficiency caused pernicious anemia that was treatable with oral liver extract. It was also noted that some cases with pernicious anemia could not be treated with vitamin B12. This finding was due to the fact that these patients had inherited defects of cobalamin absorption, transport, or intracellular metabolism. These patients were found to have an elevation of homocysteine or methylmalonic acid or both.[141,142]

Intestinal absorption and transport of cobalamin is complex. Cobalamin in the food binds to haptocorrin in saliva and the stomach. In the small intestine, cobalamin is released from haptocorrin by pancreatic proteases. Free cobalamin binds to intrinsic factor, which is produced by gastric parietal cells, to form an intrinsic factor–cobalamin (IF–Cbl) complex. The IF–Cbl complex binds to a receptor called cubam on the apical surface of epithelial cells and is internalized. Once internalized, the IF–Cbl complex is degraded in the lysosome to release cobalamin into the cytosol. Cobalamin is then transported into the blood stream by the multidrug-resistance protein, MRP1. In the portal blood, cobalamin binds to transcobalamin (TC) to form a Cbl–TC complex. Cobalamin is taken into cells through TC receptor (TCblR) mediated endocytosis of the Cbl–TC complex. Once in the cell, the Cbl–TC complex is degraded in lysosomes to release free cobalamin, that is then transported to the cytosol. Cobalamin is then converted to its active forms, methylcobalamin (MeCbl) and adenosylcobalamin (AdoCbl), through a complex process involving many proteins. MeClb is the cofactor required for the enzyme methionine synthase activity, and AdoCbl is the coenzyme required for methylmalonyl-CoA mutase activity. A number of inherited metabolic defects are known in the absorption, transportation or intracellular processing of cobalamin. Depending on the defect, elevation of homocysteine or methylmalonic acid or both are seen. There is considerable variability in both biochemical and clinical findings in patients with cobalamin defects.[141,143]

In humans, vitamin B12 is required for at least two enzyme systems. Adenosylcobalamin is a coenzyme for mitochondrial enzyme L-methylmalonyl-CoA mutase in the conversion of L-methylmalonyl-CoA to succinyl-CoA. Methylcobalamin is a coenzyme for cytosolic enzyme methionine synthetase in the conversion of homocysteine to methionine. Cobalamin metabolism and various metabolic defects are depicted in Fig. 16.6.

Clinical presentation of cobalamin deficiency results in megaloblastic anemia and neuropathy. Neurological changes may include areflexia, irritability, peripheral neuropathy, developmental regression, and poor brain growth. Methylmalonic aciduria can result in life-threatening acidosis and ketosis. There is considerable variability in clinical presentation depending on the type of defect. Cobalamin C deficiency is the most common and most severe defect, resulting in combined methylmalonic aciduria and homocystinuria. The clinical manifestations may be seen prenatally as intrauterine growth retardation, microcephaly, congenital heart disease, and dysmorphic features.

16.7.1 DIAGNOSTIC TESTS

Most cases of cobalamin deficiency are now diagnosed by newborn screening as elevated propionylcarnitine (C3) and/or methionine. In newborn screening, presumptive positive cases or in clinically suspected cases, urine organic acid, plasma amino acid, plasma homocysteine, and plasma acylcarnitine profiles are frequently performed to evaluate for elevations of homocysteine, methylmalonic acid, and propionylcarnitine (C3). Once the defect is identified, plasma homocysteine and methylmalonic acids are generally used for long-term monitoring.

On positive cases, DNA studies are carried out for confirmation and may also involve further grouping. The grouping can provide insight into whether the disease will be severe or mild, and B12 responsive or unresponsive. Complementation analysis was a powerful technique in grouping and identification of specific genes

Table 16.2 Biotin-Related Disorders and Biochemical Changes. Other Related Disorders of Branched-Chain Amino Acids Along with Biochemical Changes Are Also Shown

Deficiency of	Biotinidase	Holocarboxylase	Acetyl-CoA Carboxylase	Pyruvate Carboxylase	HMG-CoA Lyase
Gene	BTD	HLCS	ACACA	PC	HMGCL
Pathway	Biocytin → Biotin recycling	Val-Ile metabolism, pyruvate metabolism	Long-chain fatty acid synthesis	Gluconeogenesis Lactic acid metabolism	Leucine metabolism
Ketosis	Y	Y		Y	N
Acidosis	Y	Y		Y	Y
↑ Anion gap	Y	Y		Y	
Glucose	↓to Normal	C		↓to Normal	Hypoketotic hypoglycemia
Ammonia	Normal to ↑	Normal to ↑		Normal to ↑	Normal to ↑
UOA profile					
Lactic acid	↑	↑		↑	
3-HIVA		↑			↑ to ↑↑↑
3-OH-propionic	Normal to ↑	Normal to ↑			
3-Methylglutaconic					↑ to ↑↑↑
3-Methylglutaric					↑ to ↑↑↑
3-OH-3-methylglutaric					↑ to ↑↑↑
Methylcitric		Normal to ↑			
3-Methylcrotonylglycine		Normal to ↑			Normal to ↑
Propionylglycine		Normal to ↑			
Tiglyglycine		Normal to ↑			
2-Methyl-3-hydroxybutyric					

3-MCC*	Propionyl-CoA Carboxylase	3-Oxothiolase (β-Ketothiolase)	2-Me-3-OH-Butyryl-CoA (17-β-Hydroxysteroid Dehydrogenase X)	Confounding Conditions
MCC1, MCC2	*PCCA, PCCB*	*ACAT1*	*HSD17B10*	
Leucine metabolism	Val-Ile metabolism	Val-Ile metabolism	Leucine metabolism	
±	Y	Y	Y	
±	Y	Y	Y	
±	Y	Y	Y	
↓to Normal	↓to Normal		↓	
Normal to ↑	Normal to ↑	Normal to ↑		
	Normal to ↑			Gut bacteria and bacterial contamination, short bowel syndrome, other causes of lactic acidosis, drugs, MCT oil administration
↑ to ↑↑↑				Ketosis, lactic acidosis, SCOT, MAD, valproic acid
	↑			Bacterial contamination, short bowel syndrome, lactic acidosis
				Uremia, pregnancy, respiratory chain defects, methylglutaconic aciduria, 3-methylglutaconic aciduria, carbanyl phosphate synthetase deficeincy, Smith-Lemli-Opitz syndrome
				Uremia, pregnancy, respiratory chain defects, methylglutaconic aciduria, 3-methylglutaconic aciduria, carbanyl phosphate synthetase deficeincy, Smith-Lemli-Opitz syndrome
	↑			Malnutrition
↑ to ↑↑↑				Reye (like) syndromes
	↑			MMA
		↑	↑	Reye(like) syndromes
		↑	↑	Ketosis, MAT, Pearson syndrome

(Continued)

Table 16.2 Biotin-Related Disorders and Biochemical Changes. Other Related Disorders of Branched-Chain Amino Acids Along with Biochemical Changes Are Also Shown (Continued)

Deficiency of	Biotinidase	Holocarboxylase	Acetyl-CoA Carboxylase	Pyruvate Carboxylase	HMG-CoA Lyase
Glutaric					Normal to ↑
Adipic					Normal to ↑
Sebacic					Normal to ↑
Suberic					Normal to ↑
2-Methylacetoacetic					
Other			2-Ethyl-3-keto-, 2-ethyl-3-hydroxy-, 2-ethyl-hexanoic acids, hexanoic acid	Pyruvic acid β-Hydroxybutyric acid acetoacetic acid	
Acylcarnitine profile					
C2					
C3	↑	↑			
C4					
C5:1					
C5					
C5:OH	↑	↑			↑ to ↑↑↑
C6-DC					↑ to ↑↑↑
C6-DC					↑ to ↑↑↑
Biotinidase activity	↓	Nl	Nl	Nl	Nl

3-MCC*	Propionyl-CoA Carboxylase	3-Oxothiolase (β-Ketothiolase)	2-Me-3-OH-Butyryl-CoA (17-β-Hydroxysteroid Dehydrogenase X)	Confounding Conditions
				2-Ketoglutarate degradation, bacterial metabolism, uremia, ethylene glycol poisoning, lithium
				Infection, malnutrition, seizures, liver disease, MCT oil administration, ketosis, VPA, lactic acidosis, hypoglycemia, Reye(like) syndromes
				Infection, malnutrition, seizures, liver disease, MCT oil administration, ketosis, VPA, lactic acidosis, hypoglycemia, Reye(like) syndromes
				Infection, malnutrition, seizures, liver disease, MCT oil administration, ketosis, VPA, lactic acidosis, hypoglycemia, Reye(like) syndromes
		↑		
	↑↑			
↑		↑	↑	
↑ to ↑↑↑		↑	↑	
NI	NI	NI	NI	

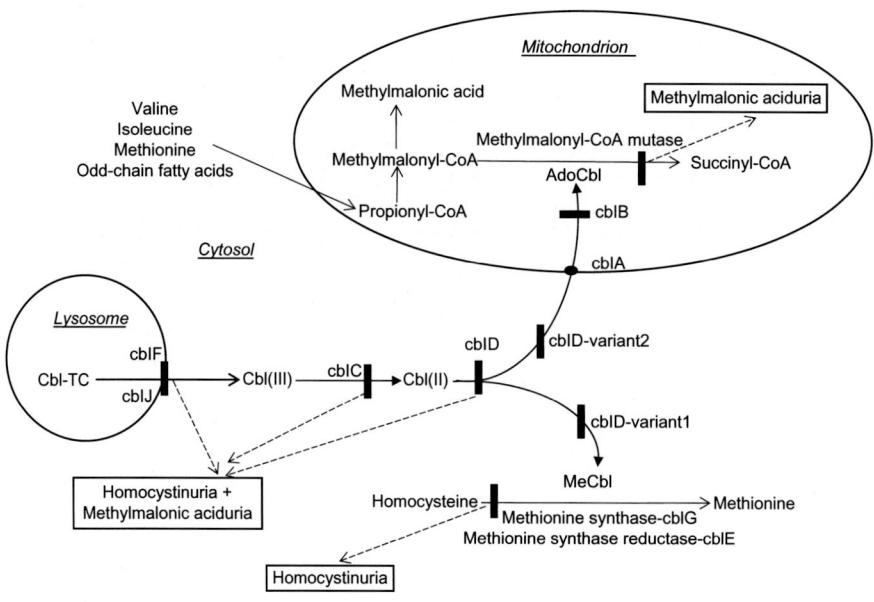

FIGURE 16.6

Cobalamin metabolism showing various forms of cobalamin. Solid bars indicate metabolic defects.

for different cobalamin defects prior to the identification of specific gene defects and the advent of whole exome analysis. In complementation analysis, fibroblast cell lines from different patients are fused to produce hybrids. A particular enzymatic defect in one cell line is corrected by the normal enzyme activity in the other cell line in a hybrid. Complementation analysis involves cobalamin requiring incorporation of radioactivity from [14C] propionate or [14C] methyltetrahydrofolate or [14C] formate to methionine and serine, and ultimately to proteins. Proteins are precipitated by trichloroacetic acid and the radioactivity is measured in the precipitate. Complementation analysis has successfully identified a number of defects in cobalamin metabolism before the identification of specific protein defects. Complementation groups, cblA, cblB, cblC, cblD (variants 1 and 2), cblE, cblF, cblG, cblJ, and mut have been described and have been associated with the synthesis or utilization of MeCbl or AdoCbl or both.[141,144] Complementation groups cblC, cblD, cblF, and cblJ correspond to defects in the synthesis of both MeCbl and AdoCbl, leading to the elevation of homocysteine and methylmalonic acid due to deficient activity of methionine synthase and methylmalonyl-CoA mutase. Complementation groups cblD (variant 1), cblE, and cblG are associated with homocystinuria due to MeCbl deficiency, and complement groups cblA, cblB, and cblD (variant 2) are associated with methylmalonic acidemia due to AdoCbl deficiency. Table 16.3 describes the biochemical changes for various cobalamin defects.

Genes associated with these complementation groups have been identified (Table 16.3). Since complementation assays are complex and not readily available, molecular testing

Table 16.3 Disorders of Cobalamin Metabolism and Associated Biochemical Findings

Defect	Biochemical Findings	Complementation Group (Gene)
Methylmalonic acidemia due to AdoCbl deficiency	Urine: Elevated methylmalonic acid, 3-hydroxypropionic acid, and methylcitrate	cblA (MMAA) cblB (*MMAB*)
	Plasma: Elevated methylmalonic acid, propionylcarnitine (C3)	cblD, variant 2 (*MMADHC*)
Homocystinuria due to MeCbl deficiency	Plasma: Elevated homocysteine, decreased methionine	cblC (MMACHC) cblD (MMADHC)
	Urine: Increased homocystine	cblF (LMBRD1) cblJ (ABCD4)
Combined methylmalonic acidemia and homocystinuria due to AdoCbl and MeCbl deficiency	Changes described above for AdoCbl and MeCbl deficiency	cblD, variant 1 (MMADHC) cblE (MTRR) cblG (MTR)

is more convenient in identifying specific cobalamin defects. Since *MMACHC* is the most common defect of cobalamin metabolism, comprising ~80% of the cases, it may be desirable to first sequence the *MMACHC* gene, although availability of multigene panel analysis tends to currently be superceding single-gene analysis.

16.7.1.1 Treatment

Treatment for cobalamin deficiency includes intramuscular or subcutaneous injections of hydroxycobalamin, oral betaine, and folate treatment in homocystinuria, and a low protein diet. Pyridoxine may also be used in homocystinuria to facilitate the conversion of homocysteine to cystathionine by cystathionine β-synthase. Levocarnitine is used in patients with methylmalonic aciduria as they can develop carnitine deficiency.

16.7.1.2 Confounding factors

Since in humans, animal products are the only source of vitamin B12, pure vegetarians are at the risk of development of vitamin B12 deficiency. Infants of mothers, who are breast-feeding and vitamin B12 deficient, are at risk for vitamin B12 deficiency. Vitamin B12 deficiency is common in patients with intestinal malabsorption, gastrectomy, and bariatric surgery. Nitrous oxide is known to activate vitamin B12 and may precipitate neurological symptoms.[145] Therefore, it is recommended that patients undergoing nitrous oxide anesthesia be checked for vitamin B12 deficiency. Many medications including phenytoin, metformin, and proton pump inhibitors are known to interfere with vitamin B12 absorption.

REFERENCES

1. Schnackenberg LK, Beger RD. Metabolomic biomarkers: their role in the critical path. *Drug Discov Today Technol* 2007;**4**(1):13–16.
2. Eggersdorfer M, Laudert D, Letinois U, et al. One hundred years of vitamins—a success story of the natural sciences. *Angew Chem Int Ed Engl* 2012;**51**(52):12960–90.
3. Brown G. Defects of thiamine transport and metabolism. *J Inherit Metab Dis* 2014;**37**(4):577–85.
4. Ganapathy V, Smith SB, Prasad PD. SLC19: the folate/thiamine transporter family. *Pflugers Arch* 2004;**447**(5):641–6.
5. Zhao R, Goldman ID. Folate and thiamine transporters mediated by facilitative carriers (SLC19A1-3 and SLC46A1) and folate receptors. *Mol Aspects Med* 2013;**34**(2–3):373–85.
6. Zhao R, Gao F, Goldman ID. Reduced folate carrier transports thiamine monophosphate: an alternative route for thiamine delivery into mammalian cells. *Am J Physiol Cell Physiol* 2002;**282**(6):C1512–7.
7. Lorber A, Gazit AZ, Khoury A, Schwartz Y, Mandel H. Cardiac manifestations in thiamine-responsive megaloblastic anemia syndrome. *Pediatr Cardiol* 2003;**24**(5):476–81.
8. Neufeld EJ, Fleming JC, Tartaglini E, Steinkamp MP. Thiamine-responsive megaloblastic anemia syndrome: a disorder of high-affinity thiamine transport. *Blood Cells Mol Dis* 2001;**27**(1):135–8.
9. Ricketts CJ, Minton JA, Samuel J, et al. Thiamine-responsive megaloblastic anaemia syndrome: long-term follow-up and mutation analysis of seven families. *Acta Paediatr* 2006;**95**(1):99–104.
10. Borgna-Pignatti C, Azzalli M, Pedretti S. Thiamine-responsive megaloblastic anemia syndrome: long term follow-up. *J Pediatr* 2009;**155**(2):295–7.
11. Alfadhel M, Almuntashri M, Jadah RH, et al. Biotin-responsive basal ganglia disease should be renamed biotin-thiamine-responsive basal ganglia disease: a retrospective review of the clinical, radiological and molecular findings of 18 new cases. *Orphanet J Rare Dis* 2013;**8**:83.
12. Debs R, Depienne C, Rastetter A, et al. Biotin-responsive basal ganglia disease in ethnic Europeans with novel SLC19A3 mutations. *Arch Neurol* 2010;**67**(1):126–30.
13. Kono S, Miyajima H, Yoshida K, Togawa A, Shirakawa K, Suzuki H. Mutations in a thiamine-transporter gene and Wernicke's-like encephalopathy. *N Engl J Med* 2009;**360**(17):1792–4.
14. Ozand PT, Gascon GG, Al Essa M, et al. Biotin-responsive basal ganglia disease: a novel entity. *Brain* 1998;**121**(Pt 7):1267–79.
15. Tabarki B, Al-Shafi S, Al-Shahwan S, et al. Biotin-responsive basal ganglia disease revisited: clinical, radiologic, and genetic findings. *Neurology* 2013;**80**(3):261–7.
16. Dakshinamurti K. Biotin—a regulator of gene expression. *J Nutr Biochem* 2005;**16**(7):419–23.
17. Ortigoza-Escobar JD, Serrano M, Molero M, et al. Thiamine transporter-2 deficiency: outcome and treatment monitoring. *Orphanet J Rare Dis* 2014;**9**:92.
18. Vlasova TI, Stratton SL, Wells AM, Mock NI, Mock DM. Biotin deficiency reduces expression of SLC19A3, a potential biotin transporter, in leukocytes from human blood. *J Nutr* 2005;**135**(1):42–7.

19. Gerards M, Kamps R, van Oevelen J, et al. Exome sequencing reveals a novel Moroccan founder mutation in SLC19A3 as a new cause of early-childhood fatal Leigh syndrome. *Brain* 2013;**136**(Pt 3):882–90.

20. Kevelam SH, Bugiani M, Salomons GS, et al. Exome sequencing reveals mutated SLC19A3 in patients with an early-infantile, lethal encephalopathy. *Brain* 2013;**136**(Pt 5): 1534–43.

21. Fassone E, Wedatilake Y, DeVile CJ, Chong WK, Carr LJ, Rahman S. Treatable Leigh-like encephalopathy presenting in adolescence. *BMJ Case Rep* 2013;**2013**:200838.

22. Banka S, de Goede C, Yue WW, et al. Expanding the clinical and molecular spectrum of thiamine pyrophosphokinase deficiency: a treatable neurological disorder caused by TPK1 mutations. *Mol Genet Metab* 2014;**113**(4):301–6.

23. Mayr JA, Freisinger P, Schlachter K, et al. Thiamine pyrophosphokinase deficiency in encephalopathic children with defects in the pyruvate oxidation pathway. *Am J Hum Genet* 2011;**89**(6):806–12.

24. Kelley RI, Robinson D, Puffenberger EG, Strauss KA, Morton DH. Amish lethal microcephaly: a new metabolic disorder with severe congenital microcephaly and 2-ketoglutaric aciduria. *Am J Med Genet* 2002;**112**(4):318–26.

25. Rosenberg MJ, Agarwala R, Bouffard G, et al. Mutant deoxynucleotide carrier is associated with congenital microcephaly. *Nat Genet* 2002;**32**(1):175–9.

26. Siu VM, Ratko S, Prasad AN, Prasad C, Rupar CA. Amish microcephaly: long-term survival and biochemical characterization. *Am J Med Genet A* 2010;**152A**(7):1747–51.

27. Spiegel R, Shaag A, Edvardson S, et al. SLC25A19 mutation as a cause of neuropathy and bilateral striatal necrosis. *Ann Neurol* 2009;**66**(3):419–24.

28. Gregersen N, Andresen BS, Pedersen CB, Olsen RK, Corydon TJ, Bross P. Mitochondrial fatty acid oxidation defects—remaining challenges. *J Inherit Metab Dis* 2008;**31**(5):643–57.

29. Hoey L, McNulty H, Strain JJ. Studies of biomarker responses to intervention with riboflavin: a systematic review. *Am J Clin Nutr* 2009;**89**(6):1960S–80S.

30. Liu D, Zempleni J. Low activity of LSD1 elicits a pro-inflammatory gene expression profile in riboflavin-deficient human T Lymphoma Jurkat cells. *Genes Nutr* 2014;**9**(5):422.

31. Mazur-Bialy AI, Buchala B, Plytycz B. Riboflavin deprivation inhibits macrophage viability and activity—a study on the RAW 264.7 cell line. *Br J Nutr* 2013;**110**(3):509–14.

32. Tu BP, Ho-Schleyer SC, Travers KJ, Weissman JS. Biochemical basis of oxidative protein folding in the endoplasmic reticulum. *Science* 2000;**290**(5496):1571–4.

33. Bosch AM, Abeling NG, Ijlst L, et al. Brown-Vialetto-Van Laere and Fazio Londe syndrome is associated with a riboflavin transporter defect mimicking mild MADD: a new inborn error of metabolism with potential treatment. *J Inherit Metab Dis* 2011;**34**(1):159–64.

34. Bosch AM, Stroek K, Abeling NG, Waterham HR, Ijlst L, Wanders RJ. The Brown-Vialetto-Van Laere and Fazio Londe syndrome revisited: natural history, genetics, treatment and future perspectives. *Orphanet J Rare Dis* 2012;**7**:83.

35. Manole A, Fratta P, Houlden H. Recent advances in bulbar syndromes: genetic causes and disease mechanisms. *Curr Opin Neurol* 2014;**27**(5):506–14.

36. Sathasivam S. Brown-Vialetto-Van Laere syndrome. *Orphanet J Rare Dis* 2008;**3**:9.

37. Sathasivam S, O'Sullivan S, Nicolson A, Tilley PJ, Shaw PJ. Brown-Vialetto-Van Laere syndrome: case report and literature review. *Amyotroph Lateral Scler Other Motor Neuron Disord* 2000;**1**(4):277–81.

38. Powers HJ. Riboflavin (vitamin B-2) and health. *Am J Clin Nutr* 2003;**77**(6):1352–60.

39. Yonezawa A, Inui K. Novel riboflavin transporter family RFVT/SLC52: identification, nomenclature, functional characterization and genetic diseases of RFVT/SLC52. *Mol Aspects Med* 2013;**34**(2-3):693–701.

40. Yao Y, Yonezawa A, Yoshimatsu H, Masuda S, Katsura T, Inui K. Identification and comparative functional characterization of a new human riboflavin transporter hRFT3 expressed in the brain. *J Nutr* 2010;**140**(7):1220–6.

41. Rhead WJ, Wolff JA, Lipson M, et al. Clinical and biochemical variation and family studies in the multiple acyl-CoA dehydrogenation disorders. *Pediatr Res* 1987;**21**(4):371–6.

42. Gallai V, Hockaday JM, Hughes JT, Lane DJ, Oppenheimer DR, Rushworth G. Ponto-bulbar palsy with deafness (Brown-Vialetto-Van Laere syndrome). *J Neurol Sci* 1981;**50**(2):259–75.

43. Foley AR, Menezes MP, Pandraud A, et al. Treatable childhood neuronopathy caused by mutations in riboflavin transporter RFVT2. *Brain 1* 2014;**137**(Pt 1):44–56.

44. Bonjour JP. Vitamins and alcoholism. V. Riboflavin, VI. Niacin, VII. Pantothenic acid, and VIII. Biotin. *Int J Vitam Nutr Res* 1980;**50**(4):425–40.

45. Fernandez-Banares F, Abad-Lacruz A, Xiol X, et al. Vitamin status in patients with inflammatory bowel disease. *Am J Gastroenterol* 1989;**84**(7):744–8.

46. Leshner RT. Riboflavin deficiency—a reversible neurodegenerative disease. *Ann Neurol* 1981;**10**:294–5.

47. Chiong MA, Sim KG, Carpenter K, et al. Transient multiple acyl-CoA dehydrogenation deficiency in a newborn female caused by maternal riboflavin deficiency. *Mol Genet Metab* 2007;**92**(1-2):109–14.

48. Ho G, Yonezawa A, Masuda S, et al. Maternal riboflavin deficiency, resulting in transient neonatal-onset glutaric aciduria Type 2, is caused by a microdeletion in the riboflavin transporter gene GPR172B. *Hum Mutat* 2011;**32**(1):E1976–84.

49. Lanska DJ. The discovery of niacin, biotin, and pantothenic acid. *Ann Nutr Metab* 2012;**61**(3):246–53.

50. Nozaki J, Dakeishi M, Ohura T, et al. Homozygosity mapping to chromosome 5p15 of a gene responsible for Hartnup disorder. *Biochem Biophys Res Commun* 2001;**284**(2):255–60.

51. Kleta R, Romeo E, Ristic Z, et al. Mutations in SLC6A19, encoding B0AT1, cause Hartnup disorder. *Nat Genet* 2004;**36**(9):999–1002.

52. Seow HF, Broer S, Broer A, et al. Hartnup disorder is caused by mutations in the gene encoding the neutral amino acid transporter SLC6A19. *Nat Genet* 2004;**36**(9):1003–7.

53. Scriver CR, Mahon B, Levy HL, et al. The Hartnup phenotype: Mendelian transport disorder, multifactorial disease. *Am J Hum Genet* 1987;**40**(5):401–12.

54. Broer S. The role of the neutral amino acid transporter B0AT1 (SLC6A19) in Hartnup disorder and protein nutrition. *IUBMB Life* 2009;**61**(6):591–9.

55. Broer S, Cavanaugh JA, Rasko JE. Neutral amino acid transport in epithelial cells and its malfunction in Hartnup disorder. *Biochem Soc Trans* 2005;**33**(Pt 1):233–6.

56. Combs GF, Combs GF. *The vitamins*, 4th ed. Amsterdam; Boston: Elsevier Academic Press; 2012.

57. Bean WB, Hodges RE, Daum K. Pantothenic acid deficiency induced in human subjects. *J Clin Invest* 1955;**34**(7, Part 1):1073–84.

58. Hodges RE, Bean WB, Ohlson MA, Bleiler R. Human pantothenic acid deficiency produced by omega-methyl pantothenic acid. *J Clin Invest* 1959;**38**(8):1421–5.

59. Hodges RE, Ohlson MA, Bean WB. Pantothenic acid deficiency in man. *J Clin Invest* 1958;**37**(11):1642–57.

60. Uchida Y, Ito K, Ohtsuki S, Kubo Y, Suzuki T, Terasaki T. Major involvement of Na-dependent multivitamin transporter (SLC5A6/SMVT) in uptake of biotin and pantothenic acid by human brain capillary endothelial cells. *J Neurochem* 2015;**134**(1):97–112.

61. Vadlapudi AD, Vadlapatla RK, Mitra AK. Sodium dependent multivitamin transporter (SMVT): a potential target for drug delivery. *Curr Drug Targets* 2012;**13**(7):994–1003.

62. Ghosal A, Lambrecht N, Subramanya SB, Kapadia R, Said HM. Conditional knockout of the Slc5a6 gene in mouse intestine impairs biotin absorption. *Am J Physiol Gastrointest Liver Physiol* 2013;**304**(1):G64–71.

63. Noda S, Umezaki H, Yamamoto K, Araki T, Murakami T, Ishii N. Reye-like syndrome following treatment with the pantothenic acid antagonist, calcium hopantenate. *J Neurol Neurosurg Psychiatry* 1988;**51**(4):582–5.

64. Pugliese A, Beltramo T, Torre D. Reye's and Reye's-like syndromes. *Cell Biochem Funct* 2008;**26**(7):741–6.

65. Zhou B, Westaway SK, Levinson B, Johnson MA, Gitschier J, Hayflick SJ. A novel pantothenate kinase gene (PANK2) is defective in Hallervorden-Spatz syndrome. *Nat Genet* 2001;**28**(4):345–9.

66. Hayflick SJ. Defective pantothenate metabolism and neurodegeneration. *Biochem Soc Trans* 2014;**42**(4):1063–8.

67. Johnson MA, Kuo YM, Westaway SK, et al. Mitochondrial localization of human PANK2 and hypotheses of secondary iron accumulation in pantothenate kinase-associated neurodegeneration. *Ann N Y Acad Sci* 2004;**1012**:282–98.

68. Hayflick SJ, Westaway SK, Levinson B, et al. Genetic, clinical, and radiographic delineation of Hallervorden-Spatz syndrome. *N Engl J Med* 2003;**348**(1):33–40.

69. Hogarth P. Neurodegeneration with brain iron accumulation: diagnosis and management. *J Mov Disord* 2015;**8**(1):1–13.

70. Sauberlich HE. *Laboratory tests for the assessment of nutritional status*, 2nd ed. Boca Raton: CRC Press; 1999.

71. Dusi S, Valletta L, Haack TB, et al. Exome sequence reveals mutations in CoA synthase as a cause of neurodegeneration with brain iron accumulation. *Am J Hum Genet* 2014;**94**(1):11–22.

72. Rosenberg IH. A history of the isolation and identification of vitamin B(6). *Ann Nutr Metab* 2012;**61**(3):236–8.

73. Cellini B, Montioli R, Oppici E, Astegno A, Voltattorni CB. The chaperone role of the pyridoxal 5′-phosphate and its implications for rare diseases involving B6-dependent enzymes. *Clin Biochem* 2014;**47**(3):158–65.

74. Clayton PT. B6-responsive disorders: a model of vitamin dependency. *J Inherit Metab Dis* 2006;**29**(2-3):317–26.

75. Albersen M, Bosma M, Knoers NV, et al. The intestine plays a substantial role in human vitamin B6 metabolism: a Caco-2 cell model. *PLoS One* 2013;**8**(1):e54113.

76. Farrant RD, Walker V, Mills GA, Mellor JM, Langley GJ. Pyridoxal phosphate de-activation by pyrroline-5-carboxylic acid. Increased risk of vitamin B6 deficiency and seizures in hyperprolinemia type II. *J Biol Chem* 2001;**276**(18):15107–16.

77. Mills PB, Struys E, Jakobs C, et al. Mutations in antiquitin in individuals with pyridoxine-dependent seizures. *Nat Med* 2006;**12**(3):307–9.

78. Brautigam C, Hyland K, Wevers R, et al. Clinical and laboratory findings in twins with neonatal epileptic encephalopathy mimicking aromatic L-amino acid decarboxylase deficiency. *Neuropediatrics* 2002;**33**(3):113–7.
79. Mills PB, Surtees RA, Champion MP, et al. Neonatal epileptic encephalopathy caused by mutations in the PNPO gene encoding pyridox(am)ine 5′-phosphate oxidase. *Hum Mol Genet* 2005;**14**(8):1077–86.
80. Whyte MP, Mahuren JD, Fedde KN, Cole FS, McCabe ER, Coburn SP. Perinatal hypophosphatasia: tissue levels of vitamin B6 are unremarkable despite markedly increased circulating concentrations of pyridoxal-5′-phosphate. Evidence for an ectoenzyme role for tissue-nonspecific alkaline phosphatase. *J Clin Invest* 1988;**81**(4):1234–9.
81. Whyte MP, Mahuren JD, Vrabel LA, Coburn SP. Markedly increased circulating pyridoxal-5′-phosphate levels in hypophosphatasia. Alkaline phosphatase acts in vitamin B6 metabolism. *J Clin Invest* 1985;**76**(2):752–6.
82. Footitt EJ, Clayton PT, Mills K, et al. Measurement of plasma B6 vitamer profiles in children with inborn errors of vitamin B6 metabolism using an LC-MS/MS method. *J Inherit Metab Dis* 2013;**36**(1):139–45.
83. Rathbun JC. Hypophosphatasia; a new developmental anomaly. *Am J Dis Child* 1948;**75**(6):822–31.
84. Whyte MP. Hypophosphatasia. In: Thakker RV, Whyte MP, Eisman J, Igarashi T, editors. *Genetics of bone biology and skeletal disease*. London: Academic Press; 2013: 337–360.
85. Whyte MP. Physiological role of alkaline phosphatase explored in hypophosphatasia. *Ann N Y Acad Sci* 2010;**1192**:190–200.
86. Greenberg CR, Evans JA, McKendry-Smith S, et al. Infantile hypophosphatasia: localization within chromosome region 1p36.1-34 and prenatal diagnosis using linked DNA markers. *Am J Hum Genet* 1990;**46**(2):286–92.
87. Harris H. The human alkaline phosphatases: what we know and what we don't know. *Clin Chim Acta* 1990;**186**(2):133–50.
88. Negyessy L, Xiao J, Kantor O, et al. Layer-specific activity of tissue non-specific alkaline phosphatase in the human neocortex. *Neuroscience* 2011;**172**:406–18.
89. Pearl PL, Gibson KM. Clinical aspects of the disorders of GABA metabolism in children. *Curr Opin Neurol* 2004;**17**(2):107–13.
90. Plecko B. Pyridoxine and pyridoxalphosphate-dependent epilepsies. *Handb Clin Neurol* 2013;**113**:1811–7.
91. Belachew D, Kazmerski T, Libman I, et al. Infantile hypophosphatasia secondary to a novel compound heterozygous mutation presenting with pyridoxine-responsive seizures. *JIMD Rep* 2013;**11**:17–24.
92. Alexion Pharmaceuticals I. FDA grants breakthrough therapy designation to asfotase alfa for perinatal-, infantile- and juvenile-onset hypophosphatasia (HPP). 05/28/2103 ed, 2013.
93. Patel M, First-in-class enzyme replacement therapy for hypophosphatasia under review, MPR March 02, 2015 http://www.empr.com/drugs-in-the-pipeline/first-in-class-enzyme-replacement-therapy-for-hypophosphatasia-under-review/article/400861/.
94. Zempleni J. Uptake, localization, and noncarboxylase roles of biotin. *Annu Rev Nutr* 2005;**25**:175–96.
95. Zempleni J, Hassan YI, Wijeratne SS. Biotin and biotinidase deficiency. *Expert Rev Endocrinol Metab* 2008;**3**(6):715–24.

96. Boas MA. The effect of desiccation upon the nutritive properties of egg-white. *Biochem J* 1927;**21**(3):712–24.

97. Gyorgy P, Melville DB, Burk D, Duv V. The possible identity of vitamin H with biotin and coenzyme R. *Science* 1940;**91**(2358):243–5.

98. Gyorgy P, Rose CS. Cure of egg-white injury in rats by the "toxic" fraction (avidin) of egg white given parenterally. *Science* 1941;**94**(2437):261–2.

99. Gyorgy P, Rose CS, Eakin RE, Snell EE, Williams RJ. Egg-white injury as the result of nonabsorption or inactivation of biotin. *Science* 1941;**93**(2420):477–8.

100. Sydenstricker VP, Singal SA, Briggs AP, Devaughn NM, Isbell H. Preliminary observations on "egg white injury" in man and its cure with a biotin concentrate. *Science* 1942;**95**(2459):176–7.

101. DU Vigneaud V, Melville DB, György P, Rose CS. On the identity of vitamin H with biotin. *Science* 1940;**92**(2377):62–3.

102. Zempleni J, Wijeratne SS, Hassan YI. Biotin. *Biofactors* 2009;**35**(1):36–46.

103. Prasad PD, Wang H, Kekuda R, et al. Cloning and functional expression of a cDNA encoding a mammalian sodium-dependent vitamin transporter mediating the uptake of pantothenate, biotin, and lipoate. *J Biol Chem* 1998;**273**(13):7501–6.

104. Said HM. Recent advances in carrier-mediated intestinal absorption of water-soluble vitamins. *Annu Rev Physiol* 2004;**66**:419–46.

105. Kohrogi K, Imagawa E, Muto Y, et al. Biotin-responsive basal ganglia disease: a case diagnosed by whole exome sequencing. *J Hum Genet* 2015;**60**(7):381–5.

106. Wolf B. Clinical issues and frequent questions about biotinidase deficiency. *Mol Genet Metab* 2010;**100**(1):6–13.

107. Wolf B. The neurology of biotinidase deficiency. *Mol Genet Metab* 2011;**104**(1–2):27–34.

108. Zempleni J, Mock DM. Biotin biochemistry and human requirements. *J Nutr Biochem* 1999;**10**(3):128–38.

109. Tsao CY, Kien CL. Complete biotinidase deficiency presenting as reversible progressive ataxia and sensorineural deafness. *J Child Neurol* 2002;**17**(2):146.

110. Wolf B, Spencer R, Gleason T. Hearing loss is a common feature of symptomatic children with profound biotinidase deficiency. *J Pediatr* 2002;**140**(2):242–6.

111. McVoy JR, Levy HL, Lawler M, et al. Partial biotinidase deficiency: clinical and biochemical features. *J Pediatr* 1990;**116**(1):78–83.

112. Wolf B, Grier RE, Allen RJ, Goodman SI, Kien CL. Biotinidase deficiency: the enzymatic defect in late-onset multiple carboxylase deficiency. *Clin Chim Acta* 1983;**131**(3):273–81.

113. Wolf B, Norrgard K, Pomponio RJ, et al. Profound biotinidase deficiency in two asymptomatic adults. *Am J Med Genet* 1997;**73**(1):5–9.

114. Wolf B, Pomponio RJ, Norrgard KJ, et al. Delayed-onset profound biotinidase deficiency. *J Pediatr* 1998;**132**(2):362–5.

115. Zempleni J, Chew YC, Hassan YI, Wijeratne SS. Epigenetic regulation of chromatin structure and gene function by biotin: are biotin requirements being met? *Nutr Rev* 2008;**66**(Suppl 1):S46–8.

116. Hassan YI, Zempleni J. Epigenetic regulation of chromatin structure and gene function by biotin. *J Nutr* 2006;**136**(7):1763–5.

117. Advisory Committee on Heritable Disorders in Newborns and Children, Services UDoHaH. Recommended Uniform Screening Panel.

118. Broda E, Baumgartner ER, Scholl S, Stopsack M, Horn A, Rhode H. Biotinidase determination in serum and dried blood spots—high sensitivity fluorimetric ultramicroassay. *Clin Chim Acta* 2001;**314**(1–2):175–85.

119. Heard GS, Secor McVoy JR, Wolf B. A screening method for biotinidase deficiency in newborns. *Clin Chem* 1984;**30**(1):125–7.

120. Pettit DA, Amador PS, Wolf B. The quantitation of biotinidase activity in dried blood spots using microtiter transfer plates: identification of biotinidase-deficient and heterozygous individuals. *Anal Biochem* 1989;**179**(2):371–4.

121. Swick HM, Kien CL. Biotin deficiency with neurologic and cutaneous manifestations but without organic aciduria. *J Pediatr* 1983;**103**(2):265–7.

122. Wolf B, Grier RE, Allen RJ, et al. Phenotypic variation in biotinidase deficiency. *J Pediatr* 1983;**103**(2):233–7.

123. Cowan TM, Blitzer MG, Wolf B. Working Group of the American College of Medical Genetics Laboratory Quality Assurance C. Technical standards and guidelines for the diagnosis of biotinidase deficiency. *Genet Med* 2010;**12**(7):464–70.

124. Wolf B. Children with profound biotinidase deficiency should be treated with biotin regardless of their residual enzyme activity or genotype. *Eur J Pediatr* 2002;**161**(3):167–8. author reply 169.

125. Pomponio RJ, Hymes J, Reynolds TR, et al. Mutations in the human biotinidase gene that cause profound biotinidase deficiency in symptomatic children: molecular, biochemical, and clinical analysis. *Pediatr Res* 1997;**42**(6):840–8.

126. Pomponio RJ, Reynolds TR, Cole H, Buck GA, Wolf B. Mutational hotspot in the human biotinidase gene causes profound biotinidase deficiency. *Nat Genet* 1995;**11**(1):96–8.

127. Wolf B, Jensen K, Huner G, et al. Seventeen novel mutations that cause profound biotinidase deficiency. *Mol Genet Metab* 2002;**77**(1-2):108–11.

128. Mardach R, Zempleni J, Wolf B, et al. Biotin dependency due to a defect in biotin transport. *J Clin Invest* 2002;**109**(12):1617–23.

129. Yang X, Aoki Y, Li X, et al. Structure of human holocarboxylase synthetase gene and mutation spectrum of holocarboxylase synthetase deficiency. *Hum Genet* 2001;**109**(5):526–34.

130. Burri BJ, Sweetman L, Nyhan WL. Heterogeneity of holocarboxylase synthetase in patients with biotin-responsive multiple carboxylase deficiency. *Am J Hum Genet* 1985;**37**(2):326–37.

131. Sakamoto O, Suzuki Y, Li X, et al. Relationship between kinetic properties of mutant enzyme and biochemical and clinical responsiveness to biotin in holocarboxylase synthetase deficiency. *Pediatr Res* 1999;**46**(6):671–6.

132. Narisawa K, Arai N, Igarashi Y, Satoh T, Tada K, Hirooka Y. Clinical and biochemical findings on a child with multiple biotin-responsive carboxylase deficiencies. *J Inherit Metab Dis* 1982;**5**(2):67–8.

133. Suormala T, Fowler B, Jakobs C, et al. Late-onset holocarboxylase synthetase-deficiency: pre- and post-natal diagnosis and evaluation of effectiveness of antenatal biotin therapy. *Eur J Pediatr* 1998;**157**(7):570–5.

134. Baumgartner ER, Suormala T. Multiple carboxylase deficiency: inherited and acquired disorders of biotin metabolism. *Int J Vitam Nutr Res* 1997;**67**(5):377–84.

135. Suzuki Y, Yang X, Aoki Y, Kure S, Matsubara Y. Mutations in the holocarboxylase synthetase gene HLCS. *Hum Mutat* 2005;**26**(4):285–90.

136. Santer R, Muhle H, Suormala T, et al. Partial response to biotin therapy in a patient with holocarboxylase synthetase deficiency: clinical, biochemical, and molecular genetic aspects. *Mol Genet Metab* 2003;**79**(3):160–6.

137. Suormala T, Fowler B, Duran M, et al. Five patients with a biotin-responsive defect in holocarboxylase formation: evaluation of responsiveness to biotin therapy in vivo and comparative biochemical studies in vitro. *Pediatr Res* 1997;**41**(5):666–73.

138. Van Hove JL, Josefsberg S, Freehauf C, et al. Management of a patient with holocarboxylase synthetase deficiency. *Mol Genet Metab* 2008;**95**(4):201–5.

139. Morrone A, Malvagia S, Donati MA, et al. Clinical findings and biochemical and molecular analysis of four patients with holocarboxylase synthetase deficiency. *Am J Med Genet* 2002;**111**(1):10–18.

140. Zeng WQ, Al-Yamani E, Acierno Jr. JS, et al. Biotin-responsive basal ganglia disease maps to 2q36.3 and is due to mutations in SLC19A3. *Am J Hum Genet* 2005;**77**(1):16–26.

141. Carrillo-Carrasco N, Adams D, Venditti CP. Disorders of intracellular cobalamin metabolism. http://www.ncbi.nlm.nih.gov/books/NBK1328/, 2013.

142. Carrillo-Carrasco N, Chandler RJ, Venditti CP. Combined methylmalonic acidemia and homocystinuria, cblC type. I. Clinical presentations, diagnosis and management. *J Inherit Metab Dis* 2012;**35**(1):91–102.

143. Froese DS, Gravel RA. Genetic disorders of vitamin B(12) metabolism: eight complementation groups—eight genes. *Expert Rev Mol Med* 2010;**12**:e37.

144. Froese DS, Gravel RA. Genetic disorders of vitamin B12 metabolism: eight complementation groups—eight genes. *Expert Rev Mol Med* 2010;**12**(e37):1–20.

145. Abels J, Kroes AC, Ermens AA, et al. Anti-leukemic potential of methyl-cobalamin inactivation by nitrous oxide. *Am J Hematol* 1990;**34**(2):128–31.

Disorders of trace metals 17

L.D. Smith[1] and U. Garg[2,3]
[1]*University of North Carolina School of Medicine, Chapel Hill, NC, United States;*
[2]*Children's Mercy Hospitals and Clinics, Kansas City, MO, United States;*
[3]*University of Missouri School of Medicine, Kansas City, MO, United States*

17.1 INTRODUCTION

Trace metals are inorganic micronutrients that are present in very low concentrations in body fluids and tissues. Their dietary requirements are in μg to mg/day. They are required for the proper functioning of many enzymes and other proteins. Their deficiency can lead to specific signs and symptoms. Sometimes the deficiency is not dietary but due to transport or recycling defects.[1] In humans, metals are obtained exogenously and require intestinal absorption and transport to the appropriate intracellular compartment for function. Various intestinal sites for metal absorption are shown in Fig. 17.1. In this chapter, metabolic disorders of several trace metals are discussed.

17.2 ZINC

Zinc is second to iron as the most abundant trace metal. It is ubiquitous, found in all tissue types and fluids, as well as being the most abundant intracellular trace element. It is an important metal cofactor, essential for the functioning of over 300 enzymes that are involved in major metabolic pathways. In addition, it participates and regulates nucleic acid and protein synthesis, and is required for the functioning of at least 3000 transcription factors.[2] A summary of zinc metabolism is given in Fig. 17.2. Elevated zinc levels are generally of little clinical consequence, although zinc and copper levels tend to be inversely related and hence high zinc levels can result in low copper levels and vice versa.[3] Copper, on the other hand, plays a critical role in physiologic redox chemistry[4] and both deficiency and excess have pathogenic consequences. Both copper and zinc affect cellular iron levels as well. Copper will be discussed in a following section.

Zinc performs many roles in the physiology of the human body including catalytic, regulatory, and structural roles. Since Zn is required for anabolic processes, zinc deficiency has a significant effect on growth, tissue integrity, and wound

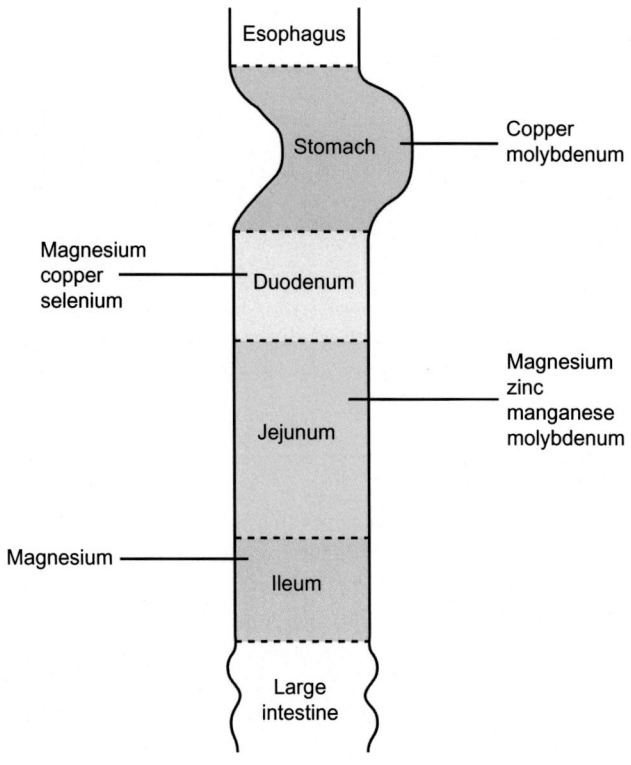

FIGURE 17.1

Various intestinal sites for metal absorption.

healing. In plasma, zinc is bound to albumin and α-2-macroglobulin. Although there is no dedicated zinc store in the body, about 10% of intracellular zinc in the liver as well as some other tissues is available as a functional pool that exchanges with the plasma pool,[5] and is important in maintaining the plasma concentration that undergoes a rapid turnover. Homeostasis is maintained via interactions between the SLC30 (ZnT) family of transporters and the SLC30 (ZIP) family of transporters. The former promote zinc efflux from cells, decreasing intracellular zinc concentrations, while the latter promote zinc influx, resulting in increased intracellular zinc concentrations. Absorption of dietary zinc occurs in the duodenum and proximal jejunum and is facilitated by the *SLC39A4-* (ZIP4) encoded zinc transporter. Absorption can be inhibited by iron as well as by fiber and phytate, which explains why the bioavailable fraction is lower in vegetarian diets that are rich in phytate. Therefore vegetarians need 50% more zinc than nonvegetarians. In the United States, Daily Reference Intake for zinc is 11 mg/day for men and 8 mg/day for women. Increased amounts are required during pregnancy and lactation. Citric acid can enhance zinc absorption. Homeostasis is maintained by intestinal absorption, gastrointestinal (GI) excretion,

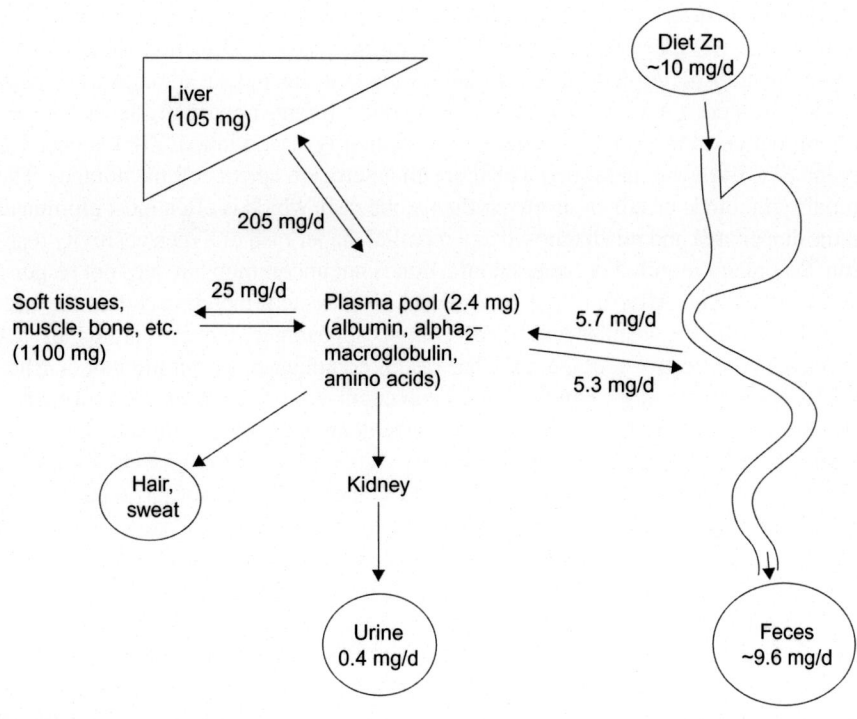

FIGURE 17.2

Summary of zinc metabolism.

Adapted from, Shenkin A, Roberts NB. Vitamins and trace metals. In: Burtis CA, Ashwood ER, Bruns DE, eds.
Tietz's textbook of clinical chemistry and molecular diagnostics. 5th ed. St. Louis, Missouri: Elsevier,
2012: 895–983.

urine excretion, and cellular retention.[6] If dietary zinc is low or there is poor absorption, excretion is diminished and circulating insulin-like growth factor-I (IGF-I) is diminished, with resultant reduction in growth. If zinc is present in excess, chelation by metallothionein occurs. In general, zinc excess has minimal medical consequences while deficiency is quite detrimental.

Zinc deficiency can result from inadequate intake, poor absorption, increased loss, or increased demand. The presenting symptoms of zinc deficiency are most obvious in the integumentary (severe acral and perioral dermatitis, alopecia, abnormal nails, nonhealing ulcers, delayed wound healing), gastrointestinal (diarrhea), immune (recurrent infections) and skeletal systems (poor growth) but can involve the central nervous system (CNS; impaired cognitive function, altered sense of smell and taste, depression), the visual system (night blindness, photophobia, blepharitis, conjunctivitis), the reproductive system (decreased testosterone levels and fertility) and fetal growth and development, if deficiency is present during pregnancy.

The inborn errors that result in zinc deficiency involve decreased function of zinc transporters. *Acrodermatitis enteropathica* results from dysfunction of ZIP4, the major zinc transporter in the intestine and insufficient zinc uptake since, as mentioned previously, there are no real zinc stores in the body. Infants are usually asymptomatic at birth but develop symptoms after breast feeding is discontinued. ZIP4 is encoded by the *SLC39A* gene and forms a channel on enterocyte apical cell membranes. The initial symptom is usually a severe erythematous rash, which is often most prominent in the diaper area and misdiagnosed as a monilial diaper rash or hypersensitivity reaction. Secondary monilial or bacterial infection is not uncommon but does not respond well to treatment. After the first year of life, if untreated, the character of the rash changes to a more pustular and hyperkeratotic appearance. Corticosteroids are not effective in the treatment of the rash. The rash is complicated by intermittent diarrhea and failure to thrive, if the condition goes unrecognized. Infection can be a severe and life-threatening consequence of prolonged zinc deficiency. Zinc deficiency in breast-fed babies can also present with a picture very similar to acrodermatitis enteropathica. This is commonly seen in premature infants as the premature gut has reduced zinc uptake capacity and the infant has increased zinc needs.[7] In other cases, this results not from an inability of the gut to absorb zinc, but rather from reduced zinc levels in breast milk secondary to heterozygous variants in the *SLC30A2* gene.[8]

While generally considered to be a benign condition, elevated plasma zinc levels with genetic inheritance have been described. The first, autosomal dominant hyperzincemia without symptoms has been described in one family and appears to be benign.[9] It is hypothesized that this condition is the result of increased binding of zinc to an altered albumin molecule. The second, hyperzincemia with hypercalprotectinemia[10,11] results in extremely high plasma zinc levels but relative zinc deficiency with concomitant persistently elevated C-reactive protein, anemia, arthritis, hepatosplenomegaly, and recurrent infections. The pathophysiology of this disorder is thought to be related to very high concentrations of calprotectin, the major zinc binding protein of phagocytic cells, and that these high levels lead to overly robust and harmful inflammation along with decreased bioavailability of zinc.[12] No gene has been identified to date as causative.

17.2.1 DIAGNOSTIC TESTS

Various laboratory tests are used for assessing zinc status. Plasma or serum levels are most commonly used for the assessment of zinc deficiency. However, it is important to keep in mind that plasma levels are insensitive to dietary zinc intake and may not correlate well with the clinical picture. Clinical responses to zinc supplementation should be used to corroborate zinc deficiency. Also it is important to measure albumin levels concomitantly since zinc levels can vary significantly with change in albumin levels. Samples for zinc should be collected in special metal-free certified tubes. The approximate reference range for plasma zinc is 60–120 µg/dL. Other assays that have been used for assessing zinc status include whole blood zinc levels, hair zinc levels, zinc-dependent enzymes, metallothionein, and urine zinc. Value of these tests is not well established.[13]

While serum zinc levels are usually low in acrodermatitis enteropathica, normal values can be seen.[14] Furthermore, the above-mentioned conditions can also result in clinical zinc deficiency; hence, zinc level alone is not diagnostic, nor is the accuracy of diagnosis improved by measuring zinc levels in other tissues (i.e., hair). Useful ancillary tests include urinary zinc excretion, low serum alkaline phosphatase activity, changes in the serum fatty acid profile, low beta-lipoprotein levels, and reduced levels of serum vitamin A. Again, these are not diagnostic tests, rather tests that confirm zinc deficiency. Small bowel biopsy is also not diagnostic, demonstrating villous atrophy and Paneth cell inclusions, which can be seen in other disorders. Testing of zinc transport is not really practical. A trial of zinc therapy with improvement while on therapy and relapse when zinc is discontinued is highly suggestive of a transporter defect rather than dietary deficiency. Identification of pathogenic variants in the *SLC39A4* gene is diagnostic.

17.2.2 TREATMENT

For infants with zinc deficiency associated with breastfeeding, dietary supplementation will result in rapid improvement and the condition resolves when breast feeding is discontinued or the diet is advanced.

17.2.3 CONFOUNDING CONDITIONS

Other conditions that can result in zinc deficiency can be classified as conditions of inadequate intake (Crohn's disease, jejunoileal bypass, bariatric surgery, small bowel resection, alcoholic pancreatitis, cystic fibrosis), reduced absorption (low dietary zinc, diets rich in phytate, sodium polyphosphate, ethylenediamine tetraacetic acid (EDTA)), increased loss (inflammatory bowel disease (IBD), diarrhea, steatorrhea, burns, trauma, sepsis, hemofiltration), and increased demand (systemic illness). A significant number of patients with sickle cell anemia have clinical signs and symptoms of zinc deficiency. These patients respond well to zinc treatment. Zinc deficiency also occurs in burn patients from losing zinc in the exudates from the burn sites. Of particular note, several medications commonly used in different medical practices can result in increased systemic loss of zinc, including thiazide diuretics, penicillamine, valproic acid, angiotensin-converting enzyme (ACE) inhibitors, EDTA-containing propofol, and cisplatin. Excessive dietary supplementation of cysteine and N-acetylcysteine can also result in increased losses. The role of elevated homocysteine levels in zinc deficiency has not been adequately studied and remains unclear.[15]

17.3 COPPER

As with zinc, copper is also an essential metal required for growth and development. It is associated with a number of metalloproteins and is required by all tissues for proper cellular metabolic function. Control of its levels is critical to avoid deficiency or excess, both of which are detrimental. Copper can adopt both an oxidized

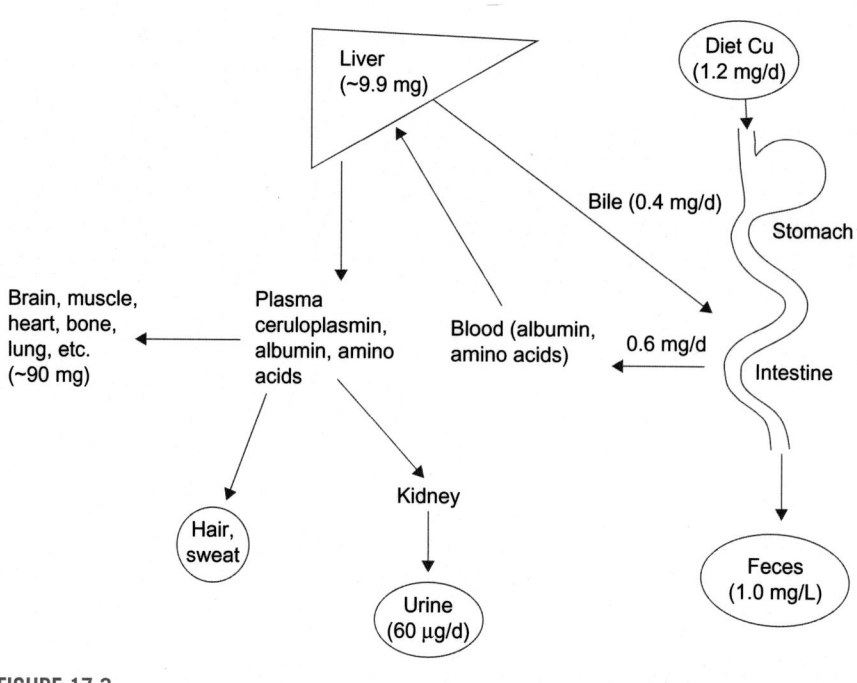

FIGURE 17.3

Summary of copper metabolism.

Adapted from, Shenkin A, Roberts NB. Vitamins and trace metals. In: Burtis CA, Ashwood ER, Bruns DE, eds. Tietz's textbook of clinical chemistry and molecular diagnostics. 5th ed. St. Louis, Missouri: Elsevier, 2012: 895–983.

(Cu^{2+}) and reduced (Cu^+) configuration and hence, is a catalytic cofactor in oxidation–reduction reactions and is vital for proper functioning of enzymatic pathways involved in energy production and antioxidant activity. A summary of copper metabolism is given in Fig. 17.3.

The median copper intake in the United States is approximately 1.0–1.6 mg/day. The majority of dietary copper absorption takes place in the duodenum via the high affinity transporter, hCTR1 (human copper transport protein 1), in the basolateral membrane of the intestinal epithelial cell.[16–18] Transport is regulated by the intracellular C-terminal domains of the homotrimer while actual transport is mediated by the extracellular and transmembrane domains.[16] It is postulated that CTR1 is needed for the release of dietary copper from subapical vesicles for delivery to copper chaperone proteins, mitochondrial cytochrome C oxidase, and Cu-ATPases. Reductases in the apical membrane are necessary for the reduction of Cu^{2+} to Cu^+, the ion that is recognized by the transporter. Divalent metal transporter I[19,20] and endocytic/pinocytic processes are postulated to be involved in the transport across the apical membrane. A low-affinity transporter, CTR2, has also been identified, the exact function of which, has not been elucidated but likely facilitates movement of copper across the apical (luminal) membrane.[21] Cu-ATPase ATP7A is then responsible for the transport of copper into intracellular vesicles and secretion of copper across the basolateral membrane into the bloodstream.[21] Copper is then transported in the blood bound to albumin, ceruloplasmin, transcuprein, and low molecular weight copper–histidine complexes for delivery to tissues. It is readily taken up by hepatocytes via hCTR1. After uptake, it is stored via chelation by metallothionein, is bound to chaperone proteins for intracellular trafficking to copper-requiring enzymes or is bound to reduce glutathione. ATP7B is necessary for the efflux of excess copper, particularly in the liver. It is also postulated to result in copper sequestration and storage in other tissues, such as in the kidney and intestine.[21] Both ATP7A and ATP7B are localized perinuclearly and thought to be targeted to the trans-Golgi network under basal conditions. They both receive copper, which binds to an N-terminal metal binding site, from a chaperone protein, Atox1. Precise control of copper homeostasis is necessary and disruption thereof results in disease. Two pools of circulating copper exist. The first pool is copper that is tightly bound to ceruloplasmin, which includes about 85–90% of circulating copper and is thus not freely available to cells and tissues. The remaining 10–15% of circulating copper is less tightly bound to albumin and other small molecules in the blood and is more freely available to cells.[22]

Copper deficiency can affect the hematologic, immunologic, neurologic, skeletal, and vascular systems. It is an under-recognized cause of hematologic and neurologic system dysfunction.[23] Furthermore, copper deficiency has been shown to result in impaired myocardial contractility, cardiac conduction defects, and neurobehavioral symptoms.[4] Excessive copper results in two distinct inborn errors of copper metabolism: Menkes disease and Wilson disease, both caused by abnormalities in specific copper transporters.

Other inherited inborn errors of copper metabolism include occipital horn syndrome and distal hereditary motor neuropathy. Another disorder, aceruloplasminemia does result in low serum copper levels as it is the major copper-carrying protein in the blood but is technically a defect in iron transport and processing that results in low serum iron levels and tissue iron deposition.

17.3.1 WILSON DISEASE

This rare autosomal recessive disorder results from homozygosity or compound heterozygosity for mutations in *ATP7B*. It occurs in about 1 in 30,000 births. First described in 1912, the presenting symptoms include nonspecific liver disease, neurologic symptoms, psychiatric illness, hemolytic anemia, skeletal anomalies, and renal Fanconi syndrome.[24] Neurologic and psychiatric presentation tends to occur sometime between the first and fifth decade of life and almost invariably has the hallmark finding of Kayser–Fleisher rings. Other eye findings include "sunflower" cataracts due to copper accumulation in the lens. Liver disease tends to be a presenting symptom in individuals less than 30 years of age, although some degree of liver dysfunction is present in all affected individuals. Transporter dysfunction leads to copper accumulation in the liver and brain. As noted above, ATP7B functions primarily in the excretion of hepatic copper into bile.[25] In addition to liver dysfunction (jaundice, hepatomegaly, edema, ascites), secondary endocrine effects can be seen, including delayed puberty or amenorrhea. Affected individuals may have electrolyte abnormalities due to urinary losses of amino acids, calcium, phosphate, glucose, and other electrolytes, which can manifest as osteoarthritis, osteoporosis, or rickets. Rapid hemolytic anemia with consequent severe effects has been observed.

Other conditions can be confused with Wilson disease. The liver dysfunction may be attributed to autoimmune chronic active hepatitis, viral hepatitis, cirrhosis, hereditary hemochromatosis, hepatocellular adenoma, or α1-antitrypsin deficiency. Neurologic symptoms may be attributed to CNS pathology (multiple sclerosis, Huntington disease, Parkinson disease, Leigh disease, leukodystrophy, or other neurodegenerative disorders), aceruloplasminemia, psychiatric illness (depression, anxiety, schizophrenia, bipolar disorder, antisocial personality disorder), or CNS vasculitis. The psychiatric manifestations can be confused with either overt psychiatric illness or drug abuse. Anemia may be erroneously attributed to other etiologies of chronic anemia and arthritis may be attributed to other rheumatologic conditions.

17.3.1.1 Diagnostic tests

Most commonly used tests are plasma copper and ceruloplasmin. In Wilson's disease both plasma copper and ceruloplasmin levels are low. The approximate reference range for plasma copper is 70–140 µg/dL. Other laboratory findings include abnormally elevated hepatic transaminases, hemolytic anemia, plasma electrolyte abnormalities, and abnormally increased urinary amino acid levels. Although serum copper levels are low, the pool of free copper is actually expanded in untreated patients with Wilson disease and copper toxicity.[22] Increased urinary excretion of copper (>100 µg/24 hours) is diagnostic as is a positive penicillamine challenge. The latter includes a pretreatment of 24-hour urine collection, followed by oral administration of 500 mg of penicillamine at the start of and 12 hours into a second 24-hour urine collection. Increased copper excretion in the second sample is suggestive of the diagnosis. Hepatic copper levels of >200 µg/gram of dry weight, measured by atomic absorption spectrometry, are characteristic of the condition with the normal level ranging from 20 to 50 µg/gram of dry weight.[26] While considered the gold standard, if the diagnosis is highly suspected, DNA sequencing may be a less invasive method although phasing of variants by examining parental DNA sequences may be necessary.

17.3.1.2 Treatment

Wilson disease can successfully be treated using a copper chelation strategy by the provision of penicillamine, which enhances urinary excretion, although it does little for impaired biliary excretion of copper. Copper overload is thus prevented. Chronic treatment with penicillamine can lead to pyridoxine deficiency; hence, pyridoxine is usually administered as well. Penicillamine use is associated with several side effects resulting in drug intolerance. These include a rash of the neck and axillae (elastosis perforans serpinginosa), nephrotoxicity, hematologic abnormalities, and paradoxical worsening of the clinical signs and symptoms. Trientine (triethylenetetramine dihydrochloride) is often used as a second line therapy in individuals who do not tolerate penicillamine. Zinc acetate, which induces intestinal epithelial cell production of metallothionein and subsequent increased binding and decreased absorption of dietary copper, can also be effective. It tends to be much slower at restoring copper balance than either penicillamine and trientine and thus, is often used as maintenance therapy. Tetrathiomolybdate can also be used to decrease copper absorption and decrease circulating copper levels, via formation of stable protein, copper, and tetrathiomolybdate complexes. To date, there are few studies comparing relative efficacy of these treatments. The current literature suggests that penicillamine is most effective for those with acute hepatic presentations, while zinc compounds are preferred for the management of presymptomatic individuals or those with a neurologic presentation.[27]

Since this disease is highly amenable to pharmacologic management, with favorable prognosis if treatment regimens are followed, liver transplantation is only performed in the case of delayed diagnosis with irreversible liver damage, or in the case of poor compliance with treatment and subsequent liver damage.[24]

17.3.1.3 Confounding conditions

While highly suggestive of the disorder, elevated urine copper levels are not completely diagnostic: elevated urine copper levels can also be seen in Menkes disease, hemochromatosis, biliary cirrhosis, thyrotoxicosis, nephrotic syndrome, and acute and/or chronic malignancies. Increased urinary copper levels can also be found in individuals taking contraceptives or on estrogen treatment as well as during pregnancy. In addition, urinary copper excretion of $>60\,\mu g/day$ can be observed in individuals taking megadoses of zinc or who are undergoing chelation therapy for other reasons. Since 90% of the copper is bound to ceruloplasmin, which is an acute phase reactant, false increases in plasma and urine copper may occur during acute infections and illness.

17.3.2 MENKES DISEASE AND OCCIPITAL HORN DISEASE

Menkes disease (MD) was first described in 1962 by Menkes et al.[28] who reported on five male infants, normal at birth, who developed seizures, developmental regression, and neurologic degeneration, along with failure to thrive and unusual hair. Death occurred between 7 and 42 months of age. It was later noticed that the hair of the affected infants had a very similar texture to the brittle wool of copper-deficient sheep.[29,30] Australian veterinarians had previously recognized a demyelinating disease in ataxic, copper-deficient lambs as well as anemia in copper-deficient ewes, highlighting the role of copper in mammalian neurodevelopment and hematopoiesis.[31] Cellular copper uptake is normal, but defective functioning of the ATP7A transport protein results in defective efflux of copper from intestinal cells to the circulatory system. Systemic copper deficiency results in defective functioning of cuproenzymes and the subsequent appearance of clinical features.

Although phenotypically normal in appearance at birth, affected males generally present at about 2–3 months of age with developmental regression, hypotonia, seizures, and poor growth. This can be missed during the newborn period as serum copper levels are generally low in normal neonates and other findings such as premature birth, large cephalohematomas, hypoglycemia, jaundice, and hypothermia are not pathognomonic for the disorder. Boys affected with this X-linked condition, have a jowly appearance with loose, redundant skin folds most prominent at the nape of the neck, the axillae, and on the trunk. Inguinal hernias may be present. Scalp hair is described as being kinky or like steel wool, and may be hypopigmented with a white, gray, or silver appearance. Microscopically, pili torti (180 degree twisting of the hair shaft), trichoclasis (transverse fracturing of the hair shaft) and trichoptilosis (longitudinal splitting of the hair shaft) are seen, with the former being pathognomonic for the disorder.[24] Despite profound truncal hypotonia, hyperactivity of the deep tendon reflexes is often present along with cortical thumbs (adducted thumbs). Signs and symptoms are related to specific enzymatic defects. For example, neurodegeneration is likely related to defective processing of neuropeptides by peptidylglycine monooxygenase and lack of catecholamine biosynthesis is due to the lack of dopamine β-hydroxylase activity. Although it would be predicted that the lack of Cu/Zn superoxide dismutase might also contribute to neurodegeneration, its dysfunction is apparently compensated for by increased activity of manganese superoxide dismutase. The unusual hair pigmentation is related to diminished tyrosinase activity, which is involved in melanin formation and the loose skin is caused by defective functioning of lysyloxidase, which is required for collagen cross-linking.

There is allelic heterogeneity at the ATP7A locus, with milder molecular variants resulting in the occipital horn disease (OHD) phenotype. This disorder derives its name from the pathognomonic X-ray finding of symmetric exostoses protruding downward from the occipital bone that may be present between 1 and 2 years of age, but is most commonly observed between 5 and 10 years of age. Infants may have a persistent open anterior fontanel as well as soft skin and joint laxity. Hypothermia, jaundice, hypotonia, and feeding problems may develop soon after birth, although symptom onset can be recognized any time from infancy to adulthood. Chronic diarrhea or recurrent urinary tract infections along with bladder diverticula can be presenting symptoms. Skeletal involvement is extensive. Elongated tortuous carotid arteries with intracranial arterial narrowing can also be seen. Hair, while coarse, does not have the classic pili torti. The prognosis, while variable, is better than Menkes disease, with longer survival. Intelligence is generally preserved. Serum copper and ceruloplasmin levels may also be normal in this disorder, although decreased levels are the norm.

Interestingly, deep intronic mutations that activate ATP7A pseudoexons have recently been described in two patients with OHD and one with classic Menkes disease who appeared to be mutation negative.[32] Wild-type transcripts were also identified in all three patients, although as might be expected, those with the OHD phenotype had more than the patient with classic Menkes disease.

17.3.2.1 Diagnostic tests

If the diagnosis is suspected, measurement of serum copper and ceruloplasmin levels is helpful, although not definitive. Levels of copper $<77\,\mu g/dL$ and ceruloplasmin of $<200\,mg/L$ suggest the diagnosis but are also within the low normal range for infants during the first 3 months of extrauterine life. Measurement of the catecholamines and their metabolites tends to be more specific for diagnosis: elevated ratios of dihydrophenylalanine (DOPA) to dihydroxyphenylglycol (DHPG), homovanillic acid (HVA) to vanillylmandelic acid (VMA), and dihydroxyphenylacetic acid (DOPAC) to DHPG in either plasma or cerebrospinal fluid correspond to the expected high levels of dopamine and low levels of norepinephrine due to enzyme deficiency. It has been proposed that not only can these ratios be used for diagnosis, but also as a biochemical marker for response to proposed therapeutic interventions.[33] Typical DOPA:DHPG ratios in affected individuals are in the range of 13 ± 6.6, while unaffected individuals have ratios in the range of 1.5 ± 0.4. In addition, the plasma ratio of dopamine to norepinephrine is useful for early diagnosis.[34] Unaffected individuals have DOPA:NE ratios in the range of 0.04 ± 0.03, while affected individuals have much higher ratios in the range of 0.83 ± 0.71. Demonstration of pathogenic variants within *ATP7A* located on the X-chromosome is critical for confirmation of the diagnosis. While no common mutations have been identified in Menkes disease, OHD tends to result with splice-site or missense mutations.[35]

An additional allelic condition has also been described: X-linked distal hereditary motor neuropathy (XDHMN).[36] This condition tends to have later onset and is limited to progressive weakness and wasting that starts distally but has no sensory involvement. Diagnosis can be difficult as there are at least seven subgroups of distal hereditary motor neuropathy with alterations in at least eight different genetic loci. The allelic heterogeneity is quite interesting as neither Menkes nor OHD have overt motor neuropathy, although both have neuromuscular involvement. Onset of symptoms ranges from 2 to 60 years of age. Molecularly, it is postulated that missense mutations that result in XDHMN incompletely disrupt trafficking rather than affecting critical functional domains, splicing or ATP7A protein levels. Hence, there are no plasma copper or ceruloplasmin abnormalities in XDHMN and diagnosis depends on clinical suspicion from family history with an X-linked pattern of inheritance and molecular confirmation.

17.3.2.2 Treatment

While historically considered to be a diagnosis refractory to treatment, it is now apparent that early diagnosis, within the first 2 weeks of life and rapid provision of intramuscular copper (copper chloride, copper gluconate, copper histidine, copper sulfate) can improve survival and decrease seizure frequency in boys with Menkes disease.[37] Normalization of neurodevelopment has been reported but is dependent upon some residual ATP7A function[34,38] or in individuals who carry mutations that selectively affect copper export with retention of the ability to perform copper incorporation into cuproenzymes.[39] Treatment is not curative but does allow for survival beyond 3 years of life.

There are currently no specific interventions for OHD or XDHMN other than supportive interventions.

17.3.2.3 Confounding conditions

Diagnosis is most difficult in the newborn period when serum copper and ceruloplasmin are typically low and can overlap levels seen in Menkes disease (MD) and OHD. Other conditions that can be associated with low plasma copper levels include excess zinc or iron ingestion, dietary copper deficiency, malnutrition, hypoproteinemia, and malabsorption. While Wilson disease also has low serum copper levels, its presentation is significantly different from MD and OHD, that there is little chance for confusion. Aceruloplasminemia can also have low serum copper levels, but usually presents in adulthood with movement disorders, diabetes, anemia, and retinal iron deposition.

Low serum ceruloplasmin levels are predominantly present in the copper transport disorders but can also be seen in conditions with significant protein loss, liver cell dysfunction, or aceruloplasminemia.

Since gadolinium, barium, and iodine interfere with metals testing, administration of contrast media within 96 hours of testing may falsely lower serum copper levels.

Table 17.1 provides biochemical abnormalities found in various disorders of copper metabolism.

Table 17.1 Biochemical Abnormalities in Various Copper Metabolism Defects

Disorder	Biochemical Abnormalities
Wilson disease	↓ Plasma copper
	↓ Plasma ceruloplasmin
	↑ Urine copper
Menkes disease	↓ Plasma copper
	↓ Plasma ceruloplasmin
	↑ DOPA/DHPG ratio
	↑ HVA/VMA ratio
	↑ DOPAC /DHPG ratio
Occipital horn syndrome	↔↓ Plasma copper
	↔↓ Plasma ceruloplasmin
	↔↑ DOPA/DHPG ratio
	↔↑ HVA/VMA ratio
Aceruloplasminemia	↓ Plasma copper
	↓ Plasma ceruloplasmin
	↓ Serum iron

DOPA: Dihydrophenylalanine; DHPG: Dihydroxyphenylglycol; HVA: Homovanillic acid; VMA: Vanillylmandelic acid; DOPAC: Dihydroxyphenylacetic acid.

17.4 MOLYBDENUM

Molybdenum is an essential metal that is used in the synthesis of molybdenum cofactor (MoCo), a modified pterin. The cofactor is required for the activity of several enzymes. As with many of the other trace mineral deficiency disorders, MoCo deficiency has a primarily neurologic presentation. While a MoCo was hypothesized in the mid-1960s, the first human case of MoCo deficiency was not identified until the late 1970s.[40] All molybdenum-containing enzymes (aldehyde oxidase, mitochondrial amidoxime reducing component, xanthine oxidase, and sulfite oxidase) use MoCo, the synthesis of which is by a highly conserved pathway among all organisms. While excess molybdenum may be toxic to ruminants, toxicity is not seen in humans.[41] Molybdenum is quite abundant in foodstuffs. Dietary deficiency has only been described in one case, in a patient with Crohn's disease on prolonged total parental nutrition without added molybdenum.[42] MoCo must be synthesized *de novo* and all genes involved in its biosynthesis are autosomally encoded. As with most autosomal recessive conditions, carriers of mutations have no obvious phenotype and mutation of both alleles is necessary. Given that MoCo is needed for the function of four MoCo-dependent enzymes, activity of all four is abrogated by any deficiency of MoCo synthesis.[43–46] There have been no identified cases of isolated aldehyde oxidase or mitochondrial amidoxime-reducing component to date. Isolated xanthine oxidoreductase deficiency results in classic xanthinuria type I.[47] Xanthinuria type II results from deficient human molybdenum cofactor sulfurase (*MCOS*) activity, which is necessary for the insertion of MoCo into xanthine oxidoreductase and aldehyde oxidase.[48] Isolated sulfite oxidase deficiency has also been described but is quite rare.[49]

17.4.1 XANTHINURIA TYPE I AND II

The xanthinurias tend to be non-life-threatening, autosomal recessive conditions that present as xanthinuria and xanthine stone formation. However, xanthine stones can result in hydronephrosis and pyelonephritis. A myopathy has also been described in xanthinuria type I. Both conditions present biochemically as xanthinuria with low serum and uric acid levels. Patients with type I xanthinuria retain the ability to metabolize allopurinol while those with type II cannot.

17.4.1.1 Diagnostic tests

In addition to urinalysis to determine if crystalluria is present, a 24-hour urine collection to measure calcium, oxalate, uric acid, and creatinine is generally part of the diagnostic workup. Serum and urine levels of uric acid are low or undetectable. Stone analysis as well as determination of urinary xanthine and hypoxanthine levels, generally measured by chromatographic methods, confirm the presence of xanthinuria. Gene sequencing, if indicated, can differentiate between type I, caused by mutations in the *XDH* (xanthine dehydrogenase) gene and type II, which results from mutations in the *MOCOS* gene.

17.4.1.2 Treatment

The mainstay of treatment is to avoid dehydration and to increase fluid intake to 1.5–2 times daily maintenance along with drinking water in the evening to avoid overly concentrated urine. A diet low in purines may be helpful (cheese, eggs, grains, fruits, nuts, vegetables). Since both xanthine dehydrogenase and aldehyde oxidase are important enzymes in drug metabolism, care should be taken with certain drugs to avoid toxicity. The former is involved in the metabolism of azathioprine and 6-mercaptopurine while the latter is necessary for the metabolism of allopurinol, cyclophosphamide, methotrexate, and quinine.

17.4.1.3 Confounding conditions

Any condition that results in radiolucent renal calculi can be confused with xanthinuria, although most will have less benign presentations. Crystal structure and stone color can be used to distinguish cystine (hexagonal, pink), uric acid (pleomorphic, red-yellow) and struvite (prism-like or coffin-lid, white) stones from xanthine (amorphous, brick red) stones.

17.4.2 MOLYBDENUM COFACTOR (MOCO)/SULFITE OXIDASE DEFICIENCY

Similar to the classic presentation of the inborn errors of the intoxication type, the major symptoms of MoCo deficiency, whatever the underlying genetic cause, are not present at birth but develop within the first week of life.[50] Combined deficiency of MoCo-dependent enzymes secondary to MoCo deficiency may not be clinically differentiated from isolated sulfite oxidase deficiency, although patients with MoCo deficiency may have facial dysmorphism (frontal bossing, micro- or macrocephaly, widely spaced eyes with long palpebral fissures, long face). Also they may have symptoms of renal stones from xanthinuria. Both MoCo deficiency and isolated sulfite oxidase deficiency can present with dislocated lenses. Neurologic involvement is present in both, with feeding difficulties, refractory seizures, opisthotonus, and exaggerated startle reflexes being prominent.[46] Cerebral atrophy with microgyria and enlarged ventricles is seen in MoCo deficiency. Brain anomalies are felt to possibly contribute to the dysmorphic features associated with condition and to result from sulfite (and derivatives) toxicity.[51,52] Biochemical parameters do not correlate with disease severity.[53,54]

Combined deficiency has been found to result from homozygous or compound heterozygous mutations in one of three genes involved in the MoCo synthesis pathway: *MOCS1* (molybdenum cofactor synthase-1), *MOCS2* (molybdopterin synthase) or *GPHN* (gephyrin).[55] Both *MOCS1* and *MOCS2* have a bicistronic architecture resulting in two different proteins from different open reading frames. This is achieved either by alternative splicing or independent translation of bicistronic mRNA.[46] MOCS1 is required for the synthesis of cyclo pyranopterin monophosphate (cPMP) from guanosine-5′-triphosphate (GTP) while MOCS2 is required for the synthesis of molybdopterin and encodes both a small and large enzyme subunit. Adenylation of MPT and insertion of molybdenum into active MoCo requires an assembly cofactor, gephyrin. A fourth gene product, a protein required for adenylation and generation of a thiocarboxylate group at the C-terminus of the smaller subunit of molybdopterin synthase, is encoded by MCOS3, although mutations have not been implicated in disease processes.[46]

17.4.2.1 Diagnostic tests

Combined deficiency of MoCo-dependent enzymes results from homozygous or compound heterozygous mutations in *MOCS1, MOCS2,* or *GPHN*. Enzyme deficiencies lead to the accumulation of hypoxanthine, xanthine, methionine, cysteine, taurine, S-sulfocysteine, cystine, sulfite, and thiosulfate. Sulfate and uric acid levels are low. Elevated urinary sulfite levels can be detected on fresh samples using urine test strips although false negatives can occur, usually because of insufficient time for sulfite accumulation soon after birth or nonenzymatic oxidation of sulfite to sulfate. Mutation analysis of all three genes confirms the diagnosis, although the majority of identified patients, to date, have had mutations in *MOCS1*. In isolated sulfite oxidase deficiency, urine hypoxanthine and xanthine are normal.

17.4.2.2 Treatment

Historically, most affected individuals did not survive beyond early childhood and treatment was palliative. Provision of high-dose inorganic molybdenum has not been shown to be effective, although there is some research evidence that this might be somewhat effective in individuals with *GHPN* mutations. Diets that restrict sulfur-containing amino acids have led to reduced levels of sulfur metabolites but have not resulted in neurologic improvement.[56] Recently, several cases of treatment with daily intravenous cyclic pyranopterin monophosphate have been reported. The first such patient began treatment at day of life 36 and 18 months of age was seizure-free but had static quadraplegic cerebral palsy and improvement in biochemical parameters.[57] Two additional patients were reported by Bowhay[58] with early treatment beginning between days of life 1 and 4. At 2 years of age, one child, per report, has had near normal neurologic development while the second is severely neurologically impaired.

17.4.2.3 Confounding conditions

Sulfite oxidase is required for the oxidation of the sulfur atom in cysteine to inorganic sulfate and thus, isolated deficiency does not represent a true defect of molybdenum metabolism. It cannot, however, be clinically differentiated from MoCo deficiency. Deficiency leads to accumulation of sulfite, thiosulfate, S-sulfocysteine, and reduced sulfate. Urinary sulfite on fresh samples using urine test strips will be elevated but false negatives are common, especially soon after birth (when there has been insufficient time for sulfite accumulation) or sulfite is nonenzymatically oxidized. Urinary and plasma S-sulfocysteine can also be detected by electrophoretic or chromatographic methods. Homocysteine levels may be reduced. Plasma and urine cystine levels are low. Xanthinuria is not observed and normal blood uric acid levels and excretion are present, differentiating isolated sulfite oxidase deficiency from combined deficiency. Mutation analysis of the *SUOX* gene and identification of homozygous or compound heterozygous mutations confirms the diagnosis, although enzymatic activity in cultured fibroblasts can also be performed. Both MoCo deficiency and isolated sulfite oxidase deficiency have overlap in clinical findings with hypoxemic-ischemic encephalopathy[59] and neonatal hyperekplexia,[60] but can be differentiated on biochemical testing, if ordered.

17.5 MANGANESE

Manganese (Mn) is necessary for healthy connective tissue and bone development. As with other trace metals, Mn is required for metabolic function as it acts as a cofactor for a number of enzymes including Mn-specific glycosyltransferases, superoxide dismutase, pyruvate carboxylase, arginase, and phosphoenolpyruvate carboxykinase. Approximate daily requirement for Mn of 1–6 mg is readily supplied by a normal diet. Mn deficiency has not been definitively documented in humans although deficiency in other animals, particularly cattle, results in ataxia and skeletal abnormalities.[61] Prolidase deficiency that leads to skin ulceration, mental retardation, increased urinary excretion of iminopeptides, and recurrent infections has been associated with Mn deficiency. Ingestion rarely leads to toxicity as intake via enterocytes and excretion by biliary duct cells is tightly regulated.[61–63] Excess Mn, however, is quite toxic and usually results from occupational inhalation exposure, although cases of hypermanganesemia have been reported with ingestion of contaminated drinking water.[64] Toxicity results in biphasic physical decline with initial psychiatric symptoms followed by a progressive dystonic gait, akinetic rigidity, and bradykinesia.[65,66] The majority of experimental work elucidating the effects of Mn has been focused on genes associated with the development of Parkinson's disease because of the link between Mn toxicity and dopaminergic neurodegeneration.[67] Recently, mutations in *SLC30A10*, which encodes a Mn transporter, have been identified resulting in autosomal recessive dystonia with brain Mn accumulation, polycythemia, and hepatic cirrhosis.[68–71]

17.5.1 DIAGNOSTIC TESTS

Diagnosis requires suspicion of the disorder, which can have either childhood or adult onset. The former presents with four-limb dystonia and the dystonic "cockwalk" gait or spastic paraparesis. The latter presents with Parkinsonism that does not respond to provision of L-dopa. In addition to the neurologic findings, whole blood Mn is elevated and is greater than 110 ng/mL with normal being less than 18 ng/mL. In comparison, levels associated with environmentally acquired hypermanganesemia, while elevated, are typically less than 110 ng/mL. Polycythemia and hepatomegaly with cirrhosis or fibrosis are also present. T1-weighted magnetic resonance imaging demonstrates hyperintensity of the basal ganglia (globus pallidus, putamen, caudate, subthalamic, and dentate nuclei) with sparing of the thalamus and ventral pons.

Confirmation of the diagnosis requires demonstration of biallelic mutations in the *SLC30A10* gene. Mn deficiency can be assessed through whole-blood Mn or better by measuring superoxide mutase and arginase activities.

17.5.2 TREATMENT

Chelation therapy with IV disodium calcium edetate and oral iron supplementation has been shown to normalize blood Mn levels; it is possible that early treatment may prevent progression of symptoms but CNS damage is probably not completely reversible.[68,70,72] Foods high in Mn (cloves, saffron, wheat, nuts, dark chocolate, mussels, and pumpkin/sesame/sunflower seeds) should be avoided.

17.5.3 CONFOUNDING CONDITIONS

While other conditions can symptomatically present as movement disorders (cerebral palsy, organic acidurias, Wilson disease, Parkinson's disease, etc.), the presence of polycythemia and elevated Mn levels suggests the diagnosis of hypermanganesemia. Other conditions that can present with hypermanganesemia include those related to environmental exposure (mining, welding, potassium permanganate contamination of methcathinone, total parenteral nutrition (TPN)), advanced hepatic cirrhosis, and portosystemic shunting.[73–76] In addition, Mn levels may be intermittently only minimally elevated; thus a single measurement may not be adequate to make the diagnosis and remeasurement may be necessary.[68]

17.6 SELENIUM

Although dietary selenium deficiency and toxicity have been recognized in the past, only recently have inborn errors of selenium metabolism been elucidated. Like many other essential elements, selenium is involved in multiple pathways through more than 30 biologically active selenocysteine-containing proteins. Selenium enters the body through food mainly as selenomethionine from plants. Average daily intake in the United States ranges from 80 to 220 µg. The reference range for plasma selenium is about 60–150 ng/mL.

Selenium deficiency (serum concentration <40 ng/mL) is rare and is associated with loss of glutathione peroxidase activity. Dietary selenium deficiency is generally seen in hospitalized patients or with the use of TPN. Selenium deficiency tends to be associated with either cardiomyopathy or symptoms of hypothyroidism, whereas excess causes hair loss, nail abnormalities, dermatitis, nausea, diarrhea, fatigue, peripheral neuropathy, and an unusual garlic breath odor. Toxic levels have not yet been well defined.

Selenoproteins are unique in that they contain the amino acid selenocysteine. To generate these proteins, UGA triplets, which are usually stop codons, must be recoded and recognize a specific serine/selenocysteine tRNA. In this process, serine is charged onto this tRNA by Ser-tRNA synthase and then converted to selenocysteine by selenocysteine synthase (SEPSECS). A specific elongation factor (EF-Sec) is also required to carry this tRNA to the ribosome, which upon interacting with translation factors allows for the insertion of selenocysteine into the protein rather than resulting in translation termination.[77,78] To date, 25 genes encoding selenoproteins are known,[79] all of which catalyze oxidation-reduction reactions. Regulation of biosynthesis of selenoproteins depends upon selenium availability, mRNA levels, and translational control mechanisms. Inflammation and chronic illness as well as statin and aminoglycoside use may lead to decreased levels of selenoproteins, but little data is available, particularly for infants and children.[80–83]

Of the selenoproteins, selenoprotein N (SEPN) is highly expressed in muscle tissue and necessary for proper muscle function and calcium handling. Mutations in *SEPN1* result in rigid spine muscular dystrophy 1 or multiminocore disease. This infantile onset, non-, or slowly progressive disorder presents with spinal rigidity, joint contractures, diffuse muscle weakness, nocturnal hypoventilation, and a restrictive respiratory syndrome. The diagnosis is made by muscle biopsy and gene sequencing.

Two recessive inborn errors of selenoprotein biosynthesis have recently been reported. Individuals with mutations in *SECISBP2*, present with growth retardation and delayed bone age, along with partial resistance to thyroid hormone. Myopathy and hearing loss may also be present. SECISBP2 encodes selenocysteine insertion sequence-binding protein 2, which is necessary for the generation of tRNA$^{[Ser]ThiamineSec}$. Symptoms are partially caused by decreased deiodinase 1–3 activities, which play a role in thyroid hormone metabolism and cochlear development. In addition to the physical symptoms, affected individuals have elevated T4, elevated rT3, high/normal thyroid-stimulating hormone (TSH), and low T3 levels, distinguishing it from partial resistance to thyroid hormone (caused by mutations in thyroid hormone receptor, beta), which has elevations of all thyroid hormones. Defective SECISBP2 activity is predicted to be independent of dietary selenium intake as supplementation does not correct the condition.[84]

A second disorder of selenocysteine synthesis has been identified: progressive cerebello-cerebral atrophy caused by mutations in the *SEPSECS* (selenocysteine synthase) gene.[85] Dysfunction of this synthase results in profound cognitive impairment, progressive microcephaly, intractable seizures, and spasticity.[86] Intractable seizures in some were responsive to selenium supplementation.

17.6.1 DIAGNOSTIC TESTS

Distinguishing selenium deficiency from an inborn error of selenium biosynthesis can be done by measuring serum selenium concentrations as well as plasma or serum glutathione peroxidase 3 activity or selenoprotein P (SePP) levels. Serum selenium is generally measured by atomic absorption or inductively coupled plasma mass spectrometry (ICP-MS). SePP levels are measured through immunoassays. The inborn errors of selenium biosynthesis will have normal selenium levels and reduced GPx3 activity or SePP levels.

17.6.2 TREATMENT

There are currently no treatments for the inborn errors of selenoprotein biosynthesis as they are generally selenium concentration–independent. However, response to selenium supplementation of seizures associated with SEPSECS deficiency has been reported.

17.6.3 CONFOUNDING CONDITIONS

Selenium deficiency is rare in healthy individuals but can be seen in conditions with impaired intestinal function. Keshan disease, a potentially fatal cardiomyopathy with myocardial necrosis results from a combination of selenium deficiency from poor dietary intake and secondary viral infection (often coxsackie virus). Kashin–Beck disease, a severe osteochondropathy seen mostly in China and related to ingestion of foods grown on selenium-deficient soil, results from combined dietary selenium and iodine deficiency, which can be alleviated by supplementation. Treatment with statins or aminoglycosides have also been reported to cause selenium deficiency. Selenium deficiency can be confused with primary hypothyroidism since it is necessary for conversion of T4 to T3. The acute phase response or infection can lower the levels of selenium, glutathione peroxidase 3 activity, and SePP.

17.7 MAGNESIUM

Although magnesium is not a trace metal, it is covered in this chapter since it is one of the most important metals in the body. In fact it is the fourth most abundant cation in the body and second-most abundant intracellular cation after calcium. It is a cofactor for more than 300 enzymes in the body. Despite its physiological importance and the necessary maintenance of high intracellular concentrations, relatively little is known about magnesium transport in humans. While hypomagnesemia is quite common, it is not often diagnosed as serum magnesium levels are not routinely monitored. Furthermore, serum magnesium levels do not really reflect total body magnesium since only 1–2% of total body magnesium is found in the blood and extracellular space, with the remainder being distributed between soft tissues (~19%), skeletal muscle (~20%), and bone (~60%).[87,88] Magnesium is a cofactor in all ATP-dependent reactions and acts as a calcium channel antagonist where it acts to modulate processes dependent upon intracellular calcium flux, such as muscle contraction and neurotransmitter release in addition to insulin and other hormone release. It is necessary for parathyroid hormone release and maintenance of 1,25 (OH)2-vitamin D levels and hence, plays a role in the development of osteopenia and osteoporosis. It is also important for proper cardiac contractility as well as for the maintenance of membrane potentials in all mammalian cells, as it is a cofactor for the Na-K-ATP pump.[87–89]

Magnesium concentrations are maintained as a balance between intake, uptake, resorption, and excretion. Approximately 300 mg of magnesium is ingested daily in the average American diet. Dietary magnesium uptake can occur anywhere along the intestinal tract with absorption being inversely proportional to the amount of magnesium in the diet. Absorption is by either paracellular mechanisms or transporter molecules, depending upon the site. Magnesium is then transported to the blood where it is found in both protein-bound and unbound states. Magnesium that is not taken up by tissues or bone is filtered by the kidney, which plays a major role in magnesium homeostasis. Approximately 80% of magnesium is ultrafilterable, most of which is resorbed in the proximal tubule, the loop of Henle, and the distal tubule. Resorption is affected by glomerular filtration rate, volume status, hormones (parathyroid hormone (PTH), calcitonin, antidiuretic hormone (ADH), glucagon, insulin), acid-base status, hypophosphatemia, hypercalcemia, and diuretic use.[87] Hypophosphatemia and hypercalcemia both result in increased urinary excretion of magnesium; hypomagnesemia may be primary or secondary in cases of either condition. Hypermagnesemia is not generally considered to result from a heritable defect in Mg^{2+} transport, but rather is suggestive of renal insufficiency, parenteral infusion, oral ingestion, or enema overuse. Lithium therapy can also result in hypermagesemia as can hypocalciuric hypercalcemia.

While Mg^{2+} absorption in the small intestine is considered to be paracellular, absorption in the cecum and large intestine is carried out by a transcellular mechanism with luminal expression of TRMP6 and TRMP7 (transient receptor potential cation channel subfamily M member 6 and 7, respectively) coupled with ENaC sodium transport. Transport across the basolateral membrane is mediated by CNNM4 (cyclin and CBS domain divalent cation transport mediator 4), postulated to be a sodium/magnesium exchanger, which is also coupled with Na-K-ATPase activity. Renal resorption is somewhat more complicated: in the proximal tubule, where approximately 10–25% of magnesium is resorbed, this paracellular process is requires Na and water resorption by NHE3 (sodium-hydrogen exchanger 3, SLC9A3) and AQP1 (aquaporin 1), along with Na-K-ATPase. The majority of Mg^{2+} reuptake occurs in the thick ascending loop of Henle. While uptake of Mg^{2+} and Ca^{2+} are paracellular, Na-K-Cl cotransporter and renal outer medullary potassium channel function, along with ClC-Kb, the basolateral chloride channel in the nephron and Na-K-ATPase, is essential. In this portion of the tubule, tight junction permeability relies on claudins, of which claudins 16 and 19 are important for permeability to Mg^{2+}. Claudin 14 and claudin 10 have been implicated as nonspecific cation blockers that may also be important in Mg^{2+} homeostasis.[87] Final urinary Mg^{2+} is determined by the distal convoluted tubule, where about 10% of Mg^{2+} is resorbed. This resorption is transcellular and tightly regulated with TRPM6 mediating luminal Mg^{2+} uptake. Membrane levels of TRMP6 are regulated by the PI3K-Akt-Rac1 signaling pathway via insulin and epidermal growth factor activation. Potassium channels are required for Mg^{2+} uptake and homeostasis in conjunction with other gated channels (for review see Swaminathan[87]).

Monogenic causes of hypomagnesemia are listed in Table 17.2.

17.7.1 DIAGNOSTIC TESTS

Hypomagnesemia often goes undetected, despite the fact that the physiologic need for it is ubiquitous. There are 15 identified heritable disorders of magnesium homeostasis, all of which affect either the thick ascending loop of Henle or the distal convoluted tubule (Table 17.2). All currently identified disorders that affect the distal loop

Table 17.2 Monogenic Causes of Hypomagnesemia

Gene & Gene Product	Disorder	Onset	Inheritance	Serum Mg²⁺	Serum Ca²⁺	Serum K⁺	Urine Mg²⁺	Urine Ca²⁺	Comments
CLCNKB CLC-Kb chloride channel	Bartter syndrome Type 3 MIM 607364	Variable	AR	N or ↓	N	↓↓	N or ↓	Variable	Ocular involvement Polyuria No nephrocalcinosis Hypokalemic metabolic alkalosis ↑ plasma renin ↑ plasma aldosterone Low blood pressure
SLC12A3 Thiazide-sensitive Na-Cl cotransporter	Gitelman syndrome MIM 263800	Variable	AR	↓	N	↓↓	↑	↓	Muscle cramps/ episodic paralysis Tetany/seizures Hypokalemic alkalosis Polydipsia ↑ plasma renin
CLDN16 Paracellin-1 Tight junction protein	Familial hypomagnesemia Renal Hypomagnesemia 3 MIM 248250	Childhood	AR	↓	N	N	↑	↑	Polydipsia/polyuria Hematuria, abacterial leukocyturia Nephrocalcinosis/ nephrolithiasis Renal failure ↑ Parathyroid hormone
TRPM6 TRPM6 ion channel	Hypomagnesemia with secondary hypocalcemia MIM 602014	Infancy	AR	↓↓	↓	N	↑	N	Tetany/Seizures

(Continued)

Table 17.2 Monogenic Causes of Hypomagnesemia (Continued)

Gene & Gene Product	Disorder	Onset	Inheritance	Serum Mg^{2+}	Serum Ca^{2+}	Serum K^+	Urine Mg^{2+}	Urine Ca^{2+}	Comments
CLDN19 Tight junction protein	Renal hypomagnesemia 5 with ocular involvement MIM 248190	Infancy	AR	↓	N	N	↑	↑	Ocular involvement Nephrolithiasis Nephrocalcinosis Progressive renal failure
EGF Epidermal growth factor	Renal hypomagnesemia 4 MIM 611718	Childhood	AR	↓	N	N	N	N	Seizures Psychomotor retardation Increased fractional excretion of Mg^{2+}
CNNM2 Cyclin M2 defect in renal tubular Mg^{2+} resorption	Renal hypomagnesemia 6 MIM 613882	Variable	AD	↓↓↓	N	N	N	N	Low levels of serum Mg^{2+} in the absence of other electrolyte disturbances
KCNJ1 K⁺ inwardly rectifying channel, subfamily J, member 1	Bartter syndrome Type 2 MIM 241200	Antenatal Neonatal	AR	N or ↓	N	↓↓	N	↑↑	Nephrocalcinosis Polydipsia, dehydration Hypokalemic metabolic alkalosis ↑ plasma renin/ aldosterone Tetany/Seizures
FXYD2 Na⁺K⁺ ATPase γ-subunit	Isolated dominant hypomagnesemia MIM 154020	Childhood	AD	↓	N	N	↑	↓	Seizures N parathyroid hormone

of Henle are inherited in an autosomal recessive fashion. The majority of these disorders present with hypomagnesemia, nephrocalcinosis, and renal failure (FHHNC1–2; Bartter syndrome types 1–4). Specific disorders may also have visual impairment (FHHNC2) or sodium wasting, hypokalemic alkalosis, and high renin/aldosterone (Bartter syndrome types 1–4). Underlying clinical suspicion is key for obtaining the diagnosis. Serum levels are preferred to plasma levels, as anticoagulants added to the collection tube can either interfere with the assay or can have magnesium as a contaminant. Again, serum magnesium levels, while a starting point for diagnosis, are difficult to accurately determine using current methods and, if found to be low (<1.2 mg/dL), require further evaluation. While measurement of ionized magnesium may become routinely available in the future, the most helpful test currently is the magnesium tolerance test, which measures the percentage of retained magnesium after parenteral administration. If deficiency is present, the amount retained is increased and is inversely related to the bone magnesium concentration. If a heritable genetic condition is suspected, then confirmation by DNA sequence analysis is necessary.

17.7.2 TREATMENT

Total body magnesium in the face of low serum magnesium is difficult to assess. Furthermore, oral magnesium tends to be poorly absorbed. Thus, in the symptomatic patient, prompt administration of intravenous magnesium sulfate is recommended as a bolus of 8 mmol over one minute, followed by 40 mmol over the ensuing 5 hours. For less critical situations, 0.5 mmol/kg/24 hours is recommended. Serum magnesium concentrations should be monitored, although normalization does not necessarily equate to repletion and continued treatment for 3–7 days is recommended.[87] Mild asymptomatic hypomagnesemia can be treated with a magnesium-rich diet. In any patient with hypomagnesemia, renal function should also be monitored as hypermagnesemia can result in toxicity manifested as hypotension and bradycardia, along with diminished deep tendon reflexes.

17.7.3 CONFOUNDING DIAGNOSES

For the early-onset heritable disorders, the major confounding diagnoses are most likely to be gastrointestinal, renal, or endocrine in nature. Chronic diarrhea and malabsorption commonly result in hypomagnesemia. Chronic renal failure can lead to renal magnesium loss and hypomagnesemia. Hypercalcemia, hyperthyroidism, hyperparathyroidism, and hyperaldosteronism are endocrine causes of hypomagnesemia. In the disorders with more variable age of onset, one must consider diabetes mellitus, alcoholism, and chronic liver disease or pancreatitis with steatorrhea. Malabsorptive conditions such as IBD and celiac disease commonly lead to decreased magnesium absorption and hypomagnesemia. Hypomagnesemia can also be a complication of medication use including diuretics, cisplatin, carboplatin, aminoglycosides, cyclosporin, theophylline, amphotericin, foscarnet, and pamidronate.[87]

REFERENCES

1. Schnackenberg LK, Beger RD. Metabolomic biomarkers: their role in the critical path. *Drug Discov Today Technol* 2007;**4**(1):13–16.
2. Vallee BL, Falchuk KH. The biochemical basis of zinc physiology. *Physiol Rev* 1993;**73**(1):79–118.
3. Malavolta M, Piacenza F, Basso A, Giacconi R, Costarelli L, Mocchegiani E. Serum copper to zinc ratio: Relationship with aging and health status. *Mech Ageing Dev* 2015; 151:93–100.
4. Hordyjewska A, Popiolek L, Kocot J. The many "faces" of copper in medicine and treatment. *Biometals* 2014;**27**(4):611–21.
5. Miller LV, Hambidge KM, Naake VL, Hong Z, Westcott JL, Fennessey PV. Size of the zinc pools that exchange rapidly with plasma zinc in humans: alternative techniques for measuring and relation to dietary zinc intake. *J Nutr* 1994;**124**(2):268–76.
6. Hambidge M, Krebs NF. Interrelationships of key variables of human zinc homeostasis: relevance to dietary zinc requirements. *Annu Rev Nutr* 2001;**21**:429–52.
7. Stevens J, Lubitz L. Symptomatic zinc deficiency in breast-fed term and premature infants. *J Paediatr Child Health* 1998;**34**(1):97–100.
8. Chowanadisai W, Lonnerdal B, Kelleher SL. Identification of a mutation in SLC30A2 (ZnT-2) in women with low milk zinc concentration that results in transient neonatal zinc deficiency. *J Biol Chem* 2006;**281**(51):39699–707.
9. Smith JC, Zeller JA, Brown ED, Ong SC. Elevated plasma zinc: a heritable anomaly. *Science* 1976;**193**(4252):496–8.
10. Gustafsson D, Breimer LH, Isaksson HS, Nilsson TK. Tissue zinc levels in a child with hypercalprotectinaemia and hyperzincaemia: A case report and a review of the literature. *Scand J Clin Lab Invest* 2012;**72**(1):34–8.
11. Sampson B, Fagerhol MK, Sunderkotter C, et al. Hyperzincaemia and hypercalprotectinaemia: a new disorder of zinc metabolism. *Lancet* 2002;**360**(9347):1742–5.
12. Sampson B, Kovar IZ, Rauscher A, et al. A case of hyperzincemia with functional zinc depletion: a new disorder? *Pediatr Res* 1997;**42**(2):219–25.
13. Shenkin A, Roberts NB. Vitamins and trace metals. In: Burtis CA, Ashwood ER, Bruns DE, editors. *Tietz's textbook of clinical chemistry and molecular diagnostics* 5th ed. St. Louis, Missouri: Elsevier; 2012. pp. 895–983.
14. Van Wouwe JP. Clinical and laboratory diagnosis of acrodermatitis enteropathica. *Eur J Pediatr* 1989;**149**(1):2–8.
15. Jing M, Rech L, Wu Y, Goltz D, Taylor CG, House JD. Effects of zinc deficiency and zinc supplementation on homocysteine levels and related enzyme expression in rats. *J Trace Elem Med Biol* 2015;**30**:77–82.
16. Maryon EB, Molloy SA, Ivy K, Yu H, Kaplan JH. Rate and regulation of copper transport by human copper transporter 1 (hCTR1). *J Biol Chem* 2013;**288**(25):18035–46.
17. Zimnicka AM, Maryon EB, Kaplan JH. Human copper transporter hCTR1 mediates basolateral uptake of copper into enterocytes: implications for copper homeostasis. *J Biol Chem* 2007;**282**(36):26471–80.
18. Nose Y, Kim BE, Thiele DJ. Ctr1 drives intestinal copper absorption and is essential for growth, iron metabolism, and neonatal cardiac function. *Cell Metab* 2006;**4**(3):235–44.
19. Przybylkowski A, Gromadzka G, Wawer A, Grygorowicz T, Cybulska A, Czlonkowska A. Intestinal expression of metal transporters in Wilson's disease. *Biometals* 2013;**26**(6):925–34.

20. Zimnicka AM, Ivy K, Kaplan JH. Acquisition of dietary copper: a role for anion transporters in intestinal apical copper uptake. *Am J Physiol Cell Physiol* 2011;**300**(3): C588–99.

21. Gupta A, Lutsenko S. Human copper transporters: mechanism, role in human diseases and therapeutic potential. *Future Med Chem* 2009;**1**(6):1125–42.

22. Brewer GJ. Zinc and tetrathiomolybdate for the treatment of Wilson's disease and the potential efficacy of anticopper therapy in a wide variety of diseases. *Metallomics* 2009;**1**(3):199–206.

23. Chhetri SK, Mills RJ, Shaunak S, Emsley HC. Copper deficiency. *BMJ* 2014;**348**:g3691.

24. Kaler SG. Inborn errors of copper metabolism. *Handb Clin Neurol* 2013;**113**:1745–54.

25. Bull PC, Thomas GR, Rommens JM, Forbes JR, Cox DW. The Wilson disease gene is a putative copper transporting P-type ATPase similar to the Menkes gene. *Nat Genet* 1993;**5**(4):327–37.

26. Whyte MP. Physiological role of alkaline phosphatase explored in hypophosphatasia. *Ann N Y Acad Sci* 2010;**1192**:190–200.

27. Wiggelinkhuizen M, Tilanus ME, Bollen CW, Houwen RH. Systematic review: clinical efficacy of chelator agents and zinc in the initial treatment of Wilson disease. *Aliment Pharmacol Ther* 2009;**29**(9):947–58.

28. Menkes JH, Alter M, Steigleder GK, Weakley DR, Sung JH. A sex-linked recessive disorder with retardation of growth, peculiar hair, and focal cerebral and cerebellar degeneration. *Pediatrics* 1962;**29**:764–79.

29. Danks DM, Campbell PE, Stevens BJ, Mayne V, Cartwright E. Menkes's kinky hair syndrome. An inherited defect in copper absorption with widespread effects. *Pediatrics* 1972;**50**(2):188–201.

30. Danks DM, Campbell PE, Walker-Smith J, et al. Menkes' kinky-hair syndrome. *Lancet* 1972;**1**(7760):1100–2.

31. Bennetts HW, Fe C. Copper deficiency in sheep in western Australia: A preliminary account of the aetiology of enzootic ataxia of lamns and an anaemia of ewes. *Australian Veterinary Journal* 1937;**13**(4):138–49.

32. Yasmeen S, Lund K, De Paepe A, et al. Occipital horn syndrome and classical Menkes Syndrome caused by deep intronic mutations, leading to the activation of ATP7A pseudo-exon. *Eur J Hum Genet* 2014;**22**(4):517–21.

33. Kaler SG, Goldstein DS, Holmes C, Salerno JA, Gahl WA. Plasma and cerebrospinal fluid neurochemical pattern in Menkes disease. *Ann Neurol* 1993;**33**(2):171–5.

34. Kaler SG, Holmes CS, Goldstein DS, et al. Neonatal diagnosis and treatment of Menkes disease. *N Engl J Med* 2008;**358**(6):605–14.

35. Kodama H, Fujisawa C, Bhadhprasit W. Inherited copper transport disorders: biochemical mechanisms, diagnosis, and treatment. *Curr Drug Metab* 2012;**13**(3):237–50.

36. Kennerson ML, Nicholson GA, Kaler SG, et al. Missense mutations in the copper transporter gene ATP7A cause X-linked distal hereditary motor neuropathy. *Am J Hum Genet* 2010;**86**(3):343–52.

37. Kaler SG, Liew CJ, Donsante A, Hicks JD, Sato S, Greenfield JC. Molecular correlates of epilepsy in early diagnosed and treated Menkes disease. *J Inherit Metab Dis* 2010;**33**(5):583–9.

38. Kaler SG. ATP7A-related copper transport diseases-emerging concepts and future trends. *Nat Rev Neurol* 2011;**7**(1):15–29.

39. Kim BE, Smith K, Petris MJ. A copper treatable Menkes disease mutation associated with defective trafficking of a functional Menkes copper ATPase. *J Med Genet* 2003;**40**(4):290–5.

40. Duran M, Beemer FA, van de Heiden C, et al. Combined deficiency of xanthine oxidase and sulphite oxidase: a defect of molybdenum metabolism or transport? *J Inherit Metab Dis* 1978;**1**(4):175–8.
41. Novotny JA, Turnlund JR. Molybdenum intake influences molybdenum kinetics in men. *J Nutr* 2007;**137**(1):37–42.
42. Abumrad NN. Molybdenum--is it an essential trace metal? *Bull N Y Acad Med* 1984;**60**(2):163–71.
43. Havemeyer A, Bittner F, Wollers S, Mendel R, Kunze T, Clement B. Identification of the missing component in the mitochondrial benzamidoxime prodrug-converting system as a novel molybdenum enzyme. *J Biol Chem* 2006;**281**(46):34796–802.
44. Havemeyer A, Lang J, Clement B. The fourth mammalian molybdenum enzyme mARC: current state of research. *Drug Metab Rev* 2011;**43**(4):524–39.
45. Ott G, Havemeyer A, Clement B. The mammalian molybdenum enzymes of mARC. *J Biol Inorg Chem* 2015;**20**(2):265–75.
46. Reiss J, Hahnewald R. Molybdenum cofactor deficiency: Mutations in GPHN, MOCS1, and MOCS2. *Hum Mutat* 2011;**32**(1):10–18.
47. Ichida K, Amaya Y, Kamatani N, Nishino T, Hosoya T, Sakai O. Identification of two mutations in human xanthine dehydrogenase gene responsible for classical type I xanthinuria. *J Clin Invest* 1997;**99**(10):2391–7.
48. Ichida K, Matsumura T, Sakuma R, Hosoya T, Nishino T. Mutation of human molybdenum cofactor sulfurase gene is responsible for classical xanthinuria type II. *Biochem Biophys Res Commun* 2001;**282**(5):1194–200.
49. Tan WH, Eichler FS, Hoda S, et al. Isolated sulfite oxidase deficiency: a case report with a novel mutation and review of the literature. *Pediatrics* 2005;**116**(3):757–66.
50. Bayram E, Topcu Y, Karakaya P, et al. Molybdenum cofactor deficiency: review of 12 cases (MoCD and review). *Eur J Paediatr Neurol* 2013;**17**(1):1–6.
51. Reiss J, Bonin M, Schwegler H, et al. The pathogenesis of molybdenum cofactor deficiency, its delay by maternal clearance, and its expression pattern in microarray analysis. *Mol Genet Metab* 2005;**85**(1):12–20.
52. Salman MS, Ackerley C, Senger C, Becker L. New insights into the neuropathogenesis of molybdenum cofactor deficiency. *Can J Neurol Sci* 2002;**29**(1):91–6.
53. Hughes EF, Fairbanks L, Simmonds HA, Robinson RO. Molybdenum cofactor deficiency-phenotypic variability in a family with a late-onset variant. *Dev Med Child Neurol* 1998;**40**(1):57–61.
54. Mize C, Johnson JL, Rajagopalan KV. Defective molybdopterin biosynthesis: clinical heterogeneity associated with molybdenum cofactor deficiency. *J Inherit Metab Dis* 1995;**18**(3):283–90.
55. Reiss J, Johnson JL. Mutations in the molybdenum cofactor biosynthetic genes MOCS1, MOCS2, and GEPH. *Hum Mutat* 2003;**21**(6):569–76.
56. Johnson JL, Waud WR, Rajagopalan KV, Duran M, Beemer FA, Wadman SK. Inborn errors of molybdenum metabolism: combined deficiencies of sulfite oxidase and xanthine dehydrogenase in a patient lacking the molybdenum cofactor. *Proc Natl Acad Sci U S A* 1980;**77**(6):3715–9.
57. Veldman A, Santamaria-Araujo JA, Sollazzo S, et al. Successful treatment of molybdenum cofactor deficiency type A with cPMP. *Pediatrics* 2010;**125**(5):e1249–54.
58. Bowhay S. Two years experience of the treatment of molybdenum cofactor deficiency. *Arch Dis Child* 2013;**98**:e1.

59. Topcu M, Coskun T, Haliloglu G, Saatci I. Molybdenum cofactor deficiency: report of three cases presenting as hypoxic-ischemic encephalopathy. *J Child Neurol* 2001;**16**(4): 264–70.

60. Macaya A, Brunso L, Fernandez-Castillo N, et al. Molybdenum cofactor deficiency presenting as neonatal hyperekplexia: a clinical, biochemical and genetic study. *Neuropediatrics* 2005;**36**(6):389–94.

61. Keen CL, Ensunsa JL, Watson MH, et al. Nutritional aspects of manganese from experimental studies. *Neurotoxicology* 1999;**20**(2–3):213–23.

62. Dorman DC, Struve MF, James RA, McManus BE, Marshall MW, Wong BA. Influence of dietary manganese on the pharmacokinetics of inhaled manganese sulfate in male CD rats. *Toxicol Sci* 2001;**60**(2):242–51.

63. Dorman DC, Struve MF, Wong BA. Brain manganese concentrations in rats following manganese tetroxide inhalation are unaffected by dietary manganese intake. *Neurotoxicology* 2002;**23**(2):185–95.

64. Bouchard MF, Sauve S, Barbeau B, et al. Intellectual impairment in school-age children exposed to manganese from drinking water. *Environ Health Perspect* 2011;**119**(1):138–43.

65. Calne DB, Chu NS, Huang CC, Lu CS, Olanow W. Manganism and idiopathic parkinsonism: similarities and differences. *Neurology* 1994;**44**(9):1583–6.

66. Olanow CW. Manganese-induced parkinsonism and Parkinson's disease. *Ann N Y Acad Sci* 2004;**1012**:209–23.

67. Benedetto A, Au C, Aschner M. Manganese-induced dopaminergic neurodegeneration: insights into mechanisms and genetics shared with Parkinson's disease. *Chem Rev* 2009;**109**(10):4862–84.

68. Quadri M, Federico A, Zhao T, et al. Mutations in SLC30A10 cause parkinsonism and dystonia with hypermanganesemia, polycythemia, and chronic liver disease. *Am J Hum Genet* 2012;**90**(3):467–77.

69. Stamelou M, Tuschl K, Chong WK, et al. Dystonia with brain manganese accumulation resulting from SLC30A10 mutations: a new treatable disorder. *Mov Disord* 2012;**27**(10):1317–22.

70. Tuschl K, Clayton PT, Gospe Jr SM, et al. Syndrome of hepatic cirrhosis, dystonia, polycythemia, and hypermanganesemia caused by mutations in SLC30A10, a manganese transporter in man. *Am J Hum Genet* 2012;**90**(3):457–66.

71. Tuschl K, Mills PB, Parsons H, et al. Hepatic cirrhosis, dystonia, polycythaemia and hypermanganesaemia--a new metabolic disorder. *J Inherit Metab Dis* 2008;**31**(2): 151–63.

72. Lechpammer M, Clegg MS, Muzar Z, Huebner PA, Jin LW, Gospe Jr SM. Pathology of inherited manganese transporter deficiency. *Ann Neurol* 2014;**75**(4):608–12.

73. Chalela JA, Bonillha L, Neyens R, Hays A. Manganese encephalopathy: an under-recognized condition in the intensive care unit. *Neurocrit Care* 2011;**14**(3):456–8.

74. Meissner W, Tison F. Acquired hepatocerebral degeneration. *Handb Clin Neurol* 2011;**100**:193–7.

75. Racette BA, Aschner M, Guilarte TR, Dydak U, Criswell SR, Zheng W. Pathophysiology of manganese-associated neurotoxicity. *Neurotoxicology* 2012;**33**(4):881–6.

76. Stepens A, Logina I, Liguts V, et al. A Parkinsonian syndrome in methcathinone users and the role of manganese. *N Engl J Med* 2008;**358**(10):1009–17.

77. Hatfield DL, Gladyshev VN. How selenium has altered our understanding of the genetic code. *Mol Cell Biol* 2002;**22**(11):3565–76.

78. Schweizer U, Dehina N, Schomburg L. Disorders of selenium metabolism and selenoprotein function. *Curr Opin Pediatr* 2011;**23**(4):429–35.

79. Kryukov GV, Castellano S, Novoselov SV, et al. Characterization of mammalian selenoproteomes. *Science* 2003;**300**(5624):1439–43.

80. Diamond AM, Jaffe D, Murray JL, Safa AR, Samuels BL, Hatfield DL. Lovastatin effects on human breast carcinoma cells. Differential toxicity of an adriamycin-resistant derivative and influence on selenocysteine tRNAS. *Biochem Mol Biol Int* 1996;**38**(2):345–55.

81. Handy DE, Hang G, Scolaro J, et al. Aminoglycosides decrease glutathione peroxidase-1 activity by interfering with selenocysteine incorporation. *J Biol Chem* 2006;**281**(6):3382–8.

82. Kohrle J, Jakob F, Contempre B, Dumont JE. Selenium, the thyroid, and the endocrine system. *Endocr Rev* 2005;**26**(7):944–84.

83. Renko K, Hofmann PJ, Stoedter M, et al. Down-regulation of the hepatic selenoprotein biosynthesis machinery impairs selenium metabolism during the acute phase response in mice. *FASEB J* 2009;**23**(6):1758–65.

84. Schomburg L, Dumitrescu AM, Liao XH, et al. Selenium supplementation fails to correct the selenoprotein synthesis defect in subjects with SBP2 gene mutations. *Thyroid* 2009;**19**(3):277–81.

85. Agamy O, Ben Zeev B, Lev D, et al. Mutations disrupting selenocysteine formation cause progressive cerebello-cerebral atrophy. *Am J Hum Genet* 2010;**87**(4):538–44.

86. Ben-Zeev B, Hoffman C, Lev D, et al. Progressive cerebellocerebral atrophy: a new syndrome with microcephaly, mental retardation, and spastic quadriplegia. *J Med Genet* 2003;**40**(8):e96.

87. Swaminathan R. Magnesium metabolism and its disorders. *Clin Biochem Rev* 2003;**24**(2):47–66.

88. Topf JM, Murray PT. Hypomagnesemia and hypermagnesemia. *Rev Endocr Metab Disord* 2003;**4**(2):195–206.

89. Long S, Romani AM. Role of Cellular Magnesium in Human Diseases. *Austin J Nutr Food Sci* 2014;**2**:10.

Index

Note: Page numbers followed by "*f*" and "*t*" refer to figures and tables, respectively.